D1466149

The
Biologic and
Clinical Basis
of
INFECTIOUS
DISEASES

GUY P. YOUMANS, M.D., Ph.D.

Professor and Chairman, Department of Microbiology

PHILIP Y. PATERSON, M.D.

Samuel J. Sackett Professor of Medicine and Microbiology

HERBERT M. SOMMERS, M.D.

Professor of Pathology

all of Northwestern University Medical School, Chicago, Illinois

W. B. SAUNDERS COMPANY / Philadelphia / London / Toronto

W. B. Saunders Company: West Washington Square
Philadelphia, PA 19105

1 St. Anne's Road
Eastbourne, East Sussex BN21 3UN, England

1 Goldthorne Avenue
Toronto, Ontario M8Z 5T9, Canada

Library of Congress Cataloging in Publication Data

Youmans, Guy P.

The biologic and clinical basis of infectious diseases.

Includes index.

I. Communicable diseases. I. Paterson, Philip Y., joint author.
II. Sommers, Herbert M., joint author.   III. Title. [DNLM:
1. Communicable diseases. WC100 Y67b]

RC111.Y68   616.9   74–25484

ISBN 0–7216–9650–3

ISBN 0–7216–9649–X pbk.

Illustration on the front cover is an electron photomicrograph of
a segmented neutrophil $\times$ 25,300.

Illustration on the back cover is an electron photomicrograph of
an alveolar macrophage $\times$ 11,000.

*Electron photomicrographs furnished by Dr. Eva F. Leake and
Dr. Quentin N. Myrvik, Department of Microbiology, The Bowman
Gray School of Medicine, Wake Forest University, Winston-Salem,
North Carolina.*

616.9
Y 83

The Biologic and Clinical
Basis of Infectious Diseases   ISBN 0–7216–9649–X

© 1975 by W. B. Saunders Company. Copyright under the International Copyright Union. All rights
reserved. This book is protected by copyright. No part of it may be reproduced, stored in a retrieval
system, or transmitted in any form or by any means, electronic, mechanical, photocopying, recording, or
otherwise, without written permission from the publisher. Made in the United States of America. Press
of W. B. Saunders Company. Library of Congress catalog card number 74–25484.

Last digit is the print number: 9   8   7   6   5   4

CONTRIBUTORS

BYRON S. BERLIN, M.D.

Laboratory Diagnosis of Viral and Mycoplasmal Infections; Nonbacterial Upper Respiratory Tract Disease; Influenza; Viral Hepatitis

Associate Professor of Medicine and Pathology, Northwestern University Medical School; Chief, Clinical Virology Laboratory, Northwestern Memorial Hospital; Consulting Staff, Veterans Administration Research Hospital, Chicago, Illinois.

MARY M. CARRUTHERS, M.D.

Viral Meningitis and Encephalitis

Assistant Professor of Medicine, Northwestern University Medical School; Chief, Infectious Diseases Section, Veterans Administration Research Hospital; Consulting Staff, Northwestern Memorial Hospital, Chicago, Illinois.

JOHN W. CORCORAN, Ph.D.

Molecular Biology of Sensitivity and Resistance to Antimicrobial Agents

Professor and Chairman, Department of Biochemistry, Northwestern University Medical School, Chicago, Illinois.

DAVID P. EARLE, M.D.

Acute Glomerulonephritis; Pyoderma

Professor of Medicine, Northwestern University Medical School; Staff Physician, Northwestern Memorial Hospital, Chicago, Illinois.

TERRY C. JOHNSON, Ph.D.

Host-Virus Interaction; Oncogenic Viruses; Slow Virus Disease

Professor of Microbiology, Northwestern University Medical School, Chicago, Illinois.

PHILIP Y. PATERSON, M.D.

Introduction; Slow Virus Disease; Fever; General Considerations of Upper Respiratory Tract, Lower Respiratory Tract, Urinary Tract, and Central Nervous System Infections; Streptococci; Streptococcal Pharyngitis-Tonsillitis; Rheumatic Fever; Neisseria meningitidis and Meningococcal Disease; Bacterial Endocarditis; Infection in the Compromised Host

Samuel J. Sackett Professor of Medicine and Microbiology; Chief, Infectious Diseases – Hypersensitivity Section, Department of Medicine, Northwestern University Medical School; Consulting Staff, Northwestern Memorial Hospital and Veterans Administration Research Hospital, Chicago, Illinois.

121054

BORIS REISBERG, M.D.

Cystitis and Pyelonephritis; Antimicrobial Therapy

Assistant Professor of Medicine, Northwestern University Medical School; Staff Physician, Northwestern Memorial Hospital; Consulting Staff, Veterans Administration Research Hospital, Chicago, Illinois.

HERBERT M. SOMMERS, M.D.

Indigenous Microbiota of Human Host; Laboratory Diagnosis of Bacterial and Fungal Infections; Syphilis; Gonorrhea; Infectious Diarrhea; Anaerobic Bacterial Disease; Drug Susceptibility Testing in Vitro

Professor of Pathology, Northwestern University Medical School; Staff Pathologist, and Chief of Clinical Microbiology Laboratories, Northwestern Memorial Hospital; Consulting Staff, Veterans Administration Research Hospital, Chicago, Illinois.

GUY P. YOUMANS, M.D., Ph.D.

Host-Bacteria Interaction; Diphtheria; Streptococcus pneumoniae; Haemophilus influenzae and Klebsiella pneumoniae; Mycobacteria; Tuberculosis; Histoplasmosis, Coccidioidomycosis, Blastomycosis; Staphylococci; Rickettsial Diseases; Zoonoses

Professor and Chairman, Department of Microbiology, Northwestern University Medical School; Staff Physician, Northwestern Memorial Hospital, Chicago, Illinois.

PREFACE

The decision to write a textbook must stem from strong motives. Our determination to undertake this ambitious challenge sprang from the experience we had over the last nine years with an interdepartmental course in Infectious Diseases for medical students. This new program was designed and initiated because of the strong feelings on the part of a number of us on the faculty from the Departments of Microbiology, Medicine, and Pathology that the information provided on the medical aspects of microbiology in the traditional type of microbiology course did not have great meaning for prospective physicians. In our former course this lack of meaning derived from the fact that much of the information provided was almost completely divorced from the clinical situations in which it could be applied to the problems of patient care. It appeared reasonable to us that the basic aspects of medical microbiology, and in particular the fundamentals of host-parasite interaction, would be more relevant and therefore more interesting to students if presented in closer relation to clinical settings.

As reflected by the organization of this book, we teach Infectious Diseases along organ system lines and make no pretense of covering all aspects of medical microbiology. Most patients with infectious disease problems have involvement of only one organ system. This, along with the fact that a relatively few microorganisms acount for most of the infections commonly seen by practicing physicians in our society, made this approach seem logical.

Medical students who use this textbook should have experienced some contact with patients and should have acquired a rudimentary knowledge of how to take a history and at least fragmentary knowledge of normal and abnormal clinical signs and laboratory values. There is little value in discussing bacterial meningitis, for example, if the student has never experienced how a supple neck feels and, therefore, what nuchal resistance or rigidity might be like. Similarly, there is little value in describing a patient with lobar pneumonia, showing chest roentgenograms and illustrating a pulmonary density, if the student is not familiar with examination of the chest, the normal response to percussion, and vesicular breath sounds. Others who study Infectious Diseases, such as students of medical laboratory technology, nursing, and public health, may approach this book with much different needs and background, but still use it successfully.

v

Brief case presentations and discussions, which may be of particular value to interns and residents, have been appended to many of the chapters. In certain chapters, e.g., Syphilis and Gonorrhea, important historic background has been included. In others, e.g., Zoonoses, epidemiologic considerations of importance are featured. All chapters are designed to stress the practical biomedical basis of coping with clinical problems.

Our experience in planning and teaching this material to medical students has strengthened two major convictions which were part of our initial desire to attempt a new teaching format. First, as a formal subspecialty of clinical medicine, Infectious Diseases can be intelligently applied to problems of the diagnosis and management of disease processes in patients only when it includes an understanding of fundamental interactions between microbial parasite and infected host; second, in the teaching of contemporary infectious disease medicine, traditional methods must be constantly reviewed and revised, and new approaches adopted. The student will more readily accept the importance and significance of basic microbiologic information if this is presented to him in close relationship to current clinical situations in which the information is relevant. This condition assumes greater importance when considered in the light of the condensed medical school curriculum of today, in which the issues of relevance of basic sciences and their applicability to the clinical arena remain in sharp focus.

Encouraged by the continued success of our new approach to the teaching of infectious diseases, and impressed by the need for an accompanying book, we have proceeded to create this volume. We sincerely hope it accurately reflects our perspectives and our approach to the teaching of medical microbiology and infectious disease and that it can be successfully used in other academic centers.

We would like to express our gratitude to Mr. Jack Hanley of W. B. Saunders Co., for his wholehearted support and thoughtful guidance, to Ms. Karen Comerford for her editing of the manuscript, and to Mr. Herb Powell for managing its production.

Our thanks also go to Mrs. Geane Kraus, Miss Victoria Monasterio, Ms. Lola Rivero, Miss Veronica Skowonski, and Miss Sharon Stafford who provided invaluable help in the preparation of typescript for chapters in the textbook.

GUY P. YOUMANS

PHILIP Y. PATERSON

HERBERT M. SOMMERS

CONTENTS

V   GENITOURINARY TRACT INFECTION

X   ANTIMICROBIAL THERAPY

Chapter 1

INTRODUCTION TO INFECTIOUS DISEASES

Infectious Diseases as a Discipline

Relationship to Microbiology

From a clinical standpoint, the specialty of infectious diseases is usually considered to be a subspecialty of internal medicine and for this reason is based within a Department of Medicine. Infectious disease consultants evaluate complex problems presented by patients in the hospital and the clinic. Important decisions regarding antimicrobial drug selection and usage are made. In this sense, infectious disease is a clinical discipline.

Fundamentally, however, the subspecialty of infectious diseases deals with problems of microbial parasites in human hosts. It brings to the clinic and the bedside specific information about the pathogenic characteristics of microorganisms and the different mode of action of various antimicrobial agents. More importantly, it brings to the clinical arena basic concepts pertaining to host defensive mechanisms and infecting microbes that are essential to an enlightened approach to management of clinical infections. Especially vital to the understanding of infectious disease is current knowledge of all of the specific humoral and cellular immune responses that must be mobilized by the host and how these responses interact with the infecting microbe before recovery from an infection can occur. It is this focus that makes clinical infectious diseases a subdivision or extension of microbiology.

Divorced from its scientific foundations, the discipline of infectious medicine quickly becomes a superficial descriptive clinical activity preoccupied with measuring body temperature, searching for "pathogens" in body fluids and secretions, and dispensing antimicrobial agents as the

1

penultimate act. By erroneously focusing on antimicrobial therapy, physicians may prescribe multiple antimicrobial agents when only one would be more advantageous, or select the "newest one" being promoted by multicolor advertisements in medical journals. The "newest" antimicrobial drugs are *not* necessarily the most effective, are often the most expensive and, because they are new and usually have had limited use, may be responsible for unexpected and serious side effects.

Role of the Host in Recovery

Many clinicians believe that identification of an infecting microorganism and knowledge of its in vitro susceptibility to antimicrobial agents are the essence of effective management of infectious diseases. Unfortunately, this "bug-drug" orientation totally ignores the infected host and the critical issue of his defense mechanisms. Because of this omission, therapeutic measures often fall short of the mark. No matter how well an infecting microorganism is characterized in terms of species and antimicrobial drug susceptibility or how promptly appropriate antimicrobial therapy is initiated, the eradication of microbes, a process essential for recovery from infection, must be accomplished by the host. Antimicrobial agents do not completely destroy bacteria. In most instances, they exert their beneficial effects merely by curtailing proliferation of the microbial population. Antimicrobial therapy, therefore, "buys time" and gives the host an opportunity to marshal whatever immune defenses are available to first restrain and then eradicate the infecting microbial parasites. This textbook emphasizes this important contribution of the host and illustrates how knowledge of host defense mechanisms is essential for effective diagnosis, prevention, and treatment of infectious disorders. Selected case abstracts provide examples of how the interrelationships between microbes and host-immune defenses can be directly applied to specific infectious disease problems.

Changing Patterns of Infectious Diseases

Resistance to Antimicrobial Drugs

The last three decades have provided painful testimony that bacteria may develop extraordinary resistance to antimicrobial drugs. Since the introduction of penicillin in 1941, the staphylococcus has persistently displayed the potential to develop resistance to virtually every new antistaphylococcal antimicrobial agent discovered. The common enteric bacteria now pose formidable antimicrobial drug resistance problems, and because of, or coincidental with, this problem, serious gram negative bacillary infections are becoming more common. Among the shigella, episomal "R" factors have led to the sudden emergence of strains resistant to as many as five different antimicrobial agents. Typhoid fever now is being observed owing to the appearance of strains of *Salmonella typhi* that are resistant to chloramphenicol, which in the past has been the best antimicrobial agent for treating this serious infection. Even the meningococcus and the gonococcus, once exquisitely susceptible to sulfonamide derivatives and penicillin, now pose serious drug resistance problems. One can summarize the situation this way: "Although man can build a better mouse trap, nature always seems to build a better mouse."

Infections Stemming from "Medical Progress"

For several decades, particularly in the last 20 years, there has been a decline in the prevalence of infectious diseases caused by certain highly pathogenic microorganisms, e.g., pneumococci, streptococci, and staphylococci. This decline has been more than offset, however, by a steady increase in the incidence of infections caused by microorganisms, previously considered to be much less pathogenic or even nonpathogenic. Many of these microorganisms constitute the normal flora of the body. When host defenses are diminished for any reason, these "indigenous" microorganisms may produce systemic life-threatening infection. Altered host defensive mechanisms may be associated with underlying disease processes, e.g., multiple myeloma, Hodgkin's disease, and leukemia. More commonly, host defenses may be compromised by the "fruits of medical progress." The indwelling intravenous polyethylene catheter offers a great advantage for long-term delivery of life-supporting fluids, electrolytes, nutrition, and therapeutics. However, it is also a foreign body which favors implantation and growth of bacteria or yeast within the vascular system. Irradiation employed in cancer therapy, immunosuppressive drugs used to enhance allograft survival, and corticosteroids which suppress inflammation represent therapeutic "advances" which may decrease host responses to infection. In many cases in which the clinician is faced with an intractable infection, successful management depends much more on pinpointing and correcting specific deficiencies in host defense, if possible, than on the selection of the "right" antimicrobial agent.

Antimicrobial drugs, themselves a classic example of medical progress, may impair host defenses and predispose to superinfections. Most antimicrobial agents will alter the normal microbial flora of the body in some fashion. Such alterations are particularly well recognized to occur in the oropharynx. Within a few days, bacteria constituting the normal oropharyngeal microbial flora begin to be replaced by microorganisms resistant to whatever antimicrobial agent the patient is receiving. The resistant bacteria, because of their new-found numerical advantage, are in a position to invade the host and cause a second infection which is superimposed on the first one still under treatment. Such secondary infections stemming from microbial flora alterations induced by antimicrobial therapy are usually designated "superinfections."

Prophylactic use of antimicrobial drugs, e.g., to prevent postoperative wound infections, may actually increase the incidence of the very type of infections which they supposedly were to have prevented. The explanation, in large part, lies in disturbances of normal microbial flora. Antimicrobial agents also may have potential sensitizing and toxic properties which can lead to protracted morbidity or even death. For these reasons, the medical student should seriously question the often repeated phrase: "Antibiotics can't do him any harm and will cover the situation until we know what's going on."

New Microbes and New Concepts

New microbes continue to be recognized, and some display almost unbelievable characteristics. A new class of infectious agents, which resemble classic viruses but yet differ from them and consequently are called "viroids," elicit no demonstrable immune response, withstand boiling in water and formaldehyde treatment, and may even survive short periods of autoclaving. Because of these properties and production of diseases with incubation periods of a year or more, viroids have many characteristics of "slow viruses." Slow viruses are responsible for a number of well-defined diseases in animals and are etiologically linked to at least three chronic, progressive, degenerative, neurologic diseases of man, viz., kuru, Creutzfeldt-Jakob disease, and a demyelinating disorder called progressive multifocal leukoencephalopathy (see Chap. 6).

More traditional microorganisms have increasingly been associated with diseases which were formerly not even considered to be infectious in nature. *Mycoplasma pneumoniae,* the cause of what was called "virus pneumonia" in the 1940s and 1950s, now is thought to play a role in Stevens-Johnson syndrome.

Mounting evidence from several quarters suggests that viruses may be important in chronic degenerative diseases. Electron microscopic studies have revealed viruslike structures or virions in the kidneys of nearly 90 per cent of patients with systemic lupus erythematosus, a chronic connective tissue disease traditionally believed to have an immunologic pathogenesis. The virus responsible for serum hepatitis, viz., hepatitis B virus, has been demonstrated in the lesions of polyarteritis nodosa, a disease usually considered to be a form of hypersensitivity vasculitis. The virus causing measles (rubeola) is now etiologically linked to a progressive and fatal neurologic disease of children called subacute sclerosing panencephalitis (SSPE). Although possessing all of the physical characteristics and antigenic properties of "wild" strains of measles, the SSPE agent is a defective virus and can be isolated from the brains of fatal cases only by using the relatively new technique of cocultivation or cell fusion. These techniques have also been used to uncover other types of defective viruses. Recent evidence suggests that paramyxo-viruses may be implicated in multiple sclerosis. Electron microscopic studies indicate that virions or nucleocapsid structures are demonstrable in specimens of brain tissue from multiple sclerosis patients. Parainfluenza type 1 virus has been isolated from two brains, using techniques for cultivating defective viruses. Finally, SV40 virus has been isolated from brain tissue of patients with progressive multifocal leukoencephalopathy, another progressive degenerative neurologic disease closely associated with malignant lymphoma (see Chap. 6).

It is intriguing that to date the best examples of viral infections causing chronic disease are those involving the nervous system. Is it the lack of regenerating capacity of neurons that allows these host cells to be persistently infected with virus? Is the nervous system a "privileged sanctuary" for a virus because host-immune defense mechanisms do not penetrate the blood-brain barrier?

Significance of Infectious Diseases

Prevalence and Economic Aspects

Acute respiratory disease, i.e., "the flu," "cold," or "sore throat," is the most common illness of man. In one superbly conducted prospective study, viral respiratory infections accounted for approximately 60 per cent of all illness experienced by a group of families in Cleveland. Acute infection of the respiratory tract is the principal reason for a patient consulting a physician.

Venereal disease has reached epidemic proportions in the United States (see Chap. 30). More than 600,000 cases of gonorrhea were reported in 1970. Since a significant percentage of clinically recognized infections are never reported for various reasons and because a significant proportion of infections remain asymptomatic and unrecognized and therefore cannot be reported, the actual number of new cases of gonorrhea in any one year is far greater than the number reported. For 1970, it is estimated that something of the order of 2,500,000 new gonorrhea infections actually occurred – a sizable proportion of our country's population, and an even greater proportion of that population which is sexually active. And the incidence-prevalence curves are still pointing upward as data for the period 1971 to 1974 are compiled (see Fig. 30–1).

According to a national health survey, at least 49,310,000 reported cases of acute infectious and parasitic diseases occurred in the United States in 1969. This represents an incidence of 250 per 1000 population or 1 out of every 4 people in our country. These statistics indicate 199,701,000 days of bed disability and 21,164,000 days of work lost. Therefore, the economic impact of infectious disease on our country's gross national product, to say nothing of the population's personal comfort, is highly significant.

Relevance to Practice of Medicine

Each of us lives in a germ-filled world. Microbes of infinite variety and complexity colonize our body surfaces and orifices. The microorganisms constituting the normal bacterial flora of the lower gastrointestinal tract are present in almost unbelievable numbers and account for nearly half of the dry weight of feces. Infectious diseases will continue to plague man as long as he lives in the world we know. Infectious problems cut across every discipline and subdiscipline of medicine. No matter how "specialized" the medical practitioner, he will see patients with infections. The task of the physician is to meet this challenge with confidence born of increased understanding of the principles of microbiology and immunology and how these principles are essential for rational decision making in the clinical arena.

References

Book

Dingle, J. H., Badger, G. F., and Jordon, W. S.: Illness in the Home. A Study of 25,000 Illnesses in a Group of Cleveland Families. Cleveland, The Press of Western Reserve University, 1964.

Symposium Volumes

Berlin, B. S., and Hilbert, M.: Control of Infections in Hospitals. Ann Arbor, Michigan, University of Michigan, Continuing Series No. 138, 1964.
Wolfgang, Z., Lennette, E. H., and Brunson, J. G.: Slow Virus Diseases. Baltimore, Williams and Wilkins Co., 1974.

Original Articles

Davies, J. E., and Rownd, R.: Transmissible multiple drug resistance in enterobacteriaceae. Science *176:*758, 1972.
Diener, T. O.: Viroids: the smallest known agents of infectious disease. Ann. Rev. Microbiol. *28:*23, 1974.
Editorial: The specialty of infectious diseases. Lancet *2:*1051, 1974.
Lawrence, R. M., Goldstein, E., and Hoeprich, P. D.: Typhoid fever caused by chloramphenicol-resistant organisms. J.A.M.A. *224:*861, 1973.
Paterson, P. Y.: Multiple sclerosis and other immunologic nervous system diseases: Clinical and laboratory considerations. *In* Friedman, H. (ed.): Immunologic Diagnosis of Autoimmune Diseases. Springfield, Illinois, Charles C Thomas, 1975 (in press).
Simmons, H. E., and Stolley, P. D.: This is medical progress? Trends and consequences of antibiotic use in the United States. J.A.M.A. *227:*1023, 1974; and Kunin, C. M.: In comment. J.A.M.A. *227:*1030, 1974.
Sprunt, K., and Redman, W.: Evidence suggesting importance of role of interbacterial inhibition in maintaining balance of normal flora. Ann. Intern. Med. *68:*579, 1968.

I

HOST-MICROBE INTERACTION

Chapter 2

CHARACTERISTICS OF HOST-BACTERIA INTERACTION: EXTERNAL DEFENSE MECHANISMS

Introduction

This chapter is concerned primarily with host-bacteria interaction. Very little attention is paid to animal parasites, either multicellular or unicellular, or to fungi. This selection is based not only upon the relative frequency of infection with these microorganisms in the Western Hemisphere at this time but also upon the fact that many host-animal parasite or host-fungus interactions involve the same mechanisms as do host-bacteria interactions. Since bacterial infection is much more common, these mechanisms and principles can more easily be defined by using the host-bacteria model. Host-virus interaction is dealt with separately. (See Chap. 4.)

As we review host-parasite interactions, we try to emphasize certain principles which a student of medicine should understand before he can properly diagnose or manage a patient with an infectious process.

Traditionally, bacteria have been divided into two broad categories: pathogenic (disease producing) and nonpathogenic (non-disease producing). Pathogens have usually been regarded as owing their disease-producing power to some unique characteristics. It is true that certain microorganisms do depend upon unique characteristics to produce disease. For example, *Clostridium tetani*, which causes tetanus, does so because it elaborates a potent exotoxin (poison) in the infected animal, and the toxin will then produce disease by damaging the nervous sytem. A microorganism such as *Streptococcus (Diplococcus) pneumoniae* can produce infection and disease because it is protected from phagocytosis by the presence of a large polysaccharide capsule. Other examples can be mentioned and are given at appropriate places in this book, but it must be emphasized that such special disease-producing characteristics of bacteria and fungi are probably the exception rather than the rule. It is now recognized that many bacteria not ordinarily regarded as pathogens have the capacity to produce infection and disease, and this capacity will depend more upon host defense mechanisms than upon any special characteristic of the microbial cell. Therefore, the distinction between pathogen and nonpathogen, or between virulent and avirulent microorganisms, has become less meaningful. It is more meaningful to speak of parasites (organisms which live at the expense of other organisms) and nonparasites (saprophytes). All microorganisms which are human parasites have the capacity to produce infection and disease in human beings, and may, therefore, be pathogenic, providing host defense mechanisms become inadequate. We must recognize though, that many physicians use the terms *pathogen* and *nonpathogen* or *virulent* and *nonvirulent* to indicate the relative capacity of parasites to cause disease. Such is the case in many sections of this book.

Many saprophytes can also produce infection if they encounter a weakened host. Therefore, in our study of host-parasite interaction, our emphasis shifts from the traditional primary consideration of the factors enhancing pathogenicity of the parasite to that of host defenses and the reaction of the host to the parasite. We do this because acquisition of infection, like eradication of infection, ultimately comes down to an issue defined by the host rather than by the microbial parasite.

Our Microbial Environment and Reservoirs of Infection

Human beings, as well as other animals, live in a microbial environment. A human being is inhabited by a host of microorganisms which compose what is called his indigenous microbiota (normal microbial flora). All of these microorganisms are parasites since they live upon the skin or mucous membrane or within the lumen of the gut at the expense of the host, or, in some cases, actually within cells in tissue. All of these microorganisms are potentially disease producing, depending upon the state of host defense (see Chap. 7).

Human beings are also in contact with a large exogenous microbial population. This population consists of the multitudes of bacteria and fungi and other microorganisms that are found in soil and water, in the air on dust particles, and in and upon our food. Most of these latter are saprophytes and do not cause disease. However, some of these are primary disease-producing bacteria, e.g., *Clostridium tetani, C. botulinum* (food poisoning), and *Bacillus anthracis* (causative agent of anthrax). In addition, many saprophytes can produce infection if host defense mechanisms are sufficiently faulty.

Another large microbial population is found in lower animals. Many of these microorganisms produce disease not only in lower animals but also in man if man comes in contact with an infected lower animal under appropriate circumstances. Moreover, the microorganism may be transmitted from animal to man by a vector such as an arthropod. Thus, there is a whole group of infectious diseases of man which are classified as zoonoses, diseases of animals transmissible to man. Some of the more important zoonoses are described in Chapter 42.

Of the three general sources of infection for man previously outlined, the most important by far is man himself. Members of the normal microbial flora may seize the opportunity when host resistance is lowered to invade and multiply; these microorganisms are then frequently referred to as opportunists. (Special attention is given to opportunistic infections in Chapter 43.) On the other hand, certain bacteria or fungi of potentially greater capacity to produce disease may be harbored only by a few persons and be transmitted from these persons to other more susceptible individuals in whom they may produce infection and disease. Persons harboring such potential disease-producing microorganisms are called carriers. For example, a man suffering from active pulmonary tuberculosis may be excreting tubercle bacilli in his sputum. He is called a diseased carrier. A person may recover from typhoid fever and retain *Salmonella typhi* in the form of a chronic infection in the gallbladder and thus become a chronic carrier, even though the immunity he developed while suffering from the disease will now prevent systemic infection and symptoms of disease in himself. A child may harbor virulent *Corynebacterium diphtheriae* in his upper respiratory tract for weeks or months after recovering from the disease; this child then becomes a chronic respiratory carrier of *C. diphtheriae*.

Transmission of Microorganisms

Since the major source of microorganisms capable of producing infection and disease in human beings is man himself, it is clear that any conditions or factors which increase the rate of contact between human beings will promote the transmission of microorganisms from person to person and therefore increase the chance of development of disease. Crowded conditions obviously will encourage transmission of microorganisms through coughing and sneezing, whether these microorganisms are part of the normal microbial flora or are temporary residents in carriers. Mucous droplets laden with bacteria are expelled from the respiratory tract into the air. These droplets usually dry rapidly and become what are called droplet-nuclei; the droplet-nuclei may remain suspended in the atmosphere for considerable periods of time and may be inhaled.

We should emphasize here the importance of hands of medical attendants, including physicians, dentists, dental hygienists, and nurses, in the transmission of microorganisms. Hand washing represents the best, and often most neglected, preventive measure in the home and the hospital environment.

Intimate forms of contact, such as kissing and sexual intercourse, promote the transfer of potential disease-producing microorganisms. The high and increasing incidence of this country's most common venereal diseases, syphilis and gonorrhea, attest to the efficacy of sexual intercourse in the transmission of bacteria.

Bacteria can also be spread from person to person by more indirect means; e.g., through food contaminated by a food handler who is an intestinal carrier of Shigella or Salmonella species. Water can become contaminated with fecal material from patients with typhoid or from typhoid carriers. Waterborne epidemics of this disease, although rare in Western countries because of the high level of sanitation, still occasionally occur. It has been correctly stated that Western civilization with its large cities could not exist in its present form without adequate sewage disposal and water purification systems. These enormously expensive installations have been developed to prevent the epidemic infectious diseases such as typhoid fever and cholera which ravaged populations of human beings in the Western world in the Middle Ages.

Infection of human beings may occur from nonhuman sources by the sullying of wounds with naturally contaminated soil or with soil contaminated by the excreta of animals or man. Direct contact with infected lower animals may also result in severe infection; e.g., a hunter may shoot a rabbit infected with *Francisella tularensis*, take the rabbit home, skin it, and then acquire tularemia as a result of direct contact with the microorganisms in the carcass of the infected rabbit. As previously noted, infection also may be transmitted to man from infected lower animals, or from other infected human beings, by arthropod vectors. These include the blood-sucking arthropods such as mosquitoes, mites, flies, and ticks. This form of transmission will be enlarged upon later. It is of particular importance in the transmission of many viral and protozoal diseases (see Chap. 42).

General Attributes of Pathogenic Bacteria

There are terms that are used to describe certain characteristics of the disease-producing power of bacteria. For example, the term *pathogen* merely means that the microorganism can, under certain circumstances, produce disease. Pathogens are also frequently referred to as being virulent (poisonous). Most bacteriologists, however, maintain that, while a pathogen is a disease-producing microorganism, the term *virulence* should refer to the degree of pathogenicity. For example, two bacterial strains may be pathogenic but one is said to be more virulent than the other because it requires fewer microorganisms to produce infection under a particular circumstance, or a microorganism may be pathogenic but it is more virulent for mice than for guinea pigs since it has been found to produce disease more readily in mice. We believe that this usage is unnecessarily confusing and cumbersome; preferably the terms *pathogenic* and *virulence* should be used as synonyms. We need only to refer to a microorganism as being more or less pathogenic under particular circumstances, or more or less virulent, as one prefers.

Tradition also postulates that in order to be pathogenic a bacterium must possess a characteristic known as *communicability*. This term means that the microorganism is readily communicated from some source, usually an infected individual, to a human being in whom it will produce disease. Therefore, a microorganism involved in a highly efficient animal-to-animal transmission system would be regarded as more communicable than a microorganism which had to depend upon a much less efficient system. It should be obvious that in this sense communicability has little or nothing to do with the microorganism. The role of the microorganism is passive since its fate is dependent upon conditions over which it has no control. The use of the term *communicability* as an attribute of a disease-producing microorganism, in our opinion, should be discarded.

In addition, bacteria supposedly possess a property referred to as *invasiveness.* Just what invasiveness consists of in any given case has not been well defined. Basically, the term refers to the capacity of a microorganism to multiply in or upon the tissues of a host; therefore, this potential for multiplication is in large part dependent upon those properties of the microorganism which permit it to resist host defense mechanisms. The term *invasiveness* implies an active, even a burrowing process on the part of the parasite and should be avoided, especially since resistance to host defense mechanisms is a passive process as far as the parasite is concerned.

One must remember that there is a wide variation between the capacity of different species to produce progressive infection and disease. With certain species, a single viable cell may be sufficient (*Rickettsia tsutsugamushi*); with others, a million or more may be required (*Salmonella typhi*).

In general, there are only two attributes which are required by the parasite for the production of disease. First, it must be able to metabolize and multiply in or upon host tissues; i.e., the oxygen tension must be satisfactory, the hydrogen ion concentration appropriate, the temperature suitable, and a favorable nutritional milieu available. Second, assuming all conditions are suitable for metabolism and multiplication, the pathogen must be able to resist host defense mechanisms for a period sufficient to reach the numbers required to produce overt disease. Once a microorganism begins to multiply and metabolize, it may produce metabolic products which injure host tissue and thus promote further extension of the infection. It should go without saying that any concomitant impairment of host defense mechanisms will aid the establishment of a microbial infection.

Because the capacity to withstand host defense mechanisms is probably the most important bacterial characteristic contributing to disease-producing capacity, the following classification of bacterial parasites based upon their ability to resist host defense mechanisms becomes more meaningful than any other to the physician and student of infectious diseases.

Classification of Disease-Producing Microorganisms

Extracellular Parasites

These are bacteria or fungi which produce infection by multiplying primarily outside of phagocytic cells. In fact, when phagocytized by neutrophils or other phagocytic cells, these bacteria are usually readily destroyed. They produce infection and disease in man only under two general circumstances. First, when the bacteria possess a structure or a mechanism which prevents their being readily phagocytosed; e.g., the possession of a polysaccharide capsule by *Streptococcus (Diplococcus) pneumoniae.* Conversely, any impairment of phagocytosis or impairment of host mechanisms for intracellular killing of bacteria would promote disease production by extracellular parasites. Both of these conditions have been encountered in actual practice and are discussed in more detail in subsequent sections of this chapter and in Chapter 3.

Facultative Intracellular Parasites

These are bacteria or fungi which can usually be readily phagocytosed by neutrophils and other phagocytic cells but are resistant to intracellular killing by these cells. A majority of these are parasites of the reticuloendothelial system, since these are the cells within which, in the normal course of events, such highly resistant parasites finally lodge. A classic example of a facultative intracellular parasite is *Myobacterium tuberculosis.*

Obligate Intracellular Parasites

These parasites are bacteria which cannot multiply unless they are within cells. They usually utilize part of the metabolic apparatus of the host cell either for nutritional purposes or to supply energy. Such parasites are frequently found in reticuloendothelial cells but other cells also may be invaded. For example, members of the family Rickettsiaceae, which produce diseases such as typhus fever and Rocky Mountain spotted fever, are found primarily in the endothelial cells lining blood vessels. On the other hand, *Mycobacterium leprae,* the causative agent of leprosy, can be found in voluntary muscle cells as well as macrophages.

The pathogenesis of a given infectious disease depends in large part upon which type of parasite is producing the disease. In addition, the proper appreciation of the three categories of disease-producing microorganisms just mentioned is important in the diagnosis, prognosis, and therapy of infectious diseases. Table 2-1 gives a partial list of some of the common disease-producing bacteria and fungi, listed under headings which indicate whether they are thought to be extracellular, facultative intracellular, or obligate intracellular parasites. It should be added here that all viruses are obligate intracellular parasites.

External Defense Mechanisms

It is convenient to divide host defense mechanisms against infection into those which operate externally and those which operate internally. It must be realized, however, that this is not an absolute division because many of the defense mechanisms usually regarded as being internal also may play a role in external defense against infection. Among those which function both

TABLE 2-1. Classification of Parasites

Genus	Species	Extracellular Parasite	Facultative Intracellular Parasite	Obligate Intracellular Parasite
Bacteria				
Actinobacillus	mallei	+		
Actinomyces	israeli		+	
Bordetella	pertussis	+		
Bacillus	anthracis	+		
Brucella	abortus		+	
Brucella	canis		+	
Brucella	melitensis		+	
Brucella	suis		+	
Clostridium	botulinum	+		
Clostridium	perfringens	+		
Clostridium	tetani	+		
Corynebacterium	diphtheriae	+		
Escherichia	coli	+		
Francisella	tularensis		+	
Haemophilus	aegyptius	+		
Haemophilus	ducreyi	+		
Haemophilus	influenzae	+		
Klebsiella	pneumoniae	+		
Listeria	monocytogenes		+	
Mycobacterium	avium		+	
Mycobacterium	bovis		+	
Mycobacterium	intracellulare		+	
Mycobacterium	kansasii		+	
Mycobacterium	leprae			+
Mycobacterium	marinum		+	
Mycobacterium	scrofulaceum		+	
Mycobacterium	tuberculosis		+	
Mycobacterium	ulcerans		+	
Mycoplasma	pneumoniae	+		
Neisseria	gonorrhoeae	+		
Neisseria	meningitidis	+		
Nocardia	asteroides		+	
Nocardia	brasiliensis		+	
Pasteurella	multocida	+ ?		
Proteus	(all species)	+		
Pseudomonas	aeruginosa	+		
Pseudomonas	pseudomallei	+		
Salmonella	(all species)	+ ?	+ ?	
Serratia	(all species)	+		
Shigella	(all species)	+		
Staphylococcus	aureus	+		
Staphylococcus	epidermidis	+		
Streptococcus	agalactiae	+		
Streptococcus	durans	+		
Streptococcus	equi	+		
Streptococcus	faecalis	+		
Streptococcus	liquefaciens	+		
Streptococcus	mutans	+		
Streptococcus (Diplococcus)	pneumoniae	+		
Streptococcus	pyogenes	+		
Streptococcus	salivarius	+		
Streptococcus	zymogenes	+		
Vibrio	cholerae	+		
Yersinia	pestis	+		

(Table continued on next page.)

TABLE 2-1. Classification of Parasites *(Continued)*

Genus	Species	Extracellular Parasite	Facultative Intracellular Parasite	Obligate Intracellular Parasite
		Chlamydia		
Chlamydia	psittaci			+
Chlamydia	trachomatis			+
		Fungi		
Blastomyces	dermatitidis		+	
Candida	albicans		+	
Coccidioides	immitis		+	
Cryptococcus	neoformans		+	
Epidermophyton	(all species)	+ ?		
Histoplasma	capsulatum		+	
Microsporum	(all species)	+ ?		
Monosporium	apiospermum	+ ?		
Sporotrichum	shenckii	+ ?		
Trichophyton	(all species)	+ ?		
		Rickettsia		
Coxiella	burnetii			+
Rickettsia	akari			+
Rickettsia	conori			+
Rickettsia	prowazeki			+
Rickettsia	quintana			+
Rickettsia	rickettsii			+
Rickettsia	tsutsugamushi			+
Rickettsia	typhi			+
		Spirochaetes		
Borrelia	duttonii	+		
Borrelia	novyi	+		
Borrelia	recurrentis	+		
Leptospira	(icterohaemorrhagiae) interrogans	+		
Treponema	pallidum	+		
Treponema	pertenue	+		

internally and externally are lysozyme, phagocytes, and secretory antibody (IgA), and perhaps other serum factors such as betalysin.

External defense depends upon anatomic, biochemical, and mechanical factors. The operation of these factors in defense against infection varies depending upon the tissue or the organ system involved. Therefore, it is convenient to discuss briefly the operation of these mechanisms in connection with each tissue or organ system that is exposed to the external environment.

Skin

Skin, with its stratified and cornified epithelium, presents a mechanical barrier to penetration of microorganisms. Penetration of skin by bacteria is appreciably more difficult than is the penetration of mucous membrane epithelial surfaces. Therefore, infection of the skin, or of the body by way of the skin, usually takes place only when the continuity of the skin has been mechanically breached. A few bacteria, e.g., *Francisella tularensis,* are so pathogenic that they can penetrate through abrasions in the skin which are too small to be visible to the naked eye. Certain pathogens, i.e., many fungi, will readily produce skin infections, especially if the skin becomes moist and soft, e.g., interdigital ringworm infection (athlete's foot).

The skin possesses an indigenous microbiota as do many of the other external surfaces of the body (see Chap. 7). These microorganisms are for the most part nonpathogenic, and the most common are staphylococci and *Proprionibacterium acnes.* Most of the staphylococci are nonpathogenic species, but *Staphylococcus aureus* may be found on skin and will on occasion produce infection and disease. This is more likely to occur when a hair follicle or a sebaceous gland which usually contains indigenous skin bacteria becomes mechanically blocked; the common pimple or a furuncle (boil) may result.

Most pathogenic bacteria which encounter the skin do not survive for any length of time. The skin usually has an acid pH and this tends to inhibit the growth of most disease-producing bacteria. In addition, long chain fatty acids which are quite bactericidal occur in sebaceous gland secretions. Moreover, the resident microflora not only helps maintain the low pH but also probably produces germicidal substances such as organic acids.

Respiratory Tract

The respiratory tract, and in particular the upper respiratory tract, is continually exposed to a wide variety of particulate material, including microorganisms contained in droplet-nuclei and dust particles. The nasal hairs induce turbulence in the inhaled air, and the majority of the particles are trapped by the mucous secretions which cover the mucous membranes of the upper respiratory tract, especially the nasal turbinates, which provide a large trapping surface. Once trapped, the particles are transported by means of the mucous stream to the base of the tongue where the accumulated material is periodically swallowed. The ciliated epithelium of the upper respiratory tract is responsible for maintaining and directing this mucous flow. It is estimated that over 90 per cent of inhaled particles may be removed by this filtering system of the upper respiratory tract. Smaller particles may pass into the lower respiratory tract. Some are taken out in the trachea, and some land on the mucous membranes of the bronchi and bronchioles. Only the smallest particles, those under 10 μ in diameter, will reach the alveoli, and the smaller the particle, the more likelihood that it will reach an alveolus. Those particles which do reach the alveoli are rapidly phagocytosed and disposed of by alveolar macrophages. Those particles which impinge upon the mucous membranes of the trachea, bronchi, or bronchioles are removed by the mucociliary stream which, owing to the beating action of the cilia, flows up and into the pharynx where the material is swallowed.

The nasal secretions also contain antimicrobial substances such as lysozyme and secretory IgA antibody; in addition, phagocytes can be found in these secretions. All undoubtedly play a significant role in destroying bacteria and thereby preventing infection.

The upper respiratory tract possesses a large indigenous microbiota (see Chap. 7). This bacterial population also plays a role in preventing infection in the upper and lower respiratory tracts. This is dealt with at greater length in a later section.

Alimentary Tract

The mouth is repeatedly exposed to microorganisms, since a major portion of the food that we eat contains a variety of bacteria. These bacteria, for the most part, are non-disease producing and are disposed of by swallowing. The mouth also contains a large number of resident micro-organisms which are continually being depleted in number by the washing effect of saliva and by swallowing.

The stomach is ordinarily sterile because of the very low pH. Most bacteria, except certain acid-resistant species, are readily destroyed owing to the hydrogen ion concentration found in the stomach. Some bacteria, however, may be protected within partially digested food particles and will pass on into the small intestine. In certain pathologic conditions which produce achlorhydria, the stomach may develop a thriving microbial population.

The upper portion of the small intestine does not contain many bacteria, but as the distal end of the ileum is approached, the microbial flora increases and enormous numbers of microorganisms can be found in the colon.

The external defense mechanisms of the host against both this indigenous bacterial flora and disease-producing bacteria that might enter by way of the mouth are the mucous secretions and the integrity of the mucosal epithelium. The peristaltic motions of the gut propel the intestinal contents downward, and as a result enormous numbers of microorganisms are evacuated daily in the feces. It has been estimated that as much as 50 or 60 per cent, dry weight, of fecal material may consist of bacteria and other microorganisms. Thus, mechanical factors are very important in defense of the intestinal tract against infection. In addition, secretory antibody and phagocytic cells may appear in the gut and undoubtedly play a large role. The important role of the indigenous bacterial flora in the protection of the host against enteric infection with certain pathogens is considered later in this chapter.

Genitourinary Tract

Under normal circumstances, the genitourinary tract in the male contains no bacteria above the urethrovesicular junction. The frequent flushing action due to the evacuation of urine, and certain bactericidal substances found in prostatic fluid, largely account for this freedom from microorganisms. Other factors are (1) the pH of the urine may be bacteriostatic; (2) bladder mucosal cells may be phagocytic; and (3) urinary secretory IgA may play a role in local defense.

In adult females, the vagina has a large microbial population consisting predominantly of lactobacilli. These microorganisms maintain a very low pH owing to the breakdown of glycogen produced by the mucosal cells which is inhibitory to the growth of most disease-producing bacteria.

Eye

In the eye, infection is effectively controlled by the flushing action of tears which drain through the lacrimal duct and deposit bacteria in the nasopharynx where the mechanisms already described for the upper respiratory tract bring about disposal of contaminating microorganisms. Tears also contain a high concentration of lysozyme, which is particularly effective against gram positive bacteria.

Attachment of Bacteria to Epithelial Surfaces

It is clear from the preceding discussion of external host defense mechanisms that if all microorganisms encountered by an animal host are either killed or eliminated by these mechanisms, infection and disease will not occur. Infection can appear, however, as the result of failure of operation of one or more external defense mechanisms, or, not infrequently, in the presence of what seems to be normally functioning external defense mechanisms. Regardless of which situation prevails, a requisite for the production of infection is that a microorganism become *attached to epithelial surfaces.* We have already pointed out that, with the exception of *Staphylococcus aureus,* pathogens are rapidly eliminated from the skin. Therefore, except for certain fungi, epithelial attachment probably is not of primary importance in infections of, or through, the skin. On the other hand, most infections of man and lower animals occur by way of the respiratory tract, the gastrointestinal tract, or the genitourinary tract. Here, mucosal surfaces are of primary importance as sites of attachment for infection-producing microorganisms. On the basis of rather recently acquired knowledge, it is possible to conclude that most bacterial pathogens which infect animals by way of mucosal surfaces preferentially attach to certain epithelial cells as a preliminary step to the induction of disease. Obviously, if a microorganism cannot successfully perform this preliminary step it cannot produce infection.

It also appears that these microorganisms attach to epithelial cells through rather specific surface interactions. Examples of such specific attachment have been studied using certain streptococci which are normal inhabitants of the mouth. *Streptococcus sanguinis* and *S. salivarius* will readily adhere to epithelial cells of the cheek and tongue but will not adhere to teeth. On the other hand, *S. mutans* will preferentially attach to tooth surfaces but will not attach readily to mucosal cells of the cheek and tongue. In fact, specific attachment (sometimes called adherence) of bacteria to mucous surfaces can probably account for the nature of the indigenous microbial flora found in the upper respiratory tract and the intestinal tract. Extensive studies on lower animals have shown that the indigenous microbial flora of the intestinal tract varies markedly but is constant at different intestinal levels. Specific attachment is a probable cause of this selectivity.

It is possible that the pathogenicity of such bacteria as *Salmonella typhi* and *Corynebacterium diphtheriae* for the intestinal mucosa and the pharyngeal mucosa, respectively, may be accounted for on the same basis. There is preliminary experimental evidence which suggests that it is the M-protein of *Streptococcus pyogenes* which accounts for the propensity of these microorganisms to attach to and infect the pharynx of human beings. This experimental evidence also indicates that antiprotein M secretory antibody can prevent adherence of *S. pyogenes* by blocking the specific receptor site on the bacterium. This theory, if correct, provides an explanation for the protective effect of immunization with M-protein against Group A streptococcal pharyngitis. Also, the "stand-fast" pili found on *Neisseria gonorrhoeae* may be responsible for its attachment to epithelial cells (see Chap. 30) and thus largely account for its capacity to produce disease.

Consequences of Attachment to Epithelial Surfaces

Several times we have indicated that the indigenous microbiota can play an important role in the prevention of infection in human beings. The indigenous bacterial flora of human beings is described in detail in Chapter 7. Here, we will establish only that the normal bacterial flora is of importance in the prevention of infection and suggest some mechanisms whereby this resident population of bacteria may function to protect against infection.

If a person is treated with penicillin to the point where the normal bacterial flora of the upper respiratory tract (mostly alpha-hemolytic streptococci) is markedly reduced, fungi, such as *Candida albicans,* may attach and colonize the mucous membranes of the mouth and pharynx and produce serious disease. This can occur within four to five days after initiation of penicillin therapy. In the same manner, if a person is treated with a broad-spectrum antibiotic such as tetracycline to the point where the normal bacterial flora of the gut is markedly reduced, staphylococci may colonize the gut and produce a severe exudative disease which may be fatal. These two examples clearly show the important role of the indigenous bacterial flora in the prevention of infection and also demonstrate one of the reasons why discretion is needed in the administration of antibiotics.

The mechanisms whereby the normal bacterial flora prevents infection by other bacteria have not been completely defined. Physicians have assumed, for the most part, that the determining factors include bacterial competition for nutrients, maintenance by normal inhabitants of conditions such as pH and oxidation-reduction potential which are unsuitable for multiplication of pathogenic bacteria, and production of factors by the nonpathogenic normal residents which exert an inhibitory effect on the growth of pathogens. The particular importance of this last factor is underlined by studies showing that viridans streptococci, which constitute a major portion of the normal oropharyngeal flora, secrete a potent factor(s) which inhibits the growth of a variety of gram negative microorganisms, including the "coliforms," normally inhabiting the intestinal tract. Reduction in density of viridans streptococci as a consequence of antibiotic therapy and decreased production of the growth inhibition factor(s) could well explain the emergence of gram negative bacteria in the oropharynx within a few days.

While the factors just mentioned undoubtedly are important, our realization that bacterial attachment to epithelial cells is a prerequisite for the induction of infection adds a new dimension to our understanding of the phenomenon of the prevention of infection by the indigenous bacterial flora.

The nature of the normal bacterial flora is dependent upon the capacity of certain bacteria to attach firmly to epithelial cells. After attachment, in order to become a significant part of the microbial flora, these bacteria must find the conditions suitable for metabolic activity and multiplication. Finally, these bacteria must be innocuous to the extent that they do not significantly affect the normal economy of the animal host. The presence of these relatively innocuous bacteria upon the surface of epithelial cells of the gut or pharynx may prevent attachment of disease-producing bacteria by covering up specific attachment sites required by the pathogenic cells. Thus, the initiating event of infection by highly pathogenic bacteria may be prevented. We have already emphasized that prohibiting attachment cannot be the only factor involved in the prevention of infection by the normal bacterial flora, but it may well be one of the most important.

Although the normal bacterial flora may prevent attachment of potentially disease-producing bacteria to epithelial cells of mucous membranes, infection, especially with certain disease-producing bacteria, can occur even in the presence of what appears to be an adequate indigenous bacterial flora. The requirements for the initiation of infection under such conditions are not known, but certainly attachment of pathogenic bacteria to the epithelial cells is the first step. Following attachment, three disease-producing processes can be recognized.

1. The parasite may multiply upon the surface of the epithelial cell without penetrating into the cell or deeper tissues. Disease in this instance is caused by the elaboration by the parasite of a soluble toxic substance which is absorbed through the mucous membrane, producing local or distant tissue damage. A classic example of this process is *Corynebacterium diphtheriae,* the causative agent of diphtheria. This microorganism attaches to the epithelium of the pharynx where it elaborates a potent toxin which is absorbed and transported to other tissues, where the major manifestations of the disease occur (see Chap. 17). Another example is *Bordetella pertussis,* the bacterium which causes whooping cough. This microorganism multiplies in the mucociliary blanket of the bronchi without entering the epithelial cells. The causative agent of cholera, *Vibrio cholerae,* attaches to epithelial cells at the base of the villi in the small intestine, where it elaborates a potent exotoxin.

Seldom, if ever, does the *V. cholerae* penetrate into or through the epithelial cells of the gut.

2. The parasitic bacteria may attach to epithelial cells, then penetrate into these cells where they multiply and produce disease by destroying the epithelial cell layer. An excellent example is bacteria of the genus Shigella, all of which may produce dysentery in human beings without penetrating into submucosal tissues. Some bacteria that produce infection in this way also may elaborate toxins which damage cells. The manner by which bacteria of this type penetrate into epithelial cells is not well understood, but apparently they enter by a process resembling phagocytosis. Since such epithelial cells are not actively phagocytic, one can speculate that these pathogens may somehow stimulate or activate a phagocytic process.

3. Certain pathogenic bacteria, after attachment to epithelial cells, may enter these cells and pass through them into submucosal tissues, often without significant damage to the mucosal cells. The factors and forces involved in this phagocytosis and transport of the parasite through epithelial cells are not known. Results of studies using electron microscopy, however, indicate that the phagocytic vacuole containing the disease-producing microorganism may pass directly through the cell and into the lamina propria. From the submucosa, the bacteria may spread to other organs in the body. There are many examples of disease-producing bacteria of this type, some of which are extracellular parasites, some facultative intracellular parasites, and some obligate intracellular parasites. Considerable attention to many of these microorganisms is given in later chapters; therefore, no examples are given here.

References

Books

Bellanti, J. A.: Immunology. Philadelphia, W. B. Saunders Co., 1971.
Davis, B. D., Dulbecco, R., Eisen, H. N., Ginsberg, H. S., and Wood, W. B.: Microbiology. New York, Hoeber Medical Division, Harper and Row, 1973.
Olitzki, A.: Enteric Fevers. Basel, S. Karger, 1972.
Weiser, R. S., Myrvik, Q. N., and Pearsall, N. N.: Fundamentals of Immunology. Philadelphia, Lea and Febiger, 1969.

Symposium Volumes

Smith, H., and Pearce, J. H.: Microbial Pathogenicity in Man and Animals. New York, Cambridge University Press, 1972.

Original Articles

Freter, R.: Experimental enteric shigella and vibrio infections in mice and guinea pigs. J. Exp. Med. *104:*411, 1956.
Freter, R.: Studies on the mechanism of action of intestinal antibody in experimental cholera. Tex. Rep. Biol. Med. *27* (Suppl. 1):299, 1969.

Mortimer, E. A., Jr., Wolinsky, E., Gonzaga, A. J., and Rammelkamp, C. H.: Role of airborne transmission in staphylococcal infections. Br. Med. J. *1:*319, 1966.

O'Brien, W.: Acute miliary tropical sprue in Southeast Asia. Am. J. Clin. Nutr. *21:*1007, 1968.

Savage, D.C., Dubos, R. J., and Schaedler, R. W.: The gastrointestinal epithelium and its autochthonous bacterial flora. J. Exp. Med. *127:*67, 1968.

Savage, D. C., McAllister, J. S., and Davis, C. P.: Anaerobic bacteria on the mucosal epithelium of the murine large bowel. Infection and Immunity *4:*492, 1971.

Sprunt, K., and Redman, W.: Evidence suggesting importance of role of interbacterial inhibition in maintaining balance of normal flora. Ann. Intern. Med. *68:*579, 1968.

Ward, M. E., and Watt, P. J.: Adherence of Neisseria gonorrhoeae to urethral mucosal cells. J. Infect. Dis. *126:*601, 1972.

Chapter 3

CHARACTERISTICS OF HOST-BACTERIA INTERACTION: INTERNAL DEFENSE MECHANISMS

Internal Defense Mechanisms

Inflammation

The inflammatory response, whether acute, chronic, or granulomatous, constitutes an important and primary internal defense mechanism. Once bacteria have penetrated into or through epithelial surfaces they act as foreign bodies and therefore stimulate an inflammatory response on the part of the host. A number of the events which occur during inflammation are important in defense against infection, but the single most important one is the accumulation of large numbers of phagocytic cells at the inflammatory site. Initially, these cells are predominantly neutrophils but, if the inflammatory process persists, macrophages will predominate. These phagocytic cells first attach themselves to the endothelial lining cells of venules and capillaries; they then can pass through the blood vessel wall by a process known as diapedesis. In the infected tissue, the phagocytes engage the bacteria and frequently bring about rapid control of the infection by phagocytosis and killing of the pathogen. Some bacteria, however, are resistant to phagocytosis because of the presence of a capsule or some specific cell wall antigen. In such situations, another inflammatory event, increased blood vessel permeability, which allows the passage of plasma proteins into the affected tissue, may become an important asset to the defense. The plasma may contain antibody which, acting as an opsonin, will promote phagocytosis of bacteria. The blood

24

also contains complement which, together with specific antibody, will powerfully promote the phagocytosis of microorganisms. In addition, blood may possess a number of other antimicrobial substances (discussed later in this chapter). During inflammation, soluble chemotactic substances are produced by white cells which assist in the accumulation of leukocytes.

The overall protective effect of the inflammatory process against infection is dramatically revealed by the finding that anti-inflammatory agents such as corticosteroids markedly reduce resistance to infectious agents. More specifically, corticosteroids delay attachment of leukocytes to endothelium and therefore interfere with diapedesis. These agents reduce chemotaxis and are antiphagocytic. They also tend to stabilize lysosomes and may produce involution of lymphoid tissue.

The consideration of the role of inflammation in infection would not be complete, however, without emphasizing that, while the early inflammatory response is protective, under those conditions in which inflammation persists and extensive necrosis occurs, the effect may be to increase susceptibility of tissue to the infectious agent. Since thrombosis of blood vessels is a common finding in areas of inflammation due to bacteria or other infectious agents, situations in which resistance is decreased are encountered frequently. There are many examples of this phenomenon, and a number are described in a later chapter. It will be sufficient to point out here that phagocytes cannot function well in avascular necrotic areas.

Phagocytosis

In order to have a reasonable picture of host-parasite interaction it is necessary to have some understanding of the nature of the phagocytic cells involved, the phagocytic process, and the mechanisms for killing of bacteria within phagocytes.

Neutrophils (polymorphonuclear leukocytes) and macrophages (reticuloendothelial system cells) are the principal cells involved in the ingestion and killing of bacteria. Neutrophils constitute the first line of defense for the host. These cells are produced in large numbers in the bone marrow. When mature, the neutrophils leave the bone marrow and circulate in the blood for six or seven hours. They then penetrate blood vessel walls by squeezing through endothelial cell junctions. The neutrophil is a short-lived cell which does not divide after leaving the bone marrow; it survives in tissue for only a few days. Enormous numbers of neutrophils are produced in the bone marrow. It has been estimated that in the human adult there are 60×10^{11} neutrophils circulating at any given time; equal numbers, at least, are present in tissue, and the bone marrow carries a reserve pool of about 30×10^{11} cells which can be mobilized rapidly. The neutrophil turnover rate is about 10^{11} cells daily. Since neutrophils are end cells which cannot divide, they come from the bone marrow equipped with numerous enzymes and antimicrobial substances which can be used for the degradation and killing of bacteria. These substances are contained in membrane-limited granules which are called lysosomes.

Macrophages are also formed in the bone marrow from a precursor cell but, in contrast to the neutrophils, are long lived and can persist in tissue for weeks or months. Most macrophages which are found in tissue, in the peritoneal cavity, or within the alveoli of the lung apparently come from blood monocytes which migrate from the blood into these areas. Macrophages are not end cells and under certain conditions can synthesize new DNA and multiply. They are also capable of considerable differentiation; e.g., in tissue they are frequently called tissue histiocytes, in the liver Kupffer cells, and in the lung alveolar macrophages. Such macrophages may present both morphologic and physiologic differences, although all these cells are recognizable as macrophages. In general, two types of mature macrophages can be recognized: (1) those wandering in tissues and body spaces (i.e., alveolar and peritoneal macrophages, skin macrophages, tissue histiocytes), and (2) those fixed to vascular endothelium (i.e., the Kupffer cells of the liver and the fixed macrophages of the spleen and lymph nodes).

Macrophages also contain lysosomes and bactericidal substances. However, most of the lysosomes, instead of being formed during the bone marrow maturation period, are produced by the mature macrophage when "activated" by contact with bacteria or other foreign material.

The phagocytic process can be divided into two stages; (1) attachment (adherence) of the bacterium to the cell membrane, and (2) ingestion. Not too much is known about the nature of the attachment of bacteria or other particles to phagocytic membranes. It is probable that many of the same factors are involved that govern the attachment of bacteria to epithelial membranes. Some bacteria readily attach to phagocytes, e.g., *Mycobacterium tuberculosis* or *Listeria monocytogenes*. These two microorganisms apparently have some specific chemical affinity for constituents of the cell membrane. These bacteria, therefore, are readily phagocytosed. On the other hand, many bacteria will not attach to phagocytic cell membranes and can be phagocytosed only with great difficulty. Many of the bacteria of this latter group are those which possess large polysaccharide capsules, i.e., *Streptococcus pneumoniae* and *Klebsiella pneumoniae*. Bacteria of this category can be phagocytosed only by one of two mechanisms: (1) if the phagocyte traps the bacterium on a rough surface where it can not slide away from the phagocytic cell, ingestion occurs without prior attachment; this process is known as surface phagocytosis, and (2) if the slippery bacterial surface is coated with specific antibody which also has a certain affinity for leukocyte membranes through the Fc portion, attachment to the phagocyte cell membrane and ingestion more readily occurs. The process of promoting attachment of bacteria to phagocytic cell membranes by antibody is known as opsonization (see Opsonic Action, later in this chapter).

Once bacteria become attached to the phagocytic cell membrane phagocytosis will occur by a process in which the phagocyte extends small pseudopods around the bacterium. These fuse and form a pouch which contains the bacterium surrounded by cell membrane. This structure is now called a phagosome. The ingestion process is an energy-requiring one in which the energy is furnished in neutrophils and in most macrophages by glycolysis. Certain macrophages, such as alveolar macrophages, however, utilize aerobic oxidative mechanisms for production of energy.

A process known as degranulation then takes place within the phagocyte. The lysosomes containing the hydrolytic enzymes and bactericidal substances fuse with the phagosome and discharge their contents. This structure is now called a phagolysosome. Within the phagolysosome, most bacteria (the extracellular parasites) are usually killed within a few minutes, although the complete degradation of the bacterium may take several hours. The exact mechanisms of bacterial killing within phagocytes are not clear. The hydrolases include cathepsins, acid hydrolases, and lysozyme; the antimicrobial substances include lactic acid, basic polypeptides, and lactoferrin. There are probably other as yet undefined germicidal substances that also play a role.

One intracellular bactericidal system that has recently received a great deal of attention is the myeloperoxidase system. Neutrophils produce hydrogen peroxide during the phagocytic process. These cells also manufacture a peroxidase which, in the presence of a halogen (chloride or iodide), will bring about the rapid killing of certain pathogenic bacteria. Apparently, in the presence of hydrogen peroxide and peroxidase, iodine or chlorine is bound to the bacterial cell and death of the bacterium will ensue.

Our knowledge of the activity of the myeloperoxidase system has come from the investigation of neutrophils obtained from patients suffering from a condition known as chronic granulomatous disease of childhood. This is a sex-linked genetic defect in which the neutrophils of these patients cannot kill microorganisms of low disease-producing power such as *Staphylococcus epidermidis, Enterobacter aerogenes, Serratia marcescens,* or *Candida albicans.* It has been shown that these neutrophils have a lowered metabolic activity and are either unable, or have a very low capacity, to produce hydrogen peroxide. The exact metabolic pathways which lead to this deficiency have not been determined, but the effect in the child is repetitive acute or chronic infection which leads to death at an early age. It is of interest that bacteria such as streptococci or pneumococci, which do not produce catalase, are still readily killed by leukocytes from such patients. The streptococci produce hydrogen peroxide and thus activate the bactericidal myeloperoxidase system since they compensate for the metabolic deficiency of the neutrophil. This has been called a form of "bacterial suicide."

Antibody Defense Mechanisms

The defense mechanisms considered up to this point, both external and internal, have been essentially nonspecific. Antibody defense mechanisms, on the other hand, are highly specific, since antibody will combine only with the antigen which induced its formation, or with antigen which is closely related chemically. Another unique feature of the immune state for which antibody is responsible is that it must be acquired (a possible exception may be the normal opsonins, discussed later). Immunity due to antibody can be acquired in two ways — actively or passively. Actively acquired immunity is mediated by antibody which is produced by an animal in response to the presence of a microorganism or microbial products. This exposure to a microorganism or its products occurs during actual infection, or it may occur following the injection of a suitable vaccine. The most important thing to remember about actively acquired immunity is that the person or animal must produce his own protective antibody in response to exposure to an external antigen.

Immunity is acquired passively when the protective antibody is transferred from an actively immunized animal to a nonimmunized one; the animal does not form its own protective antibody. The outstanding example of passively acquired immunity in human beings is the transfer of protective antibody (IgG) across the placenta from the mother to the fetus. This antibody provides the infant with a measure of protection against a variety of infectious agents for several weeks or months following birth. In some species of lower animals, antibody is not transported across the placental barrier; instead, antibody is secreted by the mother in high concentration in the colostrum. The suckling infant swallows this and it is rapidly absorbed from the intestinal tract into the bloodstream. Immunity can also be passively acquired by injecting serum obtained from an actively immunized animal into a nonimmunized one; e.g., diphtheria antitoxin produced by active immunization of horses can be injected into persons who are deficient in this protective antibody.

There are a number of types of antibody involved in resistance to infection and a number of mechanisms by which they act to protect against infection. These are described briefly below.

Toxin Neutralization

Many pathogenic bacteria produce exotoxins. These exotoxins are proteins and therefore are antigenic. The antibodies produced against toxins will neutralize the toxicity and are called antitoxins. The major diseases in which the causative organisms produce an exotoxin that is the sole or major factor in the pathogenesis of the disease are diphtheria, tetanus, botulism, gas gangrene, and cholera. It is possible to vaccinate persons against diphtheria and tetanus with a formalinized preparation of the toxin. The formalin treatment detoxifies the toxin but does not affect antigenicity. The high effectiveness of these vaccines is attested by the fact that routine vaccination of infants and children against diphtheria and tetanus is regarded as correct medical practice. As already noted, antitoxin produced in lower animals can also be used to passively protect exposed human beings, and antitoxin, when available, is useful for therapy.

Opsonic Action

A large variety of so-called normal opsonins are found in the serum of animals. These were originally called "normal" because there was no obvious antigenic stimulation which could account for their presence. It is now believed that the majority of these normal opsonins probably result from the antigenic stimulation provided by different but antigenically related bacteria. On the other hand, even inert substances such as carbon particles seem to require some opsonin found in serum, and it may be that a normal protein constituent can opsonize a wide variety of particles including many bacteria. The normal opsonins, regardless of origin, are present only in low concentration and consist for the most part of 19S antibody molecules.

Specific antibody (IgG and IgM) are potent opsonins, especially for the promotion of phagocytosis of bacteria such as the pneumococci, which have protective capsules. The function of the opsonin is apparently to promote the attachment of the bacterium to the phagocyte, a necessary preliminary to ingestion and internalization of the particle. Promotion of phagocytosis by opsonins is greatly enhanced by complement. Complement apparently further aids the adherence of the particle to the phagocytic cell membrane.

Complement is normally present in serum and consists of a number of different proteins. These are labeled C1 (with subunits C1a and C1b), C2, C3, C4, C5, C6, C7, C8, and C9. Complement has a number of functional activities; these are listed in Table 3–1, along with the subunits responsible for the various biologic properties noted.

Before complement will function in any way it must be fixed and activated. This can be done by a variety of substances, but apparently the major condition for fixation and activation is that the activating substance be in an aggregated form. The size of the aggregated particle is also of importance. For example, an aggregate of at least four protein molecules is usually required before complement will be activated. Expressed in another way, in order for complement fixation and activation to occur, the size of the particle must be such that it will have a sedimentation value of 18S or greater.

When an antigen combines with specific antibody, aggregates of antigen and antibody form. For this reason, antigen-antibody complexes are excellent complement fixing and activating agents. Of all the antibody classes, only IgM and IgG will function in this manner. IgM is far more effective than is IgG, since one molecule of IgM combined with antigen will suffice for activation whereas several hundred molecules of IgG in combination with antigen are required.

TABLE 3-1. Principal Activities of Activated Complement (C)
Proteins and Their Fragments*

Activity	C Protein or Fragment
Anaphylatoxin: Histamine release from mast cells and increased permeability of capillaries	3a; 5a
Chemotaxis: Attract polymorphonuclear leukocytes	5a; 5b, 6, 7; ?3a
Immune adherence and opsonization: Adherence of Ab-Ag-C complexes to leukocytes, platelets, etc., increasing susceptibility to phagocytosis by leukocytes and macrophages	3b; 5b
Membrane damage: Lysis of red cells; leakiness of plasma membrane of nucleated cells; lysis of gram negative bacteria	8; 9

*From Davis, B. D., Dulbecco, R., Eisen, H. N., Ginsberg, H. S., and Wood, W. B.: Microbiology. New York, Hoeber Medical Division, Harper and Row, 1973.

Following fixation, the activation of complement proceeds in a series of sequential steps. The classic steps in the activation of complement, eventually leading to cell lysis by C8 and C9, are as follows: The C1 component of complement joins with the complement-combining site on the Fc portion of the antibody. The Cl unit component actually consists of three subunits, Clq, Clr, Cls, which are held together by a calcium ion. When the Clq subunit becomes bound to antibody, this complex becomes enzymatically active and in turn activates C4. Activated C4 then combines with a Cls subunit and as a result the C4 breaks into two parts, C4a and C4b. The C4b portion then binds to the cell surface. In turn, the C2 component of complement is activated by Cls and is broken into two fragments. The C2a fragment will combine with C4b to form an enzyme which splits C3; the C3b fragment then also binds to the surface of the cell. This C3b fragment, when bound to the cell surface together with the C4b, 2a enzyme, brings about the binding of C5. Again, in turn, C6 and C7 bind with C5b. This C5b, 6, 7 complex binds to the cell surface at another site. When the C8 fraction combines with the C5b, 6, 7 complex the enzyme which has been activated produces a small hole in the cell membrane. This permits the passage of water and ions into the cell. When C9 finally combines with this complex, the hole in the membrane becomes larger, greatly accelerating the flow of water and ions into the cell. Eventually, because of the flow of water and ions into the cell, it swells and bursts. This is the mechanism of cell lysis by complement, whether the cell be a mammalian cell or a bacterial cell.

During the activation process, the various components and subfractions of the complement system produce the other effects listed in Table 3-1. From the standpoint of protection from infection, one of the most important of these properties of complement is its capacity to opsonize and thereby promote phagocytosis of microbial cells. Fraction C3b and C5b are the active opsonizing components of complement.

Complement may also be activated by substances other than classic antigen-antibody complexes. This process is frequently referred to as the alternate pathway (properdin pathway) for complement activation. Certain substances such as inulin, zymosan, bacterial lipopolysaccharides (endotoxin), and even aggregated antibodies such as IgG, IgA, and IgE will bring about activation. This pathway does not require the activation of C1, C4, and C2; instead, the C3 component is activated directly in a manner which is not clearly understood. However, when activated in this way, the C3b and C5b components also function as opsonins. The alternate pathway for activation of complement is more important than the classic pathway in those situations in which complement is involved in host-cell injury (Fig. 3-1).

Bacteriolysis

Specific antibody can promote killing of certain bacteria, particularly gram negative species, and in some cases lysis of the cell. Complement is required for this effect.

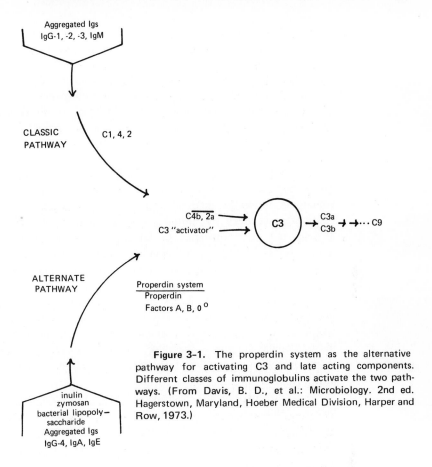

Figure 3-1. The properdin system as the alternative pathway for activating C3 and late acting components. Different classes of immunoglobulins activate the two pathways. (From Davis, B. D., et al.: Microbiology. 2nd ed. Hagerstown, Maryland, Hoeber Medical Division, Harper and Row, 1973.)

Viral Neutralization

Defense against viral infection will be taken up in a later chapter. It is necessary here, for the sake of completeness, to mention that antibody which combines with a viral capsid may ward off infection by preventing attachment of the virus to mammalian cell membranes.

Prevention of Bacterial Attachment

The role of secretory antibody (IgA) in the prevention of attachment of pathogenic bacteria to mucous membranes has already been discussed (see Chap. 2).

Cellular Immunity to Infection

The major defense of animals to infection with extracellular parasites is specific antibody operating through one or more of the mechanisms previously described. There is, however, a large group of bacteria which are either facultative intracellular parasites or obligate intracellular parasites to which a host may develop a high degree of immunity without a recognizable antibody being involved. The immunity appears to reside in cells of the reticuloendothelial system, and in thymus-derived lymphocytes, or both. Two of the pathogens which have been used for much of the experimental work on cellular immunity to infection are *Mycobacterium tuberculosis* and *Listeria monocytogenes.* Both of these bacteria are facultative intracellular parasites and both characteristically parasitize reticuloendothelial cells, i.e., macrophages. In both of these infections, the evidence is clear that immunity cannot be transferred from immunized to nonimmunized animals using serum containing antibodies directed against microbial antigens, nor is there any relationship between the antibody content of the serum of the immunized animals and their resistance to infection with the parasite. In contrast, lymphocytes obtained from animals immunized against *Listeria monocytogenes* will transfer to nonimmune animals resistance to infection with virulent listeria. In experimental tuberculosis, evidence has been obtained from a study of infected macrophages in tissue culture that lymphocytes from immunized animals produce a substance that facilitates the control of multiplication of the virulent tubercle bacillus within the infected macrophage. Cellular immunity, therefore, appears to involve two cell types — the thymus-derived lymphocyte (affector cell) and the macrophage (effector cell).

It is known that when macrophages encounter foreign substances such as bacteria, they may become activated. An activated macrophage is more motile and phagocytoses particles more readily than does the lymphocyte; in addition, it has an increased metabolic rate and quite rapidly forms lysosomal granules containing hydrolases. These activated macrophages phagocytose and control the rate of multiplication of facultative intracellular parasites more effectively than do nonactivated cells. One theory of cellular immunity to infection suggests that the lymphocytes of the immunized animal produce a soluble substance which activates macrophages and thereby promotes disposal of intracellular bacteria. At the moment, there is no direct evidence supporting this possibility. It is known that the macrophages in a tuberculous focus in an immune animal, for example, are certainly activated, but whether the lymphocytes present in the lesion are responsible for the activation is unknown at this time.

Another phenomenon which many researchers feel is related to cellular immunity to infection is delayed hypersensitivity. Tuberculin hypersensitivity occurs concomitantly with cellular immunity to tuberculosis in all animals infected with *M. tuberculosis* and in animals vaccinated with attenuated mycobacterial cells. This close association has led certain investigators to conclude that cellular immunity to infection is mediated by delayed hypersensitivity, apparently through macrophage activation. The key role of thymus-derived lymphocytes in induction of delayed hypersensitivity further strengthens the close relationship between the two phenomena. However, there is also convincing evidence that mycobacterial components such as ribonucleic acid or a mycobacterial polysaccharide can induce cellular immunity to tuberculous infection without the development of detectable tuberculin hypersensitivity. Conversely, Wax-D from the tubercle bacillus, together with tuberculoprotein, can stimulate the development of tuberculin hypersensitivity in guinea pigs without the appearance of cellular immunity to infection.

While the specificity of the induction of cellular immunity to infection is not in doubt (i.e., in an animal previously immunized against tuberculosis, the immunity can be recalled only by the introduction into the animal of tubercle bacilli), the specificity of the effector limb of the immune response has been questioned. It is clear that if cellular immunity to infection depends solely upon macrophage activation, specificity would not be manifest; once activated, a macrophage would handle all bacteria more effectively. In fact, it can be shown that animals immunized against tuberculosis with BCG vaccine (bacillus Calmette Guérin) become more resistant to infection with *L. monocytogenes* or *Brucella abortus.* Other examples of such lack of specificity have been described. However, evidence on this point is conflicting. Animals immunized with BCG vaccine may become more resistant to *L. monocytogenes,* but these animals do not appear to be nearly as resistant as are similar animals immunized with attenuated listeria cells. In addition, while macrophages within animals immunized with BCG do show increased resistance to *L. monocytogenes,* they will show no increased resistance to a disease-producing bacteria such as *Pasteurella tularensis.*

Further discussion and some amplification of the developing picture of cellular immunity to infection can be found in Chapter 24.

Multiplication of Bacteria In Vivo

Thus far we have been dealing in rather general terms with factors concerned with bacterial pathogenicity and with external and internal host defense mechanisms. We shall now discuss in somewhat more detail the multiplication and fate of bacteria within the infected host.

In order to produce disease, a pathogenic bacterium, once it has escaped the external defense mechanisms and gained access to subepithelial tissue, must multiply, since the number of pathogenic bacteria which ordinarily infect man is too small to produce disease. Bacteria multiply by binary fission; therefore, the increase in numbers of bacteria in the tissues of the host is exponential.

The rate of multiplication in vivo, where it has been accurately measured in experimental animals, has usually been found to be significantly less than the maximal rate which can be observed in artificial culture media in the test tube. It is important to emphasize that this exponential rate of multiplication is independent of the size of the infecting inoculum. In other words, given a bacterium capable of initiating infection when only a single viable cell gains access to subepithelial tissue (i.e., certain rickettsial, pasteurella, or mycobacterial species), the rate of in vivo multiplication will be the same whether the animal, or human being, is infected with one or with a million viable cells. This is represented purely diagrammatically in Figure 3-2. It has been established experimentally that animals infected with highly virulent bacteria, such as is arbitrarily represented in Figure 3-2, will die (or show some clinical

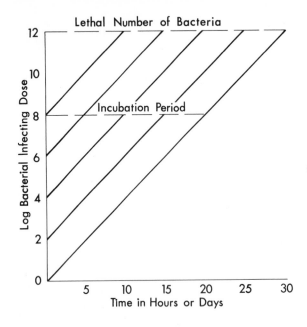

Figure 3-2. The rate of multiplication of bacteria producing infection.

manifestation of infection) only when a certain bacterial population has been reached in the infected animal. This is called the lethal number of bacteria, and in Figure 3-2 we have arbitrarily assigned this a value of 10^{12} viable bacterial cells. Examination of Figure 3-2 reveals that the only effect of varying the infecting inoculum between wide limits is upon the time of death — those animals receiving the smallest inoculum live the longest. Let us assume a parallel situation in which human beings have been exposed naturally to different infecting doses of an equally potent pathogen. We can reason that a symptom of infectious disease (i.e., fever) will occur only when a certain minimal bacterial population has been reached. It is clear from Figure 3-2 that the only effect of varying the infecting dose in natural infection of human beings is to lengthen or shorten the incubation period. Such an assumption is completely compatible with what is seen in certain infectious diseases of human beings.

Most bacteria require far more than one viable cell to produce infection and disease in man or lower animals. Experimentally, it is possible to measure quite accurately the number of pathogenic bacteria necessary to produce disease. The usual procedure is to inject a suitable susceptible species of animal with graded doses of a culture of the pathogenic bacterium and then record the number of animals which die from each infecting dose. From these data it is possible to calculate the number of bacterial cells required to kill 50 per cent of the experimental animals. This number is called the lethal dose 50 (LD_{50}). In this manner it is possible to show that different strains of the same pathogenic bacterial species may vary widely in their capacity to produce disease. For example, one strain of *Salmonella typhimurium* may have an LD_{50} for mice of 100 cells and another strain an LD_{50} of 1000. The first strain can be said to be about 10 times more pathogenic than the second. The relative virulence of different species of bacteria can also be compared in this manner. Conversely, when the LD_{50} of a bacterial strain is known, it is possible to measure and compare the resistance of different species of animals by experimentally determining the number of LD_{50}'s required to produce disease or kill the animals. By using the above procedures, or suitable modifications, much valuable data have been obtained concerning the relative virulence of microbial species, the nature of bacterial virulence, the effectiveness of chemotherapeutic agents for the treatment of infection, the factors involved in host resistance, and the effectiveness of vaccines for the prevention of infection.

Obviously, the above experimental methods cannot be employed for the exploration of the response of human beings to microbial infection. A great deal of data, however, have been recorded concerning the response of human beings to natural infection and these show that the response of human beings parallels that of lower animals. Different strains of a bacterial species may vary in virulence for human beings; e.g., the mortality rate in man from lobar pneumonia caused by type III pneumococcus is appreciably greater than that from lobar pneumonia caused by other types. The susceptibility of humans to different species of bacteria also varies greatly; to illustrate, the mortality rate may be 50 to 70 per cent of persons who become infected with *Yersinia pestis* (bubonic plague) and only 5 to 10 per cent of those who become infected with *Brucella abortus*. Thus, bacteria may vary in virulence for human beings, and human beings may vary in their capacity to resist infection.

Regardless of the rate of mortality which occurs from disease caused by a bacterial species, there remains a question of paramount importance. Why, in persons infected with the same strain of the same bacterium, do some die and others recover? There is no single answer to this question because the factors involved in recovery from an infectious disease are numerous and complex. There is, however, one factor which plays a major role in determining the outcome of an infectious disease. Simply stated, the favorable outcome of an infectious disease process depends primarily upon whether the infected person will be able to mount a specific immune response in time to bring the infection under control by antibody or cellular immune processes. With few exceptions, and even when potent antimicrobial agents (antibiotics) are employed for treatment, final cure of an infectious process depends upon immune mechanisms generated by the infected animal. With an infectious disease that has a high mortality rate, the microorganisms may multiply so rapidly that the lethal number is reached before the immune response is adequate. The person who by chance receives a large infecting dose of a less lethal pathogen may die because the lethal number of microorganisms develops before the 5 to 10 days it may take for his immune response to become adequate. Any circumstance, and there are many, which may suppress the specific immune response contributes to an unfavorable outcome. Conversely, any agent or circumstance which will hinder the multiplication of bacteria in vivo will favor recovery because more time is allowed for the development of specific forces of acquired immunity. Most antimicrobial agents act in this way. The importance of the development of host immunity for the control of an infectious process is emphasized and reemphasized in later chapters. For the moment, it is sufficient to obtain a firm grasp of the principle involved.

It is apparent from an examination of Figure 3-2 that a person may become infected with a small number of bacteria, have a vigorous immune response, and control the infection before the number of bacteria required to produce symptoms is reached. Thus, a person can be infected by bacteria which multiply in his tissue but he will not necessarily develop disease. Such infections are referred to as "inapparent" or "subclinical." Inapparent infection with a wide variety of bacteria undoubtedly occurs frequently during a person's lifetime. In fact, the high degree of resistance shown by adult human beings to a variety of disease-producing bacteria is most likely the result of previous inapparent infection. Therefore, an animal may acquire a bacterial infection without suffering from clinically apparent infectious disease. It is important to understand this distinction between "infection" and "infectious disease."

Spread of Infection

Depending upon the effectiveness of the external and internal defense mechanisms, an infection may remain localized or spread. Spread may occur by direct extension to contiguous tissue or by way of the lymphatics (lymphatic spread) and into the bood via the thoracic duct. Occasionally, bacteria enter the blood directly (hematogenous spread) through a blood vessel eroded by the necrotizing effect of the infection and the accompanying inflammatory process

Fate of Pathogens in Host

In most infections caused by extracellular parasites, when recovery occurs, all the pathogenic bacteria are killed and the patient is free of the invader. In some infections caused by facultative intracellular parasites (e.g., tuberculosis) not all the microorganisms may be killed. Instead, although the mulitplication of the parasite may be completely inhibited by cellular immune forces, the tubercle bacilli may remain viable but dormant within tissue (usually within macrophages) for weeks, months, or years. These microorganisms which persist in tissue for long periods of time may again produce disease if the immune forces which hold them in check wane or are depressed. Chapters 24 and 40 provide a fuller discussion of this situation.

References

Books

Bellanti, J. A.: Immunology. Philadelphia, W. B. Saunders Co., 1971.

Burnett, M., and White, D. O.: Natural History of Infectious Disease. New York, Cambridge University Press, 1972.

Davis, B. D., Dulbecco, R., Eisen, H. N., Ginsberg, H. S., and Wood, W. B.: Microbiology. New York, Hoeber Medical Division, Harper and Row, 1973.

Furth, R. V.: Mononuclear Phagocytes. Blackwell Scientific Publications, Oxford and Edinburgh, 1970.

Olitzki, A.: Enteric Fevers. Basel, S. Karger, 1972.

Pearsall, N. N., and Weiser, R. S.: The Macrophage. Philadelphia, Lea and Febiger, 1970.

Weiser, R. S., Myrvik, Q. N., and Pearsall, N. N.: Fundamentals of Immunology. Philadelphia, Lea and Febiger, 1969.

Symposium Volumes

Dunlop, R. H., and Moon, H. W.: Resistance to Infectious Disease. Sasketoo Modern Press, 1970.

Mudd, S. (ed.): Infectious Agents and Host Reactions. Philadelphia, W. B. Saunders Co., 1970.

Review Article

Youmans, G. P.: Relation between delayed hypersensitivity and immunity in tuberculosis. Am. Rev. Resp. Dis. *111:*109, 1975.

Original Articles

Frenkel, J. K., and Caldwell, S. A.: Specific immunity and nonspecific resistance to infection: Listeria, protozoa, and viruses in mice and hamsters. J. Infect. Dis. *131:*201, 1975.

Ley, H. L., Jr., Smadel, J. E., Diercks, F. H., and Paterson, P. Y.: Immunization against scrub typhus. V. The infective dose of Rickettsia tsutsugamushi for men and mice. Am. J. Hygiene *56:*313, 1952.

Mackaness, G. B.: The behavior of microbial parasites in relation to phagocytic cells in vitro and in vivo. *In* Smith, H., and Taylor, J. (eds.): Microbial Behaviour in Vivo and in Vitro. London, Cambridge University Press, 1964.

McCabe, W. R.: Immunization with R mutants of S. minnesota. I. Protection against challenge with heterologous gram-negative bacilli. J. Immunol. *108:*601, 1971.

A proposed new classification of macrophages, monocytes and their precursor cells. Nature (New Biol.) *240:*65, 1972.

Robbins, J. B., Myerowitz, R. L., Whisnant, J. K., Argaman, M., Schneerson, R., Handzel, Z. T., and Gotschlich, E. C.: Enteric bacteria cross-reactive with Neisseria meningitidis Groups A and C and Diplococcus pneumoniae Types I and III. Infec. Immun. *6:*651, 1972.

Youmans, G. P.: The role of lymphocytes and other factors in antimicrobial cellular immunity. J. Reticuloendothel. Soc. *10:*100, 1971.

Chapter 4

HOST-VIRUS INTERACTION: GENERAL PROPERTIES OF ANIMAL VIRUSES

Introduction

There is little question that viral diseases constitute the most common and yet the most puzzling infectious diseases that a physician encounters. With few exceptions, our inability presently to offer more than prophylactic measures to combat viral diseases has been frustrating and has only added to the apparent mystery that is too often associated with the multitude of infectious diseases that are mediated by viral agents.

It is assumed here that the reader has already been exposed to the general survey of the virus world and the mechanism of viral replication at a cellular level. An initial study of virology gives the student a glimpse at the fascinating aspects of viral replication at the biochemical level where these obligate intracellular parasites are capable, with a surprisingly small amount of genetic information, of subverting host cell metabolism to their own end and replicating at the expense of the host. Although these molecular events are central to our understanding of viruses as obligate intracellular parasites, they are not emphasized in much of the following discussion. Instead, an emphasis is placed on virus properties and activities that are more directly associated with infectious diseases. However, one should not be misled to the conclusion that the fundamental biochemical events associated with virus replication are unimportant to the study of infectious diseases. Unfortunately, these concepts are too often considered to be only tangential to the more clinically oriented professional. A considerable degree of caution must be exercised with any generalizations which may underestimate the significance of the biochemical activities of viruses, since a continual oversimplification will soon detract from a balanced understanding of viral agents and the infectious process. In addition, a thorough understanding of the biochemical events involved in the host-parasite relationship is necessary to the development and use of effective antiviral compounds in the future.

Physical-Chemical Properties of Animal Viruses

Size

That animal viruses are relatively small in size is a well-known fact. In general, the size of the physical particles (virions) of animal viruses ranges from approximately 10 nm to 300 nm. These small dimensions obviously do not allow the use of differential staining and light microscopy, procedures that have been so valuable to other areas of diagnostic microbiology. Whenever adequate quantities of virus particles can be obtained, electron microscopy has been utilized to determine the size and morphology of virions from either laboratory or clinical samples. Whenever applicable, morphologic studies have proved to be a valuable tool, since virions can often be visualized by electron microscopy in infected cells as well as in purified and concentrated virus preparations. Filtration techniques which employ a series of gradocol filter membranes with known pore sizes have also been used to measure the physical sizes of animal viruses. The limitations of these methods are often crucial, and the clinical virologist is frequently dependent on assays which involve biologic infectivity, serologic reactions, and in some cases, specific enzyme analyses in order to identify and characterize viral infectious agents (see Chap. 11).

Nucleic Acids

The ultimate success of any virus attempting to exist as an obligate intracellular parasite depends on its genetic capacity to direct its replication following infection of the host cells. Therefore, all viruses contain a central core of nucleic acid as their genetic information. Unlike bacteria and other complex forms of microorganisms, viruses are unique in that they possess either DNA *or* RNA as their genetic material. The nucleic acid component of some viruses appears to be limited to a single polynucleotide molecule or chromosome (picornaviruses) while other viruses appear to have several and separate chromosomes (orthomyxoviruses). Most animal viruses of clinical importance to man which contain DNA have double-stranded DNA molecules which are quite similar to those found in the chromosomes of higher forms of life. In contrast to the DNA viruses, numerous examples are available to illustrate that the genome of RNA viruses can exist as a single-stranded molecule or molecules. However, there is a unique group of viruses that cause infections in man which have a double-stranded RNA genome (reoviruses).

Probably the most striking feature of all animal virus genomes is their relatively small size. The largest of all animal viruses, the poxviruses, have the genetic capacity to code for approximately 200 to 300 proteins. However, the picornaviruses are limited to the direction of the synthesis of only five to eight polypeptides. It is obvious that a high IQ, as measured by genetic capacity, is not a prerequisite for an organism to be an efficient intracellular parasite and a dangerous infectious agent to animals and man.

In many cases, the genome of animal viruses is an important characteristic to their classification. However, there are limitations to the frequent use of this characteristic in the clinical setting. Relatively large amounts of virus in a pure state are required for the determination of the chemical properties of the gene component of animal viruses. As a result of these limitations, the nucleic acid component of several viruses that are important to man has not yet been resolved, e.g., infectious and serum hepatitis viruses (see Chap. 32).

Capsids

In addition to the nucleic acid component, all viruses appear to possess a protein coat or capsid that is quite specific to each particular virus. The viral capsid plays an important role in both the stability of the virus in the environment and the interaction of the infectious agent with the host cell. In some cases, the capsid proteins appear to be closely bound to the viral nucleic acid, and the resulting nucleocapsid material of the virus appears to have a helical symmetry. In other viruses, the capsid proteins appear to surround the nucleic acids in a manner similar to a shell which imparts a morphology that is described as icosahedral (Fig. 4-1). The capsid proteins of both helical and icosahedral viruses appear to play an important role in the stability of viruses to physical and chemical inactivation in nature. In most cases, the capsid offers a considerable degree of protection to the DNA or the RNA genome from hydrolysis by nucleases which are normally found in the environment or in the tissue fluids. In addition to a stabilizing effect, the viral capsid often plays a primary role in the ability of the virus to efficiently attach to susceptible host cells. This property, as well as the ability of the host to mobilize specific antibodies against viral capsid protein components, is discussed in more detail later in this chapter.

Envelopes

Some viruses possess an envelope that is primarily composed of lipid and protein and usually surrounds the capsid and the nucleic acid core (Fig. 4-1). When an envelope is an integral component of the virion, it apparently plays a critical role in viral attachment and in the ultimate penetration of the virus into the host cell. Since all viruses do not contain an envelope component, the presence or absence of this lipoprotein moiety can be used as a diagnostic tool in the preliminary identification of viral agents. Viruses which contain an envelope are particularly susceptible to inactivation by organic solvents, and exposure for brief periods to ether will result in a marked reduction in their infectivity.

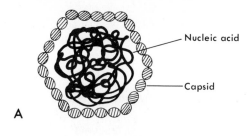

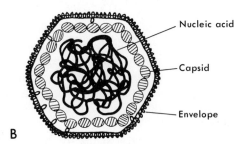

Figure 4–1. Structure of icosahedral and helical viruses. *A,* Icosahedral viruses (naked). *B,* Enveloped icosahedral viruses. *C,* Enveloped helical viruses.

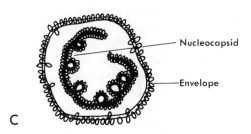

Viral Enzymes

Ever since the study of animal viruses began at a biochemical level, it has been apparent that animal viruses (virions) are characteristically devoid of most enzymes and metabolic processes that are generally associated with other forms of life. Their inert enzymatic nature even led to discussions of whether or not viruses should be considered as "living" microorganisms. Although the presence of neuraminidase in the virions of the myxoviruses was discovered long ago, the absence of detectable levels of enzymes related to energy biosynthesis and the catabolism of numerous organic substrates has been obvious.

During more recent years, the concept that the virions of animal viruses are devoid of enzyme activity has been abruptly altered. It is now apparent that many, if not most, animal viruses contain an enzyme or enzymes that are related to the replication of their nucleic acid components. This is particularly evident with the RNA viruses, since only the members of the picornavirus group appear to be lacking a viral-specific replicase in the intact virus particle. In addition, the discovery of the presence of reverse-trans-criptase molecules in all RNA-tumor viruses has caused a great deal of excitement. The significance of this latter example will be discussed in more detail in a later chapter (see Chap. 5).

Classification of Animal Viruses

The numerous suggestions and approaches that have been developed to classify animal viruses have created a great deal of confusion. At the present time, a binomial nomenclature is not available for animal viruses. The small size of virions has eliminated the use of simple staining procedures and morphologic examination with light microscopy that are central to the preliminary identification of bacteria and other microorganisms. Although at first glance the relatively simple chemical nature of animal viruses may appear to be an asset to their classification, the paucity of enzymes has not allowed the use of fermentation reactions and distinguishable metabolic products that are so familiar to the diagnostic microbiology laboratory. Therefore, the chemical simplicity of animal viruses may be more of a hindrance than an asset to attempts at classification.

An additional problem of viral classification stems from the continual evolution of viral nomenclature from the various disciplines of virology. When placed in historical perspective, most viruses were characterized long after the clinical features of their respective diseases had been described. As a result, many viruses bear the name that associates them with the clinical character-istics, e.g., measles virus, mumps virus, poliovirus, rabies virus, etc. In many cases, this is not an adequate criterion for classification, since several unrelated viruses may cause a similar clinical picture or one virus may lead to several discrete diseases. Further confusion has been added by classification schemes that are based on parameters which are too narrow for general use; this has caused a single virus to be classified simultaneously as a poliovirus, an enterovirus, a neurotropic virus, and a picornavirus.

It appears that no single classification scheme is adequate to satisfy all individuals and various disciplines of animal virology. All published classifica-tion schemes contain vestiges of the methods discussed above. Although incomplete, the viral groups listed in Table 4–1 can serve as a foundation for viral classification and aid in cataloguing many of the viruses that are of medical importance to man.

Mechanisms of Viral Infections

There are several steps of viral infection at the cellular level that are common to all animal viruses. These are (1) attachment, (2) penetration and uncoating, (3) biochemical replication, (4) assembly or maturation, and (5) release. Although these steps are common to the intracellular replication of all animal viruses, the specific kinetics and molecular mechanisms that characterize the replicative events of each virus are quite different. The numerous permutations that characterize the host-parasite relationship of specific viruses can be discussed only in generalities.

TABLE 4–1. Classification of Animal Viruses

Nucleic Acid	Symmetry	Envelope	Virion Size (nm)	Virus-Group	Examples
RNA	Icosahedral	No	18–30	Picornavirus	Poliovirus Coxsackie virus
		No	54–75	Reovirus	Reovirus
		Yes	35–80	Togavirus	Arbovirus A & B
	Helical	Yes	80–120	Orthomyxovirus	Influenza virus
		Yes	100–300	Paramyxovirus	Measles virus Mumps virus
		Yes	60–250	Rhabdovirus	Rabies virus Vesicular stomatitis
DNA	Icosahedral	No	18–24	Parvovirus	Kilham rat virus
		No	70–80	Adenovirus	Adenovirus
		Yes	110	Herpesvirus	Herpes simplex Varicella virus
	Not defined	Complex coat	200 × 300	Poxvirus	Variola virus Vaccinia virus

The mechanism of viral attachment to host cell surface membranes has been studied in considerable depth by several investigators. Attachment has been shown to be an event which involves the participation of specific receptors on the host cell surface and the macromolecules of the virion itself. The attachment process actually appears to occur in at least two discrete steps. A preliminary attachment involves an interaction between the virus and host cell which is primarily ionic in nature and is readily reversed by a shift in pH or salt concentration. The second step of attachment appears to be much more firm and is irreversible.

At one time, the penetration of animal viruses was thought to be restricted to a process of phagocytosis. This was an obvious contrast to the mechanisms of infection of bacterial cells with their respective bacteriophages. More recently, it has become clear that some enveloped viruses attach to host cells; this attachment may lead to a fusion of the viral lipoprotein envelope and the host cell surface membrane. The fusion results in the release of the viral nucleocapsid material into the cytoplasm of the host cell. The penetration of "naked" or nonenveloped viruses, such as the picornaviruses, still appears to involve a mechanism of phagocytosis whereby the intact virion gains entrance into the host cell and the stages of uncoating or removal of the capsid from the viral genome are entirely intracellular (Fig. 4–2). The uncoating of the intact poxvirus has been shown to be an intracellular event that is very complex. Evidently, the initial stages of the removal of the virus outer envelope is a cellular event while the removal of the second, or inner envelope, is directed by the virion itself.

After the capsid proteins have been dissociated from the viral genome, active replication of the nucleic acid and the synthesis of viral proteins begin. The biochemical replication of viral components is quite diverse, and simple generalizations are mostly inadequate. Obligate intracellular parasites require

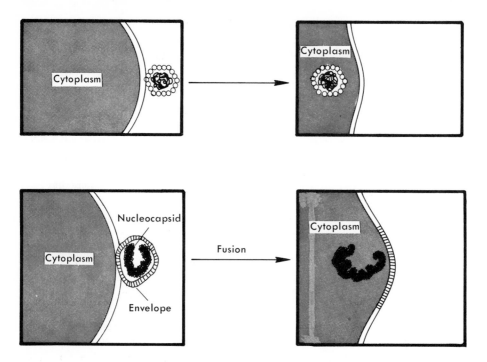

Figure 4–2. Attachment and entry of animal viruses. *Top,* Attachment and penetration by naked viruses. *Bottom,* Attachment and penetration by enveloped viruses.

a considerable amount of participation of the host cell metabolism and/or constituents for their replication. In addition to cellular ATP, viruses require the use of the cellular ribosomes, transfer RNA, enzymes, and other biosynthetic processes related to micro- and macromolecular metabolism. This intimate relationship between the biochemistry of the virus and the host cell explains certain aspects of the limited host range of animal viruses and gives some insight into the problems inherent in the development of chemotherapeutic agents to combat viral infections.

The replication of some viruses is more independent of active host cell metabolism than is that of others. For instance, poliovirus is able to replicate in the cytoplasm of cells in which DNA-dependent RNA synthesis has virtually been eliminated or the nucleus has actually been removed. However, some viruses do not appear to be so independent, and their replication requires the active gene expression of the host cell as well as the specific biochemical events directed by the viral genome.

Viruses are capable of directing the synthesis of essential components for their progeny and assembling these materials into mature virions in the nucleus and/or cytoplasm of the infected cell. The logistics and control mechanisms of viral biosynthesis and assembly are quite specific for each definite viral agent. This is also true for the mechanism of viral release. In some cases, the intracellular infection process is sufficiently injurious to result in cellular lysis with the concomitant release of both mature and incomplete virions. In other instances, the maturation and release process is relatively slow, with virions being released without the destruction of the host cell. A considerable degree of organization is associated with these replicative processes with viruses like the orthomyxo- and herpesviruses. In these examples, the events related to biochemical replication occur in both the nucleus and the cytoplasm, with the assembly of the virion initiated in the nucleus. The nucleocapsid of these viruses then migrates to the cytoplasmic membranes where the mature viruses appear to bud off from the cell surface by a process that is the reverse of the penetration step.

Cellular Responses to Viral Infections

An infection with various animal viruses can result in a wide range of cellular responses. The nature and degree of these responses are dependent on the specific viral agent and the species of the host cell that is infected. At one extreme of this spectrum are the death and lysis of the host cell as the result of major alterations in the cellular biochemical integrity. Virulent viruses apparently cause a significant depression of cellular metabolism, alterations in lysosomal stability, or changes in surface membrane properties that allow the immune surveillance system to detect and destroy infected host cells.

The infection of some cells with viruses such as herpesvirus, measles virus, or respiratory syncytial virus may lead to the formation of giant cells. These multinucleated giant cells, or syncytia, are caused by a major alteration in the properties of the surface membranes of the infected cells which leads to the fusion of several cells into one cytoplasmic mass. The presence of syncytia which can be detected by standard histologic staining and light microscopy techniques, can be an important diagnostic feature to the clinical virologist.

Cellular inclusion bodies, which can be seen by histologic staining procedures, are characteristic of several viral infections and may aid in their identification. These intracellular masses can be detected in the cell nucleus and/or cytoplasm and evidently represent either an accumulation of viruses and viral components or abnormal cellular areas which result from active virus replication. The cellular location and the staining characteristics of inclusion bodies have been useful in the diagnosis of infections with the adenoviruses, herpesviruses, measles viruses, and rabies virus.

Although agglutination of cells may not normally be considered as a typical host cell response to a viral infection in vivo, the ability of some classes of viruses to agglutinate animal cells is of considerable use in the diagnostic laboratory. A special form of cell agglutination, hemagglutination, has proved to be a rapid and simple procedure which can be employed to both quantitate and identify many viral agents. Methods of viral quantitation primarily involve a measurement of the ability of serial dilutions of a viral sample to agglutinate erythrocytes. Although the erythrocytes of several species of animals can be used for hemagglutination assays, diagnostic procedures mainly take advantage of the more sensitive erythrocytes of avian species. Identification of a viral agent that has been isolated from a clinical specimen can be aided by the use of specific antibody preparations which neutralize the ability of the viruses to attach and subsequently agglutinate erythrocytes. In addition to use of these methods for the quantification and identification of viruses, variations on these techniques have been developed to compare the antigenic relatedness of various viruses and to detect and quantitate humoral antibody in patients during the acute and convalescent stages of disease.

Not all viral infections result in an immediate and/or detectable host cell response. The intimate relationship between the biochemical requirements of the virus and the capacity of the host cell to fulfill these requirements may lead to an abortive or inapparent infection. In addition, the presence of another viral agent, which previously gained entrance to the cell, may lead to a successful interference or competition with the more virulent agent. This may cause an inapparent infection with little or no resemblance to the clinical features usually associated with an infection by the virulent agent. It should also be pointed out that dual infections, with two related or nonrelated viruses, may extensively modify the progression and clinical features of the infectious disease.

In some cases, the detection of the presence of a virus may require relatively sensitive biochemical assays which can detect specific viral antigens, alterations in host cell membrane components, or specific viral enzymes. The latter are of particular importance to the detection and identification of oncogenic viruses that lead to cellular transformation, hyperplasia, or both. In these instances, the viral infection may be characterized as being a most insidious host-parasite relationship, and the successful detection and identification of the viral agents responsible for the transformation of the cell may require biochemical and immunologic assays of a most sophisticated nature.

Resistance and Immunity to Viral Infections

Just as in infections with other microorganisms, several features of the host and the host cells provide a considerable degree of resistance to infection with many viral agents. Some of these mechanisms are quite general in nature and are not particularly unique to the study of infectious diseases caused by viral agents. For instance, skin is a barrier to the infection with many viruses, and normal body temperature and pH, as well as other physiologic aspects, establish a degree of resistance to a wide variety of viruses. Since these features are not unique to viral infections (see Chaps. 2 and 3), the following discussion is limited to the mechanisms that are most relevant or important to the host defense against viral diseases.

Receptors

Since attachment is an essential step to the efficient cycle of viral replication, the absence or unavailability of receptor material on the host cell surface membrane renders many cells resistant to viral attachment, penetration, and subsequent replication. The nature of the membrane components or their arrangement on the cell surface has been shown to be an important mechanism of cellular resistance. Chick cells have proved to be refractory to infection by poliovirus because the virions are not capable of attaching to the cells. However, it has been demonstrated that the chick cells are biochemically competent to support the synthesis of poliovirus if the cells are exposed to the poliovirus RNA. Under these circumstances, the infected cells produce mature poliovirus particles although the infection is limited to a single round of viral multiplication, since the completed progeny virions are not capable of attaching to other chick cells.

The receptors that are required for efficient virus attachment have been most thoroughly studied with the myxoviruses and some of the picornaviruses. Most viruses do not have specific organelles for attachment, and it appears that these materials are represented in multiple copies and are distributed over the virion surface. It is reasonable to assume that human beings are naturally resistant to many viruses that may infect other animals by virtue of the virions' inability to efficiently attach to the cell surface of human tissue. This restriction also explains the relatively narrow host range of many animal viruses. It should be reemphasized that the successful attachment and entry of a virion into a host cell does not necessarily result in an active cycle of viral replication. The intracellular incompatibility of the host-parasite relationship at a biochemical level or the hydrolysis of the viral genome may abort the replication cycle.

Antibodies

Humoral antibodies probably constitute one of the most important mechanisms of host resistance to viral infections. These antibody molecules primarily act by neutralizing the antigenic receptor constituents on the virion thereby preventing their attachment and subsequent penetration. Although the surface of a viral particle contains numerous repeated sequences of antigen, a single antibody molecule has been shown to be sufficient to neutralize infectivity. This is explained by the structural rearrangement of the entire viral surface which evidently occurs after the complexing of the antibody to even a single antigenic receptor. Neutralization of viruses by antibodies is usually specific since the antibody is synthesized in response to specific antigenic components (e.g., proteins or glycoproteins) of the viral capsid or envelope. As a result of this specificity, host resistance mediated by antibodies is somewhat limited in that it will not provide protection against infections with a wide variety of viruses or even to more than one antigenic type. This specificity has been a formidable problem in the production of vaccines for mass immunization. There are only three distinct antigenic types of poliovirus, and a vaccine containing types 1, 2, and 3 is sufficient to provide protection to naturally acquired poliovirus infections. However, there are over 200 antigenic types of togaviruses and it is unreasonable to expect a single vaccine to be effective against all possible encounters that an individual may have with these viruses.

Although antibodies appear to be quite effective in combating most viral diseases, this mechanism of host resistance does not cover all of the situations that one finds in infectious diseases. For instance, the mobilization of specific antibodies does not seem to explain the recovery or the recurrent nature of herpes simplex gingivostomatitis. Therefore, most virologists assume that other mechanisms, in addition to specific humoral antibodies, must play a fundamental role in resistance to viral infections.

Cellular Immunity

Although the mechanisms of this process are far from being understood, cellular immunity apparently is important to the resistance to viral infections. Observations regarding the infectious disease processes that are associated with several viruses have strengthened this theory. Case reports of children with a progressive vaccinia infection have shown that normal levels of gamma globulin and elevated titers of neutralizing antibody to vaccinia were present. In addition, the administration of massive doses of immunoglobulin offered no protection against the progression of the vaccinia infection. The disease could be arrested, however, when leukocytes from recently vaccinated donors were administered to the patients. Consistent with these observations are the reports that children with agammaglobulinemia, who are unable to mobilize detectable levels of humoral antibodies, apparently are capable of handling progressive vaccinia infections.

These observations are not restricted to vaccinia infections, since a similar picture has been associated with the complex infectious cycle of herpesvirus. The well-known latent and recurrent nature of infections with herpesvirus is not adequately explained by protection by humoral antibodies. Although neutralizing antibodies are found in individuals with either primary or secondary infections, these levels are actually reinforced by clinical and subclinical infections that occur from infancy. Despite the stable and high titers of humoral antibody in the adult, recurrent acute infections can often occur. The cellular mechanisms and/or the specific leukocyte products that play a primary role in the resistance to infections like those mentioned above are unknown. It is possible that infected cells, with viral antigens on their surface, are efficiently detected and killed by macrophages or other cellular elements of the immune system.

Interferons

The existence of interferons was first reported in 1957 by investigators who were conducting experiments on the mechanism of viral interference. During these investigations, it was found that cells infected with either live influenza virus or heat-inactivated influenza virus responded to the infection by producing a soluble substance that was capable of protecting other cells from viral infection. Although at first they were thought to be unique compounds, it is now known that interferons constitute a family of substances. Interferons are produced in response to viral infection and infections with other obligate and facultative intracellular parasites, as well as to exposure of cells to several synthetic and naturally occurring chemical compounds. In a sense, interferon production can be considered a form of cellular immunity or resistance to viral infection.

The mechanism of interferon induction by viruses appears to be related to the presence of double-stranded nucleic acids, particularly RNA molecules, during some state of viral replication. In fact, synthetic polyribonucleotides with a considerable degree of helical conformation, such as polyinosinate-polycytidylate duplexes (poly I:C), are potent inducers of interferon synthesis. On the other hand, double-stranded DNA and DNA:RNA hybrids appear to be relatively poor inducers. A considerable amount of excitement was generated by the discovery of interferons since it was soon established that, unlike antibody molecules, interferons had inhibitory activity against a wide variety of viruses. They were not restricted to an antiviral action against the specific virus that caused their synthesis. This lack of virus specificity apparently exists because interferons do not react directly with the virion but rather mediate their protective affect by an intracellular mechanism.

Although interferons do not exhibit a specificity with regard to the viral agent that initiated their synthesis, they are specific with regard to the species of cells that actually produced them. For example, interferons produced by human cells primarily protect human cells while having little protective capacity for chick cells, mouse cells, etc. The reasons for this type of specificity are related to the mode of action of interferons. Protection by interferon requires the interaction of the interferon with the host cell which leads to the formation or activation of additional intracellular substances that actually provide the cellular resistance to viral infection. Therefore, the class of compounds that are called interferons are actually inducers that mediate the synthesis of a second group of molecules. Since interferons mediate protection by an intracellular induction of host metabolism, it is not surprising that the induction and subsequent protection to viral infections are somewhat species specific.

The development of interferons for antiviral therapy has not yet reached a level of clinical significance. Several factors have provided formidable barriers to the use of interferons in clinical situations. Interferons are protein molecules, and many are relatively unstable in the tissue fluids. Therefore, passive administration of interferons has not been very successful. Even newer approaches that have utilized synthetic compounds, e.g., poly I:C, to induce the formation of interferons have proved to be rather disappointing. Although induced rapidly, interferon titers also decrease rapidly, and the animal is refractory for a period before interferon can once again be induced.

Despite the present inability to utilize purified interferons or chemical inducers in clinical situations, there is reason to believe that interferons may play a protective role during naturally acquired viral infections. It is possible that the rapid increase in interferon levels in the localized region of infection may provide a primary defense against the advancement of the disease. Although interferon levels appear to subside in a few days, the subsequent rise in antibody titers or cellular immunity may provide a secondary mechanism to limit the spread of virus from tissue to tissue. Therefore, interferon and antibody may actually work together in a two-phase form of resistance to limit viral replication in the host. Some general properties of humoral antibodies and interferons are compared in Table 4-2.

TABLE 4-2. A Comparison of Some Properties of Humoral
Antibodies and Interferons

	Humoral Antibodies	Interferons
Chemical	Protein	Protein
Synthesis restricted to the reticuloendothelial system	Yes	No
Reacts directly with virions	Yes	No
Mediate protection by induction of host cell metabolism	No	Yes
Virus specific	Yes	No
Host specific	No	Yes

Chemotherapy

Attempts to employ chemotherapeutic measures to combat viral diseases have been largely disappointing. Despite the armory of antibacterial and antimycotic agents that are available to the physician, very few compounds have been used with any degree of success against infectious diseases mediated by viruses. The intimate biochemical relationship between viral multiplication and host cell metabolism is a fundamental reason for the present failure. One must realize that any form of chemotherapy is primarily based on the concept of relative toxicity in which microorganisms are especially sensitive to the chemotherapeutic agent. Antibiotics and drugs that have been very useful to the study of molecular virology, e.g., actinomycin D, puromycin, guanidine hydrochloride, etc., are either too toxic for animals or sufficiently ineffective in the in vivo situation to be of significant clinical use.

There has been limited success in the use of chemical agents in specific instances. The substituted (halogenated) pyrimidines are probably one of the most widely used groups of compounds in clinical virology. Keratitis caused either by herpes- or vaccinia virus does respond favorably to the topical application of 5-iodo-2'deoxyuridine. Remission of the clinical features occurs rapidly with repeated administration, although recurrent infections may often follow the withdrawal of chemotherapy. Many additional compounds have been tested and periodically used in clinical circumstances. Sporadic success with several agents has been reported in the literature, although it is quite clear that considerably more investigation is necessary before a definitive answer can be made. For instance, 1-adamantanamine has been used to a limited extent for the control of influenza infections. 1-Adamantanamine apparently inhibits the penetration or uncoating of influenza virus. However, clinical use of this drug is restricted to prophylactic measures; its action is limited to the inhibition of influenza A, and toxic side effects have curtailed its general application. Restricted use has also been made of N-methylisatin-β-thiocarbazone in combating some poxvirus infections. Success in the treatment of vaccination complications such as vaccinia gangrenosa has been encouraging, but little protective activity is demonstrable in circumventing epidemics of smallpox.

It is obvious that the discovery and development of antiviral agents for clinical use will require a great deal of insight and effort. Since so many infectious diseases are mediated by viruses, this area of virology warrants an intensive investigation at both the basic science and clinical levels.

References

Books

Burrows, W.: Textbook of Microbiology. 20th ed. Philadelphia, W. B. Saunders Co., 1973.
Davis, B. D., Dulbecco, R., Eisen, H. N., Ginsberg, H. S., and Wood, B. W.: Microbiology. 2nd ed. New York, Hoeber Medical Division, Harper and Row, 1973.
Debré, R., and Celers, J.: Clinical Virology: The Evaluation and Management of Human Viral Infections. Philadelphia, W. B. Saunders Co., 1970.

Symposium Volumes

Basic Mechanisms in Animal Virus Biology. Cold Spring Harbor Symposia on Quantitative Biology. Volume XXVII. Long Island, New York, Cold Spring Harbor Laboratory, 1962.
Transcription of Genetic Material. Cold Spring Harbor Symposia on Quantitative Biology. Volume XXXV. Long Island, New York, Cold Spring Harbor Laboratory, 1970.

Review Articles

Dale, S.: Early events in cell-animal virus interactions, Bacteriol. Rev. *37:*103, 1973.
Finter, N. B.: Interferons. Amsterdam, North Holland Pub. Co., 1966.
Holland, J. J.: Enterovirus entrance into host cells and subsequent alterations of cell protein and nucleic acid synthesis. Bacteriol. Rev. *28:*3, 1964.
Smith, H.: Mechanisms of virus pathogenicity. Bacteriol. Rev. *36:* 291, 1972.
Tamm, I., and Eggers, H. J.: Biochemistry of virus reproduction. Am. J. Med. *38:*678, 1965.

Original Articles

Baltimore, D., Huang, A. S., and Stampfer, M.: Ribonucleic acid synthesis of vesicular stomatitis virus, II. An RNA polymerase in the virion. Proc. Natl. Acad. Sci. U.S.A. *66:*572, 1970.
Doyle, M., and Holland, J. J.: Prophylaxis and immunization in mice by the use of virus-free defective T particles to protect against intracerebral infection by vesicular stomatatis virus. Proc. Natl. Acad. Sci. U.S.A. *70:*2105, 1973.

Chapter 5

ONCOGENIC VIRUSES

Introduction

The present search for oncogenic viruses as possible etiologic agents of human neoplasia has generated a considerable amount of publicity in the popular press as well as in numerous scientific publications. The amount of attention that has recently been devoted to oncogenic viruses and human malignancy has led many to believe that the study of oncogenic viruses is a relatively new field of endeavor. However, the existence of oncogenic viruses was discovered in 1908 by Ellerman and Bang who demonstrated that the "spontaneous" leukemia in chickens was mediated by an infection with a filterable viral agent. Although today one can appreciate the significance of such an observation, in 1908 it appeared to many to be only a laboratory curiosity. Evidently at that time the relevance of an avian disease to human health problems was quite obscure. Three years later, in 1911, Peyton Rous reported that a viral agent was capable of inducing solid tumors, sarcomas, in chickens. These observations provided a foundation for the growth of tumor virology. The following years resulted in numerous reports of viruses that were apparently responsible for the induction of tumor growth in a wide variety of animals. A brief summary of some of these events is presented in Table 5-1. In addition to briefly outlining the progression of early tumor virology, Table 5-1 also illustrates that both DNA and RNA viruses have been associated with the induction of neoplasia and that a wide range of vertebrates are evidently susceptible to infection.

Although at the present time no one has been able to document that any human malignancy has been the direct result of an infection with an oncogenic virus, most virologists are convinced that viruses are involved with at least some forms of human malignancies, and that the lack of direct proof is primarily a technical or experimental problem. The following sections of this chapter reveal the complexity of tumor virology and the difficulty that is encountered in any attempt to document a particular virus as the etiologic agent of malignancy.

TABLE 5-1. Brief History of Oncogenic Virology

Researcher	Date	Finding
Ellerman and Bang	1908	*Leukemia of chickens
Rous	1911	*Chicken sarcomas
Creech	1929	**Bovine papilloma
Shope	1932	**Rabbit fibroma and papilloma
Lucke	1934	**Frog renal carcinoma
Bittner	1936	*Mouse adenocarcinoma
Gross	1951	*Mouse lymphatic leukemia
Stewart and Eddy	1959	**Polyoma virus, sarcomas and adenomas in mouse, hamster, guinea pig, ferret, rabbit
Sweet and Hilleman	1960	**SV40, hamster sarcomas
Trentin	1962	**Human adenovirus, hamster sarcomas

*RNA viruses
**DNA viruses

Susceptibility of Animals to Oncogenic Viruses

The host-parasite relationship that is associated with oncogenic viruses is extremely complex and has caused a great deal of difficulty in the experimental study of tumor viruses. There are many barriers inherent to the study of tumor production in animals that have been experimentally infected with viral agents suspected of having an oncogenic potential. Several physiologic parameters that affect the host-parasite relationship have been shown to either alter dramatically the form of the resulting disease or allow the animal to be refractory to the infection. In many cases it is clear that the susceptibility of animals to tumor viruses is related to the genetic composition of the host. It has been recognized for a long time that certain strains of mice are highly sensitive to the acquisition of leukemia as a result of a viral infection, while other strains appear to be refractory to the development of malignancy. This phenomenon is very likely a reflection of the intimate relationship between the expression of the host cell and viral genomes, both of which are required for the successful induction and development of malignancy. The influence of the genetic composition of humans on their susceptibility to neoplasia is not clear, although significant familial patterns have been associated with some forms of neoplasia. Whether these correlations are the result of a direct susceptibility of individuals to tumor viruses or a reflection of other physiologic factors which govern the development of neoplasia is presently not resolved.

In addition to genetic factors, host aging plays an important role in the sensitivity of animals to many tumor viruses. In most cases, newborn animals are more susceptible to infections and the subsequent development of malignancy than are either young adult or mature animals. This aspect of tumor virus transmission extends to the extreme that some viruses can only be transmitted congenitally. Hormonal factors have also been implicated in the susceptibility of animals to several tumor viruses and the progression of the disease after infection. The complexity of tumor formation is further complicated by the interaction of the host's humoral and cellular immune systems. It is suspected that the immunologic system of the host is continually surveilling tissues, destroying tumor cells shortly after they arise and before an injurious amount of proliferation can occur. An alteration in the host's immunologic capacity by disease or induced immunologic suppression can upset this balance which may result in an increased susceptibility of the individual to active tumor growth and metastasis. Some oncogenic viruses that primarily invade lymphoid tissue can severely alter the host's immune mechanism and allow an immunologic tolerance to the virus as well as a suppression of the antibody response to other antigens.

The complexity of the host-parasite relationship often causes a relatively low efficiency of tumor production in animals experimentally infected with oncogenic viruses. In addition, the tumors may take weeks or months to develop to a state in which they can be characterized pathologically. Another barrier to many studies with tumor viruses by in vivo inoculation stems from the restricted host range of many viruses. In light of the various difficulties related to the study of tumor viruses in animals, many investigators have searched for correlates between in vivo induction of tumors and the properties of cells propagated in culture after their infection with tumor viruses.

Cell Culture Systems

Several cell culture systems have been employed to investigate the host-parasite relationship between animal cells and tumor viruses. The infection of cells in culture with these viruses may lead to either a permissive or nonpermissive response. A permissive cell-virus relationship results in active viral replication which is at least superficially similar to the events associated with most productive viral replication cycles of lytic viruses. In contrast, a nonpermissive relationship does not necessarily result in active viral replication but does involve a heritable transformation or alteration of host cell growth and its metabolic and morphogenetic properties. Cellular transformation is characterized by the release of cells from the normal density-dependent control of growth, which leads to cell division and foci of cell colonies in a cellular monolayer. In addition to the induction of cell division, transformation is often accompanied by changes in cell mobility and cellular morphology and by increased synthesis and/or activation of cellular enzymes, as well as the appearance of several intracellular and surface antigens. Many of these biochemical changes are similar to the properties that are associated with neoplastic tissues. Although some caution must be taken in assuming that cellular transformation is an in vitro correlate to neoplasia in vivo, it has been shown that the introduction of transformed cells to an animal can lead to tumor production and metastasis.

The intracellular events that result in either the permissive or non-permissive host-parasite relationship are clearly a reflection of the properties of both the virus and the host cell. This is evident by the fact that the infection of one cell by a virus will lead to an active lytic cycle of viral replication while the infection of a second cell line with the same virus preparation will result in cell transformation. Examples of this phenomenon are presented in Table 5-2, which demonstrates that the cellular responses to infection with two similar DNA tumor viruses, polyoma virus and simian virus 40 (SV40), are dependent on both the virus and the species of cell line. The fact that mouse cells are permissive for polyoma virus and nonpermissive for SV40 has allowed comparisons of biochemical events that are characteristic of cell transformation to those of productive infections. These comparisons have been of considerable importance since many of the overt physical and chemical properties of polyoma virus and SV40 are very similar.

Cell culture techniques have provided a considerable amount of information regarding the molecular events that are associated with both the productive cycle of infection and the process of cellular transformation as the result of an infection with oncogenic viruses. These methods have allowed an elucidation of the host-parasite relationship at a genetic level as well as a considerable amount of insight into which biochemical events are directed by the viral genome and which are primarily the result of the host response to infection.

DNA Viruses

The oncogenic DNA (deoxyribonucleic acid) viruses are rather diverse in their chemical and physical properties and are classified within several groups: (1) the papovaviruses which include polyoma virus, SV40, papilloma viruses, and benign wart virus, (2) some adenoviruses, (3) some herpesviruses, and (4) a poxvirus. Polyoma virus and SV40 have been the most extensively studied at a genetic and molecular level. Both polyoma virus and SV40 are relatively small viruses (45 nm), do not possess an envelope, and contain a circular double-stranded DNA molecule of a molecular weight of approximately 3×10^6 daltons. It is interesting to note that despite their injurious potential, these viruses have a genetic capacity that is sufficient only to direct the synthesis of four or five average size proteins.

TABLE 5-2. Permissive and Nonpermissive Infections

	Permissive*	Nonpermissive**
Polyoma virus	Mouse	Hamster, rat
SV40	Monkey	Mouse, hamster, rat, human

*Virus replicates; lytic infection.
**Virus does not replicate; cells are transformed.

Depending on whether these viruses enter a permissive or nonpermissive relationship with the host cells, a series of biochemical events ensue that leads to either viral replication with a concomitant lysis of the cell or a process of cellular transformation. Studies involving polyoma virus and SV40 have illustrated that the events that lead to cellular transformation are of a most insidious nature. In general, the intracellular events that result in the transformation of animal cells by DNA oncogenic viruses are strikingly similar to those associated with lysogeny of bacteria by temperate bacteriophages. In both cases, a double-stranded circular DNA viral genome is integrated into a partially homologous region of the genetic apparatus of the host cell where it is maintained in a form called the provirus or prophage. The chromosomes of animal cells have multiple sites of possible integration, and several proviruses may be maintained while bacteria appear to have only one, or at least very few, areas of homology with the DNA of their respective temperate bacteriophages. In each case, the successful integration of the viral genome results in a cessation of synthesis of complete virions and accounts for the heritable features of lysogeny and transformation. Unlike similar attempts in lysogeny, numerous attempts to isolate and identify a repressor substance from animal cells that have been transformed by an oncogenic virus have been unsuccessful. It is possible that a repressor substance is not involved in cellular transformation and subsequent neoplasia but rather that another, yet unidentified, mechanism is responsible for this phenomenon.

The lack of synthesis of intact virions by cells transformed by polyoma virus or SV40 has led to a great deal of speculation concerning the mechanism of cellular transformation. Early experiments suggested that only a portion of the viral genome was required to induce cellular transformation while most, if not all, of the genetic capacity of the virus was necessary to direct a productive infection. A series of sophisticated experiments revealed that, similar to lysogeny, transcription of only a portion of the viral DNA to messenger RNA could be detected in transformed cells. More recently, investigators have shown that expression of one of the viral genes may be sufficient to maintain the heritable transformed state.

The nature of the selective mechanism which results in a restricted transcription of viral DNA is unknown. Although chemical mutagens and irradiation were successful in inducing the reversal of the prophage state to the replication of bacteriophages in examples of lysogeny, attempts to induce productive cycles of replication by these means in polyoma virus and SV40 transformed cells were unsuccessful. It is possible that these experiments failed because only a portion of the viral genome was integrated in a heritable fashion. This problem was resolved when mouse cells, transformed by SV40 virus, were experimentally fused with monkey cells which are permissive for SV40 replication (see Table 5-2). Although intact SV40 virions could not be detected over several generations of division of the mouse cells prior to fusion, the fusion process resulted in the production of infectious viral particles. This type of experiment is diagrammatically illustrated in Figure 5-1. The SV40 virus obtained from this induction was shown to be capable of transforming other mouse cells and was indistinguishable from the original parental preparation.

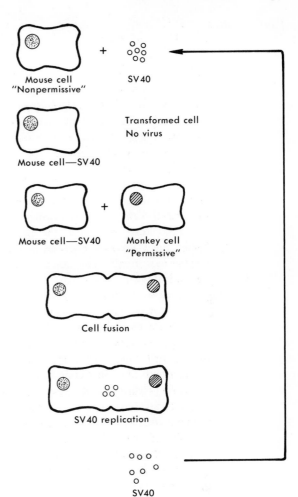

Figure 5–1. Viral rescue by cell fusion technique.

These observations illustrate that viral transformed cells, in the absence of detectable virions, contain the entire genome of the virus integrated in a stable and heritable form and that the nonpermissive host-parasite relationship restrict viral transcriptional events at a genetic level. The significance of these findings in the search for human tumor viruses is discussed later in this chapter. It should be pointed out that the mechanism of transformation previously described is primarily based on studies with polyoma and SV40 viruses. Whether other DNA tumor viruses (e.g., herpesvirus, adenovirus, etc.) mediate transformation by similar or other processes is presently not known. Certainly these latter examples contain a considerably larger DNA genome that is linear although adenoviruses have DNA molecules that can circularize. It is possible that some viruses may transform cells without the integration of the entire genome or that the viral nucleic acid can persist in the cells in a form that is similar to plasmids.

RNA Viruses

RNA (ribonucleic acid) tumor viruses (leukoviruses) are primarily associated with leukemias and sarcomas, are widespread in nature, and are found in the tissues of most, if not all, vertebrate species. These viruses are of intermediate size (80 to 120 nm) and possess an envelope and single-stranded RNA. Virions have been observed in numerous tumors from a wide range of animal species and have been described on a morphologic basis by electron microscopists as A-, B-, or C-type particles. Despite their ubiquity and the fact that they were the first oncogenic viruses described, the mechanism by which this group of viruses transform animal cells remained elusive until rather recently.

Several features of the host-parasite relationship between animal cells and the leukoviruses have made the evaluation of experimental studies difficult. Unlike the DNA tumor viruses described previously, infection of cells with leukoviruses usually does not cause a cytocidal response. The viruses appear to replicate without the destruction of the host cell, and the replication continues over extensive periods of time, possibly indefinitely, with mature virions slowly but continually being released. Moreover, when cells are transformed by leukoviruses, the host-parasite relationship that was established is not exclusively nonpermissive. In addition to their change to a transformed state, the cells synthesize viral particles and release virions during their growth. Further complications to the study of these viruses were recognized when it was learned that many leukoviruses are genetically defective and incapable of replicating without the aid of a second or helper leukosis virus. Therefore, some isolates of leukoviruses actually contain a mixture of viral particles.

In past experimental work, the mechanism by which RNA tumor viruses induce cellular transformation in a stable and heritable form posed unique problems. The direct integration of an RNA genome with the host chromosome was not feasible and several explanations were offered to provide a mechanism for this type of transformation. Since viral synthesis continued in transformed cells, it was considered possible that an integration step was not required. If the leukoviruses replicated in the nucleus of the infected cell at a rate faster than or similar to the rate of cell division, then each daughter cell could be assured of having at least one viral particle to maintain the transformed state. An example of this phenomenon was already available since mitochondria are somewhat autonomous in that they possess DNA, ribosomes, etc., and divide extrachromosomally at a rate that ensures at least one mitochondrion for each daughter cell.

The replicative properties of leukoviruses were observed to be quite unique from other RNA viruses. Treatment of infected cells with inhibitors of DNA synthesis (e.g., fluorodeoxyuridine, aminopterin, cytosine arabinoside) during early stages of infection resulted in an inhibition of leukovirus replication. However, the addition of these inhibitors at later stages of viral infection had little effect on viral yields. The reasons for this transitory requirement for DNA synthesis remained obscure for several years. In order to explain these phenomena, Temin suggested in the early 1960s that the replication and cellular transformation that resulted from leukovirus infections were a result of a provirus host-parasite relationship. Although the virions contained a RNA genome, Temin suggested that the provirus state was maintained as a viral DNA intermediate. This concept involved a transition of viral RNA to DNA during the early stages of infection, the replication of the resulting provirus DNA during cell multiplication, and the transcription of the provirus DNA to RNA during viral production. Although other experimental data supported this hypothesis, the lack of direct evidence and the inability of investigators to isolate the biochemical intermediates predicted by this hypothesis resulted in a considerable amount of skepticism.

In 1970, Temin and Mizutani, who were studying Rous sarcoma virus, and Baltimore, who was studying Rauscher murine leukemia virus, independently reported that the virions of these RNA tumor viruses possessed an RNA-dependent DNA polymerase (reverse transcriptase). Although the virions of many RNA viruses had already been shown to have RNA replicase activity (RNA to RNA), the discovery of this unique enzyme in RNA tumor viruses provided support for the provirus concept. This enzyme activity in the particles of the tumor virus also explained the requirement for DNA synthesis during the early stages of cellular infection with leukoviruses. The presence of reverse transcriptase in the virions stressed the ability of these viruses to synthesize a DNA copy of their genome which could possibly be integrated, in a stable and heritable manner, with the host cell chromosome. This discovery led to a search for reverse transcriptase activity in other RNA tumor viruses. At the present time, all RNA tumor viruses that have been surveyed, approximately 20, have been identified as having a reverse transcriptase activity. In contrast, these enzymes are not found in RNA viruses that apparently lack an oncogenic potential. An exception to this rule is visna virus, which causes a slow viral infection in sheep (see Chap. 6).

An intense effort has been initiated to characterize the physical, chemical, and enzymatic properties of these enzymes and to assess their role in the process of cellular transformation and subsequent neoplasia. For all practical purposes, the leukoviruses may actually behave genetically within the cell as DNA tumor viruses. Therefore, the reverse transcriptase activity of RNA tumor viruses may provide a universal mechanism for the oncogenicity of both DNA and RNA tumor viruses. After the infection of a host cell, the RNA tumor viruses have the potential to mediate a host-parasite relationship that is consistent with that previously described for DNA viruses.

Search for Oncogenic Viruses of Humans

Viruses and intracellular particles which morphologically resemble viruses have been observed in numerous human neoplastic tissues. A herpesvirus, the Epstein-Barr (EB) virus, has been implicated in Burkitt's lymphoma and nasopharyngeal carcinomas, and another herpesvirus has been associated with human cervical carcinoma. In addition, the observation of viruslike particles and reverse transcriptase activity in human milk has suggested that leukoviruses may be associated with at least some forms of human breast cancer.

Whether these viruses are the etiologic agents that are responsible for these malignancies or whether their presence is circumstantial has not been determined. The resolution of these problems is very complicated particularly in light of the complex host-parasite relationships that have been described for tumor virus-host cell interactions and the difficulty in reproducing neoplastic diseases with viral agents. In fact, scientists and physicians may have to form their conclusions on the weight of indirect evidence. Direct proof which substantiates that a microbial agent is responsible for a disease requires the fulfillment of Koch's postulates which have been the yardstick of medical microbiology for over 100 years. For instance, the demonstration that some adenoviruses that have been isolated from human tissues are capable of inducing tumors in other animal species does not lead to an a priori conclusion that they are responsible for human neoplasia; conversely, at the present time the evidence suggests that they are not involved in human cancer.

Several methods are now being used to obtain additional evidence regarding the possible association of various viral agents and human neoplasia. In addition to the identification of viruses in tumor tissues by electron microscopy, many of the molecular techniques that were developed in other animal-virus systems are being applied to clinical samples. Some researchers are using sensitive biochemical assays that employ radioactive precursors to discover the synthesis of viral messenger RNA molecules and the presence of viral nucleic acids in the integrated and plasmid forms in tumor tissues. Whenever leukoviruses are implicated in human cancer, investigators have attempted to detect the presence of reverse transcriptase activity. Until recently, the presence of normal DNA polymerases (DNA to DNA) in the tissues has complicated the identification of viral reverse transcriptases. However, synthetic double-stranded poly- and oligoribonucleotides have been used as templates for in vitro transcription in reverse transcriptase assays, since they have been shown to discriminate between the DNA polymerase of cells and the reverse transcriptase of RNA tumor viruses. In addition, attempts are being made to induce active viral replication by the fusion of human tumor cells to cells of other animal species in a manner similar to that described previously.

Many forms of human cancer, although caused by a viral infection, may be difficult, if not impossible, to establish. It is possible that the viral agent interacts with the host genome in a manner that derepresses specific genetic information (oncogenes) and that the presence of the virus may not be continually required to maintain the malignant state. Although the genomes of polyoma virus and SV40 are integrated in their entirety, it should be remembered that only a single viral gene appears to be sufficient to stabilize the transformed state in a heritable form. Therefore, it is possible that cellular transformation by some human tumor viruses may involve only a partial integration of the viral chromosome. Either of the two above situations would make the isolation of virions from human tumor tissues an impossible task. Even in the event of a successful induction of a productive infection which would lead to the formation of complete viral particles, the direct relationship between the microbial agent and the malignancy would be in question.

References

Books

Davis, B. D., Dulbecco, R., Eisen, H. N., Ginsberg, H. S., and Wood, B. W.: Microbiology. 2nd ed. New York, Hoeber Medical Division, Harper and Row, 1973.

Symposium Volumes

Ceglowski, W. S., and Friedman, H. (eds.): Virus Tumorigenesis and Immunogenesis. New York, Academic Press, 1973.

Clarkson, B., and Baserga, R. (eds.): Control of Proliferation in Animal Cells. Cold Spring Conferences on Cell Proliferation, Volume 1. Long Island, New York, Cold Spring Harbor Laboratory, 1974.

Colter, J. S., and Paranchych, W. (eds.): The Molecular Biology of Viruses. New York, Academic Press, 1967.

Review Articles

Black, P. H.: The oncogenic DNA viruses: A review of *in vitro* transformation studies. Ann. Rev. Microbiol. *22:*391, 1968.

Temin, H.: Mechanism of cell transformation by RNA tumor viruses. Ann. Rev. Microbiol. *25:*609, 1971.

Temin, H., and Baltimore, D.: RNA-directed DNA synthesis and RNA tumor viruses. Adv. Virus Res. *17:*129, 1972.

Original Articles

Baltimore, D.: RNA-dependent DNA polymerase of RNA tumor viruses. Nature *226:*1209, 1970.

Dmochowski, L.: Viruses and breast cancer. Cancer *28:*1404, 1971.

Dulbecco, R.: Cell transformation by viruses. Science *166:*962, 1969.

zur Hausen, H., and Schulte-Holthausen, H.: Presence of EB virus nucleic acid homology in a "virus-free" line of Burkitt tumour cells. Nature *227:*245, 1970.

Melnick, J. L., and Rawls, W. E.: Herpesvirus in the induction of cervical carcinoma. Hosp. Prac. Feb., p. 37, 1969.

Sarkar, N. H., and Moore, D. H.: On the possibility of a human breast cancer virus. Nature *236:*103, 1972.

Temin, H., and Mizutani, S.: RNA-dependent DNA polymerase of Rous sarcoma virus. Nature *226:*1211, 1970.

Chapter 6

SLOW VIRUS DISEASES

Introduction

The purpose of this chapter is to describe briefly a group of infections of animals and man called slow virus diseases. All of these diseases have extremely long incubation periods, a relentless course, and a fatal outcome. Several of the diseases appear to be caused by conventional viruses. Others are associated with atypical infectious agents which have unique physical-chemical and biologic properties.

The discovery that slow virus diseases occur in man as well as in animals has completely redefined present thinking about the role of infection as a cause of human disease. It is now clear that transmissible agents believed to be viruses are intimately associated with several chronic degenerative diseases of man formerly thought to be genetic disorders, autoimmune diseases, or degenerative consequences of aging.

Slow virus diseases in all probability result from a very special type of virus-host relationship. It seems fair to predict that elucidation of the incredibly complex virus-host interactions characterizing the slow virus diseases, as well as those interactions responsible for a variety of other infections marked by chronicity or associated with viral latency, will have an enormous impact on clinical medicine of the future.

Background, Definition, and Examples of Prototype Slow Virus Diseases

The phrase "slow infection" was first employed by the late Bjorn Sigurdsson in the early 1950s to describe several transmissible diseases he and his associates were studying in Icelandic sheep. Each disease had a remarkably long incubation period, developed insidiously, and followed a progressive, usually fatal, clinical course. The term *slow* was used to distinguish these infections from other well-known "chronic" infections that have more conventional short incubation periods, more variable clinical patterns, and do not necessarily end in death.

The criteria for a slow infection as set out by Sigurdsson include (1) an incubation period of many months or even several years, (2) clinical manifestations and histopathologic changes limited to a single organ system, and (3) a relentless protracted course terminating in death. With relatively few modifications, these are the cardinal features of those infectious processes designated today as slow virus diseases.

Slow Virus Diseases of Animals

Prototypic slow virus diseases of animal hosts and man are listed in Table 6–1. Maedi, a progressive pulmonary disease, and rida, a neurologic disorder which in all likelihood is identical to scrapie, are of historic interest because they helped shape Sigurdsson's concept of "slow infections." Visna, a demyelinating disease of the central nervous system with varying degrees of perivascular inflammation which occurs in only certain breeds of sheep, also was described by Sigurdsson and his associates and considered to be a slow virus disease.

TABLE 6–1. Prototypic Slow Virus Diseases of Animals and Man

Animal diseases

Sheep
Maedi
Rida
Visna
Scrapie

Mink
Transmissible mink encephalopathy
Aleutian disease of mink

Human diseases

Kuru
Creutzfeldt-Jakob disease
Progressive multifocal leukoencephalopathy
Subacute sclerosing panencephalitis

Scrapie is a progressive degenerative disorder of the central nervous system neurones. It is an old disease, being known to sheep herders in England and Europe at least 200 years ago. Scrapie was suspected of being a communicable disease long before it was transmitted to other animals in 1899. The disease is named for the tendency of infected sheep to rub or "scrape" against fences and other objects, presumably to seek relief from persistent, intense pruritus. Like visna, only certain breeds of sheep appear to be susceptible to infection with the scrapie agent. The basic histopathologic changes of scrapie are mainly confined to the gray matter of the brain and characterized by "status spongiosus." This term denotes a sequence of neuronal degeneration consisting of cytoplasmic vacuolation, nerve cell ballooning, and eventual complete cellular disintegration. Loss of nerve cells creates a spongelike or cystic appearance. Astrocytes in affected regions, either in response to neuronal injury or because they also are infected, undergo hypertrophy and proliferate. The activated astrocytes put out numerous fibrillary processes, leading to gliosis. Despite the fact that scrapie is an infectious process, there is little or no inflammation. Invasion of meninges and brain parenchyma by histiocytes and lymphocytes does not occur to any appreciable extent.

Transmissible mink encephalopathy is characterized by status spongiosus more striking than that seen in scrapie. Some investigators have suggested that transmissible mink encephalopathy may actually be scrapie, in which the mink acquire infection by being fed meat of scrapie-infected sheep as part of their diet.

Aleutian disease of mink, like both visna and scrapie, is dependent upon a suitable host genotype for its phenotypic expression. Only mink which are homozygous for the recessive Aleutian coat color mutation are susceptible. In contrast to the other slow virus diseases of animals, Aleutian disease of mink is not a disorder of one organ system but a systemic disease involving many organs. The identifying pathologic lesion is an intense plasmacytosis with extensive infiltration of host tissues by plasma cells. The plasma cell proliferation is associated with a profound hypergammaglobulinemia. As much as one half of the total circulating plasma protein may be gamma globulin. Glomerulonephritis and widespread vasculitis of varying degrees of severity occur concomitantly with the plasmacytosis and hypergamma-globulinemia (Figs. 6-1 to 6-3). These lesions are believed to result from circulating virus-antibody complexes and the deposition of such immune complexes in the kidneys and other target organs.

Slow Virus Diseases of Man

Kuru (Table 6-1) is the first progressive, degenerative disease of man shown to have an infectious cause. The disease was initially described in the late 1950s by Gajdusek and Zigas in members of the head-hunting, cannibalistic, primitive Fore tribe which inhabits the highlands of New Guinea. Kuru derives its name from a Fore word equivalent to "shivering." There is evidence suggesting that the incubation period can be as long as 25 years. The disease is characterized clinically by erratic myoclonic jerks, increasing tremors, incoordination, progressive ataxia eventually precluding walking or even standing, severe inanition, and tissue wasting. Death usually occurs within 9 to 12 months after onset. Histopathologically, kuru is characterized by varying degrees of status spongiosus of the brain; it is especially marked and extensive in the cerebellum (Figs. 6-4 to 6-7).

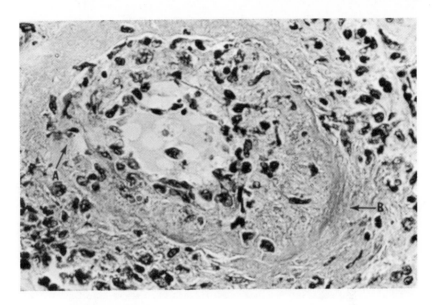

Figure 6–1. Acute inflammatory changes within an artery of a mink with Aleutian disease. Many of the infiltrating cells are neutrophils *(A);* deposits of fibrinoid material are readily demonstrable *(B).* (X 275.) (From Cheema, A., Henson, J. B., and Gorham, J. R.: Aleutian disease of Mink. Prevention of lesions by immunosuppression. Am. J. Pathol. *66:*543, 1972.)

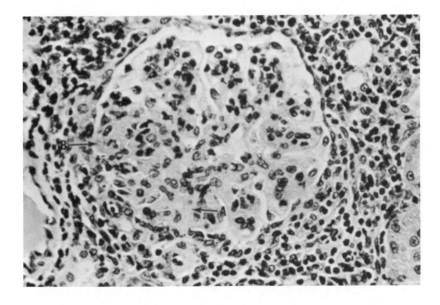

Figure 6–2. Acute inflammation involving a glomerulus in the kidney of a mink with Aleutian disease. Intraglomerular accumulation of eosinophilic material *(A),* together with a few neutrophils *(B),* is evident. Most conspicuous is the intense periglomerular accumulation of inflammatory cells. (X 400.) (From Cheema, A., Henson, J. B., and Gorham, J. R.: Aleutian disease of mink. Prevention of lesions by immunosuppression. Am. J. Pathol. *66:*543, 1972.)

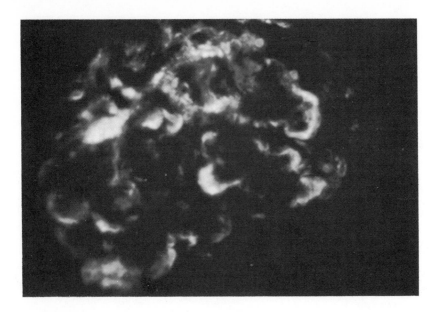

Figure 6-3. Immunofluorescence representing presence of the third complement component (C3) after staining of glomerulus of mink with Aleutian disease with fluoresceinated anti-mink C3. (× 400.) (From Cheema, A., Henson, J. B., and Gorham, J. R.: Aleutian disease of mink. Prevention of lesions by immunosuppression. Am. J. Pathol. *66:*543, 1972.)

Early studies of kuru revealed that it occurred among young boys and girls and among adult women but virtually never involved adult men. This feature, together with the absence of inflammatory changes in the central nervous system, initially suggested that the disease might be a sex-linked genetic disorder. However, successful transmission of kuru to chimpanzees and New World monkeys in the mid-1960s by Gajdusek and his associates and evidence of a replicating agent in these experimental hosts as well as in kuru-affected brain tissues indicated that kuru is an infectious disease.

It is now virtually certain that transmission of kuru among the Fore tribespeople is the result of contact with or ingestion of infected brain tissue during cannibalistic ceremonial rituals. In support of this theory, a steady

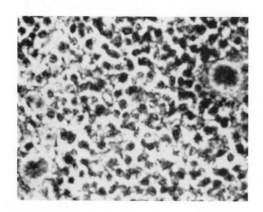

Figure 6-4. Spongiform changes in caudate nucleus of the brain of a patient with kuru. Note varying degrees of "open space" around individual cells (Approx. × 92). (From Neumann, M. A., Gajdusek, D. C., and Zigas, V.: Neuropathologic findings in exotic neurologic disorders among natives of the highlands of New Guinea. J. Neuropathol. Exp. Neurol. *23:*486, 1964.)

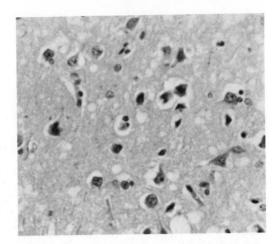

Figure 6–5. Higher magnification illustrating spongiform changes in cortex of same patient (Fig. 6–4) with kuru. (X 300.) (From Neumann, M. A., Gajdusek, D. C., and Zigas, V.: Neuropathologic findings in exotic neurologic disorders among natives of the highlands of New Guinea. J. Neuropathol. Exp. Neurol. *23:*486, 1964.)

decline in the incidence of kuru was observed after "westernization" of the Fore people led to cessation of cannibalism. The fact that adult Fore women were in charge of preparing brain and other tissues of individuals dying of kuru, often encouraging their own children to consume infected material, whereas tribal protocol precluded adult Fore men from coming into contact with the tissues, offers a reasonable explanation for the peculiar sex-linked pattern of occurrence of the disease.

In the early 1920s, Creutzfeldt and Jakob described a presenile dementia affecting middle-aged or younger individuals, the first case reported being a 23-year-old woman. This syndrome, now known as Creutzfeldt-Jakob disease, is characterized by a variety of motor or sensory symptoms and signs and is often associated with abnormal myoclonic jerking and tremors. The basic histopathologic findings consist of widespread neuronal degeneration with obliteration of normal cytoarchitecture of the brain. These changes are especially marked in the cerebral cortex. This degenerative process also leads to spongiform changes of the neurons, and astrocytes to some degree.

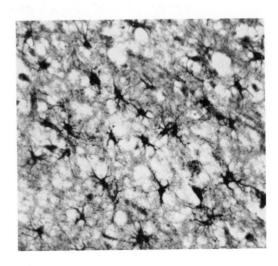

Figure 6–6. Greatly hypertrophied astrocytes in spongy cortex of same patient (Figs. 6–4 and 6–5). (X 250.) (From Neumann, M. A., Gajdusek, D. C., and Zagas, V.: Neuropathologic findings in exotic neurologic disorders among natives of the highlands of New Guinea. J. Neuropathol. Exp. Neurol. *23:*486, 1964.)

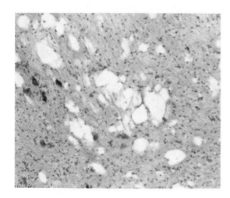

Figure 6–7. More conspicuous spongiform changes in midbrain of another patient with kuru. (X 92.) (From Neumann, M. A., Gajdusek, D. C., and Zigas, V.: Neuropathologic findings in exotic neurologic disorders among natives of the highlands of New Guinea. J. Neuropathol. Exp. Neurol. *23:*486, 1964.)

Since Creutzfeldt-Jakob disease is the only disease of man other than kuru which is associated with striking spongiform histopathologic changes, it was not surprising that Gajdusek and Gibbs and co-workers decided to extend their studies of kuru to this disease. They reported transmission of Creutzfeldt-Jakob disease to chimpanzees in the late 1960s, thereby providing evidence that presenile dementia of man can have an infectious cause.

To underline the prominence of the striking spongiform changes seen in kuru and Creutzfeldt-Jakob disease, Gajdusek has proposed that slow virus diseases with this fundamental histopathologic change be designated as "subacute spongiform encephalopathy." This suggestion has been generally adopted. Diseases constituting the "subacute spongiform encephalopathy" group include the two animal diseases, viz., scrapie and transmissible mink encephalopathy, and the two human diseases, viz., kuru and Creutzfeldt-Jakob disease.

For reasons that are not clear, transmission of each of the above slow virus diseases from their natural host to a new species of experimental animal results in a marked accentuation of the characteristic spongiform change. The question arises as to whether this common histopathologic end result of infection means that one infectious agent conceivably is responsible for the seemingly diverse diseases constituting the group of subacute spongiform encephalopathies. Could kuru and Creutzfeldt-Jakob disease reflect ingestion of or intimate contact with sheep tissue infected with scrapie virus? This possibility already has been suggested concerning the origin of transmissible mink encephalopathy. Clinical and histopathologic differences between these diseases, as well as differences in properties of their respective etiologic agents, may merely reflect long-standing residence and propagation of each agent in different hosts of different genotypes.

Progressive multifocal leukoencephalopathy is a demyelinating disease affecting individuals in the fifth and sixth decades of life. The clinical setting almost always is one of immunosuppression. Individuals developing progressive multifocal leukoencephalopathy usually have either primary disease known to be associated with an abnormality in host immune responsiveness, e.g., Hodgkin's disease, or some other primary disorder for which immunosuppressive drug therapy has been prescribed. Specific examples include hematoproliferative disorders and systemic diseases of presumed immunologic etiology such as lupus erythematosus or Wegener's granulomatosis. Progressive multifocal leukoencephalopathy also has been reported in a recipient of a renal allograft; the patient required immunosuppressive drugs to maintain function of the kidney transplant.

In contrast to most of the slow virus diseases of animals and the two spongiform encephalopathies of man, a conventional virus appears to be the causal agent in progressive multifocal leukoencephalopathy. Virions morphologically indistinguishable from SV40 virus have been observed in electron photomicrographs of brain tissue of patients with the disease (Fig. 6-8). Virus has been isolated and propagated in tissue culture from brain specimens which closely resembles SV40 (see Chap. 5).

Subacute sclerosing panencephalitis is a neurologic disease of young children and adolescents. Cases rarely occur in individuals beyond 14 years of age. The disease was originally described in the 1930s under various names,

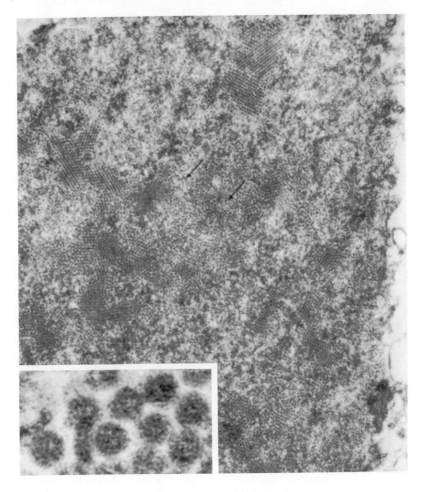

Figure 6-8. Myriads of virions almost filling nucleus of glial cell in the brain of a patient with progressive multifocal leukoencephalopathy. Arrows indicate occasional filamentous structures, possibly of viral origin. (× 23,700.) Inset shows details of virions with both spherical and elongated particles. (× 252,000.) (From ZuRhein, G. M.: Polyoma-like virions in a human demyelinating disease. Acta Neuropathol. (Berl.) *8:*57, 1967.)

including Dawson's inclusion body encephalitis and Van Bogaert's subacute sclerosing leukoencephalitis. The prominent inclusion bodies, which were the basis for Dawson's nosologic terminology, suggested from the beginning that the disease had a viral cause.

Initial clinical manifestations of subacute sclerosing panencephalitis are insidious, consisting of such changes as shortened attention span, poor performance of schoolwork, and subtle behavioral problems. More overt signs appear within a few weeks or months, e.g., mental deterioration, myoclonic jerking, and ataxia. The disease culminates in stupor, dementia, decorticate rigidity, and finally death. The cerebrospinal fluid often has a selective increase in gamma globulin content. A substantial portion of this gamma globulin has been shown to result from de novo synthesis of IgG within the central nervous system.

The histopathologic findings of subacute sclerosing panencephalitis are more varied than those of many of the other slow virus diseases, consisting of the following degenerative and inflammatory components: perivascular mononuclear cell infiltrates, proliferation of astrocytes, diffuse destruction of myelin (especially within the subcortical white matter of the cerebral hemispheres), and prominent acidophilic inclusion bodies in neuronal and glial cells which exhibit varying degrees of cellular injury and degeneration.

Epidemiologic surveys indicate that close to 85 per cent of cases of subacute sclerosing panencephalitis occur in children residing in or previously living in rural areas. A very high proportion of patients are known to have experienced an attack of measles at a very early age, i.e., before two or three years of age. This is of special interest in light of extensive data incriminating this virus as a cause of the disease. Subacute sclerosing panencephalitis is classed as a slow virus disease (see Table 6–1) because of the exceptionally long period elapsing between acquisition of measles virus infection and onset of neurologic clinical manifestations and the invariably progressive and fatal course of the disease.

As is true for progressive multifocal leukoencephalopathy, subacute sclerosing panencephalitis appears to be a slow virus disease elicited by a conventional virus. Considerable evidence indicates that subacute sclerosing panencephalitis is the direct consequence of persistent measles virus infection. Electron microscopic studies have revealed structures with all of the morphologic features of measles virus (Figs. 6–9 and 6–10). The inclusion bodies stain specifically with labeled measles antibody (Fig. 6–11). Patients with subacute sclerosing panencephalitis have extremely high titers of measles antibody in their blood and cerebrospinal fluid. Finally, a virus closely resembling measles virus has been isolated from brain tissue of some patients by the technique of co-cultivation of the explanted brain specimen with a permissive line of tissue culture cells.

One might ask why the slow virus diseases appear to affect preferentially the nervous system. There is clear evidence that comparable titers of infectious activity exist in organs other than the brain in every one of the diseases in which this point has been assessed. Therefore, the idea that susceptible host cells capable of supporting viral replication only reside in nervous tissue can be rejected. If cell repair capacity or cellular regenerative potential should prove to be a critical factor in ongoing slow virus-host

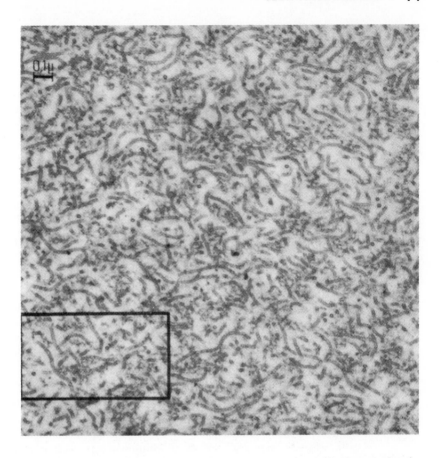

Figure 6–9. Intranuclear inclusion within nerve cell of the brain of a patient with subacute sclerosing leukoencephalitis (panencephalitis), which consists of randomly striated tubules. (X 56,000.) (From Perier, O., Vanderhaeghen, J. J., and Pelc, S.: Subacute sclerosing leukoencephalitis. Electron microscopic finding in two cases with inclusion bodies. Acta Neuropathol. *8:*363, 1967.)

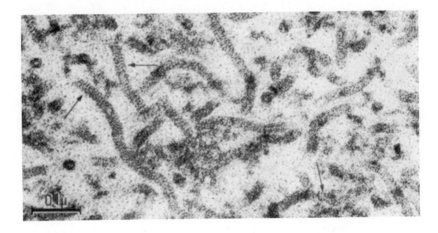

Figure 6–10. Framed portion of Figure 6–9 at higher magnification to illustrate transverse striations of the tubules. (X 150,000.) (From Perier, D., Vanderhaeghen, J. J., and Pelc, S.: Subacute sclerosing leukoencephalitis. Electron microscopic finding in two cases with inclusion bodies. Acta Neuropathol. *8:*363, 1967.)

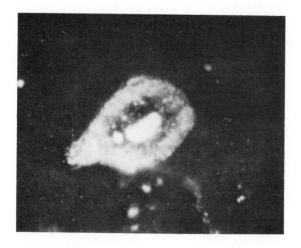

Figure 6–11. Bright fluorescence of nucleus and cytoplasm of a neuron in nervous tissue of a patient with subacute sclerosing panencephalitis indicative of the presence of measles antigen after staining with fluoresceinated measles antiserum. (From Freeman, J. M., Magoffin, R. L., Lennette, E. H., et al.: Additional evidence of the relation between subacute inclusion-body encephalitis and measles virus. Lancet 2:129, 1967.)

interactions, the well-known inability of neuronal cells to replicate might well explain the selective vulnerability of nervous tissue to slow virus disease. The extensive neuronal cell disintegration which reaches its maximum expression in the subacute spongiform encephalopathies certainly bears witness to the accumulative destructive effects slow virus infections can exert on host target tissues.

The propensity of slow virus infections to involve nervous tissue may reflect limited capacity of antibodies or immune cells to penetrate blood-brain-cerebrospinal fluid barriers and exert much influence on virus replicating within nervous tissue. Viewed in this light, the brain represents a "privileged sanctuary" in which viruses might well establish slow and relentless infection, relatively unhampered by host immune responses. In such a setting, the infectious agents might cause target cell destruction sufficient to result in clinical and pathologic manifestations of disease.

Virus-Host Relationships Characterizing Slow and Other Types of Viral Infections

Reference has already been made to the likelihood that slow virus diseases probably represent a special type of virus-host relationship. It is important to try to identify in what ways slow virus–host interactions differ from other types of virus-host interactions and viral diseases.

Various types of virus-host relationships associated with different types of viral diseases and specific examples of each are listed in Table 6–2. The viral diseases can be divided into two main categories with respect to the fate of the virus; i.e., whether the virus is eliminated or whether it persists in host tissues for long periods of time.

In acute viral infections, the infectious agent reaches its maximum level or titer in a very short period of time, i.e., days or weeks. It is then rapidly eliminated by the host concomitant with build-up of immunologic responses of one kind or another. The virus does not persist; the host usually recovers. Durable immunity provides resistance to reinfection at a later date.

TABLE 6–2. Different Types of Viral Infections and Characteristics of Their
Respective Virus-Host Relationships

Fate of Virus in Host	Type of Infection	Characteristic Virus-Host Relationships	Specific Examples
Eliminated; does not persist	Acute	Short incubation periods (2 days to 2 or 3 weeks) Virus recoverable before but not after disease onset; recovery common Recovered host immune to same or closely related viruses	Variola (usually results in disease) Poliomyelitis (rarely results in disease)
Not eliminated; persists in host tissues for months, years, or for life	Latent	Acute primary infection, recovery and subsequent relapses-remissions of disease Virus recoverable during primary and relapsing phases of infection; not recoverable from target tissue during remissions Host immune response demonstrable but ineffective in preventing relapse	Herpes simplex ("fever blisters") Varicella-zoster ("shingles")
	Chronic	Variable incubation period, outcome, and course Virus persists and regularly recoverable Host immune response demonstrable but does not influence pattern of disease.	Rubella syndrome Cytomegalovirus infection Hepatitis B (serum hepatitis) infection
	Slow	Incubation periods of months or years Relentless, progressive, and lethal course of disease Virus recoverable before onset and throughout course of disease Host immune response unpredictable: invariably absent; inconstant and weak; constant and exaggerated	Kuru Progressive multifocal leukoencephalopathy Subacute sclerosing panencephalitis (many would qualify as "chronic" infection)

If the host does not eliminate the virus, its persistence can lead to various types of virus-host relationships which translate into different types of infections, viz., latent, chronic, and slow virus infections (see Table 6–2). These three types of infections, in addition to differences in their incubation periods, are distinguished with respect to whether the virus is regularly recoverable (chronic and slow) or only intermittently so (latent), whether a host immune response is regularly demonstrable (latent and chronic) or not (slow), and whether the clinical course is relentless and lethal (slow) or variable (latent and chronic).

Properties of Viruses

Typical or Conventional Viruses

The etiologic agents of progressive multifocal leukoencephalopathy and subacute sclerosing panencephalitis appear to resemble typical viruses. Their conventional nature has allowed the use of standard biologic and biochemical procedures, which is an enormous advantage.

Of the 3 papova-like viruses associated with progressive multifocal leukoencephalopathy, the one most often isolated, designated "JC" virus (for the initials of the patient from who it was isolated), is morphologically and chemically related to other members of this group, e.g., SV40, polyoma virus, and human wart virus (see Chap. 5). Antigenically, JC virus appears to be a new papova virus which is distinct from both polyoma virus and human wart virus, although it does appear to have at least a weak antigenic relationship to SV40. Like SV40, the JC virus is able to induce brain tumors in hamsters following experimental infection. JC virus has been successfully propagated in human fetal glial cell cultures. Serologic surveys have shown that approximately 70 per cent of healthy adults have circulating antibodies to the JC virus. The ubiquity of the virus and the low incidence of progressive multifocal leukoencephalopathy suggest that infection rarely results in disease. Perhaps a significant downturn in host immune status, secondary to a primary disease or vigorous use of immunosuppressive drugs, jeopardizes a previously stable virus-host interaction which had been sufficient to maintain the virus in a latent phase. During a period of sustained immunosuppression, the virus may become activated, invade the brain, and initiate disease. Alternatively, JC virus conceivably is part of a "normal brain viral flora," and in the face of diminished immunologic host forces it can begin replicating in situ and cause neurologic disease.

A close correlation between a measles-like virus and subacute sclerosing panencephalitis has been established by a number of different investigators. Since patients with the disease typically have abnormally high titers of humoral antibodies reactive with measles virus, several researchers have suggested that impairment of cellular immune mechanisms may be directly responsible for the inability of the host to limit viral proliferation and cellular damage. Support for this theory has been provided by reports of altered cellular immune responsiveness in some patients. Recently, the measles-like virus has been isolated and shown to possess a neucleocapsid with a helical symmetry and RNA, similar to other members of the paramyxovirus group (see Chap. 4). The virus has been isolated from brain tissue of several (but not all) patients with subacute sclerosing panencephalitis and propagated in tissue culture.

A third type of conventional virus appears to be associated with Aleutian disease of mink. A picornavirus (see Chap. 4) has been isolated and purified from tissue extracts by affinity chromatographic techniques. The facts that disease in mink is associated with markedly elevated specific antibody levels and large amounts of this antibody could be secured proved to be of direct aid in efforts to purify the virus. Coupling the antibody to an inert substrate allowed the virus to be selectively absorbed. Subsequent elution of the virus provided virus-rich preparations suitable for physical and chemical characterization. Like other picornaviruses, the agent associated with Aleutian disease of mink appears to be an icosahedral virus approximately 20 nm in diameter.

The virus causing visna also behaves like a conventional virus. Several years elapsed before it was discovered that choroid plexus cultures were necessary for isolating and propagating the agent, thereby highlighting the specificity of host cell susceptibility for in vitro cultivation of an infectious agent. Since demyelination is a prominent histopathologic change in both visna and progressive multifocal leukoencephalopathy, one would suspect that, in vivo, both of the viruses causing these diseases would have a special predilection for infecting oligodendrocytes, the glial cells responsible for synthesis of myelin. Electron microscopic studies have already supplied evidence for this in the latter disease but not in the former.

Atypical Infectious Agents

The infectious agents associated with the subacute spongiform encephalopathies (kuru, Creutzfeldt-Jakob disease, scrapie, and transmissible mink encephalopathy) have not yet been isolated or characterized.

No hint of detectable specific antibody has been uncovered in these diseases despite extensive efforts to do so. Repeated attempts to isolate and propagate the agents in standard tissue culture lines have invariably proved unsuccessful. Kuru and Creutzfeldt-Jakob agents clearly do persist in high titer in explant cultures of infected chimpanzee brain in vitro. However, such cultures show no evidence of cytopathic changes indicative of infection, and demonstration of each agent in an infectious form is dependent on development of the respective diseases, i.e., kuru and Creutzfeldt-Jakob disease, following inoculation of the explant brain cultures into chimpanzees.

The unavailability of specific antibody preparations and the inability to induce cytopathic effects in cell culture leave the virologist without two of the most useful tools normally available for virologic research. Unfortunately, studies of these agents are solely dependent on the use of infectivity assays in laboratory animals. The extremely long incubation periods that elapse before clinical symptoms of the disease occur further compound the difficulty. For all of these reasons, progress has been slow, even slower than the diseases under study.

Based on limited information derived from infectious assays, the scrapie agent and probably the other atypical agents as well, are unique types of infectious units. The scrapie agent is extremely resistant to inactivation by heat and chemicals. Early studies suggested that the scrapie agent was also extremely resistant to inactivation by irradiation, and the possibility existed that these atypical agents did not have nucleic acid. However, it has been shown more recently that the scrapie agent can be inactivated by irradiation but that the size of the genome is very small. Its estimated molecular weight is approximately 1.5×10^5 daltons. This finding has led some investigators to suggest that the scrapie agent may be an extraordinarily small infectious unit, perhaps analogous to "viroids." Viroids are a new class of infectious agents which produce diseases of plants and vegetables that are of economic importance to agriculture. One of the most extensively studied viroids, potato stunt tuber agent allegedly consists of "naked RNA" and has been cited as a possible model agent for scrapie.

It should be emphasized, however, that to the best of our knowledge no RNA exists in mammalian cells as naked RNA. Even messenger RNA has been shown to have an equal amount of or more protein associated with it. Furthermore, membrane filtration data indicate that scrapie infectivity is associated with units having a size of approximately 25 to 35 nm. This size estimation clearly is in conflict with that calculated from the irradiation inactivation-target size studies. The most likely explanation for these discordant observations is that the scrapie agent is indeed small but exists in some complexed form with host cells. Recent studies indicating that scrapie infectivity is intimately associated with nerve cell membrane preparations or fragments illustrate one type of special virus-host relationship that is consonant with available information.

Prolonged Incubation Periods

The many months or even years that intervene between the time of actual infection and the point when overt clinical disease occurs has already been mentioned as a serious obstacle to study of slow virus diseases. Young, impatient research scientists are not attracted to experiments which require several years' time. However, even the older, established investigator encounters innumerable problems, e.g., proper physical facilities for maintaining often expensive animals (e.g., chimpanzees) under observation for years under conditions which exclude infection by extraneous environmental agents. In the only published account of transmission of scrapie to a primate host, the incubation period following inoculation of a Cynomolgous monkey with scrapie-infected mouse brain was five years and five months!

Once a slow virus disease has been transmitted to and serially passaged in a new species of experimental animal, the incubation period may be shortened. This has been observed with the scrapie agent in mice and with kuru in chimpanzees. Such has not been true with the Creutzfeldt-Jakob disease agent, since incubation periods still run close to two years or more in second passage chimpanzees and monkeys.

What clues can one find in explaining the remarkably long incubation periods? There is no compelling evidence that the prolonged incubation periods reflect inordinately slow replication of the agents. Those conventional type viruses which have been propagated in tissue culture, e.g., visna virus and the JC papoviruses isolated from patients with progressive multifocal leukoencephalopathy, replicate at rates no different from that of other typical animal viruses. Before concluding that there is nothing slow about the viruses, one should keep in mind that visna virus and JC papovirus may not replicate at the same rate in vivo in the nervous tissue milieu. Furthermore, nothing is known about replication rates of the agents associated with the subacute spongiform encephalopathies.

One point to consider is how do these viruses reach their central nervous system target? During the 1950s, conventional neurotropic viruses such as poliovirus were shown to appear in the bloodstream well in advance of clinical signs of neurologic disease. This finding paved the way for successful prevention of poliomyelitis by vaccines capable of inducing circulating antibody titers sufficient to neutralize the virus before it could invade the brain and spinal cord. These studies gave rise to the view that most, if not all, viruses reach the central nervous system as a consequence of viremia. Pushed to one side in the enthusiastic embrace of this concept were older observations indicating that some viruses, including polioviruses, can migrate in nerve fibers and travel in retrograde fashion toward the brain and spinal cord.

Recent studies have shown that terminal nerve fibers, i.e., motor end plates, have the capacity to "ingest" a variety of particles by endocytosis. Inert particles gaining access to terminal fibers in this fashion exhibit retrograde movement within axons. Their rate of progression can be measured with a fair degree of accuracy. It is surprising to learn that the rate of retrograde migration toward the neuraxis is only about half that of anterograde migration.

Based on observations that the histopathologic changes of scrapie in mice occur in widely different anatomic regions of the brain and that such changes may begin at very different points in time, at least one investigator has suggested that the scrapie agent gains entry to central nervous system tissues not by viremia but via the peripheral nerves.

Since the mode of entry of all of the infectious agents causing slow virus diseases in their natural hosts is unknown, it may be wise to keep an open mind on the subject. It could well be that these agents commonly gain access to peripheral nerve terminals and do so only at considerable distances from the central nervous system, e.g., through abrasions on the feet. Even more importantly, once the agents are in the peripheral nerve axoplasm they might exhibit unexpectedly slow rates of retrograde migration to the neuraxis via peripheral nerve fibers. Either circumstance might be sufficient to account for the characteristic long incubation periods.

Lack of Host Immune Responses

Mention has already been made of the conspicuous lack of any host immune response to the atypical agents associated with the subacute spongiform encephalopathies. This is an important point deserving more than passing notice.

Firstly, it seems unreasonable to think that lack of an immune response is a reflection of the small size of these agents. Using data obtained for the scrapie agent, one notes that the estimated molecular weight of this agent, 1.5×10^5 daltons, is well above that of many smaller molecular weight constitutents which are excellent antigens. The size of the scrapie infectious unit, viz., 25 to 35 nm, is not materially different from that of poliomyelitis virus, which is noteworthy for its immunogenic activity. Furthermore, if the scrapie agent is complexed to host cell membranes, as recent data suggest, such complexing should actually serve to enhance its antigenic potential, based on what is known about the immunogenicity of small molecular weight haptens, e.g., dinitrochlorobenzene, when complexed to host constituents.

Secondly, virtually all efforts to demonstrate immune responses against these agents have focused on neutralization of infectivity of the agent. As already emphasized, work on these slow virus disease agents has been hampered by the necessity of using infectivity as the sole means of assay. It is entirely possible that host immune responses are made but against antigenic determinants different from those involved in neutralization tests.

Thirdly, practically no attention has been paid to the overall immunologic responsiveness of natural or experimental hosts infected with the spongiform encephalitogenic agents. How well do patients or chimpanzees with kuru or Creutzfeldt-Jakob disease respond to unrelated antigens? What are the immunologic responses of scrapie-infected mice to a battery of antigenic stimuli? Conventional viruses are known which either potentiate or depress immunologic responsiveness of a host; there is no reason to believe that the atypical slow virus disease agents might not be endowed with similar immunoregulatory potential. One need envision only that these agents have a selective capacity to infect and activate thymus-derived lymphocytes responsible for exerting a suppressive effect on cell-mediated immune responses and antibody production. Under such circumstances, one could readily explain the apparent immunologic unresponsiveness of hosts infected with these agents. What type of response do scrapie-infected mice make to sheep red blood cells? How does their capacity to reject skin allografts compare with that of uninfected litter mate control mice?

Finally, circulating immunosuppressive factors have been reported to occur in patients with a diverse number of different infectious and malignant diseases. These immunosuppressive serum factors usually are detected by their capacity to diminish or quench proliferative responses of cultured lymphocytes of clinically well donors following stimulation with various mitogens or antigen(s) to which the lymphocyte donor is sensitized. A search should be made for such circulating immunosuppressant factors in the subacute spongiform encephalopathies.

Histopathologic and Immunologic Correlates of Slow Virus Diseases

Increasing evidence has been presented from several quarters that the characteristic inflammatory responses accompanying the tissue injury observed in infections caused by conventional viruses may in large part be due to host immune responses to the virus. According to this view, antibody produced by the host interacts with virus within the target tissue. This virus-immune response then activates, by one or more specific pathways, various inflammation cascades culminating in infiltration of host tissues with lymphocytes and histiocytes. Evidence for this theory is particularly strong in the case of lymphocytic choriomeningitis, a neurotropic viral infection of mice and other mammals.

The role of host immune responses in the development of histopathologic changes of infectious processes is illustrated by the slow virus diseases. Correlations between patterns of histopathologic changes and presence or absence of host immune responses are set out in Table 6–3.

TABLE 6-3. Histopathologic and Immunologic Correlates in Slow Virus Diseases

Slow Virus Disease	Histopathologic Change		Host Immune Response
	Degeneration	Inflammation	
Scrapie	+	0	0
Transmissible mink encephalopathy	+	0	0
Kuru	+	0	0
Creutzfeldt-Jakob disease	+	0	0
Progressive multifocal leukoencephalopathy	+	± or 0	± or +
Visna	+	+	+
Subacute sclerosing panencephalitis	+	+	++
Aleutian disease of mink	+	+++	+++

In each of the spongiform encephalopathies, the basic histopathologic change is one of cellular degeneration and destruction. Perivascular mononuclear cell infiltrates are not a feature; inflammatory responses are minimal or absent. In these four diseases, there is a total lack of any demonstrable immune response. In progressive multifocal leukoencephalopathy, immune responses to the papovavirus are often minimal at best, which is not surprising since this disease is observed only in clinical settings involving immunosuppression. A variable degree of inflammatory response is seen in lesions of this disease.

In contrast to the spongiform encephalopathies, visna and subacute sclerosing panencephalitis and Aleutian disease of mink are characterized by (in the order mentioned) increasingly more intense and widespread inflammatory changes, which occur concurrently with those changes of a degenerative nature. In each of these three diseases, respectively, immune responses of increasing magnitude are demonstrable. Circulating antibody titers appear to correlate directly with the intensity of the inflammatory responses in host target tissues.

References

Books

Persistent Infections. *In* Fenner, F., McAuslan, B. R., Mims, C. A., Samsbrook, J., and White, D. O. (eds.): The Biology of Animal Viruses. 2nd ed. New York, Academic Press, 1974.

Zeman, W., and Lennette, E. H. (eds.): Slow Virus Diseases. Baltimore, Williams & Wilkins Co., 1974.

Review Articles

Diener, T. O.: Viroids: The smallest known agents of infectious disease. Annu. Rev. Microbiol. *28:*23, 1974.

Eklund, C. M., and Hadlow, W. J.: Implication of slow viral diseases of domestic animals for human disease. Medicine *52:*357, 1973.

Fuccillo, D. A., Kurent, J. E., and Sever, J. L.: Slow virus diseases. Annu. Rev. Microbiol. *28:*231, 1974.

Gajdusek, D. C.: Slow virus diseases of the central nervous system. Am. J. Clin. Pathol. *56:*320, 1971.

Gajdusek, D. C.: Slow virus infection and activation of latent infections in aging. Adv. Gerontol. Res. *4:*201, 1972.

Holland, J. J.: Slow, inapparent and recurrent viruses. Sci. Am. *230:*33, 1974.

Lampert, P. W., Gajdusek, D. C., and Gibbs, C. J., Jr.: Subacute spongiform virus encephalopathies. Scrapie, Kuru and Creutzfeldt-Jakob disease: A review. Am. J. Pathol. *68:*626, 1972.

Original Articles

Alper, T., Haig, D. A., and Clarke, M. C.: The exceptionally small size of the scrapie agent. Biochem. Biophys. Res. Commun. *22:*278, 1966.

Blinzinger, K., and Anzil, A. P.: Neural route of infection in viral diseases of the central nervous system. Lancet *2:*1374, 1974.

Diener, T. O.: Is the scrapie agent a viroid? Nature (New Biol.) *235:*218, 1972.

Gajdusek, D. C., and Zigas, V.: Degenerative disease of the central nervous system in New Guinea. N. Engl. J. Med. *257:*974, 1957.

Gajdusek, D. C., Gibbs, C. J., Jr., and Alpers, M.: Experimental transmission of a kuru-like syndrome to chimpanzees. Nature *209:*794, 1966.

Gibbs, C. J., Jr., and Gajdusek, D. C.: Infection as the etiology of spongiform encephalopathy (Creutzfeldt-Jakob disease). Science *165:*1023, 1969.

Oldstone, M. B. A., and Dixon, F. J.: Pathogenesis of chronic disease associated with persistent lymphocytic choriomeningitis viral infection. I. Relationship of antibody production to disease in neonatally infected mice. J. Exp. Med. *129:*483, 1969.

Sigurdsson, B., Palsson, P. A., and Grimsson, H.: Visna, a demyelinating transmissible disease of sheep. J. Neuropathol. Exp. Neurol. *16:*389, 1957.

Chapter 7

THE INDIGENOUS MICROBIOTA OF THE HUMAN HOST

Introduction

Present day infection more often results from the interaction with bacteria that compose the normal flora of the host than from exogenous microorganisms. This is in sharp contrast to the epidemics of the past, when plague, cholera, or smallpox, diseases associated with microorganisms capable of causing infection in any susceptible host, were the scourges of mankind. Today, the most serious threat of infection is from our own microbiota.

In Chapter 2, the change in type of microorganisms associated with infection today from the highly contagious, virulent microbes of the past was shown to be related in part to two variables: (1) changes in host resistance, and (2) modification of host flora. Decreases in host resistance may result from multiple factors, including acquired immunologic deficiencies, nutritional deprivation, and acute and chronic illnesses. External physical agents such as trauma, irradiation for malignant tumors, or accidental exposure to nuclear irradiation can rapidly interfere with normal host defense mechanisms and predispose to infection. The intentional suppression of the inflammatory or immune response by azothioprine, corticosteroids, antilymphocyte serum, or other agents may predispose to infection by microorganisms otherwise considered to be harmless to the host.

The virulence of parasites in the normal host microbiota may change rapidly, depending on the acquisition of new phage or serotypes of bacteria. Episomes coding for genetic resistance to antimicrobial agents can be transferred to one bacterium by another within the gastrointestinal tract.

81

Bacterial populations, previously sensitive to numerous antimicrobial agents, can rapidly become resistant to many agents by episome transfer. While bacteria such as *Mycobacterium tuberculosis* and *Yersinia pestis* (plague) are capable of inducing disease in well-nourished, vigorous young adults, the serious infections seen in today's hospitals are more commonly caused by *Escherichia coli, Klebsiella pneumoniae, Staphylococcus aureus,* and *Proteus mirabilis.* All of these organisms can be recovered from one site or another from the normal human host. Inasmuch as most humans live in harmony with these bacteria without signs of infection, physicians come to regard them as "nonpathogens." However, with tissue necrosis following surgery, suppression of immune response, or modification of host defense mechanisms, the nonpathogen may quickly become a "pathogen."

Indigenous Microbiota

There are several reasons why the study of the normal human microbiota is helpful. (1) A knowledge of the different types of organisms in or on a surface of the body at various locations gives greater insight into the kind of infections that might occur following tissue injury at these sites. (2) Knowledge of bacteria native to any one part of the body helps the physician place in perspective the possible source and significance of microorganisms isolated from clinical infections. (3) Knowledge of the indigenous microbiota is important in understanding the consequences of overgrowth by microorganisms normally absent at that site. One such example is the heavy growth of yeast in the gastrointestinal tract that can occur in a patient given large doses of neomycin. Although neomycin is effective in suppressing bacteria in the Family Enterobacteriaceae, it has no effect on yeast, and administration of this drug is frequently followed by an annoying diarrhea associated with an almost pure growth of *Candida albicans.*

Interaction of Indigenous Microbiota

Little is known of the overall significance of the microbial flora in the human body. One reason for this is that the study of the microbial flora in the past has been primarily directed toward the isolation, enumeration, and classification of microbial species. While procedures for enumerating bacteria on exposed surfaces such as the skin are not difficult, considerably more effort is necessary to study the microbial flora in different segments of the gastrointestinal tract. Investigation of this type requires specialized sampling equipment and culture media, and specialized technical training for personnel. Although the enumeration and identification of bacterial species is a necessary first step, they do not provide information about the interaction between one bacterial species and another. *Bacteroides melaninogenicus,* for example, a strict gram-negative anaerobic bacillus, requires the presence of three other anaerobic bacteria to produce severe necrotizing infections of the mouth. None of the four microorganisms are capable of causing infection when used singly. One of these microorganisms, a diphtheroid, is necessary for the synthesis of vitamin K, a substance needed for growth by *B. melaninogenicus.* The interaction between the other two bacterial species, the bacteroides, and the diphtheroid that leads to a necrotizing infection is not known. It is more than likely that many similar interactions occur between different bacterial species within the body, both in diseased and normal regions.

Bacterial Nomenclature

One of the annoying problems facing the practicing physician is the constant reclassification and changing names of microorganisms. A recent example is the renaming of the bacterium associated with pneumococcal pneumonia. Until 1967, this microorganism was officially known as *Diplococcus pneumoniae* in the United States. Although taxonomists have recognized that there are similarities between the streptococci and pneumococci for many years, microbiologists in the United States preferred to separate the two by continuing to use a different genus name even though scientists in other parts of the world had decided that these microorganisms were related. In 1967, agreement by microbiologists in the United States to reclassify this organism within the Streptococceae was reflected by approval of a change in the name from *D. pneumoniae* to *Streptococcus pneumoniae.*

Although the reasons for changing the names of microorganisms are usually not relevant to the medical significance of the microorganism, physicians should be aware that nomenclature for microorganisms is constantly changing — that one should be able to recognize an old friend in new clothes. Several recent examples of nomenclature changes are the following:

> *Yersinia pestis* for *Pasteurella pestis* — the agent of plague
> *Francisella tularensis* for *Pasteurella tularensis* — the microorganism that causes tularemia
> *Acinetobacter calcoaceticus* for *Herellea vaginicola* — a gram negative bacillus

Table 7–1 lists the members of the Family Enterobacteriaceae. This group of microorganisms consists of many of the facultative anaerobic bacteria commonly associated with urinary tract infections, bacterial diarrheas, and bacterial septicemia. The recognition by taxonomists of additional characteristics facilitating separation of bacterial species will continue to result in changes in nomenclature. Therefore, it is best not to become unalterably attached to terminology used in older or even current texts.

Indigenous Microbiota by Anatomic Region

In this section, comments pertaining to different anatomic regions of the body are given to provide additional information about host-parasite characteristics and the indigenous microbiota. No attempt is made to list all factors relevant to establishing the characteristic indigenous microbiota. A knowledge of the microorganisms normally found at different regions of the body is helpful in the interpretation of reports from the Clinical Laboratory.

TABLE 7-1. Family Enterobacteriaceae*

Escherichia coli
Shigella dysenteriae
flexneri
boydii
sonnei

Edwardsiella tarda
Salmonella choleraesuis
typhi
enteritidis
1800 + other varieties
Arizona hinshawii
Citrobacter freundii
diversus

Klebsiella pneumoniae
ozaenae
rhinoscleromatis
Enterobacter cloacae
aerogenes
hafniae
agglomerans
Serratia marcescens
liquefaciens
rubidaea
Proteus mirabilis
vulgaris
morgani
rettgeri
Providence alcalifaciens
stuartii

---

*Modified from Edwards, P. R., and Ewing, W. H.: Identification of Enterobacteriaceae. 3rd ed. Minneapolis, Burgess Publishing Co., 1972.

Skin

The skin shows wide variation in structure and function from one site of the body to another. Differences in the thickness of the epidermis and number and type of dermal appendages between the eyelid, axilla, and sole of the foot will determine differences in the numbers and types of microbial population. Ecologic factors vary greatly between the desquamating surface epithelial cells and the lumen of sebaceous glands deep in the dermis. Most skin bacteria are found on the superficial squamous epithelium, colonizing keratinized, dead cells. Viruses, e.g., varicella (chickenpox), require living cells for hosts, and, therefore, infect cells found in or near the basal germinal layers of the epidermis. Lipophilic anaerobic bacteria, such as *Propionibacterium acnes* (formerly called *Corynebacterium acne*) live in the deep sebaceous glands and are not exposed to surface decontaminating solutions used prior to venipuncture. For this reason, propionibacteria are not uncommonly found in blood and cerebrospinal fluid cultures and cultures of bone marrow, presumably owing to contamination of the aspirating needle during collection of the specimen (see Table 7–2).

TABLE 7–2. Microorganisms Found in the Skin

Microorganism	Range of Incidence (Per Cent)
Staphylococcus epidermidis (albus) (coagulase negative)	85–100
Staphylococcus aureus (coagulase positive)	5–25
Streptococcus pyogenes (Group A)	0–4
Propionibacterium acnes (anaerobic corynebacteria)	45–100
Aerobic corynebacteria (diphtheroids)	55
Candida albicans	Uncommon
Other Candida species, particularly C. parapsilosis	1–15
Gram negative bacteria, e.g., Enterobacteriaceae or Pseudomonas species	Uncommon

As discussed in Chapter 2, the normal skin has several mechanisms to control overgrowth and infection from resident bacteria. Sweat glands excrete lysozyme (muramidase) which may be effective in lysing *Staphylococcus epidermidis* and other gram positive bacteria. Sebaceous glands secrete complex lipids which may be partially degraded by specific enzymes from certain gram positive bacteria. These bacteria, therefore, can change the secreted lipids to unsaturated fatty acids having strong antimicrobial activity against gram negative bacteria and certain fungi. Some of the unsaturated fatty acids resulting from bacterial degradation are volatile and may be associated with a strong odor. For this reason, deodorants have been formulated containing antibacterial substances exerting selective action against gram positive bacteria. Suppression of gram positive bacteria may then result in a shift of the skin bacterial population to predominantly gram negative bacteria. Such a shift of flora, while reducing the amount of aromatic unsaturated fatty acids and presumably making the deodorant user more socially acceptable, may predispose to colonization and possible infection by gram negative bacteria.

Prior colonization of the skin by one bacterial species may prevent or retard colonization by another. This phenomenon has been termed "bacterial interference" and may result from preferential attachment to specific receptors between the bacterium and epithelial cells (see Chap. 2). During the early antibiotic era, infection by penicillin-resistant strains of phage type 80/81 *Staphylococcus aureus* frequently appeared in newborn nurseries, where spread from mothers to infants and from infant to infant often occurred with frightening speed and disastrous results. In an attempt to reduce this threat, newborn infants were deliberately colonized with a strain of *Staphylococcus aureus* designated 502A, which seemed to prevent or at least delay colonization of the infant by a more virulent staphylococcus. The use of *Staphylococcus aureus* 502A to produce bacterial interference by intentional colonization has been of significant help in selected situations, but occasional infections have appeared in susceptible infants. The terms "pathogenic" and "nonpathogenic" are relative, depending upon the presence or absence of poorly defined host resistance factors (see Chaps. 36 and 37).

Nose and Nasopharynx

The most common bacteria found in the nose are staphylococci, usually in highest numbers just inside the nares. In this location, both *Staphylococcus aureus* and *S. epidermidis* are considered to mirror the microbiota of the skin of the face at the nasal labial fold (see Chap. 36 and 37). Obtaining a culture of the posterior nasopharynx is difficult owing to the problem of passing a culture swab or wire through the nasal passages without contamination. Although special swabs are available for this purpose, they are used infrequently, owing to the decreased need for such cultures, and are consequently hard to find. Cultures of the posterior nasopharyngeal region are indicated when surveying suspected carriers or contacts of patients with diphtheria. Diphtheroids, a large, poorly classified group of gram positive bacteria not associated with infection, are commonly found in the nose as well as in the nasopharynx. (See Table 7–3.)

TABLE 7–3. Microorganisms Found in the Nose and Nasopharynx

Microorganism	Range of Incidence (Per Cent)
Staphylococcus aureus	20–85
Staphylococcus epidermidis	90
Aerobic corynebacteria (diphtheroids)	5–80
Streptococcus pneumoniae	0–17
Streptococcus pyogenes (Group A)	0.1–5
Alpha- or nonhemolytic streptococci	Uncommon
Neisseria catarrhalis	12
Haemophilus influenzae	12
Gram negative bacteria (Enterobacteriaceae)	Uncommon

Oropharynx

Like the nose, the oropharynx contains large numbers of both *Staphylococcus aureus* and *S. epidermidis.* Recovery of *S. aureus* from either the nose or throat does *not* mean that the patient should be automatically considered as a carrier of a virulent strain of the microorganism, nor that the patient should be treated with antibiotics.

Perhaps the most important group of microorganisms native to the oropharynx are the alpha-hemolytic streptococci. Although the commonly used term for alpha-hemolytic streptococci, *Streptococcus viridans,* is still used in many texts and by clinicians with the implication that it refers to a single bacterial species, it should be noted that the term applies to a large group of poorly classified streptococci frequently having in common only the ability to produce an alpha-hemolytic reaction on sheep blood agar. Careful identification procedures can classify to a well-defined species many of these alpha-hemolytic strains of streptococci, but the general term *S. viridans* persists. Cultures from the oropharynx will also show large numbers of diphtheroids and *Neisseria catarrhalis,* small gram negative cocci, related in part to *N. meningitidis* and *N. gonorrhoeae* but without known ability to cause disease.

Cultures from patients with sore throats may show varying types of bacteria that can be associated with infection either in the throat or at other sites of the body. These include Lancefield Group A streptococci, *Neisseria meningitidis, Streptococcus pneumoniae,* and *Haemophilus influenzae* (see Table 7–4). In most instances, when these strains are studied further, they are found not to have virulence factors such as serologically distinct capsules or other surface structures that characterize similar microorganisms causing severe infectious disease.

TABLE 7–4. Microorganisms Found in the Oropharynx

Microorganism	Range of Incidence (Per Cent)
Staphylococcus aureus	35–40
Staphylococcus epidermidis	30–70
Aerobic corynebacteria (diphtheroids)	50–90
Streptococcus pyogenes (Group A)	0–9
Streptococcus pneumoniae	0–50
Alpha- and nonhemophytic streptococci	25–99
Neisseria catarrhalis	10–97
Neisseria meningitidis	0–15
Haemophilus influenzae	5–20
Haemophilus parainfluenzae	20–35
Gram negative bacteria, e.g., *Klebsiella pneumoniae*	Uncommon

One of the most interesting aspects of the microbial flora of the nasopharynx is the relationship of alpha-hemolytic streptococci to other bacteria in this region. This group of bacteria have been shown to have inhibitory effects against colonization by Group A beta-hemolytic streptococci, pneumococci, *Staphylococcus aureus,* and the gram negative Enterobacteriaceae. The mechanism of inhibition by the alpha-hemolytic streptococci varies because of differences in the mode of action of secreted toxic substances.

Factors other than the administration of antibiotics or the length of hospital stay (exposure) may also be associated with modification of the pharyngeal flora. A recent study has suggested that the most important factor of pharyngeal colonization by gram negative bacilli is related to the severity of the patient's underlying illness. It was found that seriously ill or moribund patients are more likely to have gram negative bacteria in the pharynx than those less seriously ill. Colonization of the pharynx was then considered to be associated with an increased risk of pneumonia by gram negative bacteria. The reason for colonization by gram negative bacteria in this group of patients is not yet known.

Preferential attachment of different strains of bacteria to epithelial cells was mentioned in Chapter 2 and has been shown to be of significance in suppressing colonization by *Candida albicans* in germ-free mice. Blocking of the attachment of Group A streptococci to pharyngeal epithelial cells by parotid secretions of IgA anti-M protein has already been described (see Chap. 2).

Mouth

The microbial flora of the mouth shows marked changes, depending upon the presence or absence of teeth and the presence or absence of caries. With the development of teeth in the child, different strains of streptococci appear with a predilection for tooth surfaces (*Streptococcus sanguis* and *S. mutans*) or the buccal and gingival epithelial surfaces (*S. salivarius*). The presence of these and other oral bacteria contribute to the formation of dental plaque which in turn results in a low oxidation-reduction potential (Eh) on the surface of the tooth. The reduced oxidation-reduction potential will then permit growth of strict anaerobic bacteria such as *Bacteroides melaninogenicus, B. oralis,* or *Veillonella alcalescens,* particularly between opposing teeth and the dental-gingival crevices. *S. mutans,* one of the bacterial strains showing a predilection for attachment to tooth surfaces, is commonly associated with dental caries and cavity formation in teeth. The presence of a cavity in a tooth permits increased bacterial colonization and growth with further reduction in the oxidation-reduction potential within cavities and between adjacent teeth. In this manner, uncontrolled dental caries predispose to colonization and growth of large numbers of anaerobic bacteria and oral treponemes. Patients with advanced dental caries are of particular risk of incurring anaerobic pulmonary infections should they lose consciousness and inadvertently aspirate oral-pharyngeal secretions. Upon extraction of carious teeth and removal of protected sites for bacterial colonization and growth, the number of anaerobic bacteria and treponemes in the mouth falls rapidly. (See Table 7–5.)

TABLE 7–5. Microorganisms Found in the Mouth (Saliva – Tooth Surfaces)

Microorganism	Range of Incidence (Per Cent)
Staphylococcus epidermidis (coagulase negative)	75–100
Staphylococcus aureus (coagulase positive)	Common
Streptococcus mitis and other alpha-hemolytic streptococci	100
Streptococcus salivarius	100
Peptostreptococci	Prominent
Veillonella alcalescens	100
Lactobacilli	95
Actinomyces israeli	Common
Enterobacteriaceae	65
Haemophilus influenzae	25–100
Bacteroides fragilis	Common
Bacteroides melaninogenicus	Common
Bacteroides oralis	Common
Fusobacterium nucleatum	15–90
Candida albicans	6–50
Treponema dentium and *Borrelia refringens*	Common

Stomach

Under ordinary circumstances, the stomach is not considered to contain many viable microorganisms owing to the very acid pH of gastric contents. Most bacteria are either inactivated or killed when swallowed and exposed to a pH of 2 to 3 for even a short time. Exceptions may occur if there is rapid passage of microorganisms through the stomach or if the microorganisms are particularly resistant to gastric acidity, e.g., mycobacteria. Following ingestion of food, the numbers of bacteria will increase, only to fall with gastric emptying. Changes in the gastric microflora will also occur if there is an increase in gastric pH following high intestinal obstruction, thus permitting reflux of alkaline duodenal and jejunal secretions into the stomach. The bacterial content of the stomach is then likely to reflect that of the oropharynx and in addition will include both gram negative aerobic and anaerobic bacteria. (See Table 7–6.)

TABLE 7–6. Microorganisms Found in the Stomach and Small Intestine

Microorganism	Range of Incidence (Per Cent)
Stomach – Usually sterile, owing to gastric pH of 2–3	
Jejunum – Gram positive facultative bacteria (Enterococci, lactobacilli, diphtheroids)	Small numbers
Candida albicans	20–40
Ileum – Distal portion may show small numbers of Enterobacteriaceae and anaerobic gram negative bacteria	

Small Intestine

The upper portion of the small intestine contains few bacteria. Of the bacteria present, gram positive cocci and bacilli comprise the majority. *Streptococcus faecalis* (Group D streptococci), lactobacilli, and diphtheroids are occasionally found in the jejunum (see Table 7–6). The presence of diverticula of the duodenum or small intestine may create blind pockets and may in turn be associated with the proliferation of large numbers of bacteria which can modify the microbiota of the intestine at that level. Occasionally, a duodenal diverticulum has been associated with such large numbers of bacteria that they have modified absorption of vitamin B_{12}.

Intestinal obstruction below the ampulla of Vater tends to encourage the growth of microorganisms that can tolerate a high concentration of bile, e.g., *Streptococcus faecalis, Bacteroides fragilis,* and several species of Proteus. High concentrations of bile tend to limit the types of bacteria that cause infections in the liver, bile ducts, and gallbladder. Such microorganisms, in addition to *B. fragilis,* include *Salmonella typhi* and *Clostridium perfringens,* both of which may cause acute or chronic cholecystitis. Conversely, the susceptibility of pneumococci to the surface active, detergent action of bile makes infection with these organisms in the hepatobiliary tract almost nonexistent.

Candida albicans can be recovered from the small intestine in 20 to 40 per cent of normal humans. The small intestine may be the source of yeasts that rapidly replace bacteria succumbing to orally administered, broad-spectrum antibiotics such as neomycin, which is often given in preparation for intestinal surgery. Yeast in the small intestine may also represent one source of candida frequently found in blood cultures from seriously ill and debilitated patients, particularly those with disease that may result in ulceration of the intestinal tract.

In the distal portion of the small intestine, the microbiota begins to take on the characteristics of the colon; large numbers of enterobacteriaceae and anaerobic bacteria start to appear.

Large Intestine

The colon has by far the largest microbial population in the body. It has been estimated that the number of microorganisms in stool specimens approaches 10^{12} organisms per gram. Previously, it was not appreciated that this tremendous number of microorganisms consisted primarily of anaerobic, gram negative, non-spore forming bacteria, and gram positive, spore forming and non-spore forming bacilli. Not only are the vast majority of the microorganisms anaerobic but also there are large numbers of different species involved. Several investigators have calculated the ratio of strictly anaerobic to facultative anaerobic (Enterobacteriaceae) bacteria at approximately 300 to 1. Less than 0.3 per cent of all bacteria in the stool are members of the family Enterobacteriaceae or related species.

In elaborate studies to determine the qualitative and quantitative fecal microbiota, 93 per cent of the bacteria estimated to be present by direct Gram stain of serial dilution of fecal specimens were recovered by culture. One hundred thirteen separate species of microorganisms were found, each representing at least 0.05 per cent of the flora. The frequency of bacterial species and their relative percentage of fecal population are listed in part in Table 7–7. Of interest are the five subspecies of *Bacteroides fragilis.* The most common organism in the colon, almost by a factor of two, *B. fragilis* subspecies *vulgatus* is infrequently isolated from cultures of patients with serious clinical infections. By contrast, *B. fragilis* subspecies *fragilis,* a microorganism ranked twenty-ninth in frequency and constituting only 0.6 per cent of the bacteria in the fecal population, is the most commonly isolated subspecies of *B. fragilis* isolated from blood cultures, wounds, and abscesses. In this study, various members of the family Enterobacteriaceae were isolated in equal frequency with numerous other bacterial species between ranks 76 and 113, each of which constituted approximately 0.06 per cent of the flora.

One of the most common microorganisms associated with gas gangrene, *Clostridium perfringens,* has been found in low numbers in the stools of 25 to 35 per cent of normal subjects (see Table 7–8). The true figure for colonization with *C. perfringens* is probably higher. The significant incidence of intestinal clostridial colonization helps to explain the not uncommon postmortem finding of clostridial bacteremia in patients with ulcerative lesions in the gastrointestinal tract. Preterminal clostridial sepsis is particularly prone to occur in patients with lymphomas or leukemia who have ulcerative lesions involving the gastrointestinal tract.

Table 7–8 lists a few representative species of the bacterial flora of the colon. In many instances, it is likely that the ability of these bacteria to invade tissues and cause infectious disease may be related to complex interactions between one species and another, such as that referred to previously between *Bacteroides melaninogenicus* and the anaerobic diphtheroids.

TABLE 7–7. Relative Frequency of Bacterial Species in Fecal Flora*

Rank	Per Cent	Organism(s)
1	12	*Bacteroides fragilis* subspecies *vulgatus*
2	7	*Fusobacterium prausnitzi*
3	6.5	*Bacteroides adolescentia*
4	6	*Eubacterium aerofaciens*
5	6	*Peptococcus productus II*
6	4.5	*Bacteroides fragilis* subspecies *thetaiotaomicron*
7	3.6	*Eubacterium eligens*
8	3.3	*Peptococcus productus I*
9	3.2	*Eubacterium biforme*
10	2.5	*Eubacterium aerofaciens III*
11	2.3	*Bacteroides fragilis* subspecies *distasonis*
28	.7	*Bacteroides fragilis* subspecies *ovatus*
29	.6	*Bacteroides fragilis* subspecies *fragilis*
59–75	.13	*Streptococcus faecalis*
76–113	0.06	*Escherichia coli, Klebsiella pneumoniae,* and 37 other bacterial species

*Adapted from Moore, W. E. C., and Holdeman, L. V.: The human fecal flora of 20 Japanese-Hawaiians. Appl. Microbiol. *27:*916, 1974.

Factors associated with establishing colonization of certain strains of bacteria at different sites in the body have already been discussed in Chapter 2. Briefly, indigenous microorganisms in the gastrointestinal tract can inhibit or prevent infections by *Vibrio cholerae,* shigella, or salmonella. Mechanisms for such interference include the production of antibiotics or bacteriocins by one group of organisms against a second, microbial competition for nutrients in one environment as compared to another, or susceptibility of one strain of bacteria to toxic substances produced by a second strain. An example of the latter is the inhibitory effect of volatile, short-chain, fatty organic acids produced by anaerobic bacteria on *Salmonella typhimurium,* preventing infection when only small numbers of organisms are present. Similar susceptibility by other bacteria to short-chain fatty acids — produced in large quantity by anaerobic bacteria — can significantly inhibit growth and viability of shigella, *Pseudomonas aeruginosa,* and *Klebsiella pneumoniae.* The role of bacterial-epithelial attachment has only recently been recognized as a factor in establishing infection in the gastrointestinal tract. Attachment of *V. cholerae* to epithelial cells in the small intestine can be prevented by specific IgA. Motility of the intestinal tract can also influence the composition of the intestinal microbiota. Rapid peristalsis is of significant value in maintaining low levels of indigenous flora in the small intestine. Intestinal obstruction may quickly result in bacterial overgrowth in the proximal segment.

TABLE 7-8. Microorganisms Found in the Large Intestine

Microorganism	Range of Incidence (Per Cent)
Anaerobic bacteria — 300 times as many anaerobic bacteria as facultative aerobic bacteria (e.g., *E. coli*)	
Gram negative bacilli (nonspore forming)	
Bacteroides fragilis (5 subspecies)	100
Bacteroides melaninogenicus (3 subspecies)	100
Bacteroides oralis (2 subspecies)	100
Fusobacterium nucleatum	100
Fusobacterium necrophorum	100
Gram positive bacilli (with and without spores)	
Lactobacilli	20–60
Clostridium perfringens	25–35
Clostridium innocuum	5–25
Clostridium ramosum	5–25
Clostridium septicum	5–25
Clostridium tetani	1–35
Eubacterium limosum	30–70
Bifidobacterium bifidum	30–70
Gram positive cocci	
Peptostreptococcus (anaerobic streptococci)	Common
Peptococcus (anaerobic staphylococci)	Moderate
Facultative aerobic and anaerobic bacteria	
Gram positive cocci	
Staphylococcus aureus (associated with nasal carriage)	30–50
Enterococci (Group D Streptococcus)	100
Streptococci (Groups B, C, F and G)	0–16
Gram negative bacilli	
Enterobacteriaceae	100
Escherichia coli	100
Shigella — Groups A–D	0–1
Salmonella enteritidis (1400 species)	3–7
Salmonella typhosa	0.0001
Klebsiella species	40–80
Enterobacter species	40–80
Proteus mirabilis and other Proteus species	5–55
Pseudomonas aeruginosa	3–11
Candida albicans	15–30

Genitourinary Tract

In the normal human, the kidneys, ureters, and urinary bladder do not have a microbial flora. In both the male and female, there may be a few bacteria present in the distal portion of the urethra; however, these are confined to short segments near the meatus, and the numbers of bacteria near the sphincter of the urinary bladder are usually negligible (see Table 7–9). In contrast, the adult female genital tract has a very complex microbial flora, constantly changing with the variation of the menstrual cycle. Shortly after the female is born, the vagina becomes populated with lactobacilli (Döderlein's bacilli). As the infant loses the effect of maternal progesterone stimulation, the lactobacilli disappear but return with the menarche and the development of endogenous endocrine stimulation. Lactobacilli are so named because they produce lactic acid. A large population of lactobacilli helps to maintain the pH of the vagina and external cervical os at approximately 4.4 to 4.6. At this pH, many of the gram negative bacteria found in the gastrointestinal tract will not grow. *E. coli* may be inhibited from active growth at a pH of less than 5.0, although some strains can grow, albeit poorly, in more acid environments. Microorganisms capable of proliferating at this low pH include the enterococci, *Candida albicans,* and large numbers of anaerobic bacteria.

TABLE 7–9. Microorganisms Found in the Genitourinary Tract

Microorganism	Range of Incidence (Per Cent)
Kidneys and urinary bladder normally sterile. Female and male urethra usually sterile except for short anterior segment	
Vagina and Uterine Cervix	
Lactobacilli	50–75
Bacteroides species	60–80
Clostridium species	15–30
Peptostreptococcus	30–40
Bifidobacterium	10
Eubacterium	5
Aerobic corynebacteria (diphtheroids)	45–75
Staphylococcus aureus	5–15
Staphylococcus epidermidis	35–80
Enterococci (Group D Streptococcus)	30–80
Streptococci (usually Group B)	5–20
Enterobacteriaceae	18–40
Candida albicans	30–50
Trichomonas vaginalis	10–25

As previously mentioned, the vaginal microbiota and the metabolic activity of the squamous epithelium of the vaginal mucosa are subject to cyclic fluctuations with normal hormonal variation. Progesterone tends to increase the content of glycogen in the epithelial cells which in turn increases the amount of carbohydrate available for microbial growth. During the early development of birth control pills, vaginal candidiasis (moniliasis) was an annoying problem for many patients taking pills containing relatively large amounts of progesterone. It should be noted that a pH of 5.0 to 6.0 may be selective for candida and other species of yeast.

The cervicovaginal canal has large numbers of anaerobic gram positive cocci, gram negative bacilli, and clostridia. Most of these organisms are capable of growth in the low pH of the vagina and ordinarily are not of much medical significance. They represent a considerable threat and may produce a serious infection, however, as a complication following induced abortion. Contamination of traumatized, devitalized, and partially necrotic endometrium with *Clostridium perfringens* can lead to serious and even fatal sepsis.

Summary

The objective of this section is to furnish the student with a list of names of bacterial organisms native to different regions of the body and to introduce nomenclature of the type the student can expect to see on culture reports. Most microorganisms associated with clinical infection today may be the same or similar to those constituting the patient's indigenous microbiota. This host-derived source of microbial infectious agents again emphasizes the role of host defenses in the development of infection. As defined in Chapter 2, the terms *pathogen* and *nonpathogen,* when applied to microorganisms, are relative terms and are better replaced by a concept of the continual variation of factors constituting the host defense. This complex interaction may be influenced by antimicrobial agents, normal cyclic hormonal changes, and acute and chronic disease, as well as many other factors still to be discovered.

References

Books

Rosebury, T.: Microorganisms Indigenous to Man. New York, McGraw-Hill Book Co., 1961.

Review Article

Savage, D. C.: Survival on mucosal epithelia, epithelial penetrations and growth in tissues of pathogenic bacteria. *In* Smith, H., and Pearce, J. H. (eds.): Microbial Pathogenicity in Man and Animals. New York, Cambridge University Press, 1972.

Original Articles

Aly, R., Maibach, H. I., et al.: Protection of chicken embryo by Viridans Streptococci against the lethal effect of *Staphylococcus aureus.* Infect. Immun. *9:* 559, 1974.

Freter, R.: Mechanism of action of intestinal antibody in experimental cholera. Infect. Immun. *2:*556, 1970.

Glynn, A. A., Brumfilt, W., and Howard, C. J.: K antigens of *Escherichia coli* and renal involvement in urinary-tract infections. Lancet *1:*514, 1971.

Gorbach, S.: Intestinal microflora. Gastroenterology *60:*1110, 1971.

Johanson, W. G., Pierce, A. K., and Sanford, J. P.: Changing pharyngeal bacterial flora of hospitalized patients. Emergence of gram-negative bacilli. N. Engl. J. Med. *281:*1137, 1969.

Johanson, W. G., Jr., Blackstack, R., Pierce, A. K., and Sanford, J. P.: The role of bacterial antagonism in pneumococcal colonization of the human pharynx. J. Lab. Clin. Med. *75:*946, 1970.

Levison, M. E.: Effect of colon flora and short-chain fatty acids on growth in vitro of Pseudomonas aeruginosa and Enterobacteriaceae. Infect. Immun. *8:*30, 1973.

Liljemart, W. F., and Gibbon, R. J.: Suppression of Candida albicans by human oral streptococci in gnotobiotic mice. Infect. Immun. *8:*846, 1973.

Marples, M. J.: Life on the human skin. Sci. Am. *220:*108, 1969.

Moore, W. E. C., and Holdeman, L. V.: Human fecal flora: The normal flora of 20 Japanese-Hawaiians. Appl. Microbiol. *27:*961, 1974.

Selwyn, S., and Ellis, H.: Skin bacteria and skin disinfection reconsidered. Br. Med. J. *1:*136, 1972.

Sprunt, K., and Redman, W.: Evidence suggesting importance of role of interbacterial inhibition in maintaining balance of normal flora. Am. Intern. Med. *68:*579, 1968.

Sprunt, K., Leidy, G., and Redman, W.: Prevention of bacterial overgrowth. J. Infect. Dis. *123:*1, 1971.

Turk, M., Ronald, A. R., Clark, H., Winterbauer, R. H., Atlas, E., Silverblatt, F., and Petersdorf, R. G.: Studies on the epidemiology of Escherichia coli, 1960-1968. J. Infect. Dis. *120:*13, 1969.

Winterbauer, R. H., Turck, M., and Petersdorf, R. G.: Studies on the epidemiology of Escherichia coli infections. V. Factors influencing acquisition of specific serologic groups. J. Clin. Invest. *46:*21, 1967.

II

CLINICAL AND MICROBIOLOGIC DIAGNOSTIC CONSIDERATIONS

FEVER

General Considerations

Normal Body Temperature

Body temperature under normal conditions is determined by the "set point" of the hypothalamic thermoregulatory system and a delicate balance between heat production and heat loss. Generation of body heat is derived from metabolism of all food and from body activity, especially muscle tensing and contraction. Loss of body heat occurs through radiation, convection, and vaporization. The major pathways of heat loss are peripheral blood flow in the skin, sweating, and the respiratory tract.

Although "normal body temperature" is usually considered to be 98.6°F, there is a standard deviation of at least 0.6°F around this "magic figure." In any given individual, normal temperature may vary anywhere from 97°F up to 99.6°F. In all persons, there is a diurnal variation in body temperature, maximal recordings occurring in the late afternoon or early evening, and a nadir occurring around three to five o'clock in the morning. Persons who work at night and sleep during the day have this same diurnal temperature pattern, suggesting that body exercise and food digestion are minor factors in maintenance of the diurnal gradient.

Definition of Fever

Physiologically speaking, fever results from any disturbance in hypothalamic thermoregulatory activity leading to an increase of the thermal "set point." Fever is defined clinically as any temperature above 100.5°F (37.8°C) when measured orally or above 101.5°F (38.4°C) when measured rectally. It is important to note that at any new thermal "set point" associated with fever, a balance between heat production and heat loss still obtains. The normal diurnal pattern is still observed, albeit in exaggerated form.

99

Mechanisms of Fever Production

Although endotoxin derived from gram negative microorganisms is "the classic pyrogen" and most of our information concerning mechanisms of fever has been derived from studies utilizing bacterial endotoxins, it should be stressed that there are many other clearly established pyrogenic constituents and stimuli. Virtually all microorganisms, including viruses, have the propensity for inducing fever despite the fact that most lack any discrete identifiable pyrogen. Injection of antigen into a sensitized host or injection of preformed antigen-antibody complexes into a normal host may duplicate the febrile response to bacterial endotoxin. These facts underline the importance of factors other than infection per se in production of fever and help direct our attention to a common pathway of fever generation.

It also should be stressed that injection of endotoxin elicits a number of biologic responses in addition to a rise in body temperature. There is a relatively rapid decrease in the total number of circulating polymorphonuclear leukocytes, followed by a striking increase in such cells secondary to release of polymorphonuclear leukocytes and precursor cells from the bone marrow. This sequence of neutropenia followed by leukocytosis is observed with subpyrogenic doses of endotoxin and probably is the most sensitive in vivo indicator of endotoxin activity. Other biologic effects of endotoxin include a variable decrease in the number of circulating platelets, subtle alterations in the clotting system, a precipitous decrease in serum iron, and an outpouring of adrenal cortisol and pituitary growth hormones. These and other less well-defined effects of endotoxin account for the constellation of subjective and objective manifestations experienced and exhibited by man after exposure to endotoxin. They occur in parallel with a rise in body temperature and collectively constitute the overall response to endotoxin.

Exogenous Pyrogens. The pyrogenicity of gram negative microorganisms resides in a lipopolysaccharide macromolecular constituent of their cell walls, i.e., endotoxin. The lipid moiety is responsible for the toxic and pyrogenic properties of bacterial endotoxin. The polysaccharide moieties, structurally interdigitated into the terminal portions of the lipid, carry a number of important antigenic determinants, e.g., "0" antigens, which induce production of antibodies. Some of these antibody responses are utilized in diagnosis and also provide a convenient method of classifying bacteria into different serotypes.

The typical febrile response to injection of bacterial endotoxin in the rabbit and in man is shown in Figure 8–1. In the rabbit, a rise in body temperature occurs after a latent period of 15 to 30 minutes, peaks at 90 minutes, and then begins to decline. If a sufficiently large dose of endotoxin is injected into the rabbit, a second and greater rise in temperature is observed that peaks in approximately three hours and then declines.

A different febrile pattern of response to an injection of endotoxin is observed in man (Fig. 8–1). There is a much longer latent period of approximately 60 to 90 minutes before body temperature rises. This rise in temperature has a single "monophasic" or "single hump" phase that peaks in approximately three hours and then declines.

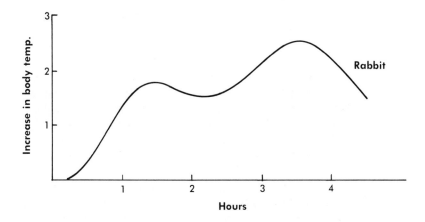

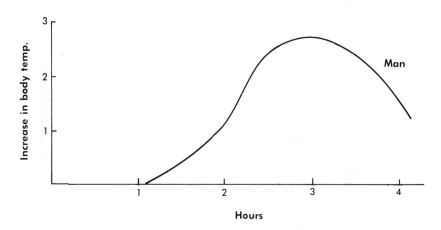

Figure 8–1. Typical febrile response to injection of bacterial endotoxin in the rabbit and in man.

The explanation for the early febrile response in the rabbit, which causes the fever pattern in this species of animal to assume a characteristic "diphasic" or "double-humped" pattern, is still not clear. There are strong clues, however, that the initial rise of temperature in the rabbit results from a direct impingement of the injected endotoxin on the temperature-regulating center of the central nervous system. Presumably receptor sites in the central nervous system of the rabbit, in contrast to those in man, are more numerous or more accessible and allow direct interaction with endotoxin.

It should be noted that the "monophasic" fever curve observed in man can be superimposed upon the later-occurring or second phase of fever in the rabbit. In both the rabbit and man, this later response is believed to be caused by endogenous pyrogen.

Endogenous Pyrogen. Evidence from several quarters indicates that all exogenous pyrogenic stimuli directly or indirectly cause the release of endogenous pyrogen and that it is endogenous pyrogen which acts on the thermoregulatory center and leads to increase in body temperature. Endogenous pyrogen exists in a precursor form in neutrophilic or polymorphonuclear leukocytes as well as in all representatives of the bone marrow–derived phagocytic cell series. The latter cells include the peripheral blood monocyte, the mobile tissue macrophages (histiocytes), the so-called fixed alveolar macrophages of the lung, and the Kupffer cells of the liver. Generation of endogenous pyrogen in active form requires active protein synthesis. Endogenous pyrogen has not been fully characterized to date, but most data indicate that it has a molecular weight of approximately 13,000, is readily heat labile, in contrast to bacterial endotoxin, and is readily inactivated by proteolytic enzymes.

The fever pattern induced by endogenous pyrogen has the shortest latent period of any known pyrogen. Maximum body temperature is reached within one hour and has no "double hump." The fever elicited by a single intravenous bolus of endogenous pyrogen is transitory, lasting no longer than two to three hours at most.

There are two mechanisms whereby exogenous pyrogens cause generation and release of endogenous pyrogen. These mechanisms are depicted in diagrammatic form in Figure 8–2. First, bacterial endotoxin or intact microorganisms stimulate phagocytosis, and the resulting phagocytic target host cells produce endogenous pyrogen. The precise sequence of events is not yet defined. Some data indicate that altered membrane permeability is an essential step. Sodium transport across phagocytic cell membranes is intimately associated with release of endogenous pyrogen; both events are inhibited by ouabain. Other evidence suggests that formation of phagolysosomal vacuoles and activation of an endogenous pyrogen precursor within the lysosomal granules of polymorphonuclear leukocytes and macrophages may play important roles. Second, fever induced by injection of antigen into a sensitized host or injection of antigen-antibody complexes probably is a reflection of activation of lymphocytes. The lymphocytes would appear to produce a "lymphokine" that is liberated into the extracellular fluid and then acts on the polymorphonuclear leukocyte to stimulate endogenous pyrogen production and release.

Endogenous pyrogen once released into the blood stream by either of the foregoing mechanisms appears to inhibit thermosensitive neurons in the anterior hypothalamus. This in turn releases the inhibitory effect of these thermosensitive neurons on the "thermal blind" neurons of the posterior hypothalamus and leads to vasoconstriction. The details of how endogenous pyrogen impingement on the hypothalamus translates into a new thermal "set point" and fever are not clear. One line of evidence, supported by considerable experimental data, suggests that once peripheral vasoconstriction occurs, the resulting drop in body surface temperature causes thermal receptors in the skin to activate somatic motor nerves which then innervate skeletal muscles, leading to increased muscle contractions, expressed as shivering or shaking chills. The net results are increased body heat and a rise in body temperature.

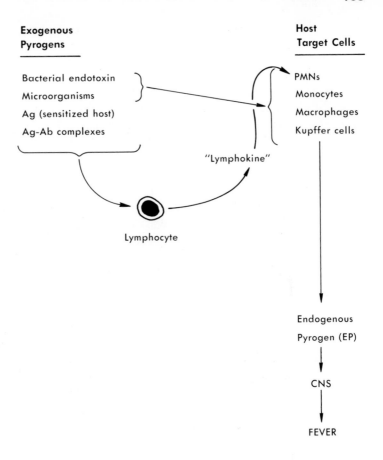

Figure 8–2. The two mechanisms by which exogenous pyrogens cause generation and release of endogenous pyrogen (EP).

Pryogen or Endotoxin Tolerance. Daily injections of relatively large doses of endotoxin produce progressively less fever until, after 7 to 10 such injections, the rabbit or human subject no longer exhibits a febrile response to even very large amounts of the pyrogen. This form of "endotoxin tolerance," induced in a relatively short time by closely spaced injections of relatively large amounts of endotoxin, has certain features: it does not persist for long after the last injection; it cannot be transferred with serum, and it exhibits no endotoxin antigenic specificity. In contrast, if rabbits or human subjects are injected less often with smaller doses of endotoxin over a longer period of time, a different form of tolerance is induced. This form of endotoxin tolerance has the following features: it is more durable and persists for a much longer time after the last injection; it can be transferred by serum, and it is as immunologically specific as the particular endotoxin used to induce it. The basis for this later-appearing, more durable, and more specific form of tolerance would appear to be antibody that is reactive with the carbohydrate 0-antigenic determinants of the endotoxin lipopolysaccharide macromolecule.

The tentative explanations for these two forms of endotoxin tolerance are as follows. Pyrogen injected intravenously localizes to a large degree within the liver where it impinges on the Kupffer cells, a major source of endogenous pyrogen. Repeated exposure of the Kupffer cells to relatively large doses of endotoxin rapidly renders them refractory and unable to release endogenous pyrogen after contact with endotoxin. This form of endotoxin tolerance does not depend on any immune response of the host. For example, it can be induced in hypogammaglobulinemic individuals. The other form of endotoxin tolerance, appearing later and following repetitive injections of small amounts of endotoxin, is caused by production by the host of antibodies which react with endotoxin 0-antigenic determinants. How such antibodies cause tolerance is still not settled. Some data suggest that the antibodies react with the injected endotoxin and in some way prevent the Kupffer cells of the liver from releasing endogenous pyrogen. For example, the antibodies may interact with specific receptor sites on the Kupffer cells, analogous to cytophilic antibody, and thereby prevent these sites from combining with endotoxin.

If a substance known to block the reticuloendothelial system, e.g., colloidal gold, is injected into a host with endotoxin tolerance, a febrile response once again is observed after injection of small amounts of endotoxin in pyrogenic doses. The termination or disruption of pyrogen tolerance associated with reticuloendothelial system blockade is explained as follows. The blocking agent allows an appreciable proportion of injected endotoxin to be trapped no longer by the Kupffer cells. Consequently, it is shunted to other tissues, e.g., the spleen, where it interacts with other cells capable of generating and releasing endogenous pyrogen after exposure to endotoxin.

Clinical Fever Patterns

Specific types of fever patterns have been recognized by clinicians for decades. *Intermittent fever* is characterized by return of body temperature to normal during the day and peak elevation in temperature during the evening. If the swings in temperature are extremely wide, this type of febrile pattern is called a "hectic" or "septic" fever. *Remittent fever,* in which the body temperature does not return to the normal base line at any time, waxes and wanes over a 2 or 3 degree temperature range. Most fevers associated with infections are of a remittent type. *Sustained fever* is characterized by relatively little variation throughout the day and night. *Miscellaneous fever patterns* include relapsing febrile states with periods of normal body temperature interspersed with bouts of fever, e.g., the Pel-Ebstein type of fever which allegedly is common in patients with lymphoma or Hodgkin's disease.

It is widely believed that these different types of fever patterns have special diagnostic significance with respect to infections due to specific microorganisms. This concept has been greatly overemphasized and from a practical standpoint does not have much merit when one moves from the textbook into the clinic. There are several "general rules," however, which most infectious disease consultants agree are worthy of serious attention.

1. A temperature above 106°F is usually not a primary result of an infectious process. The major exception is infection of the central nervous system, e.g., encephalitis or meningitis.

2. At both extremes of life, febrile responses to infection may be spectacularly disproportionate to the infection in question. Young children may have temperatures of 104° or 105°F with the most trivial type of infection. In still younger children, viz., less than three years of age, remarkably little fever may be observed in association with infections that regularly elicit brisk febrile responses in fully mature individuals. Older persons above the age of 70 also may exhibit little or no fever, despite the presence of serious suppurative disease. The lack of fever accompanying infections during very early life has been cited as evidence that delayed hypersensitivity to a variety of bacterial and viral antigens mediated by small thymic-derived lymphocytes or T cells may in part account for generation of fever during the course of infectious disorders. On this basis, lack of febrile responsiveness in older persons could be explained by the decline in T cell function that occurs with aging and that also accounts for loss of delayed hypersensitivity to microbial antigens.

3. In an adult, an oral body temperature greater than 104°F usually indicates bacterial pneumonia or pyelonephritis. Fever blisters, if present, may be a helpful differential point suggesting pneumococcal pneumonia as the diagnosis.

4. Intermittent fevers are often associated with profuse sweating, especially at night. This is why close questioning about "night sweats" may be very useful in documenting the occurrence of fever over a sustained period of time. Night sweats of significance require a change in night clothes; the mere accumulation of moisture around the neck or on the forehead does not denote night sweats.

5. Drug fevers are usually of a sustained type and out of all proportion to the clinical well-being of the patient. The patient's chart may suggest a very ill person with a severely toxic condition; observation of the patient may reveal quite the contrary.

6. Although debate continues over the relative merit of lowering body temperature and the best means to do so, there are in fact no hard data pointing to fever per se being a disadvantageous response in the patient. Many clinicians feel that in patients who do not have serious cardiovascular disease, in which elevations of body temperature might impose no significant burden on heart function, the best approach is to let the fever run its course. A single 5-grain tablet of acetylsalicylic acid (aspirin) may cause not only a plummeting of temperature but also a drop in blood pressure in some individuals, especially older patients with pneumococcal pneumonia or bacteremia due to gram negative microorganisms. Sporadic use of aspirin, with cycles of precipitous fall in body temperature and profuse sweating followed by a sharp return of fever with or without a bed-shaking chill, often makes a patient feel much worse than allowing a temperature of 102° to 104°F to continue uninterruptedly.

Fever of Unknown Origin

One of the most perplexing and special categories of febrile response is that of fever of unknown origin. This may be defined as a temperature greater than 101.5°F daily, persisting for at least two or three weeks, during which time a reasonably active search for the cause has proved unrewarding. As shown in Table 8-1, categories of fever of unknown origin most important to consider include: infection (40 per cent), neoplasms (about 20 per cent), connective tissue diseases (15 per cent), miscellaneous identifiable diseases (15 per cent), and no diagnosis (10 per cent).

TABLE 8-1. Categories of Fever of Unknown Origin*

Infection — 40%

    Systemic: tuberculosis, endocarditis and others
    Local abscess: intra-abdominal (liver, colon, pelvis) and renal

Neoplastic disease — 20%

    Lymphoma
    Hypernephroma
    Occult: colon and liver

Connective tissue disease — 15%

    Disseminated lupus erythematosus
    Rheumatoid arthritis
    Periarteritis nodosa
    Wegener's granulomatosis

Miscellaneous diseases — 15%

    Granulomatous processes of undetermined etiology
    Inflammatory bowel disease
    Cirrhosis of liver and other hepatic disorders characterized by hepatocellular necrosis
    Factitious fever

Undiagnosed — 10%

---

*Modification of classification of Jacoby and Swartz (N. Engl. J. Med. *289:*1407, 1973). Specific diseases or conditions in each category are of major diagnostic significance because of their frequency.

Specific infections often presenting as fever of unknown origin include the following: bacterial endocarditis; tuberculosis; a localized suppurative process within the biliary system, liver, or kidney; intra-abdominal abscesses; and pelvic vein suppuration. Miscellanous problems of a noninfectious nature that must be considered in any evaluation of a patient with fever of unknown origin include: multiple pulmonary emboli, regional enteritis, sarcoidosis, drug fever, and factitious fever.

In most instances, correct diagnosis in patients with fever of unknown origin rests upon securing tissue from that organ system that is primarily involved in whatever process accounts for the fever. Radioscans of lungs, liver, or spleen; lymphangiograms; and other dye contrast studies can be useful in pinpointing organ system abnormalities and leading to appropriate closed or open biopsy. After all leads have been exhausted, in view of the great frequency of intra-abdominal processes responsible for fever of unknown origin, laparotomy may be resorted to as a diagnostic maneuver.

One approach commonly taken to fever of unknown origin is the initiation of antimicrobial therapy, often including so-called broad-spectrum drugs. The basis for such therapy would appear to be a clinician's belief that antimicrobial agents will "clarify" the situation, i.e., reveal whether the fever has a bacterial cause, or a hope that an intensive course of antimicrobial therapy will be curative. Such "therapeutic trials" usually accomplish little and often complicate and delay definitive attempts to arrive at a correct diagnosis. For such reasons they are to be soundly condemned in most circumstances. As Table 8–1 indicates, more than half the conditions causing fever of unknown origin would not be influenced by antimicrobial agents. In addition, of those infectious processes responsible for the fever, a large proportion represent abscesses of one kind or another that will require surgical drainage in conjunction with antimicrobial therapy for cure. In the remaining proportion of infections, use of antimicrobial agents in specific combinations over long periods of time is often mandatory for beneficial results.

References

Review Articles

Atkins, E.: Pathogenesis of fever. Physiol. Rev. *40:*580, 1960.

Atkins, E., and Bodel, P.: Fever. *In* Zweifach, B. W., Grant, L., and McCluskey, R. T. (eds.): The Inflammatory Process. New York, Academic Press, 1974.

Original Articles

Atkins, E., and Bodel, P.: Fever. N. Engl. J. Med. *286:*27, 1972.

Deal, W. B.: Fever of unknown origin: an analysis of thirty-four patients. Postgrad. Med. *50:*182, 1971.

Greisman, S. E., and Hornick, R. B.: Mechanisms of endotoxin tolerance with special reference to man. J. Infect. Dis. *128:* Suppl. 265, 1973.

Jacoby, G. A., and Swartz, M. N.: Current concepts: fever of undetermined origin. N. Engl. J. Med. *289:*1407, 1973.

Petersdorf, R. G., and Beeson, P. B.: Fever of unexplained origin: report on 100 cases. Medicine *40:*1, 1961.

Wolff, S. M.: Biological effects of bacterial endotoxins in man. J. Infect. Dis. *128:* Suppl. 259, 1973.

Chapter 9

APPROACH TO
THE FEBRILE PATIENT

Basic Problem

Most infectious diseases follow a febrile course. Recording of body temperature is the earliest, easiest, and most objective means for recognizing an infectious process and evaluating its severity and duration. Frequently, fever may be the *only* clinical manifestation of an infectious problem.

Fever per se, as well as all symptoms and signs resulting from the febrile state, is a nonspecific physiologic response. The same signs and symptoms may be associated with a variety of noninfectious disorders, e.g., crushing injuries, immunologic diseases resulting from drug hypersensitivity, vascular disease leading to ischemic necrosis, and necrosis associated with malignant tumors. The common denominator in all of these diseases is tissue injury. Regardless of its cause, tissue injury brings about the release of a small molecular weight mediator termed *endogenous pyrogen* (see Chap. 8). Endogenous pyrogen acts on the central nervous system, alters the thermo-regulatory activity of the hypothalamus-diencephalon, and causes a rise in body temperature.

From a practical standpoint, the physician must reach a provisional or tentative diagnosis and make a decision concerning antimicrobial therapy relatively soon after he evaluates a febrile patient. Diagnostic and therapeutic decisions must be made immediately in some instances, e.g., a patient with suspected bacterial meningitis. In other cases, several days or a week can be allowed to pass while a diagnostic evaluation is in progress and data are collected before arriving at a decision, e.g., a patient with low-grade fever and a pulmonary infiltrate. The major point is that in most cases, the decision to initiate antimicrobial therapy is made well in advance of obtaining definitive bacteriologic, virologic, or serologic data. The information derived from cultures and susceptibility studies, even though it arrives after initial diagnostic and therapeutic decisions have been made, is useful in substantiating those decisions made at "zero time." The information is especially important when it invalidates those decisions and thereby provides specific guidelines for modifying the diagnosis and/or revising therapy.

Four Basic Questions

There are four questions that must be raised and answered when evaluating patients with fever.

An Infectious or Noninfectious Process?

Clues that suggest an infectious cause include the abruptness and the height of the fever pattern, the total and differential leukocyte count, and the clinical pattern of localizing symptoms and physical findings. However, most important is the *clinical setting.*

Acute bacterial pneumonia and pulmonary embolism or infarction are both characterized by relatively sudden onset of fever, dyspnea, chest pain, cough, and physical findings of pleural inflammation and/or increased lung density. Both diseases may be accompanied by marked leukocytosis. Differential diagnosis stems from considering the clinical setting. What are the patient's age and sex, his particular habits, and his immediate past history? Is it the "right" season for acute infection of the respiratory tract? Is there a good reason for thromboembolic disease to occur? Does the sputum appear purulent or does it contain evidence of fresh blood? The height of fever and the degree of leukocytosis are further guidelines. The temperature in bacterial pneumonia is usually above 102° or 102.5°F and often above 104°F, whereas fever associated with pulmonary embolism-infarction most often is below this level. Leukocytosis in bacterial pneumonia usually exceeds 15,000 cells per cubic millimeter; total leukocyte counts lower than this are more commonly found following pulmonary embolism-infarction.

Are Bacteria Responsible, and Is Antimicrobial Therapy Indicated?

Infectious disease consultants have long looked for a practical and rapid method of distinguishing those patients with febrile illnesses caused by bacterial infection from all other patients in whom the fever has a nonbacterial etiology and therefore would not be influenced by antimicrobic therapy. The nitroblue tetrazolium test may be such a discriminatory aid. It is too early in the evolution of the nitroblue tetrazolium test to determine its overall efficacy in evaluating febrile patients. It seems to be an important laboratory test, in addition to those which are already much in use, e.g., total and differential peripheral blood leukocyte count and sedimentation rate.

If a Nonbacterial Infection, Is Antimicrobial Therapy Not Indicated?

One must also think of fungal, protozoan, mycoplasmal, and rickettsial infections when specific antimicrobial therapy is available and indicated. Even in certain viral infections, therapy may be indicated, e.g., keratitis due to *Herpesvirus hominis* type 1. In this disease, topical application of idoxuridine (5-iodo-1-deoxyuridine) is highly effective in preventing irreversible corneal scarring and loss of vision in the affected eye.

If Noninfectious, What Is the Basis of Fever?

In dealing with this question, one begins to appreciate that the discipline of infectious diseases is one of the broadest subspecialties of internal medicine. An incisive approach to infectious diseases requires a large store of information about all organ systems and their respective disorders. This includes diseases of a noninfectious nature as well as those which are infectious. It should be emphasized that the last diagnosis to be entertained is "factitious or spurious fever." This situation, in which a patient willfully creates a false elevation of body temperature by manipulating the clinical thermometer, usually involves one who is associated with a hospital environment or responsible for patient care, i.e., a nurse or physician. The easiest way to detect "factitious fever" is to measure the temperature of a freshly voided urine specimen. The temperature of freshly voided urine varies directly with body temperature. There is virtually no way that a patient can manipulate the temperature of bladder urine, in contrast to the extraordinary manipulations that can be carried out with an oral or rectal mercury thermometer, even when a medical attendant is standing by the bedside.

Answering Basic Questions

Approaches to answering these questions may be summarized as follows:

1. The most important part of the initial evaluation of a febrile patient is the *clinical setting.* What pertinent data can be quickly obtained about the patient as an individual in relationship to his medical problem? What is his or her age? Where is he living? What kind of work does he do? What other disease problems or factors favoring development of infection can be identified? What other information concerning close contacts or recent travel seems epidemiologically useful?

2. The *physical findings* are then evaluated along with all initial *laboratory data,* including x-rays. Newer tests, e.g., the nitroblue tetrazolium test and counterimmunoelectrophoresis, which can generate information in a matter of a few hours, may be especially useful. At this point, a *provisional or tentative diagnosis* usually can be formulated.

The collection of appropriate material for microscopic examination can be of considerable value at this point. For example, draining purulent material when Gram stained and found to contain gram positive cocci may be important if that material later fails to yield any microorganisms on culture.

The microorganisms might well have been anaerobic streptococci which were inactivated on exposure to oxygen prior to being cultured. Pus from a brain abscess may be found on Gram stain to contain large numbers of gram negative bacilli but only occasional gram positive cocci. Culture of this material may yield streptococci within two to four days, whereas the gram negative rods, which are most likely members of the Bacteroides genus, may not appear for 10 to 12 days since anaerobic bacteria often grow slowly (see Chap. 10).

Every effort must be made to ensure that a portion of any tissue biopsy specimen is sent to the clinical microbiology laboratory for appropriate cultures. The remainder of the tissue should be processed for histopathologic sections, remembering that special stains may be required to detect microorganisms in microscopic sections. Definitive diagnosis usually requires isolation of a microorganism; therefore, material for bacteriologic culture or viral isolation must be collected and submitted promptly to the appropriate laboratories (see Chap. 10).

3. *A decision to initiate antimicrobial therapy* usually is made if the provisional diagnosis incriminates an infectious disease(s) which the physician believes is caused by *microorganisms susceptible to one or more antimicrobial agents.* Prior to starting therapy, at least two blood cultures should be drawn at least 30 minutes apart and preferably from separate sites. More than two blood cultures may be necessary in diseases in which bacteremia is inconstant. The important point is never to rely on a single blood culture. Should a single culture be reported positive for a microorganism normally residing on the skin, e.g., *Staphylococcus epidermidis,* deciding whether it is a "contaminant" or a true indication of bacteremia may be an insoluble problem.

If antimicrobial therapy is initiated, it should preferably consist of one drug directed against a specific microorganism or a limited number of microorganisms and it should be the least toxic antimicrobial agent possible. The practice of selecting a so-called broad-spectrum antimicrobial drug to give "maximum coverage" may not provide "specific coverage," however, and it increases the possibility of altering the indigenous microbial flora.

The following case abstracts are examples of the approach described in the foregoing discussion. They illustrate how the concepts outlined in this textbook can be applied to a rational means of handling febrile problems.

CASE PRESENTATION 1

A 38-year-old housewife in previously good health developed fever (as high as 103°F), frontal headache, intense generalized muscular aching, and an intermittent nonproductive cough on January 4, 1969. She was forced to take to bed and over the next five days slowly improved, using symptomatic measures. On January 9 (the sixth day of illness) she suddenly experienced severe right-sided pleuritic chest pain, a sharp rise in fever to 104°F, a marked increase in cough, and increasing breathlessness. A few hours later in the Emergency Room, she appeared acutely ill, tachypneic, and cyanotic, and was noted to be coughing up traces of purulent sputum.

Physical examination revealed a temperature of 103.8°F; pulse, 110 per minute; blood pressure, 90/60; and respirations, 32 per minute. The nail beds were dusky; the skin reflected dehydration. Coarse inspiratory rales and impaired resonance were noted over the lower right lateral-posterior chest.

Laboratory data: Hematocrit 14.5 per cent, white blood count 16,000 with 82 per cent segmented neutrophils. Urinalysis was within normal limits. Sputum smear showed many polymorphonuclear leukocytes and many gram positive cocci with occasional gram positive rods and rare gram negative coccobacilli. Chest x-ray revealed a nondescript density in the right lower lung.

The type of initial illness and its setting, i.e., winter season of the year, points to influenza. The abrupt departure from an otherwise uneventful convalescence strongly suggests complicating secondary bacterial pneumonia, viz., preceding respiratory infection, purulent sputum, pleuritic chest pain, and leukocytosis. The sputum smear is consistent with pneumococcal or staphylococcal infection. Both bacterial species are among the most common causes of bacterial pneumonia complicating influenza. Nafcillin, a semisynthetic and penicillinase-resistant derivative of penicillin, is administered, since a penicillinase-producing staphylococcus could be present. This particular semisynthetic penicillinase-resistant antimicrobial agent is highly effective against both the pneumococcus and penicillin-resistant as well as penicillin-susceptible staphylococci. Therapy is initiated only after sputum has been collected and cultured and two blood cultures drawn in rapid succession from two separate sites have been secured.

During the next three days, the patient showed gradual clinical improvement, even though there was an increase in the right lung infiltrate based on physical findings and chest x-ray examinations. Sputum culture revealed a heavy growth of *Staphylococcus aureus* reported to be susceptible to penicillin. Blood cultures were sterile. Serologic tests using paired sera showed a greater than fourfold antibody rise against influenza virus, "Asian" A_2 strain. On the fourth hospital day, defervescence, along with clearing of the pulmonary infiltration, occurred. At this time, antimicrobial therapy was changed from intravenous nafcillin to intramuscular procaine penicillin. After remaining afebrile over the next five days, she was discharged on a regimen of oral penicillin to be taken during the next two weeks of convalescence.

CASE PRESENTATION 2

A 46-year-old female with a diagnosis of lymphosarcoma established six months previously entered the hospital on February 15, 1971, with a three-day history of shaking chills and fever spiking to 105°F in association with attempts to decrease her daily prednisone dose from 60 to 20 mg per day. She appeared chronically ill and was weak and anorexic.

Physical examination revealed a temperature of 102°F; pulse, 100/m; blood pressure, 110/70; and respirations 28 per minute. Except for pale mucous membranes and a firm, nontender 3 X 3 cm size lymph node in the right axilla, the remainder of the examination was within normal limits.

Laboratory data: hematocrit, 10.5%; leukocyte count, 8000 with normal differential. Urinalysis normal. One of four blood cultures taken during the first two days of hospitalization was reported positive for a gram positive coccus, tentatively identified as Staphylococcus. Urine cultures were negative.

On the third hospital day, the patient's temperature approached 105°F and she showed signs of clinical deterioration.

This patient was known to have a primary disease, lymphosarcoma, associated with defective cellular immunity. This fact, plus the corticosteroid therapy she had received, should alert the physician to impaired host defenses and the increased likelihood of infection. The kinds of infections this type of patient experiences, however, are apt to be caused by "opportunistic microorganisms," e.g., members of the normal respiratory or intestinal microbial flora such as gram negative bacteria or *Candida albicans.* Increased susceptibility to gram positive coccal infections is *not* a feature of lymphosarcoma. Furthermore, there is no evidence of any infectious process that might explain why the single blood culture yielded a common microorganism constituting part of the normal flora of the skin. Therefore, the isolated microorganism is considered to represent a contaminant. For these reasons, no antimicrobial therapy is prescribed, even though a strong plea to "cover the patient" with an antimicrobial agent is made by the housestaff caring for the patient. The patient's prednisone dosage is increased on the premise that the fever and chills are due to increased activity of the lymphosarcomatous process in the face of decreased prednisone therapy.

Another reason for withholding antimicrobial therapy in this patient is the propensity for most antimicrobial drugs to alter the normal bacterial flora of the host in some way. In an already debilitated host receiving an anti-inflammatory drug such as prednisone, microbial "opportunists" may induce serious pneumonia or invade the bloodstream to cause systemic infection involving many different organ systems, i.e., life-threatening "superinfections." The occurrence of superinfection is one important reason for not prescribing antimicrobial therapy unless clear evidence exists for doing so.

The patient became afebrile and marked clinical improvement occurred after the daily dose of prednisone was increased to 60 mg for three days. Two additional blood cultures taken during this period were sterile.

These two case presentations highlight the clinical application of basic principles of medical microbiology and host-microbial agent interaction. The "knee-jerk reflex" approach of administering antimicrobial agents to febrile patients in hopes of "covering the patient" often fails, since it is based on emotion rather than reason. This method of dealing with a febrile patient may have harmful effects for the patient because it ignores the powerful biologic properties possessed by most antimicrobial agents.

References

Fossieck, B., Jr., Craig, R., and Paterson, P. Y.: Counterimmunoelectrophoresis for rapid diagnosis of pneumococcal meningitis. J. Infect. Dis. *126:*106, 1973.

Matula, G., and Paterson, P. Y.: Spontaneous in vitro reduction of nitroblue tetrazolium (NBT) by neutrophils of adult patients with bacterial infection. N. Engl. J. Med. *285:*311, 1971.

Chapter 10

LABORATORY DIAGNOSIS OF BACTERIAL AND FUNGAL INFECTIONS

Why Make a Diagnosis?

There are a number of reasons for making a specific diagnosis of an infectious disease. First, there is the advantage in the care of the patient. Once a diagnosis has been established, further steps to determine the cause of the illness need not be taken, thus saving the patient considerable financial expense and personal discomfort. Therapy is more easily determined and in many instances will be more specific. The prognosis for the illness of known cause will always be more apparent than for illness of unknown cause. Secondly, a specific diagnosis contributes to the education of the physician. This should result in the earlier recognition and appropriate therapy for the next patient he encounters with the same illness. Thirdly, after the cause of an infection is established as being due to a microbial agent, it is possible to use this information in preventative medicine. In many instances, vaccines can be developed such as those currently used for protection against polio-myelitis, influenza, measles, and rubella. Recognition of specific causative agents can stimulate a search for new or modified antimicrobial agents or can indicate the need for other types of control measures, such as mosquito eradication of malaria. The early recognition of specific microorganisms also can serve as a warning of epidemics and thereby provide time for taking measures to control or blunt outbreaks of infectious disease.

The diagnosis of an infectious disease is best accomplished by the isolation and identification of a specific infectious agent. Occasionally, the isolation of the agent is not possible, and the diagnosis must be established by noting an increasing titer of antibody to a specific infectious agent.

Although the isolation and identification of bacteria causing infectious disease are usually not difficult, it is essential for the student to become familiar with certain general concepts related to the collection, transporta-tion, and identification of the suspected agent. In the following section, principles for the collection and identification of microorganisms are stressed, but no attempt is made to list the details associated with different methods of isolation and identification. These and other aspects of the laboratory identification of infectious agents can be found in recent texts devoted to this subject (see References).

Recovery of Microorganisms by Culture

Culture Media and Incubation

Bacteria and fungi are usually recovered by inoculation upon artificial culture media. Most culture media are either in a liquid or solid form, with agar acting as an inert solidifying agent. Liquid culture media are preferable to solid media in that they support growth of smaller numbers of microorganisms, but if more than one microorganism is present, fastidious microorganisms may be rapidly overgrown. The advantage of a solid culture medium is that it allows isolation of individual microorganisms from mixed cultures. Enrichment or inhibitory agents may be added to either type of medium to enhance or suppress growth of different microorganisms.

Specimens for culture of bacteria or fungi may be collected either from sites normally free of bacteria such as blood and cerebrospinal fluid, or from sites which have large numbers of a mixed bacterial flora, e.g., the oropharynx, gastrointestinal tract, or cervicovaginal canal. Most often a single microorganism is present when infectious agents are found in normally sterile sites or fluids. In contrast, cultures for infectious disease involving the throat, gastrointestinal tract, or female genital tract may show many different bacterial species. To isolate disease-producing agents from regions with mixed flora may require selective culture media and specialized isolation pro-cedures. For recovery of certain fastidious bacteria, it may be necessary that specimens be collected in a manner which provides special requirements for suspected microorganisms. Different types of bacteria and fungi may need specific culture media or unique incubation conditions or both for growth. Failure to provide these conditions will result in lack of recovery of the microorganism, even though it may be present in large numbers. One such example, *Neisseria gonorrhoeae*, the bacterium causing gonorrhea, is very sensitive to sudden changes in temperature. If the specimen to be cultured is inoculated to a cold agar plate just removed from a refrigerator, the organisms may not grow, even though a large number of bacteria are present in the specimen. Other kinds of bacteria, such as *Neisseria meningitidis*, will grow very poorly or not at all if not incubated under an increased atmosphere of CO_2. Pneumococci may be recovered in only 45 to 55 per cent of sputum specimens from patients with pneumococcal pneumonia who have blood cultures positive for *Streptococcus pneumoniae*. Although pneumonocci are known to be present in the sputum of such patients, there is strong evidence that these microorganisms are inhibited by products of the oral pharyngeal flora that contaminate sputum (Fig. 10–1). Anaerobic bacteria also need a special environment for culture. These microorganisms will not grow in the presence of oxygen, and failure to provide an adequate oxygen-free environment results in a culture negative for growth despite large numbers of microorganisms.

Many microorganisms have specific temperature requirements, and this fact can affect recovery. *Mycobacterium marinum* and *Mycobacterium ulcerans* are microorganisms that cause ulcerating skin infections in humans. Both microorganisms have an optimum temperature range of 30° to 33°C, growing slowly or not at all at 37°C. Preference for growth at these lower temperatures is probably related to the fact that skin temperature is closer to 30°C than to 37°C. The same temperature preference is shown for fungi that inhabit skin (dermatophytes).

Collection of Specimens

Recovery of Microorganisms at Differing Intervals during Infection

The type of specimen and stage during an illness when a culture is taken may determine whether or not the microorganism will be isolated. In typhoid fever, the bacillus can be isolated first from the blood and shortly afterward from the urine. Although a few typhoid microorganisms can be found in the stool early in the disease, large numbers do not appear until 10 to 20 days after first ingesting the microorganisms (Fig. 10–2). Isolation of *Neisseria*

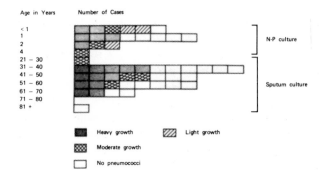

Figure 10–1. Recovery by culture of pneumococcus from the respiratory tract of 51 patients with bacteremic pneumococcal pneumonia. *N-P*, nasopharyngeal. (From Barrett-Conner, E.: The non-value of sputum culture in the diagnosis of pneumococcal pneumonia. Am. Rev. Resp. Dis. *103:*845, 1971.)

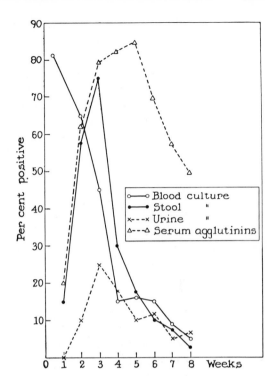

Figure 10–2. Results of serum agglutination tests and of blood, stool, and urine cultures on patients during the course of typhoid fever. (From Morgan, H.: The Salmonella. *In* Dubos, R. (ed.): Bacterial and Mycotic Infections of Man. 3rd ed. Philadelphia, J. B. Lippincott Co., 1958.)

meningitidis from patients with acute meningitis may be erratic when the cerebrospinal fluid has large numbers of neutrophils. Occasionally, *N. meningitidis* will be recovered by culture when there are no more than 25 to 50 cells per cubic millimeter, while on other occasions the microorganism may not be recovered when the cell count is as high as 3000 to 4000 per cubic millimeter of spinal fluid. In the first instance, it may be postulated that isolation of the microorganism occurred because the cerebrospinal fluid was obtained early during infection, presumably prior to the mobilization of a significant neutrophil response. Failure to isolate the organism when many white blood cells are present may be related to phagocytosis of the bacteria by the neutrophils with intracellular killing.

For the diagnosis of tuberculosis, it is recommended that the collection of specimens be carried out daily for a minimum of four to six days. Because of the slow, chronic course of the disease, there may be irregular shedding of *Mycobacterium tuberculosis* resulting from sporadic ulceration and discharge of bacilli from submucosal bronchial foci. The intermittent release of these microorganisms explains the clinical pattern of positive and negative cultures collected on successive days and the need to collect specimens for a minimum of four to six days (see Chap. 24).

Collection of cultures after starting antimicrobial therapy may also affect recovery of bacteria. Small amounts of certain antimicrobial agents, while not having a bactericidal effect, may cause suppression of growth of bacteria and result in a false sense of security to the physician following the failure to isolate an infectious agent.

Isolation of Infectious Agents from Mixed Bacterial Populations

The problem of isolation of a disease-producing microorganism from a mixed microbial population may be handled in several ways. Specimens can be inoculated directly to agar plates and streaked to obtain isolated colonies which can then be studied for differential characteristics. When large numbers of contaminating bacteria are present, inhibitory agents can be included in the culture plating media. These inhibiting agents may be of many types: aniline dyes in small amounts will inhibit gram positive bacteria; increased sodium chloride content is selective for *Staphylococcus aureus*; increased agar content will reduce the spreading motility of *Proteus mirabilis*; and antibiotics can be used either alone or in combination to selectively inhibit growth of different types of microorganisms.

Need for Prompt Inoculation

The more rapidly the specimen can be inoculated to culture media, the better will be the recovery of the suspected agent. Bacteria in urine specimens may show rapid growth in the urine, depending on pH, osmolality, and urea content. *Escherichia coli* in urine specimens having optimum conditions may show a generation time of 20 to 30 minutes. A large volume of urine taken for culture will maintain body temperature for some time if held at room temperature. Failure to inoculate the urine to culture media promptly or a lack of prompt refrigeration of the specimen may result in doubling and quadrupling the number of viable bacteria within 40 to 60 minutes of voiding.

Culture Swabs

There is a large variety of methods for collecting specimens for culture, and unfortunately no one method can best be applied for the recovery of all infectious agents. Swabs made of differing types of material are useful, and perhaps the most commonly used is cotton. Although cotton swabs are inexpensive and readily available, some contain small amounts of lipoproteins that may be inhibitory to fastidious bacteria. To avoid this problem, culture collection swabs made of polyester fibers (Dacron) are available. Polyester swabs are said to be particularly effective in the recovery of Group A beta-hemolytic streptococci in throat culture surveys when mailed to receiving laboratories in envelopes containing a dehydrating agent (Table 10–1). Another type of culture swab uses a fiber of calcium alginate, a material which is nontoxic to bacteria and has the added advantage of dissolving in sodium hexametaphosphate. By dissolving the calcium alginate, the microorganisms drawn into the fibers by capillary action are released and more easily recovered on culture. Despite the potential advantage of the calcium alginate, this material is not widely used, perhaps because of high cost and the extra effort required to dissolve the fibers.

TABLE 10-1. Comparative Agreement and Disagreement of Group A
Streptococcal Isolations from Four Swab Types after 4 and 72 Hours*

	Agreement				Disagreement				
	4-hour +		−		+		−		
	72-hour +		−		−		+		
Group A Streptococci	No.	%	No.	%	No.	%	No.	%	Total Number of Specimens
Dacron with silica gel	131	82	638	96	13	10	16	8	798
Dacron without silica gel	69	62	527	93	37	5	5	33	638
Cotton with silica gel	104	72	549	93	21	13	19	15	693
Cotton without silica gel	49	60	575	92	49	0	0	50	673

*From Hosty, T. S., Johnson, M. D., et al.: Evaluation of the efficiency of four
different types of swabs in the recovery of Group A streptococci. Health Lab. Sci.
*1:*163, 1964.

Transport Media

A transport medium should be used for sending cultures to the laboratory
when the specimen cannot be inoculated within a few minutes after being
taken. Transport media do not contain carbohydrate or nitrogen sources
necessary for replication, thereby preventing overgrowth of fastidious
organisms by contaminating flora. Transport media are buffered, have
sufficient agar to be semisolid, and may contain a variety of compounds
designed to favor the survival of specific microorganisms. The main purposes
of the medium are to prevent the microorganisms from drying and to inhibit
overgrowth by contaminants. Charcoal has been used in certain types of
transport media to neutralize the possible effect of toxic lipoproteins on
cotton swabs. Several similar types of transport media are in common use,
and one, Cary-Blair, has been used successfully for recovery of shigella from
stool specimens after a three week journey from Thailand to Washington,
D.C. Recently, the use of polyester culture swabs in plastic tubes containing a
small ampule of a transport medium has simplified the transportation of
culture swabs to the laboratory.

The transport of material to be cultured anaerobically poses a special
problem. Exposure of these microorganisms to small quantities of oxygen
may kill or severely injure fastidious anaerobes, preventing or delaying
recovery and identification. Several systems for transport of such specimens
have been proposed. These include the use of oxygen-free vials, modified
transport medium containing strong reducing agents, and oxygen-free tubes
for transporting culture swabs (see Chap. 38).

Blood Cultures

Although recovery of bacteria from blood during episodes of septicemia is usually not difficult, an understanding of certain concepts will help in the selection of the most appropriate medium and isolation procedure. The skin at the anticipated venipuncture site must be thoroughly prepared with tincture of iodine, using a saturated sponge and starting at the center and moving in enlarging circles toward the periphery. The site should then be further cleaned with 70 per cent alcohol. Care must be taken not to let excess iodine run between skin folds, since prolonged contact with iodine may result in skin burns, particularly in the semicomatose patient. The fingers used for palpation of the anticipated venipuncture site should be disinfected with the iodine sponge to prevent contaminating the skin. For each culture, a minimum of 10 ml of blood should be removed in a syringe. Smaller amounts should be taken from children, depending on their size. Inject no more than 5 ml of blood into each of two bottles which contains at least 100 ml of culture broth. One culture bottle should be used for the recovery of aerobic and facultative anaerobic bacteria, and the second bottle for the recovery of strict anaerobic bacteria. Carefully vent the bottle for aerobic culture by disconnecting the needle from the syringe and equilibrating the vacuum in the culture bottle with the ambient air. The culture medium should include an anticoagulant, and in recent years there has been an increasing preference for sodium polyanetholsulfonate (SPS-Liquoid). Sodium polyanetholsulfonate has, in addition to its anticoagulant action, an anticomplementary and antiphagocytic effect to reduce or prevent further intracellular killing by neutrophils following injection of the blood into the culture bottle.

The rapid recovery and identification of bacteria and fungi from blood cultures provide highly useful information, since a blood culture that is positive for bacteria or fungi usually indicates a serious infection. In most instances, bacteria and yeast will grow promptly, with rapid identification of the organism following. In some cases, however, recovery of the organism may take longer, since the effect of early or incomplete antibiotic therapy may have injured the microorganism, resulting in either a delay in recovery or interruption of growth. Reversible injury to the cell wall or plasma membrane may be caused by antimicrobial therapy, exposure to complement-antibody interactions in the host, or the transient exposure of strict anaerobes to the oxygen content of the arterial blood. Because the injury may involve the cell wall or cell membrane, recovery may occur more rapidly if the organism is placed in a hypertonic, osmotically buffered culture medium containing 10 to 15 per cent sucrose. Once the injured organisms have made several divisions, subculture to a standard medium will result in rapid growth. Culture media containing 10 to 15 per cent sucrose may also promote the recovery of yeast, which may infect prosthetic heart valves or colonize indwelling intravascular plastic catheters.

Dilution of the blood sample in culture media will contribute to a reduction of humoral and cellular host defense mechanisms that may be active at the time the blood is taken for culture. Some bacteria will still be inhibited from growth by human serum after a 20-fold dilution of blood with culture broth (Table 10–2). Frequently, blood cultures are only diluted

10-fold, and this may be insufficient to prevent continued complement-antibody interaction on susceptible organisms. A 1:20 dilution of blood to culture broth may be sufficient to eliminate the effect of small amounts of antimicrobial agents in the blood at the time of culture. Penicillinase or cephalosporinase can be added to the culture if the patient had been given one of these agents before the blood culture was taken. Unless there is a clear history of administration of one of the penicillins or cephalothin, it is best not to add inactivating enzymes to blood cultures because of the possibility of bacterial contamination from the enzymes. Dilution of blood taken for culture in a large volume of culture medium with prompt subculture will frequently have the same effect as the inactivating enzymes.

TABLE 10–2. Growth From Small Inocula in Blood-Broth Mixtures*

a		b	
Growth from Small Inocula of Streptococcus viridans in Blood-Broth Mixtures*		Growth from Small Inocula of Escherichia coli in Blood-Broth Mixtures†	
Blood-Broth Ratio	Positive/Total Bottles Inoculated	Blood-Broth Ratio	Positive/Total Bottles Inoculated
1/60	17/18	1/60	16/16
1/50	18/18	1/50	14/16
1/40	18/18	1/40	14/16
1/30	18/18	1/30	15/16
1/20	14/18	1/20	12/16
1/10	9/18	1/10	9/16
1/5	9/18	1/5	8/16
1/2	4/18	1/2	3/16
1/1	7/18	1/1	1/16

*From Roome, A. P. C. H., and Tozer, R. A.: Effect of dilution on the growth of bacteria from blood cultures. J. Clin. Pathol. *21:*719, 1968.
**Average number of organisms inoculated per experiment varied from 2 to 14.
†Average number of organisms inoculated per experiment varied from 2 to 3.

Urine Cultures

One of the most common sites of clinically significant infection is the urinary tract. Infection may occur within the interstitial tissue of the kidney, tubules, or pelvis, or at any point along the ureters, urinary bladder, or urethra. Studies relating clinical infection to the number of bacteria in voided urine have suggested that one of the best ways to determine the presence of infection in the urinary tract is to demonstrate at least 100,000 viable bacteria per milliliter of urine on culture (Fig. 10–3).

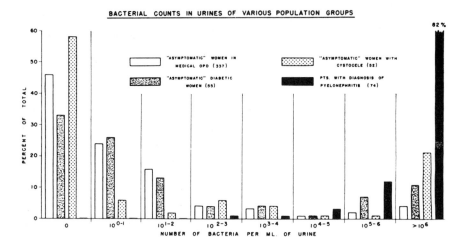

Figure 10–3. Bacterial counts in urines of various population groups. From Kass, E. H.: Asymptomatic infections of the urinary tract. Trans. Assoc. Am. Physicians *69:*56, 1956.)

The microorganism associated most frequently with urinary tract infection is *Escherichia coli,* which under ideal conditions may undergo a doubling in numbers every 20 to 30 minutes. Many bacterial species are able to utilize urine as a culture medium, and although generation times may not always be as short as 20 minutes, they can be brief and may divide every 30 to 40 minutes. Factors influencing growth of bacteria in urine include pH, which is significantly higher in women and therefore more friendly to bacterial growth; osmolality, lower in females and again more likely to support bacterial growth (Fig. 10–4); and urea content of urine – the higher the urea content, the more inhibitory it is to bacterial growth.

Although the rate of replication following collection of a urine specimen can be reduced by prompt refrigeration, the best method to determine the number of bacteria in a freshly voided specimen is to inoculate culture media promptly.

Collection of the urine specimen should be done in a way that minimizes the possibility of external contamination which may result in counts higher than those in the bladder at the time the specimen was voided. The procedure

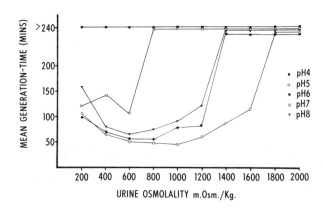

Figure 10–4. The effect of variation of urine pH and osmolality on the growth rate of *Escherichia coli.* (From Asscher, A. W., Sussman, M., Waters, W. E., et al.: Urine as a medium for bacterial growth. Lancet *2:* 1037, 1966.)

least likely to result in contamination of bladder urine is suprapubic puncture of the distended urinary bladder with a long aspirating needle. Inasmuch as suprapubic aspiration does not appeal to most patients (or physicians), alternative methods for collecting urine are commonly used. Urethral catheterization of the urinary bladder is not recommended for initial cultures because of the possibility of introducing bacteria into the bladder which might previously have been sterile. The simplest and most practical method is the collection of a midstream urine sample during voiding. Collection of the midstream urine specimen involves starting the urine stream to dislodge and wash out bacterial growth that may have occurred in the urethra since the last voiding. Five to ten ml is then collected prior to the voiding of the latter part of the urine. The specimen should not contain urine collected during the terminal phase of voiding because prostatic secretions or urethral sphincter contractions may dislodge small clumps or microcolonies of bacteria and artificially increase the bacterial count. Although it may not be possible to exclude all contamination during collection — with the exception of suprapubic aspiration — midstream specimens will probably give the most accurate reflection of the number of bacteria in the urine.

Collection of urine specimens for culture from women poses a special problem because of the increased possibility of contamination. The procedure should be carefully reviewed with the patient in order to explain why precautions must be followed. The patient should be instructed concerning the careful cleaning of the labia and external urethral meatus and prevention of the labia from contaminating the urine stream during voiding. A midstream specimen with prompt inoculation to culture media usually will provide an adequate reflection of the number of bacteria in the urine (Fig. 10–5).

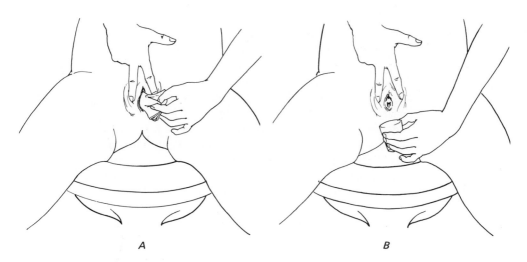

A   *B*

Figure 10–5. Collection of a urine sample from women. *A,* With the labia held apart, washing is done from high up front toward the back with gauze soaked in soap. *B,* The cup is held so that it does not touch the body, and a sample is obtained only while the subject is urinating with the labia held apart. (From Kory, M., and Waife, S. O. (eds.): Kidney and Urinary Tract Infections. Eli Lilly and Company, 1971.)

Prompt delivery of the specimen to the laboratory is important, since all too frequently the specimen may be left in a Nursing Service Room until a series of specimens are collected and then taken to the laboratory.

Sputum Cultures

The success of the collection of sputum for culture depends on the type and extent of pulmonary disease in the patient. Most sputum specimens have been heavily contaminated with oropharyngeal secretions and bacteria and may contain only small amounts of secretions from the lower respiratory tract. Many sputum specimens contain only salivary and oropharyngeal secretions and frequently represent only an honest but ineffective effort by patients to raise secretions from the lower respiratory tract. In one study, collection of sputum by expectoration and culture for pneumococci by standard procedures resulted in isolation of *Streptococcus pneumoniae* in only 55 per cent of patients with clinical pneumonia and pneumococcal bacteremia (Fig. 10–1). Similar results were found when sputum was injected intraperitoneally in mice, a procedure known to be more sensitive than culture for recovery of pneumococci. Although the reasons for the poor recovery of *S. pneumoniae* by culture are not known, there is evidence that interaction with other organisms or products from organisms found in the oropharynx may suppress growth of the pneumococcus.

Another method for collection for culture of material from the lower respiratory tract is the induction of sputum by ultrasonic or heated saline nebulization. This procedure increases the moisture content of the air going to the lower respiratory tract and improves the ability of the tracheobronchial cilia to bring up otherwise thick, viscid, or partially dehydrated secretions. Nebulization is particularly well suited for the recovery of *Mycobacterium tuberculosis* but can also be used for inducing sputum in other types of pulmonary infection.

Tracheal cannulation, bronchoscopy, or bronchial brushing guided by fluoroscopy are additional methods for the collection of specimens from the lower respiratory tract. All of these procedures suffer from some degree of oropharyngeal microbial contamination.

One of the best ways to collect a specimen for culture from the lower respiratory tract is translaryngeal aspiration. In this procedure, a large bore needle is passed percutaneously between the cricothyroid and thyroid cartilages, and a small, plastic catheter is introduced into the trachea. Saline is administered through the catheter and then aspirated along with tracheobronchial secretions (Fig. 10–6). The tracheobronchial tree below the larynx is sterile, and any organisms found usually reflect bacterial or fungal agents associated with infection in the lower respiratory tract. Translaryngeal aspiration may cause considerable discomfort to the patient, who may be seized with intense coughing spasms following injection of saline into the trachea. The procedure should be done only after careful consideration of the potential advantages and disadvantages.

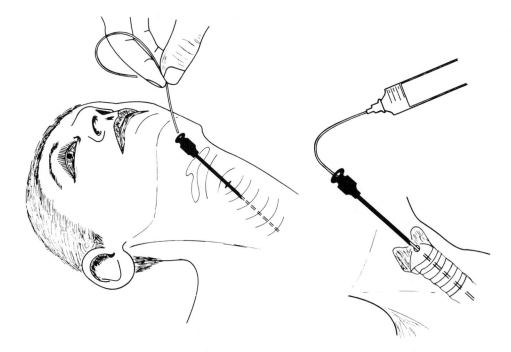

Figure 10–6. Technique of translaryngeal aspiration. The neck is hyperextended by placing a pillow under the shoulders. The skin over the cricothyroid membrane is cleansed (isopropanol) and anesthetized (lidocaine). Using a large-size, commercial, intravenous catheter set, a 14-gauge needle is inserted through the skin into the trachea. While pointed caudad, the polyethylene catheter is passed into the trachea; the steel needle is withdrawn, leaving the catheter in place. Two to 4 ml of sterile 0.9 per cent NaCl solution is injected rapidly through the catheter. A paroxysm of coughing invariably results. Suction is immediately applied, and tracheobronchopulmonary secretions and exudates are aspirated into the catheter-syringe. The catheter is withdrawn, and pressure is applied over the puncture site. (From Hoeprich, P. D.: Infectious Diseases. New York, Harper and Row, 1972.)

Cerebrospinal Fluid Cultures

Cerebrospinal fluid drawn from patients with suspected meningitis should be taken directly to the laboratory for prompt Gram staining and inoculation to culture media. Certain strains of *Neisseria meningitidis* may be very sensitive to decreases in temperature below 35°C. Therefore, the spinal fluid must be kept warm during transportation to the laboratory, and any culture media used for inoculation should be warmed to 37°C. If the cerebrospinal fluid is not cloudy, any microorganisms present should be concentrated by centrifugation. The supernatant spinal fluid should be saved in a sterile tube, and the sediment should be used to make smears for Gram staining and inoculation to culture media. All cerebrospinal fluid not used for stains or culture inoculation should be incubated separately along with the inoculated media at 37°C under 5 to 10 per cent CO_2. Cerebrospinal fluid serves as a growth medium for a number of bacteria causing acute meningitis and should be stained again the following day for evidence of bacterial growth. If invasion of the meninges by the bacterium has occurred only shortly before taking the spinal fluid and the microorganism is not found on the initial Gram stain or culture, growth in the cerebrospinal fluid following incubation may provide both a larger number of microorganisms and an increased amount of bacterial polysaccharide that can be detected by counterimmunoelectrophoresis the following day (discussed later in this chapter).

Wound Cultures

Specimens for culture from infection at different sites of the body may require a wide range of media, procedures, and techniques for recovery of microorganisms, depending on the part of the body involved and the type of infection suspected. Cultures of skin infections may only require inoculation to a few simple media, but drainage from postoperative wounds, from ascitic, pleural, and joint fluids, or from deep sinus tracts may all harbor anaerobic bacteria. All such cultures should be taken in a manner which minimizes or excludes exposure to oxygen. If infection from mycobacteria or a fungus is suspected, portions of exudate or tissue should be collected rather than a swab. Few microorganisms are shed in these types of infection, and recovery from a swab is usually disappointing. Again, prompt delivery of the specimen to the laboratory will reduce the effect of overgrowth or suppression by contaminating microorganisms and facilitate recovery of the organism.

Direct Stains of Clinical Specimens

Gram Stains

One of the most useful and rapid procedures in the diagnosis of bacterial or fungal infections is the Gram stain. A Gram stain can be quickly and easily made on exudates, fluids, aspirates, and tissue impressions — in short, from any specimen suspected of being the site of a bacterial, fungal, or, in some cases, viral infection. In the preparation and interpretation of Gram stains, several points should be emphasized. Lack of familiarity with the staining procedure or with the appearance of Gram stains may lead to errors in interpretation. Such errors can often be avoided by the simultaneous staining of previously prepared control slides containing both gram positive and gram negative bacteria. If slides with unstained bacteria are not available, gram positive and gram negative bacteria can readily be found in saliva. Some bacteria decolorize more readily than others and may appear gram negative when they are really gram positive. It is also important to know that when gram positive bacteria die, they may lose their ability to retain crystal violet, thereby appearing gram negative. Dead bacteria may also decrease in size. The phenomenon of both gram positive and gram negative bacteria of varying sizes may occasionally be seen when stains are made on 18-hour broth cultures of pure cultures. Chains of gram positive cocci or bacilli may show a sharp transition to a gram negative appearance in a contiguous chain correlated with a decrease in size of the bacteria. Occasionally, the decrease in size of the microorganism that can develop with the loss of viability may lead the microscopist to the erroneous conclusion that there are two types of bacteria present.

In addition to looking for bacteria in a Gram stain, the presence and type of inflammatory cells should be noted. Neutrophils in large numbers may denote an infection controlled primarily by phagocytosis and intracellular killing, such as the obligate extracellular parasites (e.g., pneumococci, meningococci, gonococci, or *Haemophilus influenzae*). If neutrophils are present, the size and shape of phagocytosed intracellular bacteria can help in the presumptive identification of pneumococci, meningococci, or gonococci. Smears taken from clinical specimens showing bacteria without accompanying inflammatory cells should be interpreted with caution, as they may represent colonized microorganisms not associated with an invasive infection. Gram stains may be helpful in the rapid, presumptive identification of a number of acute infections, e.g., staphylococcal enterocolitis, gonorrheal urethritis, meningococcal meningitis, nocardial abscesses, or other types of infections in which the shape and staining reaction of the microorganism, in association with the type of inflammatory cell response and clinical pattern, are consistent with a well-defined infectious disease. One exception to the need for correlation of inflammatory cell types with the presence of bacteria is the watery diarrhea of cholera; this disease is caused by a toxin which does not incite an inflammatory cell response (see Chap. 31).

A Gram stain should be made as soon as a culture is taken from a wound. Correlation of the Gram stain with the cellular and morphologic characteristics of the exudate and the bacterial or fungal organisms recovered on culture may show a discrepancy that would suggest that an anaerobic bacterium had been present but not recovered on culture.

Acid-Fast Stains

Mycobacteria are frequently called "acid-fast microorganisms." This term refers to the fact that these microorganisms have such a strong affinity for certain stains that they resist destaining with strong acids. Classically, "acid-fast" refers to the ability of the microorganism to retain carbolfuchsin following decolorization with 4 per cent hydrochloric acid, a procedure which will readily decolorize most other types of bacteria. The best known acid-fast stain is the Ziehl-Neelsen, which requires that the stain be applied to the smear or tissue section over a steaming water bath. Another carbolfuchsin acid-fast stain is the Kinyoun stain, comparable in reliability but easier to prepare than the Ziehl-Neelsen stain. The Kinyoun stain does not require steaming and can be used "cold."

During the past 10 years, acid-fast fluorochrome stains for mycobacteria have become increasingly popular. Auramine, sometimes used in combination with rhodamine, is the most commonly used of the fluorochrome stains. Most laboratories employing auramine for identification of mycobacteria in smears or within tissues find it to be slightly more sensitive than the carbolfuchsin stains. Although auramine is no more specific for mycobacteria than carbolfuchsin, the organisms are more easily seen, staining bright yellow to gold against a contrasting dark background. Because of this contrast it is possible to screen larger areas of the slide using a lower magnification objective than the oil immersion objective required for examination of carbolfuchsin acid-fast stains. Examination of fluorochrome stains usually requires special high intensity light sources with strong monochromatic lighting derived from mercury vapor or halogen light sources. Light of the proper wavelength excites the fluorochrome stain to emit the yellow color characteristic of auramine. Fluorochrome stains are *not* fluorescent antibody stains and should not be confused with them. Fluorescent antibody stains for different species of mycobacteria have been developed but have had little practical use. For additional information regarding aids to establishing the diagnosis of tuberculosis, see Chapters 23 to 25.

Other Stains

Fluorescein-tagged antibodies to specific bacteria have been developed and are used in both research and clinical microbiology laboratories to identify bacteria. Perhaps the most widely used application of fluorescein-tagged antisera is for Group A beta-hemolytic streptococci. Fluroescent antibody stains have also been employed in the identification of entero-pathogenic strains of *Escherichia coli, Neisseria gonorrhoeae,* and a number of Salmonella species. The use of specific, fluorescein-tagged antisera provides a rapid, sensitive technique for screening salmonella from mixtures of enteric organisms.

Polychromatic stains for malaria and microfilaria are of great help in the rapid identification of protozoa and hemoflagellates in blood smears. Stains giving characteristic reactions for fungi include the periodic acid-Schiff stain and the methenamine silver stain. The latter stain is particularly helpful in the identification of *Pneumocystis carinii.*

Hyphal forms of fungi associated with infection in skin or nails can be easily identified after warming epithelial scrapings or nails gently in 10 per cent potassium hydroxide, which acts as a keratolytic agent. The use of potassium hydroxide for the identification of fungi from nonkeratonized specimens (e.g., sputum) is inappropriate.

Negative staining techniques may be of great help in the visualization of organisms having translucent capsules, e.g., *Cryptococcus neoformans, Streptococcus pneumoniae,* or *Haemophilus influenzae.* For this purpose, a dilute solution of India ink or methylene blue may be used. The presence of a capsule is indicated by a clear halo around the organism (Fig. 10–7). Reaction with specific antisera increases the size of the capsule in pneumococci and *H. influenzae* and is the basis of the "quellung reaction" for serotyping of pneumococci. Care should be taken that the final solution used for contrast to study the smear is not so strong as to exclude all transmitted light. The India ink or other contrast material should also be checked to exclude any endogenous yeast or bacteria.

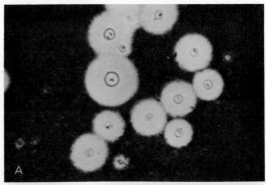

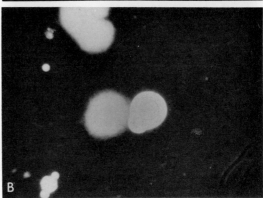

Figure 10–7. Cryptococcosis. *A,* India ink preparation of spinal fluid showing yeast cells surrounded by large capsule. *B,* Budding yeast cell within capsule. (From Rippon, J. W.: Medical Mycology. Philadelphia, W. B. Saunders Co., 1974.)

Identification of Isolated Microorganisms

Gram Stain

Once a culture has shown growth, the first step in identification of a microorganism is a Gram stain. Although it is usually not difficult to tell the staining reaction and shape of the microorganism, occasionally microorganisms may best be described as "gram-variable coccobacilli." The shape of a microorganism may change slightly depending upon the culture medium used. A Gram stain made from a broth culture may show one form, while a stain made from an agar medium may show a slightly different shape.

Biochemical Identification

With few exceptions, the identification of a bacterium is established by determining the presence of different enzymes known to be characteristic for individual species. In most instances, this is done by inoculation to various culture media containing substrates for the enzymes which have been found to be useful in taxonomic characterization. Most such tests result in a decrease in pH following production of acid, but some cause an increase in pH, e.g., urease. Standard acid-base indicators are incorporated in the culture media to indicate various end points. The number of characteristics necessary for accurate identification of microorganisms is variable, but sufficient differential tests should be inoculated to exclude closely related species. Table 10–3 is an example of a currently used set of identification characteristics. Identification of species of any one microorganism may require from 3 to 25 tests, depending on the microorganism.

Gas Chromatography

In a search for more rapid and specific methods for separating bacteria having similar characteristics, gas chromatography has been used to detect short chain volatile organic acids. This procedure has been found to be of significant help in identification of anaerobic bacteria (Figs. 10–8 and 10–9). Propionibacteria will produce propionic acid; lactobacilli will produce lactic acid. The hope that this technique might have application for species identification of bacteria other than anaerobes has not been fulfilled, partially because of significant variability in the composition of different lots of culture media which results in a wide variation of end products. Spontaneous mutants of bacteria showing slightly different metabolic activity also cause variable production of different end products. Application of gas chromatography to clinical specimens, e.g., serum, urine, or cerebrospinal fluid, in the hope of rapid specific identification of infection has not yet been of significant help. Further development of this procedure may overcome the present restrictions.

Detection of Microbial Products or Antigens

Immunodiffusion and Counterimmunoelectrophoresis

The recent recognition that antigenic substances from microbial organisms can be detected in tissue fluids has opened a new approach to the diagnosis of infectious disease. One of the first applications of this principle was the demonstration of soluble polysaccharide from *Cryptococcus neoformans* in cerebrospinal fluid of patients with cryptococcal meningitis. The same principle has been applied to other infectious agents in the central nervous system, e.g., the capsular polysaccharide antigens of pneumococci, meningococci, and hemophilic bacteria. Soluble antigen may be present wherever the microorganism is replicating or where the antigen may be cleared from the body. Cryptococcal antigen can usually be found in the serum and urine as well as in the cerebrospinal fluid in patients with cryptococcal meningitis. Cryptococcal polysaccharide in the urine may represent either renal infection or clearance of the antigen from a focus of infection elsewhere in the body. Similarly, type-specific pneumococcal polysaccharide may be found in cerebrospinal fluid, serum, pleural fluid, or the urine of patients with pneumococcal meningitis, pneumonia, or septicemia. The chemical composition of pneumococcal polysaccharide in the

BIOCHEMICAL REACTIONS OF ENTEROBACTERIACEAE (INCL. YERSINIA), AEROMONAS, AND VIBRIO*

	ESCHERICHIEAE			SALMONELLEAE				KLEBSIELLEAE								PROTEEAE						Yersinia			Aeromonas	Vibrio
						Citrobacter		Kleb-siella	Enterobacter				Serratia			Proteus				Providencia						
	Escherichia	Shigella	Edwardsiella	Salmonella	Arizona	freundii	diversus	pneumoniae	cloacae	aerogenes	hafniae	agglomerans	marcescens	liquefaciens	rubidaea	vulgaris	mirabilis	morganii	rettgeri	alcalifaciens	stuartii	Y. entero-colitica	Y. pseudo-tuberculosis	Y. pestis	A. hydrophila (other sp. vary)	V. cholerae
Oxidase Test	−	−	−	−	−	−	−	−	−	−	−	−	−	−	−	−	−	−	−	−	−	−	−	−	+	+
Indol	+	−or+	+	−	−	−or+	+	−or+	+	−	−	−or+	−	−or+	−	+	−	+	+	+	+	−or+	−	−	+	+
Methyl Red	+	+	+	+	+	+	+	−or+	−	−	+	−	−	−or+	−	+	+	+	+	+	+	+	+	+	+	+
Voges-Proskauer	−	−	−	−	−	−	−	+	+	+	+	−or+	+	+	−or+	−	−or+	−	−	−	−	−	−	−	−or+	−or+
Simmons'Citrate	−	−	−	d	+	+	+	+	+	+	+	d	+	+	+	d	+or(+)	−	+	+	+	−	−	−	+or−	(+)or−
Hydrogen Sulfide (TSI)	−	−	+	+	+	+or−	−	−	−	−	−	−	d	d	−	+	+	−	−	−	−	−	−,d	−,d	−	−
Urease	−	−	−	−	−	d	d	+	d	d	−	d	dʷ	dʷ	dʷ	+	+	+	+	−	−	+	+	+	−	−
KCN	+or−	−	−	+	−	+	+	+	+	+	+	+	+	+	−or+	+	+	+	+	+	+	−	−	−	−	−
Motility	+or−	−	+	+	(+)	+	+	−	+	+	+	d	+or(+)	+or(+)	+or(+)	+	+	+	+	+	+	−or+	−	−	+or−	+
Gelatin (22 C)	−	−	−	−	−	−	−	−	+	−	−	d	+	+	−	+	+	−	−	−	−	−	−	−	+	+
Lysine Decarboxylase	d	d	+	+	+	−	−	+	−	+	+	d	+	+	−	−	+or−	−	−	−	−	−	−	−	+	+
Arginine Dihydrolase	d	d	−	+or(+)	+or(+)	+or(+)	−	−	+	−	−	d	−	−	−	−	−	−	−	−	−	−	−	−	+	−
Ornithine Decarboxylase	d	dⁱ¹¹	+	+	+	d	+	−	+	+	+	d	+	+	−	−	+	+	−	−	+or(+)	+or(+)	−	−	+	+
Phenylalanine Deaminase	−	−	−	−	−	−	−	−	−	−	−	−	−	−	−	+	+	+	+	+	+	−	−	−	−	−
Malonate	−	−	−	−	+	d	+	+	+or−	+	+or−	d	−	−	+or−	−	−	−	−	−	−	−	−	−	−	−
Gas from Glucose	+	−⁽¹⁾	+	+	+	+	−or+	+	+	+	+or−	d	+	+	+	+or−	+	+	−or+	+or−	−	−	−	−	+or−	(+)
Lactose	+	−⁽¹⁾	−	−	d	d	−or+	+	+	+	+or−	d	−	d	+	−	−	−	−	−	−	+or−	+	+	−or+	−
Sucrose	d	−⁽¹⁾	−	−	−	d	−or+	+	+	+	−	d	+	+	+or(+)	+	d	−	d	d	d	+	+	+	+	+
Mannitol	+	+or−	+	+	+	+	+	+	+	+	+	+	+	+	+	−	−	−	+	d	d	+	+	+	+	+
Dulcitol	d	d	−	d⁽²⁾	−	+or−	+or−	−or+	−or+	−or+	−	d	−	−	−	−	−	−	d	d	−	−	−	−	−	−
Salicin	d	−	−	−	−	d	(+)or+	+	+or(+)	+	+	d	−	+	+or(+)	+	d	−	d	d	−	−	−,d	−	+	−
Adonitol	−	−	−	−	−	−	+	+	−or+	+	−	d	+	−	+or(+)	−	−	−	+	+	+or−	−	−	−	−	−
Inositol	−	−	−	d	−	−	−	+	d	+	−	d	d	d	d	−	−	−	−	+or−	d	+	−	−	−	−
Sorbitol	d	d	−	+	+	+	+	+	+	+	+	d	+	d	−	−	+	−	d	d	−	+	−	+	−	−
Arabinose	+	d	−or+	+	+	+	+	+	+	+	+	+	−	+	+	+	−	−	+	+	+	+	+	+	+	−
Raffinose	d	d	−	−	−	d	−or+	+	+	+	d	d	d	+	+or(+)	−	−	−	−	−	−	−	−	+	−	−
Rhamnose	d	d	−	+	+	+	+	+	+	+	+	+or(+)	−	d	−	−	−	−	+or−	−	−	+	+	+	−	−

(1) Certain biotypes of S. flexneri produce gas; cultures of S. sonnei ferment lactose and sucrose slowly and decarboxylate ornithine.
(2) S. typhi, S. cholerae-suis, S. enteritidis bioser. Paratyphi-A and Pullorum, and a few other ordinarily do not ferment dulcitol promptly; S. cholerae-suis does not ferment arabinose.
(3) Gas volumes produced by cultures of Serratia, Proteus, and Providencia are small.

+, 90 percent or more positive. −, 90 percent or more negative. d, different biochemical types [+, (+), −], −], (+) delayed positive (decarboxylase reaction, 3 or 4 days). + or −, majority of cultures positive.
− or +, majority negative. w, weakly positive reaction.

*Compiled by: A.C. Sonnenwirth, November 1973.
Data on Enterobacteriaceae from: "Differentiation of Enterobacteriaceae by biochemical tests", Enteric Bacteriology Laboratories Chart, DHEW-PHS-CDC, Atlanta, Ga. 30333, July, 1973.

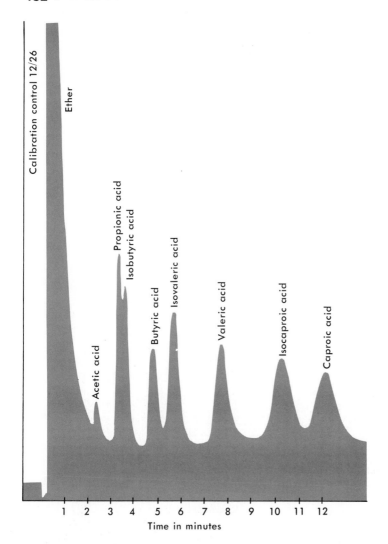

Figure 10–8. Calibration curve for organic acids detected by gas chromatography.

urine differs slightly from that found in the serum, presumably as a result of partial degradation of the polysaccharide prior to clearance by the kidney.

Several different immunologic techniques are available for detection of microbial antigens in clinical specimens. Ouchterlony gel diffusion for antigen-antibody precipitin reactions has been used, but with the intro- duction of counterimmunoelectrophoresis, the advantages of simplicity, speed, and increased sensitivity resulting from concentration of the antigen and antibody in a small reaction zone have made counterimmunoelectro- phoresis preferable to Ouchterlony gel diffusion in the detection of precipitin reactions. Counterimmunoelectrophoresis has been found useful in the rapid identification of antigens from bacteria associated with meningitis, septicemia, pneumonia, and septic arthritis. In some instances, the amount of antigen present in a specimen can be quantitated by comparison against purified polysaccharide (e.g., *Neisseria meningitidis*) or polyribose phosphate

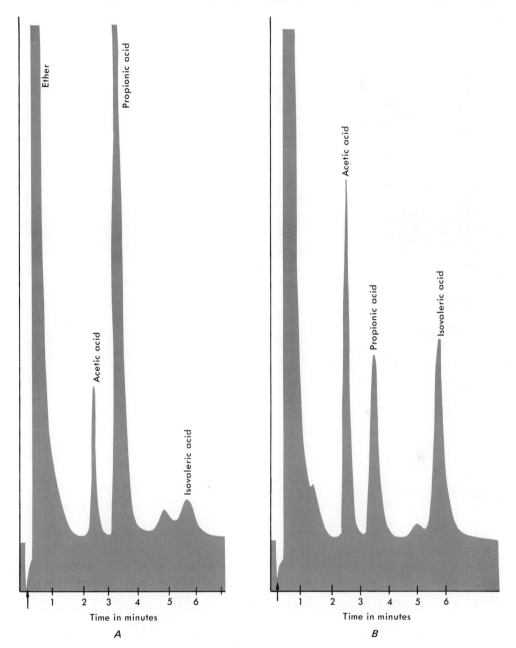

Figure 10–9. *A,* Gas chromatography from pure culture of Propionibacterium species. *B,* Gas chromatography from pure culture of *Bacteroides fragilis.*

(*Haemophilus influenzae*). Using counterimmunoelectrophoresis, it has been possible to determine levels of *N. meningitidis,* type C antigen associated with irreversible sepsis, disseminated intravascular coagulation, and death (Fig. 10-10). The rapid identification and quantitation of microbial antigen in cerebrospinal fluid or serum can provide important prognostic information, thereby giving the clinician advanced notice that aggressive therapy is mandatory.

+   −

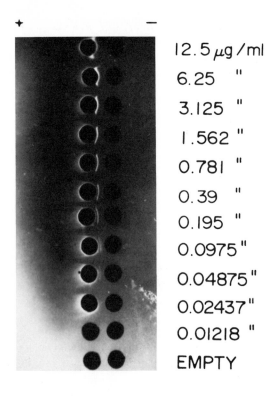

12.5 µg/ml

6.25 "

3.125 "

1.562 "

0.781 "

0.39 "

0.195 "

0.0975 "

0.04875 "

0.02437 "

0.01218 "

EMPTY

Figure 10–10. Sensitivity of counter-immunoelectrophoresis in detecting *Neisseria meningitidis* group-specific polysaccharide antigen. Each well contained 10 µl of reagent. Anode side contained *N. meningitidis* group C antiserum. Cathode side contained dilutions of meningococcal polysaccharide antigen. (From Edwards, E. A.: Immunologic investigations of meningococcal disease. I. Group-specific *Neisseria meningitidis* antigens present in the serum of patients with fulminant meningococcemia. J. Immunol. *106:*314, 1971. © 1971 The Williams & Wilkins Co., Baltimore.)

Latex Agglutination

In addition to counterimmunoelectrophoresis, several other methods can be used for detecting microbial antigens in clinical specimens. Antibody to cryptococcal polysaccharide can be adsorbed to latex particles which agglutinate in the presence of the polysaccharide. *Haemophilus influenzae* polyribose phosphate can also be detected by latex particles adsorbed to antibody. Red blood cells sensitized by exposure to tannic acid have been described as indicator particles for bacterial antigens when adsorbed to specific antibody.

Limulus Lysate Assay for Endotoxin

A process whereby the detection of unique products from microorganisms establishes the diagnosis of an infectious agent without the recovery and identification of the organism has been sought for many years. Recently, a method has been described in which minute quantities of endotoxin cause the gelation of an extract from the amoebocyte lysate of *Limulus polyphemus.* The test has been used as a means of detecting clinical septicemia due to gram negative bacteria. Analysis of serum for endotoxin by the Limulus assay has been received with mixed response, some investigators appearing to have more success with the test than others. The Limulus assay has also been used in the diagnosis of acute meningitis resulting from gram negative bacteria. In this application, it appears to be a sensitive indicator of the presence of endotoxin in cerebrospinal fluid that can result from gram-negative bacteria, including *Escherichia coli, Neisseria meningitidis,* and *Haemophilus influenzae.* The Limulus assay is not as specific for microorganisms as are counterimmunoelectrophoresis or latex agglutination procedures. With additional experience, the Limulus assay test may become better standardized and provide an additional diagnostic tool for establishing the cause of infection.

Demonstration of Change in Specific Antibody Titer

Not infrequently, attempts to recover the infecting microorganism are not successful, owing to premature therapy, host response, inadequate material for culture, or other reasons. In many instances, an infection by a specific agent can be established by demonstrating a rise in antibody titer against one or more antigens from the infecting agent. Such an approach requires that serum from the patient be obtained early in the course of the illness with a second, or convalescent, serum collected after 10 to 12 days. The interval between collection of the sera may vary, depending on the length of time the patient has been sick. The objective of such studies is to demonstrate an antibody rise following an interval during which the host can respond to antigenic stimulation with a rise in titer of specific antibody. The antibody may be directed against a specific microorganism, e.g., Group C *Neisseria meningitidis* or to a product of a specific microorganism, e.g., streptolysin O, an extracellular protein produced by the Group A beta-hemolytic streptococcus. For this reason, it is good practice to collect a serum sample from all patients with serious infections as soon as they are admitted to the hospital and keep it for later use.

There are many different immunologic procedures available for demonstrating changes in antibody titer, and the technique used will vary, depending on the type of antibody formed. Antibodies may be demonstrated by agglutination, precipitin, complement-fixation, or hemagglutination, or by bactericidal or other methods.

References

Books and Laboratory Manuals

Bailey, W. R., and Scott, E. G.: Diagnostic Microbiology. 3rd ed. St. Louis, C. V. Mosby Co., 1970.

Bodily, H. L., Updike, E. L., and Mason, J. (eds.): Diagnostic Procedures for Bacterial, Mycotic and Parasitic Infections. 5th ed. New York, American Public Health Association, 1970.

Edwards, P. R., and Ewing, W. H.: Identification of Enterobacteraceae. 3rd ed. Minneapolis, Burgess Publishing Co., 1971.

Hoeprich, P. D. (ed.): Infectious Diseases. New York, Harper and Row, 1972.

Holdeman, L. V., and Moore, W. E. C. (eds.): Anaerobic Laboratory Manual. Blacksberg, Virginia, Virginia Polytechnic Institute and State Laboratory, 1972.

Lennette, E. H., Spaulding, E. H., and Truant, J. P. (eds.): Manual of Clinical Microbiology. 2nd ed. Washington, D.C., American Society for Microbiology, 1974.

Rippon, J. W.: Medical Mycology. Philadelphia, W. B. Saunders Co., 1974.

Original Articles

Asscher, A. W., Sussman, M., Waters, W. E., et al.: Urine as a medium for bacterial growth. Lancet *2:*1037, 1966.

Barret-Connor, E.: The nonvalue of sputum culture in the diagnosis of pneumococcal pneumonia. Am. Rev. Resp. Dis. *103:*845, 1971.

Ehrenkranz, N. J., Elliot, D. F., and Zarco, R.: Serum bacteriostasis of *Staphylococcus aureus.* Infect. Immun. *3:*664, 1971.

Gaines, S., Ul Hague, S., Paniom, W., et al.: A field trial of a new transport medium for collection of feces for bacteriologic examination. Am. J. Trop. Med. Hyg. *14:*136, 1965.

Hoeprich, P. D.: Etiologic diagnosis of lower respiratory tract infections. Calif. Med. *112:*1, 1970.

Johnson, W. G., Blackstock, R., Pierce, A. K., et al.: The role of bacterial antagonism in pneumococcal colonization of the human pharynx. J. Lab. Clin. Med. *75:*946, 1970.

Kaye, D.: Antibacterial activity of human urine. J. Clin. Invest. *47:*2374, 1968.

Nachum, R., Lipsey, A., and Siegel, S. E.: Rapid detection of gram negative bacterial meningitis by the limulus lysate test. N. Engl. J. Med. *289:*931, 1973.

Rathbun, H. K., and Govani, I.: Mouse inoculation as a means of identifying pneumococci in the sputum. Johns Hopkins Med. J. *120:*46, 1967.

Roome, A. P. C. H., and Tozer, R. A.: Effect of dilution on the growth of bacteria from blood cultures. J. Clin. Pathol. *21:*719, 1968.

Chapter 11

LABORATORY DIAGNOSIS OF VIRAL AND MYCOPLASMAL INFECTIONS

Introduction

Viruses and mycoplasma are small infectious agents that are capable of passing through bacteria-retaining filters. This property resulted in viruses and mycoplasma being classed together as "filterable agents" well before their respective distinguishing characteristics were recognized. Although smallness is, for practical purposes, the only property they have in common, viruses and mycoplasma are often handled in the same diagnostic laboratory because both cause "nonbacterial" illnesses that may be indistinguishable from each other on clinical grounds alone and because both are frequently found

137

together as a double infection. Moreover, serologic procedures that are commonly used in diagnostic virology can also be used successfully for diagnosis of mycoplasmal infections.

The laboratory diagnosis of viral or mycoplasmal infections is as fundamental to an accurate clinical diagnosis of viral or mycoplasmal illness due to these agents as the laboratory diagnosis of bacterial infection is to accurate clinical diagnosis of bacterial infection. The overall principles that govern the laboratory diagnosis of infection with viruses and mycoplasma are strikingly similar to those for diagnosis of bacterial infections, but the methods used for diagnosis of each class of infectious agent may differ considerably. The criteria for laboratory diagnosis of infection with mycoplasma or viruses are more stringent. Under some circumstances, the diagnostic criteria are met only by both isolating the infective agent and demonstrating by serologic means that the host responded immunologically to the infection.

The diagnosis of a viral or mycoplasmal infection should be approached in a systematic fashion, i.e., collecting appropriate clinical specimens, transporting them rapidly to the clinical laboratory, observing the findings in the diagnostic laboratory, and finally interpreting the results carefully. Although the laboratory has responsibility for the proper conduct of the laboratory phase of the study, it is the physician who has the responsibility for interpreting the laboratory data. For this reason, he should know how the specimen was collected and processed in the laboratory if the results are to be applied to patient care.

Collection of Specimens

Principles

Diagnosis of a particular mycoplasmal or viral illness in a patient can be translated into specific questions. Is there evidence that the patient has been infected with the particular agent? Is infection with the agent associated with the particular clinical disease in a causal manner? Is the temporal relationship between the illness and infection in the patient consistent with development of the clinical disease? Thus, the strategy for diagnosis is to collect specimens which can both establish the fact of infection and permit an estimate of the stage of the infectious process at the time specimens are collected. As a rule, this strategy is translated into obtaining specimens for both isolation of the infectious agent and measurement of the immunologic response to the infection, since information derived from these specimens can be used to estimate the stage of the patient's illness. For example, in the case of self-limited viral infection (Table 11–1), laboratory isolation of virus and an absence of antibody in serum taken at the same time would be expected in an acute illness but would not be consistent with convalescence. Obviously, specimen collection must be started early in the course of the illness, on the one hand to obtain samples which contain infectious virus or mycoplasma and, on the other, to secure acute phase serum which is low in antibody.

Furthermore, since one of the objectives is demonstration of a change in the immune status resulting from infection, a serum sample should also be obtained during convalescence.

TABLE 11–1. Course of Infection in Self-Limited Viral Infections

Stage of Illness	Level of Virus in Infected Tissue	Level of Antiviral Antibody
Prodrome	High	Low to absent
Acute	Moderate	Low
Defervescence	Low	Moderate
Convalescence	Low to absent	High

The need for obtaining clinical specimens early cannot be over-emphasized. Viral infections are not easily differentiated from bacterial infections on clinical grounds alone. If specimens are initially sent only to a bacteriology laboratory, a minimum of two days may pass before an illness will be recognized as nonbacterial. The time taken to exclude bacterial infection by waiting for negative results of bacterial cultures could engender a delay which would seriously reduce chances for successfully developing confirmatory laboratory data. Therefore, it is important to send specimens not only to the bacteriology laboratory but also to the virology laboratory. Specimens are also sent later at appropriate intervals, i.e., defervescence and convalescence. If the infection is recurrent, clinical specimens should also be sent during and after each flare-up.

Practice

General Considerations

In practice, the type of specimens submitted to the diagnostic laboratory for viral isolation depends on the tissues and organs involved in the illness (Table 11–2). Mucosal surfaces, i.e., nose, throat, mouth, trachea, bronchi, eye, and rectum, are sampled most frequently, since they are the customary points for entry and exit of infectious agents. An effort is also made to obtain samples of diseased tissue, since isolation of virus would be strong evidence of a direct relationship between the agent and the disease. The types of samples submitted for viral isolation may be as varied as cerebrospinal fluid in aseptic meningitis, corneal scrapings in keratitis, and vesicle fluid in bullous or vesicular dermatitis.

The equipment for collecting samples for the diagnostic laboratory is available in all medical facilities. Blood can be collected in a sterile manner by Vacutainer or collected by syringe and put into a sterile tube. If the patient can tolerate the loss, 15 to 20 ml of clotted blood should be sent to the

TABLE 11–2. Appropriate Specimens for Viral Isolation

Clinical Problem	Specimen
Upper respiratory infection	Throat swab, gargle, nasal swab, nasal wash, feces
Lower respiratory infection	Throat swab, gargle, sputum, lung tissue, feces
Meningitis, encephalitis	Cerebrospinal fluid, throat swab, feces, brain tissue
Myositis	Feces
Myocarditis	Throat swab, feces, pericardial fluid
Dermatologic conditions	Vesicle fluid, feces
Keratitis	Corneal scraping
Peripheral neuritis	Cerebrospinal fluid, feces
Fever of unknown origin	Urine, feces, cerebrospinal fluid, biopsy

laboratory. The blood should remain unrefrigerated until the serum is separated from the clot to avoid loss of cold agglutinins which will be removed from the serum if they adsorb onto the red cells. If the blood sample cannot be delivered to the laboratory within 24 hours, the serum should be removed, placed in a sterile tube, and refrigerated until subsequent transmittal to the laboratory. (Do not refrigerate whole blood, since hemolysis may result and cold agglutinins may be lost.)

The equipment for collecting samples for viral or mycoplasmal isolation is equally simple. Usually, a cotton-tipped applicator stick and a tube with 1 to 2 ml of sterile broth, such as brain-heart infusion broth or trypticase soy broth, are all that is needed. Some laboratories suggest that 0.5 per cent concentration of bovine serum albumin be added to the broth. The cotton-tipped applicator is used as a swab for gently abrading mucosal surfaces from which samples are obtained. The cotton tip is first moistened in the culture medium, the mucosal surface is scraped, and the tip is rinsed in the collection tube. Usually, the surface is swabbed two to three times.

Samples of tissues and body fluids should also be placed in sterile containers. Cerebrospinal fluids, urine, and exudates can be put into tightly capped tubes and refrigerated until they are sent to the virology laboratory. Tissue samples, biopsy specimens, etc. should be placed in small tubes or containers and covered with sterile tissue culture media or with bacterial culture broth and refrigerated. Tissues must be sent to the laboratory immediately. Fluids and exudates can be frozen if a delay is anticipated before they reach the laboratory. However, biopsy specimens should not be frozen, since freezing destroys the tissue and ruins whatever chance there might be to culture cells obtained directly from the patient.

Specific Examples

Specimens from Upper Respiratory Tract. Samples from the respiratory tract usually do not present a problem in collection. Throat swabs are obtained by wiping a cotton-tipped applicator stick firmly over the tonsillar and posterior pharyngeal regions twice. After each wipe, the cotton tip is rinsed vigorously in the same 1 ml volume culture media. Nasal swabs can be obtained with small swabs and a gentle touch. Satisfactory sampling of the oropharyngeal flora can also be obtained by gargles with simple culture media such as brain-heart infusion broth or trypticase soy medium. This procedure is simple but requires the active participation of the subject. First, the patient is instructed to cough and then to gargle 15 ml of collecting fluid. On completion of the gargle, the fluids are collected in a cup and the cycle of "cough, gargle, and spit" is repeated with a second 15 ml aliquot of medium.

Some virologists advocate collection of nasal secretions. This is not routinely done, however, because it causes more discomfort than the collection methods previously described. In this procedure, the patient should be carefully positioned so that the culture medium which is instilled in the external nares will flow into the nasal cavity. Satisfactory results are obtained when the patient is placed in a recumbent position with a pillow under the shoulders to hyperextend the neck or when the patient lies across a bed with his head over an edge. A partial reclining position with hyperextension of the neck is less satisfactory. The patient is instructed to hold his breath as 2 ½ to 3 ml of sterile broth is instilled into each nostril. The patient is then quickly returned to an upright position and instructed to expectorate and catch all drippings from the nose in a sterile receptable. The method is recommended only for highly cooperative patients.

Specimens from Lower Respiratory Tract. Swabbing the throat or gargling not only is used to collect materials from the upper respiratory tract but also is a useful means for collecting specimens from patients with diseases of the lower respiratory tract. Sputum provides sampling of the lower respiratory tract but is contaminated by oral secretions. Sputum should be collected after coughing and then sent quickly to the laboratory. Material obtained from bronchi and lungs by transtracheal aspiration or bronchial brushing usually gives a truer sampling of the lower respiratory tract, since there is less risk of contamination by oral secretions.

Cerebrospinal Fluid. At the time a spinal tap is done for diagnosis of an illness, 5 ml or more of spinal fluid should be obtained and sent directly to the virology laboratory. Cerebrospinal fluid can also be used for serologic study if additional amounts of spinal fluid are supplied. Extra spinal fluid can often be obtained from the chemistry and cytology laboratories by asking that samples in excess of the needs of their examinations be sent to the Clinical Virology Laboratory.

Feces. Fecal samples should be limited to 1 to 2 gm samples and should be placed in a test tube with 1 to 2 ml of sterile broth. It is also convenient to collect a small quantity of feces on the tip of a cotton-tipped applicator stick and to place it in 1 to 2 ml of broth. Fecal samples can also be obtained from an obstipated patient by wiping feces from the examining finger onto a cotton-tipped applicator stick after a digital rectal examination. Rectal swabs or anal swabs done immediately after defecation are useful for obtaining fecal samples in children.

Tissue Specimens. Before a biopsy is performed on a patient with a suspected viral infection, the hospital virologist should be consulted. The virologist should provide an appropriate transport medium and help to arrange rapid transport to the clinical laboratory. If special studies are requested, e.g., growing cells from the specimen in tissue culture, the virologist is consulted a day or two before the tissue specimen is actually obtained. Tissue specimens should not be rinsed with disinfectants nor placed in formalin if they are to be sent to the virology laboratory.

Transport to Laboratory

One key to effective use of the viral and mycoplasmal diagnostic facility is shortening the interval between collecting clinical materials from the patient and inoculating the specimen onto media or susceptible cells and animals. The need for rapid transport of specimens to the laboratory arises from the fact that the number of recoverable infectious units in specimens decreases with time. The loss of infectivity is due to heat, pH effects, and enzymes in secretions which singly or together inactivate viruses. Some delay may be unavoidable if specimens are obtained when the virology laboratory is closed or when the patient is not on the same premises as the laboratory. If there will be a delay of less than 24 hours in inoculating the specimen onto susceptible cells, the wisest course is to refrigerate the specimen until it reaches the laboratory. For transporting the specimen, adequate cooling can be obtained by placing the specimen container into a small, precooled, insulated bag or box containing ice. If a longer delay is anticipated, the materials should be frozen in airtight containers, preferably below $-60°C$, and transported to the virology laboratory in a frozen state. Freezing and thawing viral suspensions tends to reduce viral infectivity and, as a rule, freezing specimens is avoided unless prolonged delay is anticipated and the specimens can be transported in a frozen state. Specimens must be in an airtight container, preferably glass-sealed if solid CO_2 ice is used as a refrigerant, since viral infectivity is also reduced by pH changes which result when CO_2 dissolves in the transport medium. Finally, delay in getting a specimen to the virology laboratory can be further reduced if the laboratory is informed by telephone when to expect the material.

Approach to Viral Isolation and Identification

Principles

Isolation of viruses is similar to isolation of bacteria except that the complexity of the problem in the virology laboratory is greater because viruses are obligate intracellular parasites. Thus, the basic problem that must be solved in the diagnostic laboratory, if a virus is to be isolated from a clinical specimen, is to find a suitable host that will support viral replication. Early virologists inoculated clincial materials into susceptible animals such as mice, ferrets, and chicken eggs and looked for the appearance of overt illness or pathologic effects. These older methods resulted in isolation of a few viruses, e.g., those causing smallpox, vaccinia, Herpes simplex, influenza, mumps, and yellow fever, but were laborious and were not suited to most clinical laboratories.

Advances in tissue culture methods have led to isolation of a number of new viral agents and development of many new techniques for identification of viral isolates. Yet, even tissue culture methods appear to have limited use for diagnostic purposes because most tissues or cells are capable of supporting growth of only relatively few viruses and, conversely, because most viruses have a limited tissue tropism. Tissue culture methods led to major advances in diagnostic virology and development of several new techniques that depend intimately on growth of viruses in cells, e.g., hemadsorption, viral interference, biochemical characterization of viruses, etc. However, there are still too few useful approaches available for isolation and identification of viruses.

Practice

Cell Culture Methods

Isolation in Cell Culture. In practice, cell cultures which are susceptible to the broadest range of viruses should be used, since they are most likely to detect the greatest variety of viruses in clinical materials.

Cells used in the virology laboratory are designated by their source and by their characteristics. *Primary cell* cultures are outgrowths of cells obtained directly from tissue fragments which have been treated with trypsin to disperse cells enzymatically into a cell suspension. The suspension is placed in a nutrient growth medium and the cells are permitted to attach to the walls of the tube. Primary monkey kidney cells, human amnion cells, or human embryonic kidney cells are representative types employed for isolation of virus; they are susceptible to a wide variety of viruses (Table 11–3). Primary cell cultures can be subcultured as secondary cell cultures for only a few generations. On the other hand, *semicontinuous cell lines,* e.g., WI-38 cells and human diploid fibroblast cells, derived from an outgrowth of cells from fetal lung tissue, can be subcultured for many generations. *Continuous cell lines* are transformed or neoplastic cells which have been derived from cancer tissue, e.g., Hep-2 cells, which were derived from a human laryngeal carcinoma. Continuous cell lines can be subcultured for an indefinite number of generations.

In preparation for inoculation into tissue culture, clinical specimens are suspended in a culture medium and lightly centrifuged to reduce the amount of cellular debris. In addition, specimens may also be passed through a bacteria-retention filter to reduce the number of bacteria. As a rule, penicillin and streptomycin are added to the medium to suppress multiplication of bacterial contaminants. Tissue specimens obtained by biopsy are ground with sterile sand to release intracellular virus or are treated with trypsin for recovery of infected cells.

The precise manner of handling each specimen is individualized and depends on the clinical problem and the presumed causative agent. For example, a throat swab from a patient with influenza viral infection can be rinsed in brain-heart infusion broth or other simple bacterial culture and

TABLE 11–3. Susceptibility of Cells to Human Viruses

Cell Culture Type		DNA Viruses			RNA Viruses				
		Adeno-virus	Herpesvirus HS and HZ CMV	Poxvirus Vaccinia and Smallpox	Picornavirus Rhino-virus	Picornavirus Entero-virus	Myxo-virus	Rubella	Toga-virus
HEK	P*	+	+	+	+	+			
RMK	P	+		+		+	+		
WI–38	C**		+	+	+				
HeLa	C	+	+			+	+		
HEp–2	C	+	+	+		+	+		
RK–13	C							+	
BS–C–1	C							+	+
BHK–21	C		+	+				+	
HuAm	P	+	+				+		
CETC	P			+					

Abbreviations: HS, Herpes simplex virus; HZ, Herpes zoster virus; CMV, Cytomegalovirus; HEK, Human embryonic kidney; RMK, Rhesus monkey kidney; WI–38, Human embryonic lung; HeLa, Carcinoma of the human cervix; HEp–2, Carcinoma of the human larynx; RK–13, Rabbit kidney; BS–C–1, Grivet monkey kidney; BHK–21, Baby hamster kidney; HuAm, Human amnion; CETC, Chicken embryo tissue culture.

*P, Primary cell.

**C, Continuous cell line.

inoculated directly onto tissue culture. Centrifugation will not much reduce infectivity of influenza specimens, as the virus is extracellular and is not sedimented with the cells. In contrast, herpesviruses are largely cell-associated, and spread of infection in a culture frequently appears to be from cell to cell. Centrifugation of clinical specimens which may contain herpesviruses is not done before inoculating the tissue culture so as not to sediment cells which may contain virus. For example, when a brain tissue biopsy is performed on a patient with a possible Herpes simplex encephalitis, the tissue is treated with trypsin and the cells which are obtained by this process are inoculated onto a cell culture monolayer which is susceptible to herpesvirus, e.g., human embryonic kidney cells.

Detection of Viral Effects. Tissue cultures which have been inoculated with clinical materials are examined for evidence of cytopathic changes induced by viral infection. Several types of cytopathic effects can be seen, and a preliminary diagnosis may be suggested by the observed pattern. For example, Herpes simplex virus and adenoviruses cause primary human cells to swell, become refractile, and lose their ability to adhere to the culture tube (see Table 11–4). Yet, the two infections can be distinguished; cells infected with advenovirus look like bunches of ripe grapes on a vine; cells infected with Herpes simplex virus are scattered over the monolayer. Several

TABLE 11-4. Cytopathic Effects of Viruses

Type	Viruses										
	HSX	HVZ	CMV	ADEN	INF	MV	RESY	MEAS	POLIO	ECHO	COXB
Cell lysis											
Focal		x	x							±	
Generalized	x			x	x				x	±	x
Giant cells	x	x									
Syncytia						x	x	x			

HSX, Herpes simplex; HVZ, Herpes varicella-zoster; CMV, Cytomegalovirus; ADEN, Adenovirus; INF, Influenza virus; MV, Myxovirus; RESY, Respiratory syncytial; MEAS, Measles; POLIO, Poliovirus; ECHO, Echovirus; COXB, Coxsackie B.

paramyxoviruses, e.g., those of mumps and rubeola, and respiratory syncytial virus, induce snycytia formation, an easily recognizable cytopathic effect which is due largely to cell fusion. Herpes simplex virus causes giant cell formation possibly due to fusion of cells, but large and extensive syncytia are not seen.

Most cultures are observed for 10 to 14 days and are subcultured by passage onto fresh tissues if evidence of viral infection is seen. The actual time before development of cytopathologic findings depends on both the properties of individual viruses and the concentration of virus inoculated onto the monolayer. Considerable variation is seen. For example, with Herpes simplex virus, infection of human amnion or human kidney cells, in large dose, results in evident cytopathologic findings in less than 24 hours, but in small dose may take three to four days to produce evident cytopathologic findings. In contrast, cytomegalic viral infection in human fibroblast cells, WI-38, may take as long as three weeks for development of cytopathologic effects. The cytopathic effect of some viruses, e.g., those causing herpes varicella-zoster, and cytomegalovirus, is focal in nature, giving rise to localized plaques of infected cells. Other viruses, e.g., those causing influenza, and polioviruses, produce diffuse cytopathic effects in ordinary tissue cultures. Viral agents which normally give rise to a diffuse cytopathic effect can often be forced to give plaques if they can be prevented from diffusing through the tissue culture medium to remote uninfected cells. The customary method of limiting spread of virus in a tissue culture is to layer Agar-gel which contains culture medium over the cell layer. The Agar-gel effectively limits the spread of virus and results in characteristic *plaques* which can be seen by the unaided eye (Fig. 11-1).

Other viruses cause little obvious cytopathology, and infection with these viruses is detected by indirect means, e.g., *hemadsorption* and *interference* testing. The principle underlying the hemadsorption phenomenon is based on the fact that viral infection may alter the surface of an infected cell so as to enable adsorption of red blood cells onto specific virus-induced membrane-bound receptors (Fig. 11-2).

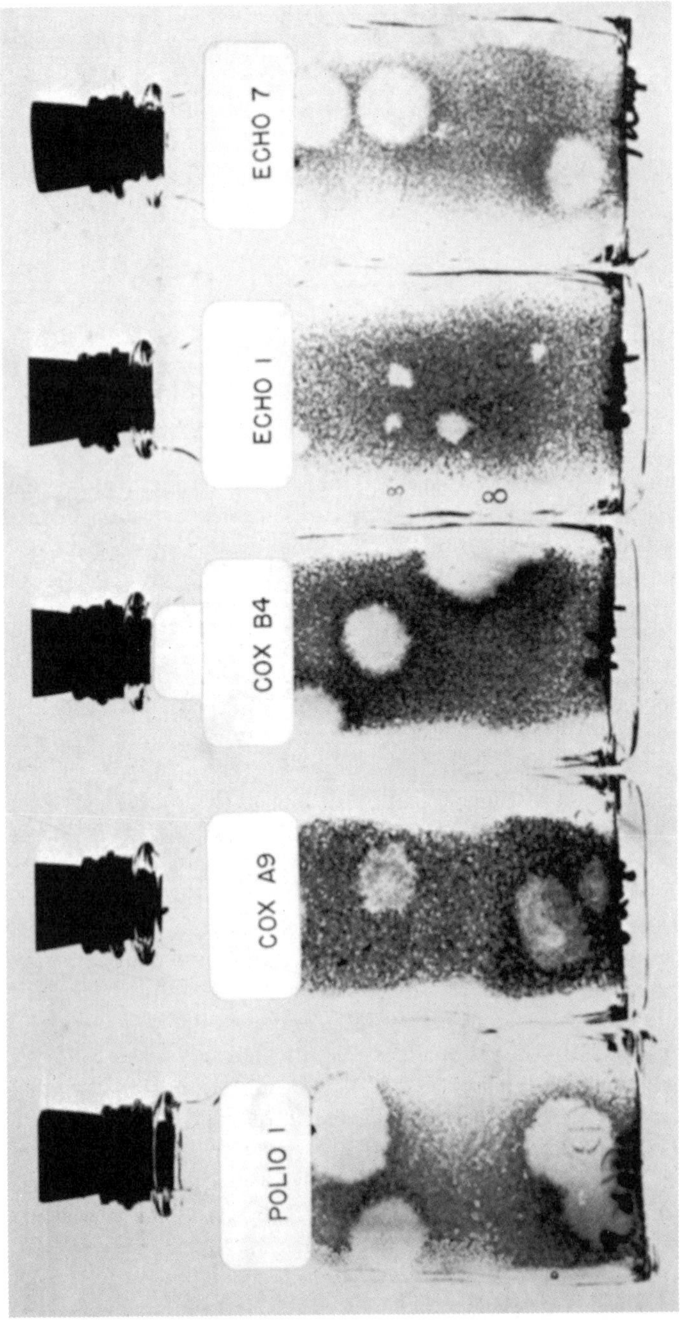

Figure 11-1. Plaques are visible in these tissue cultures which have been covered by a layer of Agar-gel. (From Hsiung, G. D.: Applications of primary cell cultures in the study of animal viruses. III. Biological and genetic studies of enteric viruses of man (enteroviruses). Yale J. Biol. Med. 33: 359, 1961.)

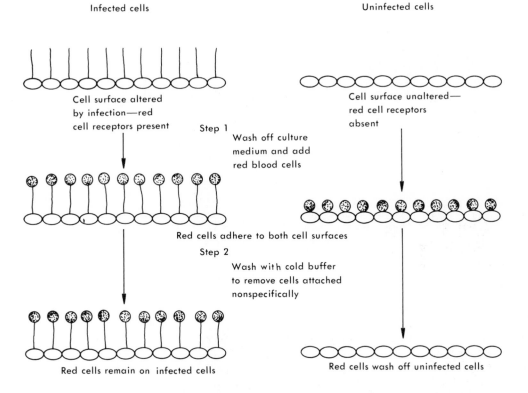

Infected cells   Uninfected cells

Cell surface altered
by infection—red
cell receptors present   Step 1

Cell surface unaltered—
red cell receptors
absent

Wash off culture
medium and add
red blood cells

Red cells adhere to both cell surfaces

Step 2

Wash with cold buffer
to remove cells attached
nonspecifically

Red cells remain on infected cells

Red cells wash off uninfected cells

Figure 11–2. Method for showing hemadsorption phenomenon.

Hemadsorption (HAds) is associated with viral infection with hemagglutinating viruses, e.g., those causing influenza and mumps, and parainfluenza viruses, and reflects viral antigens on the cell surface. In the case of the parainfluenza group of viruses, the test is performed by exposing the infected monolayer to a 1 per cent suspension of washed guinea pig red cells and after an appropriate time rinsing nonadherent cells from the monolayer. Hemadsorption is detected microscopically by seeing red cells adhering to the cell monolayer. Uninfected cells do not show hemadsorption; specific antiviral serum can prevent hemadsorption. The *interference* test, which has been used for detection of rubella virus in cell cultures, operates on a different basis. Infection of African green monkey kidney cells with rubella virus, for example, gives a persistent infection without obvious cytopathic effect. In contrast, infection of African green monkey kidney cells with coxsackie A9 virus results in cell lysis and death. However, if African green monkey kidney cells are first infected with rubella virus and then later exposed to 100 to 1000 infectious doses of coxsackie A9 virus, the cells survive the lethal challenge (Fig. 11–3).

Hemagglutination (HA) of red cells is another device for detecting viruses in tissue culture. Many viruses, including species from myxoviruses, adenoviruses, and enteroviruses, have the ability to cause red cells from a variety of vertebrate species to agglutinate. The presence of the virus in tissue culture

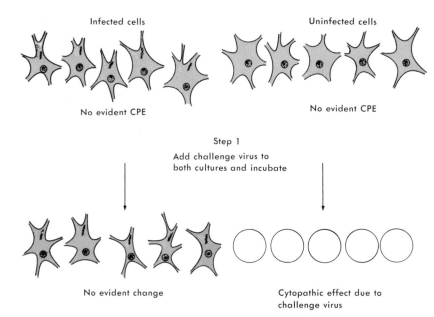

Figure 11-3. Method for showing interference phenomenon.

can be demonstrated by adding supernatant tissue culture fluid from infected cells to low concentrations (0.5 to 2 per cent) of red cells. The method has limited usefulness in a clinical virology laboratory because virus which agglutinates cells from one animal may not agglutinate cells from another species. The hemagglutination phenomenon requires that fresh red cells be employed to attain highest sensitivity.

Biochemical Classification of Viruses. Viral isolates are efficiently classified by three relatively simple procedures (see Table 11-5) which reveal important biochemical properties. Deoxyribonucleic acid (DNA) viruses are unable to replicate in tissue culture with a medium containing 5-iodo-2-deoxyuridine (IUDR), a base analogue of pyrimidine nucleoside. Exposing unenveloped viruses, e.g., adenoviruses, reoviruses, picornaviruses,

TABLE 11-5. Identification of Viruses by Physical and Chemical Properties

Property (Test)	Poxvirus	Herpesvirus	Adenovirus	Orthomyxovirus	Reovirus	Enterovirus
Nucleic acid (IUDR)	DNA (−)*	DNA (−)	DNA (−)	RNA (+)**	RNA (+)	RNA (+)
Envelope (Ether)	Yes (−)	Yes (−)	No (+)	Yes (−)	No (+)	No (+)
Susceptible to acidity	Yes (−)	Yes (−)	Yes (−)	Yes (−)	Yes (−)	No (+)

*No growth (−)
**Growth (+)

to ether or chloroform does not appreciably reduce their infectivity for susceptible tissue culture, and exposing enteroviruses to medium with pH less than 3.0 does not reduce their infectivity for cell cultures. Rhinoviruses are characterized as IUDR-resistant and ether-resistant viruses which lose infectivity in buffer at a pH of 3.0. (See Chap. 4.)

Individual species within each group are identified by several serologic techniques, such as complement-fixation (discussed later in this chapter) and neutralization of viral infectivity with specific antisera. Because of the great number of known viruses, serologic methods would be inefficient and expensive without preliminary grouping according to biologic and biochemical features. For example, if the isolate is an adenovirus, it may have to be tested against as many as 33 antisera before identification can be made by the neutralization method (see Table 11–6). If the isolate is an enterovirus, it may be necessary to test it against as many as 60 antisera.

TABLE 11–6. Etiologic Classification of Human Viruses

Family	Antigenic Types	Total Number	Representative Viruses
DNA Viruses		43	
Poxvirus	3		Vaccinia virus, smallpox virus
Herpesvirus	5		Herpes simplex virus, herpes varicella-zoster virus, cytomegalovirus
Adenovirus	33		Adenovirus, type 7
Papovirus	2		Human wart virus
RNA Viruses		250	
Myxovirus			
Orthomyxovirus	5		Influenza virus
Paramyxovirus	8		Measles, mumps, parainfluenza, and respiratory virus, and syncytial virus
Togavirus			
Alphivirus	20		Venezuela equine encephalitis virus
Flavivirus	30		Yellow fever virus, dengue virus
Unclassified	20		Sandfly virus
Arenavirus	3		Lymphocytic choriomeningitis virus
Corona virus	>1		(Respiratory viruses)
Rhabdovirus	>1		Rabies virus
Reovirus	3		(Respiratory and enteric orphan viruses)
Picornavirus			
Enterovirus	80		Poliomyelitis virus, coxsackievirus A and B, echovirus
Rhinovirus	100		(Common cold virus)
Unclassified Viruses	6	6	Rubella virus, infectious hepatitis virus
		>299	

Other Hosts for Viral Detection

Embryonated Eggs. While tissue or cell culture methods provide the most sophisticated approach to viral isolation, some earlier methods continue to be used either because viral isolation is more rapid or because the viruses cannot be grown in cell culture. Embryonated chicken eggs can be used for isolation and growth of several viruses (Fig. 11–4). Influenza, parainfluenza, and mumps viruses usually can be isolated by inoculating the chick amniotic cavity and then testing the amniotic fluid two to three days later for its capacity to agglutinate fresh chicken red cells. Data based on tests in eggs and cell culture (see Table 11–7) permit differentiation between numbers of the myxoviruses.

TABLE 11–7. Differentiation Between Various Myxoviruses

Viral Property	Influenza	Parainfluenza	Mumps	Measles	Respiratory Syncytial
Growth in chick egg (amnion)	+	±	+	–	–
Syncytia formation in tissue culture	–	±	+	+	+
Hemadsorption in tissue culture	+	+	+	±	–

Members of the poxvirus and herpesvirus families multiply in eggs when they are inoculated directly onto the chorioallantoic membrane, where they form somewhat characteristic lesions, called pocks. By combining the results obtained in eggs with those seen in tissue culture, members of the group can be identified. For example, herpes simplex (*Herpes hominis,* types 1 and 2) viruses can be differentiated from other members of the herpes family by their ability to produce pocks on chorioallantoic membranes of chicken eggs and by their resistance to pH of 3.0 (see Table 11–8). *Herpes hominis* type 2 produces larger pocks on egg membranes than does *Herpes hominis* type 1. Herpes varicella-zoster (V-Z) virus can be differentiated from cytomegalovirus (CMV) by the capacity for varicella-zoster virus to grow on human kidney or human amnion cell cultures. Smallpox produces fairly typical large pocks with necrotic centers.

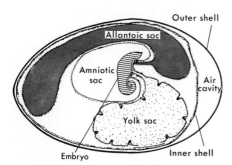

Figure 11–4. Diagrammatic representation of chicken embryonated egg (8 to 12 days).

TABLE 11–8. Differentiation Between Poxviruses and Herpesviruses

Susceptible Host	Smallpox and vaccinia virus	Herpes simplexvirus	Herpes varicella-zoster virus	Cytomegaloviruses
Chorioallantoic membrane	+*	+	–**	–
Human embryonic kidney	+	+	+	–
Diploid fibroblast (WI–38)	+	+	+	+

*Growth (+)
**No growth (–)

Smallpox is a serious infection which requires that expert help be obtained immediately if the disease is a likely diagnostic possibility. Certain identification of smallpox virus requires considerable experience; therefore, local and state health departments should be contacted immediately in order that the full weight of the diagnostic service of the National Center for Disease Control may be applied to identifying the virus, and in order that national health authorities may be aware of the possible presence of this infection in a community.

Mice. Mice continue to serve a useful function in a viral diagnostic laboratory, particularly for primary isolation and characterization of enteroviruses. Mice are used for primary isolation of coxsackieviruses, type A, since only coxsackie A9 has been consistently isolated in tissue culture among this group of viruses. The clinical specimen is inoculated intracerebrally and intraperitoneally into suckling mice, which are then observed for development of paralysis, tremors, and convulsions, and they may be examined microscopically for histopathologic evidence of myositis. Various members of the enterovirus group can be differentiated on the basis of their effects in mice and tissue culture (see Table 11–9).

TABLE 11–9. Differentiation Between Various Enteroviruses

Susceptible Host	Poliomyelitis virus	Echovirus	Coxsackievirus A	Coxsackievirus B
Suckling mice	Paralysis +	– (Echo 9+)*	Seizures Myositis +	Seizures +
Tissue culture Rhesus monkey kidney cells	+	+	– (Coxsackie A9, 21)*	–
Human embryonic kidney	+	+	–	+

*Exception

Newer Approaches to Viral Isolation

Cell Fusion. New virologic methods should increase the probability of recovering viruses in diseases of suspected viral etiology. One such example is *cell fusion* or *hybridization,* a phenomenon in which single cells from the same or disparate species are fused into multinucleated giant cells. The method of cell fusion is based on the observation that Sendai virus, a parainfluenza virus of mice, can induce cells to form syncytia independent of its capacity to multiply in these cells. When Sendai virus is used for cell fusion, it is first treated with ultraviolet light to prevent its multiplication in the hybridized cells. The inactivated virus is then added to a mixture of nonpermissive cells which are thought to be infected with a latent form of the suspect virus and uninfected permissive cells. Although presumably infected with the suspect virus, the nonpermissive cells are not capable of supporting its multiplication. In contrast, the permissive cells would support growth of the suspected virus if they became infected. Fusion of the permissive and nonpermissive cells appears to activate the latent virus, and the cell hybrid is then capable of supporting multiplication of the virus. This method was recently used for recovery of a papova-like virus from brain tissues of patients with progressive multifocal leukoencephalopathy. Cell fusion can also be obtained with lysolecithin in lieu of Sendai virus. (See Chap. 5.)

There are three assumptions underlying the use of Sendai virus for cell fusion in a search for suspected viral agents: (1) that the virus causing the disease exists in a latent state in cells which for one reason or another are not capable of yielding the virus in an infectious state; (2) that the uninfected cell which is fused with the cell containing the latent virus can supply one or more factors that will permit growth of the virus; and (3) that the recovered virus does not engage in genetic recombination with inactive Sendai virus. It takes little imagination to appreciate the exciting possibilities suggested by this fundamental biologic observation.

Co-Cultivation. The method of co-cultivation is less sophisticated than cell fusion. In this procedure, a tissue specimen from the patient is treated with trypsin to disperse the cells which presumably contain virus. The cells are inoculated onto several types of cells in monolayer culture and observed for an indefinite period as the double cell culture is subcultured according to its nutritional state. It is possible that cell fusion also occurs during co-cultivation but at a lower frequency than that obtained by inducing cell fusion with virus. Co-cultivation was initially used to isolate a measles-like virus from brain tissue of patients with subacute sclerosing panencephalitis.

Immunologic Viral Identification

Strain Identification. Biochemical and biologic properties provide a basis for classifying viral isolates under broad group headings but do not furnish adequate data for distinguishing between individual serotypes, i.e., distinguishing echovirus, type 3, from echovirus, type 9. A definitive identification is usually made by the serum *neutralization test.* In this test, infectious virus is mixed with specific antiviral serum. The mixture is incubated and then inoculated onto susceptible cells. If the antiserum is directed against the virus, the recipient cells will not be infected. As a control, cells are also inoculated with mixture of the virus and normal serum to show that the neutralization reaction is specific. Strain identification is essential when there is interest in identifying patients who are infected with some specific microorganism, e.g., as in an epidemiologic study. However, for most clinical situations, classifying the viral isolate into one of the groups listed in Table 11–6 is sufficient.

Newer Methods for Identifying Viral Antigens. Other methods have been employed in special circumstances to identify viral antigens in clinical materials. For example, immunofluorescence has proved useful for detection of (1) influenza viral antigens in nasal mucosal cells, (2) rabies and herpes simplex viral antigens in brain tissue, (3) vaccinial antigens in skin scrapings, and (4) Epstein-Barr antigen(s) in leukocytes from patients with infectious mononucleosis. Several fluorescent antibody methods have been proposed as a means for rapid diagnosis of viral infection. In most of these procedures, cells obtained from a patient are washed and then incubated with specific fluorescent antibody or with appropriate controls and examined within a few hours. Fluorescent methods permit high efficiency when a laboratory is engaged only in study of specific agents and can ignore other viral antigens in which it has no interest. However, the high degree of specificity of the fluorescent technique, which is so highly desired when studying a viral infection with a single strain of virus, becomes a disadvantage when the objective is to find all viruses, since the laboratory would be required to stock a bewildering array of specific antisera, each directed against one type of virus. Immunodiffusion methods and radioimmunoassay procedures efficiently demonstrate Australian antigen in sera of patients with viral hepatitis, type B, and are adaptable to automation techniques. However, here again a high degree of specificity associated with these procedures is a disadvantage because it would be necessary to test each isolated virus against a confusing array of antisera.

Electron microscopic study of viral particles in tissues and secretions also has been suggested as a possible diagnostic tool since it presumably would permit direct visualization of noninfectious forms of virus as well as infectious virus. However, results have so far been discouraging because of the lack of specific findings and problems of distinguishing viral particles from nonviral debris. For example, it was initially believed that smallpox virus — which has a distinctive cuboid form — would be easily recognized; however, even experienced workers have had difficulty in distinguishing smallpox virus from artifacts that arise in preparing a specimen for study. Possibly, the development of new electron microscopic methods which use antibodies tagged with electron-dense substances such as ferritin or horseradish peroxidase will aid in distinguishing specific viral particles, a technique called *immune electron microscopy.*

Serologic Approach to Viral Diagnosis

Principles

The serologic approach to diagnosis of viral infections depends on demonstrating that the patient has had an immunologic response to the viral antigen. The immune response is usually measured in terms of a serologic response achieved from a variety of methods, e.g., serum neutralization tests, hemagglutination-inhibition tests, complement-fixation, and other means of measuring antibody in sera and other body fluids. In principle, in each test, some specific biologic acitivity of the virus is interfered with or neutralized by serum containing antibody to the virus. The diagnosis of infection in each test depends on the demonstration of an increase in antibody levels occurring between the time when serum was first taken, during the acute phase of the illness, and when a second serum was obtained, approximately 10 to 14 days later. It is essential to test both sera together as a control for variability inherent in serologic procedures.

Commonly used serologic tests in a diagnostic virology laboratory estimate antibody content of a serum by determining the greatest dilution of serum which shows the desired immunologic activity. The reciprocal of the dilution of the serum at the end point is called the titer of the serum. For example, a serum which will neutralize poliovirus type 1 infectivity when diluted 320 times but which fails to show neutralizing activity when diluted 640 times would be said to have a titer of 320 against type 1 poliovirus. Most serologic procedures are performed with serial dilutions of serum, e.g., 1/10, 1/20, 1/40, etc. Data accumulated by a large number of workers indicate that the error in serial dilution procedures is approximately one dilution on either side of the end point. Consequently, a diagnostic increase is defined as a difference of at least two serial dilutions between the titers of two sera. For example, if the dilution series is made by twofold steps, a fourfold or greater rise in antibody titer will be required.

Practice

Serum Neutralization

The serum neutralization test, which was previously described in this chapter as an aid to strain identification of a virus (see Biochemical Classification of Viruses), can also be employed to ascertain the capacity of a serum to neutralize or interfere with viral infectivity in susceptible hosts. The test is performed by mixing dilutions of patients' sera with a predetermined amount, usually 100 to 1000 infectious doses, of a known virus. The serum-virus mixtures are allowed to react during a period of incubation and are then inoculated onto a susceptible host. The highest dilution of serum which prevents viral-induced changes in the host defines the end point. Serum neutralization is a highly specific virus-antibody reaction and therefore is limited in use to measuring antibody levels against a specific virus, either the virus isolated from the patient or one of particular interest to the investigator.

Hemagglutination-Inhibition

The hemagglutination-inhibition test is restricted for use to viruses which have a demonstrable agglutinin for red cells. The test is similar to the neutralization test except that the test measures the ability of serum to neutralize or inhibit a standard amount of viral hemagglutinating activity, usually four to eight units. Hemagglutination-inhibition reactions also show high specificity and have been helpful in showing antibody titers against rubella virus and several myxoviruses. The usefulness of hemagglutination-inhibition tests may be limited by the presence of nonspecific inhibitors of hemagglutination which normally appear in sera. Nonspecific inhibitors are a problem in the diagnostic laboratory, since they may mask the presence of specific antibody and consequently obscure the fact of an antibody rise. Most nonspecific inhibitors are lipoproteins or glycoproteins and must be removed or destroyed by special treatment of the sera in a way which does not destroy antibody.

Hemadsorption-Inhibition

The hemadsorption-inhibition test, which is similar in principle to the hemagglutination-inhibition test, measures the capacity of serum to interfere with the hemadsorption reaction which was previously described for detection of myxoviruses. This test has chiefly been used in epidemiologic studies of parainfluenza and mumps viral infections, but is not commonly employed in a clinical virology laboratory.

Complement-Fixation

The complement-fixation test depends on the fact that antibody-antigen complexes bind serum complement and leave insufficient amounts of complement (C) for hemolysis of sensitized sheep red blood cells. In this test, dilutions of patient serum are mixed with a standard amount of viral antigen and incubated to permit the formation of antibody-antigen complexes. A standard amount of complement in the form of fresh guinea pig serum is added to the serum-antigen mixture, which is again incubated to permit a reaction between complement and immune complexes which may have formed by the antigen-antibody reaction. This reaction depletes the amount of complement that is available for the hemolytic reaction which would be expected when red cells which are coated with anti–red blood cell antibody are added. The end point signifying specific complement binding or fixation is an absence of red cell hemolysis. In the absence of an antibody-antigen reaction and consequent formation of immune complexes, complement is not depleted and the hemolysis-sensitized red cells are hemolyzed with release of hemoglobin. The highest dilution of serum which prevents erythrocyte hemolysis is the end point. The complement-fixation test can be used to measure antiviral antibody to a variety of viruses. Moreover, the total number of viral complement-fixation antigens needed is less than the number of viruses which can be detected; e.g., a single adenovirus antigen is sufficient to detect 23 adenoviruses, and one influenza A virus antigen is a common intrafamily antigen for all type A influenza viruses. However, the breadth of the complement-fixation reactivity usually obviates speciation of virus within a large family. With some myxovirus infections, the complement-fixation test is of special use for diagnosis, because infection is associated with the appearance of a complement-fixing antibody specifically directed against internal or ribonucleoprotein (S) antigens of the virus. In these infections, the occurrence of a complement-fixation titer of 1:80 or higher with the ribonucleoprotein antigen of influenza or mumps viruses is presumptive evidence for recent infection. A disadvantage of the test is that sera may become anticomplementary with storage.

Other Methods

Fluorescent antibody methods and counterimmunoelectrophoresis offer additional in vitro measurements of antibody response. An indirect method for fluorescent antibody is commonly used. Tissue cultures are inoculated with known viruses. The infected cells are exposed to the patient's serum, the cells are washed and then exposed to fluorescent antibody directed against human immunoglobulins. If the patient's serum has antibody against the virus which infects the cells, the tissue will be stained by the fluorescent anti-human gammaglobulin. In the absence of antibody, specific staining will not occur. The fluorescent antibody method is time consuming and thus is not customarily used to ascertain serum titers against specific agents.

Use of *counterimmunoelectrophoresis* as a diagnostic laboratory test is new and, at present, confined to demonstrating antibody to influenza type A virus, adenovirus, and the hepatitis-associated antigen seen with viral hepatitis type B. In this method, the viral antigen is placed in a small hole punched into an agar gel coating which overlays a glass microscope slide. The patient's serum is placed into a second hole which is about 3 mm from the antigen hole. An electrical current is applied parallel to a line joining the two depressions. A precipitin line develops when an antibody-antigen reaction occurs between the serum and viral antigen. The method is simple and has the advantage of rapidity over other methods for showing antiviral antibody.

Interpretation of Results

Considerable care must be taken in the interpretation of serologic data because of the many factors that can influence the outcome of a test. Comparison of antibody titers of serum taken during acute and convalescent stages of illness must be limited to sera which are tested concurrently, since there is usually sufficient variation between results when sera are tested separately to obviate apparent differences that might be seen. It is important to inquire of the laboratory personnel whether it is their practice to run paired sera in the same test.

The interval between paired sera should, as a rule, be 10 to 14 days, but practical considerations concerned with the collection of clinical specimens recommend collection of sera at weekly intervals and on the day of discharge from the hospital. In this manner, collection of acute phase and convalescent phase sera can be assured. Although paired sera should always be obtained, it is not always necessary to wait for the results procured with the second serum. As previously indicated, in the first serum sample, high titers of complement-fixing antibodies against cytomegalovirus, adenovirus, and most myxoviruses are presumptive evidence of recent infection in adults. The second serum should be run along with the first serum to confirm the initial finding and to ascertain whether additional rise or fall in antibody titer occurs.

Isolation of Mycoplasma pneumoniae

Principles

The approach to isolation of mycoplasma in the laboratory is practically the same as that for isolating bacteria, since mycoplasma grow extracellularly. *Mycoplasma pneumoniae,* which is regarded as a prototype of the six species that infect man, is the only mycoplasma generally acknowledged as a human pathogen. *M. pneumoniae* can multiply in enriched liquid and solid media under either aerobic or facultative anaerobic conditions. Mycoplasma medium is usually enriched with horse serum or bovine ascitic fluid and yeast cell extract, and consistent results in growing mycoplasma depend on obtaining freshly prepared media. Although most mycoplasma require an atmosphere of 5 per cent carbon dioxide in 95 per cent nitrogen, *M. pneumoniae* can grow in 5 per cent carbon dioxide in air. Mycoplasma media are supplemented with penicillin, thallium acetate, and Fungizone to suppress overgrowth of less fastidious bacteria. Approximately three weeks are needed for colonies to grow to a size that can be detected with a simple magnifier.

Practice

The opportunity for isolation of *M. pneumoniae* from a patient's specimen is enhanced if the agar plate is taken to the bedside and the sample is directly inoculated. The plate should be returned to the laboratory and incubated for 30 days at least.

Mycoplasma colonies can be recognized under 20 to 40 X magnification as small colonies which have a lenticular appearance on the surface of the agar. Transfer of *M. pneumoniae* from plate to plate is more difficult than the passage of bacteria, since the colonies are not so easily removed from the agar surface. Instead, a small piece of agar bearing a colony is rubbed over the surface of a fresh plate. Subcultures of *M. pneumoniae* are made either on enriched agar or in biphasic medium which consists of a combined liquid and semisolid medium.

M. pneumoniae colonies can be identified by their biochemical properties. *M. pneumoniae* produces beta hemolysis of sheep or guinea pig red blood cells which have been spread in a thin agar sheet over the mycoplasma colonies. Hemolysis is generally ascribed to the action of hydrogen peroxide which is produced by metabolically active *M. pneumoniae*. *M. pneumoniae* can also be identified by its ability under aerobic conditions to reduce colorless 2,3,5-triphenyl-2H-tetrazolium to triphenylformazan, which is red. None of the other mycoplasma can reduce the dye, and a positive reaction is so specific that a neutralization test with specific antiserum is not necessary.

Serologic Diagnosis of M. pneumoniae Infection

Several kinds of antibody are found at different stages of an *M. pneumoniae* infection, and a significant rise in any one is strong evidence for a presumptive diagnosis. *Cold agglutinins,* which appear during the acute illness, demonstrate the ability of the patient's serum to react with the large "I" antigen which is in the "I-i" erythrocyte antigen system. The presence of anti-I antibody is shown by agglutination at 4°C of adult human type 0 red cells which have the I antigen on their surface. The specificity of the reaction is shown by the failure of the serum to agglutinate human cord blood cells which lack the I antigen. Cold agglutinins have been regarded as nonspecific antibodies because they do not react directly with intact *M. pneumoniae.*

Most laboratories use a *complement-fixation* test for detecting antibody activity. Complement-fixing antibodies appear in 85 per cent of patients with *M. pneumoniae* infections. In adult groups, complement-fixing antibody titers of 1:80 or greater are unusual; therefore, titers at or higher than the 1:80 dilution are accepted as presumptive evidence for infection. A *metabolic inhibition* test for *M. pneumoniae* also can be used to measure antibody levels. In this test, dilutions of a patient's serum are incorporated into the medium customarily used to demonstrate the tetrazolium reduction activity. In the presence of specific antiserum, growth of the agent is inhibited and the consequent reduction of the tetrazolium salt is inhibited. Metabolic-inhibition antibodies appear later than complement-fixing antibodies and remain elevated for a longer time. Performance of this test depends on growing *M. pneumoniae* in the laboratory; therefore, it is usually restricted to laboratories with special interests in this area. Most diagnostic laboratories depend on the complement-fixation test.

Clinical Interpretation of Laboratory Data

What is the significance of finding a virus or demonstrating an immunologic response in any particular patient? For the clinician, the principal question is whether the findings are related to the patient's illness. The association between a virus and a particular illness rests on fulfilling Koch's postulates as far as possible or on accumulating sufficient epidemiologic information that points to a reasonable conclusion. The relationship between viruses and specific clinical pictures is not a neat one-to-one correspondence, and this fact sometimes makes difficult a clear demonstration of a causal relationship. The situation is compounded when evidence of simultaneous infection with two agents is found. The problem then is to decide whether both agents are involved in the disease process, or, as in the case of serologic increase in response to two or more agents, whether only one agent caused the disease, with the second immune response being due to a booster effect of cross-reacting or shared antigens. In all instances, the judgment as to whether a patient has a particular disease is a clinical decision and, as previously indicated, the function of the laboratory is to supply data that will aid in and provide confirmation of diagnosis.

References

Andrews, C., and Pereira, H. G.: Viruses of Vertebrates. 3rd ed. Baltimore, Williams and Wilkins Co., 1972.

Blair, J. E., Lennette, E. H., and Truant, J. P. (eds.): Manual of Clinical Microbiology. Baltimore, Williams and Wilkins Co., 1970.

Grist, N. R., Ross, C. A. C., Bell, E. J., and Stoutt, E. J.: Diagnostic Methods in Clinical Virology. Philadelphia, F. A. Davis Co., 1966.

Horsfall, F. L., Jr. (ed.): Diagnosis of Viral and Rickettsial Infections. New York, Columbia University Press, 1946.

Horsfall, F. L., Jr., and Tamm, I.: Viral and Rickettsial Infections of Man. 4th ed. Philadelphia, J. B. Lippincott Co., 1965.

Hoskins, J. M.: Virological Procedures. New York, Appleton-Century-Crofts, 1967.

Hsiung, G. D.: Diagnostic Virology. New Haven, Yale University Press, 1973.

Lennette, E. H., and Schmidt, N. J.: Diagnostic Procedures for Viral and Rickettsial Infections. 4th ed. Washington, D. C., American Public Health Association, 1969.

Paul, J.: Cell and Tissue Culture. 4th ed. Baltimore, Williams and Wilkins Co., 1970.

III

UPPER
RESPIRATORY
TRACT
INFECTION
AND SEQUELAE

Chapter 12

UPPER RESPIRATORY TRACT INFECTION: GENERAL CONSIDERATIONS

Introduction

Upper respiratory tract infections include a large number of acute, inflammatory processes that involve primarily the nose, paranasal sinuses, middle ear, and, most importantly, the pharynx and tonsils. Acute respiratory tract disease is the most common reason for patients' consulting physicians, and it ranks as the most important form of acute illness in the United States (see Table 12–1). Infections of the nasal passages and/or the posterior

TABLE 12–1. Incidence and Type of Acute Illnesses in the United States in 1970*

Category of Acute Illness	Per Cent
Infectious Diseases	
Upper respiratory tract infections	31.3
Influenza	19.7
Digestive	5.7
"Virus" (unspecified)	4.6
Pneumonia	3.0
Common childhood	1.9
Others	5.4
Subtotal:	71.6
Injuries	14.6
All other acute diseases	13.8
Total:	100.0

*From Current Estimates, Health Interview Survey 1970, National Health Survey, Series 10, No. 72.

pharynx and tonsils are so frequent that laymen and physicians consider them "part of life."

Most patients do not make any distinction between infection of different regions of the upper respiratory tract. Thus, any upper respiratory tract infection is often referred to as a "cold" or "sore throat." In the case of some patients who are alerted to the importance of streptococci as an etiologic agent in upper respiratory tract disease, the phrase "strep throat" is commonly employed. Streptococcal infection of the pharynx and tonsils is the only reportable, common, communicable infectious disorder of the upper respiratory tract. Because it is a reportable disease, data are available on its prevalence. As shown in Table 12–2, streptococcal sore throat ranks second in frequency among a number of reportable infectious diseases in the United States.

TABLE 12–2. Relative Frequency of Common Infectious Diseases in the United States in 1971*

Disease	Number of Cases
Gonorrhea	670,268
Streptococcal sore throat	433,405**
Mumps	124,939
Syphilis	95,997
Measles	75,290
Tuberculosis (new, active)	35,035
Salmonellosis (excluding typhoid fever)	21,928
Amebiasis	2375
Meningococcal	2262
Poliomyelitis (paralytic)	17

*From Annual Supplement, Summary 1971, Morbidity and Mortality: Reported incidence of notifiable diseases in the United States, 1971.
**Data are for 1970 since streptococcal infection reporting not complete for 1971.

Physicians commonly lump together all clinical manifestations of upper respiratory tract infection under the term "acute URI" or, more simply, "URI." While admittedly there are frequent anatomic overlappings of many upper respiratory tract infections, it is advantageous for the physician to focus on that specific anatomic site which is initially or primarily involved. This allows him to consider different upper respiratory tract infections from the perspective of specific etiologic infectious agents which are most likely to be responsible. This approach provides a rational basis for diagnosis and management.

There are many misconceptions concerning upper respiratory tract infection which are held by both patients and physicians. This is due, in part, to the frequency of upper respiratory tract infections and to the fact that most are transitory, relatively benign, self-limited illnesses. Real problems that spring from this cavalier attitude include the following: (1) It is not widely recognized that the overwhelming majority of upper respiratory tract infections are caused by viruses, and since there is not yet available any antimicrobial agent of proven efficacy for viral disease of the respiratory tract, the frequent prescribing of antimicrobial agents for upper respiratory tract infections has no rational basis. (2) Acute pharyngitis-tonsillitis due to Group A streptococci is the most important upper respiratory tract infection because it can be and should be treated with specific antimicrobial drugs. Although physicians and some patients are aware of this, they may not realize that streptococcal pharyngitis-tonsillitis *cannot* be diagnosed on clinical grounds. Furthermore, they may not appreciate the fact that this bacterial infection represents a relatively small percentage of upper respiratory tract infections. Thus, antimicrobial agents are prescribed for "strep throat" or "sore throat" on the basis that the etiologic agent is or may be Group A streptococci, when in reality the causative agent more often than not is a virus. (3) Physicians and patients often do not appreciate the fact that distinguishing streptococcal pharyngitis-tonsillitis from all other infections of the upper respiratory tract *can be* accomplished with relative ease by means of throat culture. By using a throat culture as a means for identifying those infections due to streptococci, the informed physician can specifically prescribe antimicrobial agents for only those patients that need them.

The basic problem confronting the clinician is how to distinguish the 5 to 10 per cent of patients with upper respiratory tract infections caused by bacteria in whom specific antimicrobial therapy is indicated. In a more practical vein, the physician must be able to identify rapidly the 90 to 95 per cent of patients with nonbacterial infections of viral origin in whom antimicrobial therapy is *not* warranted and only symptomatic measures are indicated.

Spectrum of Etiologic Agents

Viruses

More than 90 per cent of acute upper respiratory infections in adults are caused by viruses (see Chaps. 4 and 11). These viruses have an extraordinary diversity and worldwide distribution. For example, at least 50 antigenically distinct rhinoviruses are known to be etiologically associated with the "common cold." Yet such rhinoviruses collectively account for only about one quarter of colds experienced by patients.

Group A Streptococci

One of the most important causes of acute infection of the upper respiratory tract is the Group A, beta-hemolytic streptococcus. Statistically, it is the most common cause of acute bacterial, exudative pharyngitis-tonsillitis. The importance of oropharyngeal streptococcal infection is based in large part on the unique etiologic role of Group A streptococcal pharyngitis-tonsillitis in the pathogenesis of rheumatic fever, especially rheumatic carditis with the possibility of irreversible and life-threatening scarring of heart valves (see Chap. 15). Every patient with an acute respiratory infection character-ized by pharyngeal inflammation must be evaluated in terms of whether or not Group A streptococci are present. If they are present, prompt eradication of the streptococci by means of antimicrobial therapy in most cases will prevent development of rheumatic fever and rheumatic heart disease. This must be the central focus in the approach to upper respiratory tract infectious diseases.

Other Bacteria

Other bacteria sometimes may cause pharyngitis-tonsillitis or infection of other regions of the upper respiratory tract. These include the pneumo-coccus, meningococcus, gonococcus, and especially the diphtheria bacillus and *Haemophilus influenzae.* Anaerobic bacteria, e.g., members of the Bacteroides genus and microaerophilic streptococci, have been strongly implicated in infection of the paranasal sinuses. Pneumococci, staphylococci, and Group A streptococci especially are important in suppurative disease of the paranasal sinuses and middle ear. These bacterial infections usually are associated with viral infections of the nose and pharynx, respectively.

Spectrum of Clinical Syndromes

Common Cold

This is the most common upper respiratory tract infection and the most frequent infectious problem experienced by man. The clinical manifestations of the common cold include sneezing, a watery discharge from the nose, which becomes thicker and assumes a yellowish or semipurulent appearance over a period of several days, and a feeling of general malaise. There is usually no fever. Cough is *not* an initial manifestation of the common cold; it usually signifies disease of the lower respiratory tract. During the early phases of a cold, the nasal mucosa is edematous and has a "boggy" appearance. Most patients complain of a "scratchiness" of their posterior pharynx and, for this reason, the patient frequently states that he has a "sore throat." The common cold runs a course of no more than several days. Persistent watery nasal discharge which continues for a period of weeks or months always suggests the possibility of allergic rhinitis. Complicating middle ear infections are especially common in children, presumably owing to inflammation of excessive lymphoid tissue which causes temporary obstruction of the eustachian tubes.

The etiologic agents most clearly associated with the common cold are the rhinoviruses, one of three genera composing the family of picornaviruses (see Chaps. 4 and 11). Based on viral isolation studies utilizing nasal secretions, rhinoviruses account for only 10 to 25 per cent of colds in adults and 5 to 10 per cent of colds in children. The etiologic agents responsible for the majority of common colds have not yet been identified. Since there are at least 50 different antigenically distinct serotypes of rhinoviruses, and since each allegedly has a capacity to infect man, it is no wonder that colds are common and have plagued man for centuries. In addition to the galaxy of antigenically distinct rhinoviruses causing the common cold, there is the additional problem of immunity to any given antigenic serotype being transitory in nature. Thus, the reason why colds are so common stems in part from the great number of known and unknown viral agents capable of causing this infectious process as well as the lack of durable immunity to a given viral serotype.

Acute Pharyngitis-Tonsillitis

"Sore throat," like the common cold, is one of the most common reasons for patients seeking medical attention. It may occur as an isolated event or appear in association with infection of other anatomic regions of either the upper or lower respiratory tract. Acute pharyngitis-tonsillitis probably is the single most often misdiagnosed and mismanaged entity in the practice of medicine.

Group A streptococci are the major cause of bacterial infection of the posterior pharyngeal mucous membranes and tonsils, or tonsillar areas in patients who have undergone tonsillectomy. Infection usually involves contiguous structures, i.e., the anterior and posterior tonsillar pillars, uvula, and soft palate. Group A streptococci may cause suppurative diseases outside the pharynx and tonsillar regions by extending into peritonsillar and parapharyngeal tissues, causing peritonsillar and parapharyngeal abscesses, or the streptococcus may invade the middle ear and set up a suppurative otitis media. On rare occasions, streptococci infecting the tonsils and pharynx may enter the blood stream and cause streptococcal septicemia with the possibility of metastatic infection of remote organ systems, e.g., joints and heart.

Another cause of pharyngitis-tonsillitis is diphtheria. However, as spelled out in detail elsewhere (see Chap. 17), the clinical manifestations of upper respiratory tract infection due to *Corynebacterium diphtheriae* are due to the potent exotoxin produced by this microorganism rather than to its invasion of host tissues per se. Although an exudate may be present in diphtheria, its characteristic appearance and location usually allows the physician to distinguish it from the exudate induced by Group A streptococcal infection (see Chap. 14).

Infection of the pharynx and/or tonsils by *Streptococcus pneumoniae*, *Neisseria meningitidis* or *N. gonorrhoeae* probably accounts for a very small percentage of acute bacterial pharyngitis. There is also some evidence that Group C and Group G streptococci can, on rare occasions, cause pharyngitis. The exact incidence of oropharyngeal infection due to these diverse bacterial species is unknown, since many laboratories do not take the steps necessary to fully identify and characterize them in throat cultures. In young children, usually less than five years of age, and also in older adults, i.e., those in the sixth to eighth decades of life, acute pharyngitis due to *Haemophilus influenzae* may occur. A far more important respiratory tract infection caused by *H. influenzae,* however, is acute epiglottitis (discussed later in this chapter).

A variety of other nonbacterial infectious agents have the capacity to infect the pharynx and/or tonsillar areas. The clinical syndrome associated with these agents is termed *nonbacterial pharyngitis.* This syndrome is discussed in detail in Chapter 18. For the sake of completeness, the viruses which are etiologically most important in this syndrome include the adenoviruses, *Herpesvirus hominis* types I and II, enteric cytopathic viruses of human origin (echoviruses), the myxo- and paramyxoviruses, Epstein-Barr (EB) virus, and cytomegalovirus (CMV virus).

Both the Epstein-Barr virus and the cytomegaloviruses are now securely linked to infectious mononucleosis from an etiologic standpoint. Infectious mononucleosis is important for three reasons. First, it can cause a clinical picture of pharyngitis-tonsillitis which is indistinguishable from that caused by Group A streptococci. Second, 20 to 25 per cent of patients with infectious mononucleosis due to Epstein-Barr virus have demonstrable Group A streptococci in their throat, based on isolation of these microorganisms from throat cultures. The number of Group A streptococci is sufficiently large to suggest that in many of these patients these microorganisms may be causing disease in concert with Epstein-Barr virus. This is a debatable point and more data are necessary. Third, infectious mononucleosis has its highest incidence among high school and college students. It affects an age group that is still quite susceptible to Group A streptococcal infection and rheumatic fever (see Chaps. 13 and 15). For these reasons, "sore throat" in a young high school or college student poses a special diagnostic dilemma. It is not sufficient to make a diagnosis of infectious mononucleosis without determining whether or not Group A streptococci are present in the throat. If Group A streptococci are present, they should be eradicated with appropriate antimicrobial therapy.

Gingivostomatitis

This entity occurs most often in young children. The buccal mucosa has a "firey red" appearance, and a grayish membrane or exudate may be present. The process may involve the gums or tongue in addition to the buccal musoca.

There are three principal etiologic agents to consider. *Herpesvirus hominis* type I produces small, 1 to 3 mm, circular ulcers on a larger erythematous base. These lesions tend to appear in the anterior portions of the oropharynx, viz., the gums, lips, and anterior buccal mucosa or anterior portion of the tongue.

Coxsackieviruses also produce similar type ulcers but they usually have a less acute appearance with less associated inflammation of the surrounding mucosa. Furthermore, the ulcers characteristically occur in the posterior regions of the oropharynx, viz., soft palate and uvula, anterior or posterior tonsillar pillars, and posterior pharynx.

The third infectious agent is *Candida albicans,* which produces an infection of the buccal mucosa and tongue, and, less commonly, other regions of the oropharynx. The infection produced by this fungus is often referred to as "thrush," a feature of which is the occurrence of small areas of snow-white or gray-white patches of exudate lying on an acutely inflamed mucosa. Such areas may coalesce to form a conspicuous membrane simulating that seen in diphtheria or infectious mononucleosis. The situation is rarely confused with the exudate of Group A streptococcal pharyngitis. Infections of the oropharynx caused by *Candida albicans* or other Candida species are especially common in neonates and infants, in patients with an altered oropharyngeal microbial flora secondary to antimicrobial therapy, and in patients with a primary immunodeficiency disease or immunologic deficits secondary to an underlying disease and/or therapy, e.g., a patient with acute lymphocytic leukemia receiving corticosteroids and cytotoxic drugs. Extension of oropharyngeal candidal infection to the lungs or dissemination of the yeast to other organ systems via the bloodstream is particularly apt to occur in patients with any significant aberration in natural and acquired host defense mechanisms, i.e., the compromised host (see Chap. 43).

Acute Epiglottitis

Acute inflammation of the epiglottis usually develops with frightening rapidity and almost invariably is or can become an emergency situation with ever-present threat of airway obstruction requiring incisive action. Although the peak incidence of this disease, often termed the *croup syndrome,* is among children one to two years of age, at least 10 per cent of cases occur in adults. Fever of moderate degree, with evidence of respiratory tract infection such as rhinitis or a cough which may be crouplike, and intermittent or constant stridor signifying a compromised airway, is the usual picture.

Precise diagnosis is made by visualization, as complete as possible, of the hypopharynx or larynx region, always performed with the patient in the sitting or upright position to decrease the hazard of sudden airway obstruction; demonstration of an enormously swollen, acutely inflamed epiglottis confirms the diagnosis. The epiglottis may be swollen to 8 to 10 times its normal size and appear bright red, resembling a maraschino cherry.

The diagnosis can be strongly suspected by obtaining a roentgenogram of the lateral neck which shows the pathognomonic changes illustrated in Figure 12–1. In acute epiglottitis, the epiglottis and aryepiglottic folds almost fill the entire hypopharynx, with ballooning of the airway above and a normal-appearing larynx and subglottic trachea region below. In acute croup, i.e., acute laryngotracheobronchitis, which may closely resemble acute epiglottitis clinically, the hypopharynx also shows ballooning; however, the supraglottic and glottic structures are normal, whereas the subglottic region is obviously constricted, representing the site of airway obstruction. The advantage of roentgenographic diagnosis lies in avoiding the need for time-consuming and hazardous repeated attempts to visualize what is a difficult anatomic region for most physicians to examine under normal or optimal circumstances. The patient with acute epiglottitis should be accompanied to the x-ray depart-ment by a medical attendant who has appropriate equipment for performing an immediate tracheostomy and the knowledge to use it. Impending or

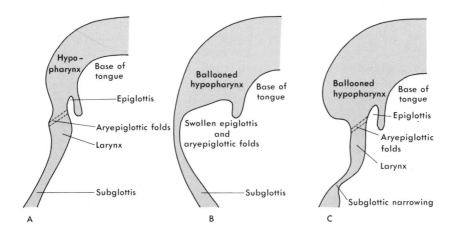

Figure 12-1. Schematic drawings of lateral neck airway roentgenograms illustrating: *A,* Normal hypopharynx and epiglottic region, larynx, and subglottic airway (the hypopharynx is here defined as that region behind and below the base of the tongue not directly visible during ordinary inspection). *B,* Pathognomonic changes of acute epiglottitis with enormous swelling of the epiglottis and aryepiglottic folds, leading to ballooning of the hypopharynx. *C,* Pathognomonic changes associated with "croup" or acute laryngotracheobronchitis with ballooning of the hypopharynx but a relatively normal epiglottic region with markedly constricted subglottic airway.

sudden airway obstruction can be anticipated in a high proportion of cases, dictating the need for lifesaving tracheostomy.

Although *Haemophilus influenzae*, type B, is implicated most often as the etiologic agent, it is quite clear from a number of studies that acute epiglottitis is a syndrome and may be caused by many other microorganisms. These include Group A streptococci, bacteria constituting the normal oropharyngeal flora such as *Streptococcus pneumoniae* and *Staphylococcus aureus,* and the paramyxoviruses (paramyxovirus types 1 to 4 or respiratory syncytial virus). Acute laryngotracheobronchitis is usually caused by one of the parainfluenza viruses (types 1 to 3) or respiratory syncytial virus.

Suppurative Complications

Mention has already been made of the fact that a number of bacterial species, e.g., pneumococci, staphylococci, Group A streptococci, and anaerobic bacteria, may initiate infection of the paranasal sinuses and middle ear. Bacterial infection of these anatomic regions usually are secondary to preceding viral infection. The inflammatory response elicited by the virus results in swelling of mucosal surfaces and obstruction of anatomic orifices. These changes cause stasis of secretions and other alterations in local host defense mechanisms. The net result allows bacteria constituting the normal microbial flora of the oropharynx to colonize these anatomic areas in numbers sufficient to cause clinically manifest disease.

Because of concern of secondary bacterial infection, some physicians routinely employ antimicrobial agents in the management of viral disease of the upper respiratory tract. This is probably unwise for several reasons. It is not known how often secondary bacterial colonization occurs or results in frank disease, but there is reasonably good evidence that this problem may be anticipated in only a small proportion of patients. This is certainly true of adults, in whom obstruction of the eustacian tubes is much less apt to occur; consequently, complicating otitis media is seen far less often in adults than in children. In addition, no single antimicrobial agent will be effective in preventing suppurative complications due to all of the bacteria that have been implicated. Finally, the risk of undesirable or even life-threatening side effects of routine antimicrobial therapy becomes significant when one considers the prevalence of viral respiratory tract disease. The best policy would appear to be conservative supportive therapy and withholding of antimicrobial therapy until clinical signs of secondary, suppurative complications become evident. At that time, antimicrobial therapy can be initiated and subsequently modified as indicated by the results of cultures of appropriate clinical specimens.

References

Bass, J. W., Steele, R. W., and Wiebe, R. A.: Acute epiglottitis. A surgical emergency. J.A.M.A. *229:*671, 1974.

Evans, A. S., and Dick, E. C.: Acute pharyngitis and tonsillitis in University of Wisconsin students. J.A.M.A. *190:*699, 1964.

Evans, A. S.: Clinical syndromes in adults caused by respiratory infection. Med. Clin. North Am. *51:*803, 1967.

Monto, A. S., and Ullman, B. M.: Acute respiratory illness in an American community. The Tecumseh study. J.A.M.A. *227:*164, 1974.

Mufson, M. A., Webb, P. A., Kennedy, H., Gill, V., and Chanock, R. M.: Etiology of upper-respiratory-tract illnesses among civilian adults. J.A.M.A. *195:*1, 1966.

Poole, C. A., and Altman, D. H.: Acute epiglottitis in children. Radiology *80:*798, 1963.

Sloyer, J. L., Jr., Howie, V. M., Ploussard, J. H., Amman, A. J., Autrian, R., and Johnston, R. B., Jr.: Immune response to acute otitis media in children. I. Serotypes isolated and serum and middle ear fluid antibody in pneumococcal otitis media. Infect. Immun. *9:*1028, 1974.

Chapter 13

GROUP A AND OTHER STREPTOCOCCI

Introduction

Classification

Group A streptococci are one subclass of several large classes of streptococci which collectively constitute a large group of microorganisms of remarkable heterogeneity. One purpose of this chapter is to clarify the commonly used classification systems for Group A and other streptococci. Another purpose is to emphasize important relationships which exist between specific classes and subclasses of streptococci and their related diseases.

Importance of Lancefield Group A Streptococci and Their Products

Streptococci classified as Group A, based on antigenic specificity of their cell wall carbohydrate as described by Dr. Rebecca Lancefield during the early 1930s, have an especially important place in infectious medicine. Group A streptococci are the most common cause of bacterial pharyngitis-tonsillitis (see Chaps. 12 and 14). They are also uniquely linked to the development of rheumatic fever and acute glomerulonephritis (see Chaps. 15 and 16). Effective management of upper respiratory tract infections and prevention of these sequelae of Group A streptococcal infection require familiarity with these important microorganisms and the various cellular and extracellular products they elaborate. A third purpose of this chapter is to briefly describe those cellular and extracellular products of Group A streptococci which have special pathogenetic and diagnostic importance.

Classification of Group A and Other Streptococci

General Properties

Gram Reaction, Morphology, and Growth

Group A streptococci, as well as all other subclasses and major classes of streptococci, are gram positive cocci with a propensity to grow in chains of variable lengths, especially when cultured in vitro. Their name is derived from Greek words meaning *necklace* and *berry.* In vivo, streptococci usually occur as single cocci, diplococci, or even tetrads, or as short chains consisting of three to six bacterial cells at most. They are smaller than staphylococci. While lacking the allegedly lancet shape and diplococcal characteristic of pneumococci, they cannot readily be distinguished from *Streptococcus pneumoniae* by morphologic characteristics.

All of the streptococci require an enriched medium for primary isolation and luxurious growth in vitro, e.g., blood agar and Todd-Hewitt broth. Some streptococci which are of increasing clinical importance can *only* be grown under conditions of markedly reduced oxygen tension or strict anaerobiasis. Even then, several days may be required for initial evidence of growth, and some strains cannot be subcultured in the microbiology laboratory following isolation. Like *Streptococcus pneumoniae,* which they resemble closely in many different ways, the Group A streptococci do not produce catalase. Those streptococcal species of medical significance almost invariably are strict microbial parasites of man.

Anatomic Loci of Cell Wall Constituents and Extracellular Soluble Products

Probably no other pathogenic microorganism has been so extensively studied and found to elaborate such an array of constituents and products as Group A streptococci. Some of these constituents and products which are of major clinical significance are shown in schematic fashion in Figure 13-1.

Recently isolated Group A streptococci possess an external capsulelike layer of hyaluronic acid, which is responsible for the mucoid appearance of discrete streptococcal colonies on an agar culture. Some strains produce considerable quantities of this capsular material so that the colonies may actually be "pushed" along the surface of a blood agar plate by gentle pressure with a bacteriologic loop. A very experienced clinical microbiologist

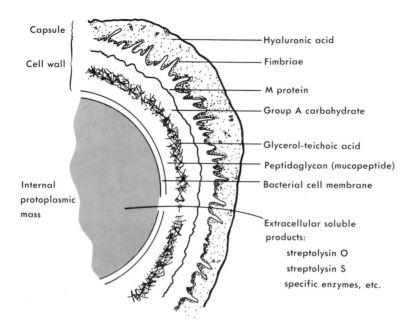

Figure 13-1. Schematic representation of a Group A streptococcal cell illustrating anatomic loci of various cell wall constituents and extracellular soluble products.

might note this feature in suspecting that the colonies are Group A streptococci.

Extending into the hyaluronic acid outer layer are the fimbriae or finger-like projections of the subsurface layer of M protein. Some evidence suggests that these fimbriae, coated with or consisting totally of M protein, may be the means by which the bacterial cells attach to host cells (see Chap. 2). The M protein is a very important constituent of the streptococcal cell wall, since it is the antigen which is responsible for the induction of immunity to streptococcal infection caused by the corresponding M serotype (see below).

Making up the remaining bulk of the bacterial cell wall is a macro-molecular complex which consists of the immunologic specific Group A carbohydrate, already noted to be the basis of the Lancefield grouping classification, and the peptidoglycan (mucopeptide) as shown in Figure 13–1. The carbohydrate and peptidoglycan are linked together through an as yet undetermined physical-chemical association and create a mosaic rather than the separate onion skin–like layers as are so often depicted in illustrations of the anatomy of the streptococcal cell wall. One of the constituents found within this mosaic is the glycerol–teichoic acid moiety (see Fig. 13–1) which, together with the carbohydrate-peptidoglycan complex, accounts for the rigidity of the bacterial cell wall. Bounding the internal protoplasmic mass is the usual cytoplasmic bacterial cell membrane.

A variety of hemolysins, e.g., streptolysin O and streptolysin S, and enzymes and other products of intracellular metabolic activity are synthe-sized within the internal protoplasmic mass, i.e., "core," of the streptococcal cell. These soluble products by a process not yet defined accumulate in the extracellular environment. More than 20 distinct soluble extracellular products of Group A streptococci have been described.

Classification Systems

Hemolytic Reactions on Blood Agar

The earliest classification system of the streptococci was based on different hemolytic reactions observed on blood agar plates. Types of hemolytic reactions are illustrated in Figure 13–2.

Typical beta hemolysis characteristically occurs around colonies of Group A streptococci. There is complete lysis of the erythrocytes in the blood agar medium. Coalescence of focal areas of beta hemolysis may result in relatively large areas of complete clearing of the blood agar through which underlying newsprint can be read. Other Lancefield groups of streptococci giving a beta-hemolytic reaction include Groups C and G.

Another very important subclass of streptococci, Group D, characteristically gives no hemolytic reaction on blood agar plates. This lack of observable hemolytic reaction traditionally has been termed "gamma hemolytic reaction," a phrase designated to imply *no* significant observable gross hemolysis. Such streptococci are better referred to as nonhemolytic streptococci. As indicated in Figure 13–2, however, not all strains of Group D streptococci are nonhemolytic. This is even more true of Group B streptococci. A significant percentage of Group D and especially Group B strains give beta-hemolytic reactions. The zones of clearing observed with such strains usually are much smaller than the large areas of typical beta hemolysis associated with Group A streptococci. In addition, occasional strains of Group D streptococci produce partial hemolysis of blood agar, i.e., an alpha-hemolytic reaction.

Those streptococci characteristically giving an alpha-hemolytic reaction, sometimes called "green hemolysis," represent an extremely diverse group of

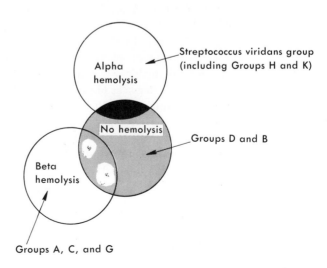

Figure 13–2. Classification of streptococci based on hemolytic reactions on blood agar.

microorganisms which are collectively termed the *Streptococcus viridans* group. It is to be emphasized that this group is a mixed bag. A few distinct species have been identified, e.g., *Streptococcus mutans,* based on unusual synthetic properties. Others can be assigned to specific Lancefield subgroups, e.g., *Streptococcus salivarius,* which produces a cell wall carbohydrate reactive with Group H antiserum. Still other strains merge with *Streptococcus pneumoniae,* elaborating carbohydrates which cross-react with antisera against some of the higher serotypes of pneumococcal capsular poly-saccharides. The great majority of the so-called viridans streptococci, however, remain uncharacterized beyond their capacity to give an alpha-hemolytic reaction on blood agar, the basis for their name.

Antigenic Properties

Lancefield Grouping. The modern era of streptococcal classification was ushered in with the discovery by Dr. Rebecca Lancefield that a large number of streptococci exhibiting beta- or alpha-hemolytic reactions, or giving no evidence of hemolysis, possessed antigenically distinct cell wall carbo-hydrates. The elaboration of such distinct carbohydrates allowed an immunologic classification to be established using antiserum. All Group A streptococci synthesize an antigenic cell wall carbohydrate, *N*-acetylglucosa-mine. It can be extracted from cell walls under suitable conditions and can be shown to react specifically with appropriate (Group A) antiserum. There are some 18 to 20 distinct subgroups lettered A through H, and K through P. Of these, Groups A, B, and D are the most important in the study of human disease.

Subgrouping. *M Serotypes.* Group A streptococci may be further subdivided based on their production of antigenically distinct M proteins. These antigens may be recognized using the same principles worked out by Dr. Lancefield, viz., extracting M protein from a heavy growth of Group A streptococcal cells and showing that it reacts with a specific M protein antiserum. Not all Group A streptococcal isolates can be serotyped since some, even when freshly isolated, do not produce sufficient amounts of M protein to be detected serologically. Serial passage of such isolates in mice may allow them to be M-typed at a later date, as mouse passage often causes enhanced production of M protein. Unhappily, serial animal passage also stimulates production of a streptococcal extracellular product, a potent protease, which degrades M protein. One often is left with a "trade-off," viz., augmented protease production matching enhanced M protein synthesis which precludes serotyping of isolates.

T Patterns. Many strains of Group A streptococci also produce cell wall proteins which are antigenically distinct from M proteins. These proteins are called T proteins. The pattern of T proteins produced by a given Group A streptococcal isolate as recognized by appropriate antisera is of epidemio-logic importance, e.g., identifying specific strains of streptococci that are responsible for outbreaks of pyoderma and acute glomerulonephritis (see Chaps. 16 and 36).

Subclasses of Streptococci and Related Diseases of Major Importance

Group A and other specific streptococci, together with related diseases of major medical importance, are listed in Table 13–1. The classes of streptococci are set out according to their expected hemolytic reaction on blood agar plates. The three most important subgroups of streptococci, Groups A, B, and D, also are listed with the names of the prototype species of each.

TABLE 13–1. Group A and Other Streptococci and Streptococcal Diseases

Hemolytic Reaction or Lancefield Group		Prototype Species	Clinical Diseases	Chapter References
Beta hemolysis,	Group A	*S. pyogenes*	Pharyngitis-tonsillitis Pyoderma Rheumatic fever Glomerulonephritis (Puerperal sepsis; acute endocarditis)	7, 12, 14–16 and 36
	(Group C)	(*S. equi*)	(Endocarditis)	41
	(Group G)	(*S. cariis*)	(Endocarditis)	41
	Group B	*S. agalactiae*	Neonatal sepsis and meningitis	7, 33
No hemolysis, (Nonhemolytic streptococci)	Group D	*S. faecalis* (*S. bovis*)	Endocarditis Urinary tract infections	7, 41
Alpha hemolysis, (viridans group)	Group K	*S. salivarius*	Endocarditis	41
	Group H	*S. sanguis*	Endocarditis	41
	?	*S. mitis*	Endocarditis	41
	?	*S. mutans*	Dental caries (Endocarditis)	
Microaerophilic and anaerobic streptococci (peptostreptococci)		?	Brain abscess Gynecologic infections Pulmonary abscess	7, 33, 39

Streptococcus pyogenes, the prototype species of Group A streptococci, is especially noted for its role in causing acute pharyngitis-tonsillitis and pyoderma (see Chaps. 14 and 36). Also listed are the two most important nonsuppurative complications of these two bacterial infections, viz., rheumatic fever and glomerulonephritis. *S. pyogenes* also can produce septicemia, as can every other streptococcus listed in Table 13–1, and this may result in endocarditis. Group A streptococci historically are associated with puerperal fever, a devastating infectious complication of childbirth and unfortunately still observed from time to time. *S. pyogenes* also is associated with two other diseases not listed in Table 13–1, viz., erysipelas and scarlet fever. For reasons that are not clear, both diseases are presently rarely encountered in the United States.

Streptococcus agalactiae, the prototype species of Group B streptococci, is associated with sepsis or meningitis of the newborn or of children only several weeks old. It is a normal constituent of the pharyngeal and vaginal microbial flora and occasionally is a cause of sepsis in adults, especially women. A syndrome of septicemia and thromboembolism with areas of ischemic necrosis of the skin has been described in diabetic women. Like *Streptococcus pyogenes,* this microorganism has also been identified as an important cause of puerperal sepsis. There is increasing evidence that specific Group B subgroups, recognized by immunologic means, are associated with these different clinical patterns of disease. Such information should prove valuable in epidemiologic investigations of Group B streptococcal infections and provide a better means for prevention and control of disease.

Streptococcus faecalis is the prototype species of the enterococci of Group D streptococci. This species, as well as four or five others possessing the Group D cell wall carbohydrate, is part of the enteric microbial flora; hence, these species are referred to collectively as enterococci. *Streptococcus bovis* and *Streptococcus equinus* produce Group D cell wall carbohydrate but are *not* part of the enteric microbial flora. They are nonenterococcal members of the Group D streptococci. *S. bovis* differs from other species of Group D streptococci in that it is highly susceptible to penicillin in contrast to the enterococci which are notoriously penicillin-resistant. This is an important distinction, since all Group D streptococci have the capacity to cause endocarditis as well as urinary tract infections, and the penicillin-resistance of the enterococcal strains causes special problems in creating effective antimicrobial therapy. Penicillin can be used when it is recognized that *S. bovis* is the causative agent.

While only three species of the alpha-hemolytic *Streptococcus viridans* group are listed in Table 13–1, it should be emphasized that many others could be included. All are characterized by producing an alpha-hemolytic reaction on blood agar. Collectively, these microorganisms represent a predominant component of the normal microbial flora of the oropharynx, gums, and teeth. *Streptococcus mitis* and *Streptococcus salivarius* are the most common causes of subacute bacterial endocarditis. *Streptococcus mutans* is a leading candidate for the most important cause of dental caries. This species of streptococcus forms a water-insoluble levan polymer by-product from sucrose fermentation. The mucinous levan allows the streptococcus to adhere to dental enamel, and the water-insoluble character of the polymer allows acid products of the metabolizing bacterial cell to accumulate and reach high concentrations within the polymer. The accumulated acid then acts on the dental enamel and produces caries.

The fourth class included in Table 13-1 are the microaerophilic and anaerobic strains of streptococci (peptostreptococci). As yet there is no prototype species, but several distinctive species are in the process of being characterized. These strains are important etiologic agents of brain abscess and pulmonary abscess and also frequently cause gynecologic infections in association with pregnancy and childbirth or following gynecologic surgery (see Chap. 39).

Group A Streptococcal Constituents and Products

Of the multiplicity of cellular and soluble extracellular synthetic end products elaborated by Group A streptococci, relatively few are of special importance from a biomedical standpoint. Those of importance are listed in Table 13–2.

TABLE 13–2. Major Constituents and Products of Group A
Streptococci of Biomedical Importance

Constituent or Product	Biomedical Importance
Capsule and Cell Wall	
Hyaluronic acid capsule	Responsible for mucoid colonies Antiphagocytic
M protein and fimbriae	Basis for serotyping Antiphagocytic Responsible for type-specific immunity Responsible for matt colonies Implicated in adherence to host epithelial cells
Group A carbohydrate (structurally linked to peptidoglycan)	Antigenic component for Lancefield grouping Cross-reactive with heart valve glycoprotein Induces uniquely persistent elevated antibody titer in patients with rheumatic heart disease
Peptidoglycan (mucopeptide; linked to Group A carbohydrate)	Responsible for bacterial form and cell wall rigidity Site of new wall synthesis (and locus of penicillin antibacterial action) Cytotoxicity for mammalian cells in vivo and in vitro
Extracellular Products	
Streptolysin O (SLO)	Causes beta hemolysis associated with subsurface colonies Anti-SLO antibody titers helpful in retrospective diagnosis (not antigenically unique for Group A streptococci)
Streptolysin S (SLS)	Causes beta hemolysis surrounding surface colonies Nonantigenic
Hyaluronidase	Antibody titers especially useful in diagnosis of streptococcal cutaneous infection May facilitate spread of streptococcal cells in host tissues
Streptokinase	Fibrinolytic activity has potential therapeutic use Basis for serosanguineous nature of exudates associated with streptococcal infections
Streptodornase (DNAse B)	Solubilizes (depolymerizes) DNA in exudates Antibody titers helpful in diagnosis
NADase	Late rise and slow decline of antibody especially helpful in diagnosis of chorea

The hyaluronic acid enveloping streptococcal microorganisms interferes with their ingestion by host phagocytic cells. Because the hyaluronic acid is identical in chemical composition to that constituting human connective tissues, it is treated as "self" and does not induce an immune response. In contrast to the situation found in other encapsulated gram positive coccal bacteria, e.g., *Streptococcus pneumoniae,* the outermost surface of Group A streptococci, therefore, cannot be coated with specific antibodies, i.e., opsonins. Phagocytosis of these microorganisms cannot be materially enhanced.

The M protein beneath the enveloping hyaluronic acid capsule and penetrating it by means of fingerlike projections is a critical antigenic constituent and virulence factor. Evidence from some quarters suggests that the M protein may be a basis for the bacterial cell adhering to specific receptor sites on host oropharyngeal epithelial cells (see Chap. 2). This postulated mechanism of adherence could be the initial step whereby Group A streptococci implant upon and colonize the oropharynx. Support for this theory is provided by the lack of ability of streptococcal cells to adhere to epithelial cells when previously exposed to specific anti-M secretory IgA from parotid gland secretions.

M protein is antigenic and represents the basis for subdividing the Group A streptococci into different serotypes. As already stated, the M protein is responsible for type-specific immunity to streptococcal infection, e.g., resistance to type 4 streptococci but susceptibility to type 12. Antibody specifically reactive with M protein might exert its protective effect by combining with antigenic determinants on fimbriae protruding into or through the hyaluronic acid capsule, thereby preventing adherence of the streptococci to epithelial cells. The most likely source for such antibody might well be the oropharyngeal secretions, i.e., secretory IgA antibody.

It would be of interest to determine how well secretory IgA antibody levels in saliva against a given M protein streptococcal serotype correlate with resistance to colonization by that same serotype. Such data may prove to be of practical importance in deciding how to best immunize individuals so that they produce maximum titers of salivary IgA reactive with those M protein serotypes represented in the vaccine.

The specific carbohydrate is the major antigenic constituent of the Group A streptococcus, accounting for almost 10 per cent of its dry weight. It is a relatively simple polysaccharide with a molecular weight of approximately 10,000 and consisting of two monosaccharides, *N*-acetylglucosamine and rhamnose. As already mentioned, this carbohydrate, together with the peptidoglycan, constitutes an important cell wall macromolecule (see Fig. 13–1). It is the synthesis of this macromolecular complex which is inhibited by penicillin and which leads to dissolution of the structurally rigid bacterial cell wall. The *N*-acetylglucosamine moiety of the complex has been implicated in the pathogenesis of rheumatic fever and carditis through two observations, viz., cross-reactivity with mammalian heart valve glycoprotein and inordinately high and persistent Group A carbohydrate antibody titers found in a large percentage of individuals with rheumatic heart disease (see Chap. 15). The mucopeptide moiety has inherent cytotoxicity for a variety of mammalian cells and membranes and also has been implicated in rheumatic inflammation (see Chap. 15).

Of the six extracellular products listed in Table 13–2, three are of great importance in the diagnosis of recent streptococcal infection. One of these,

DNAse B, together with streptokinase, also has found limited use as a debridement-solubilizing enzyme in several types of clinical settings, e.g., liquefaction of pleural exudates, cleaning of stasis ulcers, etc. Since both products are antigenic and induce antibodies, they cannot be employed for long in a given patient before febrile reactions and other evidence of antigen-antibody reactions contraindicate further use of them.

Streptolysin O, the oxygen-labile hemolysin responsible for beta hemolysis around subsurface colonies of streptococci, is widely used as an antigen in detecting rising titers of its corresponding antibody, the anti–streptolysin O (ASO) test. As is discussed elsewhere (see Chap. 14), antibodies are not induced by streptolysin O following cutaneous infections due to Group A streptococci, and the anti–streptolysin O test usually cannot be used for diagnostic purposes in patients with pyoderma.

Hyaluronidase is antigenic and immunologically specific for Group A streptococci. While *Staphylococcus aureus* produces a hyaluronidase with the same enzymatic properties, it does not cross-react with antibody raised in response to Group A streptococcal hyaluronidase and vice versa. Detection of rising hyaluronidase antibody titers is diagnostically useful in patients with pyoderma and also in the 15 to 20 per cent of patients with acute streptococcal pharyngitis-tonsillitis who do not elaborate anti–streptolysin O antibodies (see Chaps. 14 to 16 and 36).

While only a few laboratories are equipped to measure immune responses to NADase, this antibody has a very unique place in the diagnosis of rheumatic diseases. As discussed elsewhere (see Chap. 15), the diagnosis of rheumatic fever often hinges on demonstrating a rising, a very high, or, rarely, a falling titer of antibody reactive with one or more Group A streptococcal antigens. Antibody responses to most of these antigens, e.g., streptolysin O or hyaluronidase, usually reach their peak and have fallen back toward the normal range within a period of three to six months. Chorea, a rheumatic inflammatory process involving the central nervous system, in contrast to the other manifestations of acute rheumatic fever, frequently does not appear until several months after an attack of streptococcal infection. Immune responses to NADase are very late in appearing. They may not reach maximum titers until three to six months after streptococcal infection. Demonstration of a rising NADase antibody titer may be the only means of documenting antecedent Group A streptococcal infection that occurred several months previously and providing support for the diagnosis of chorea.

Isolation and Identification of Group A Streptococci

Blood Agar Streak Plates

Practical Aspects

Irrespective of what type of clinical specimen is cultured (other than blood), streaking of a properly prepared blood agar plate is essential for recognition of most streptococci. In the differential diagnosis of sore throat (see Chaps. 12 and 14), the most common clinical setting where Group A streptococci are looked for specifically, a blood agar plate is the only type of culture medium routinely employed.

There are a few technical points to be emphasized in preparation and use of blood agar plates. Blood agar must be made using sheep blood as a source of the erythrocytes. The proportion of blood to agar must be correct so that the erythrocytic substrate does not exceed the lytic activity of hemolysins diffusing into the medium by growing streptococci. The plates must be poured to a critical depth, thin enough to permit complete clearing should beta hemolysis occur and yet thick enough to permit "stabbing" of the agar with the streaking device to ensure subsurface growth of bacterial cells. Some strains of Group A streptococci elaborate streptolysin O but do not produce streptolysin S. Beta hemolysis by such strains will be recognized only around submerged colonies growing in the depths of the agar where oxygen-labile streptolysin O can exert lytic activity.

To save money or for other reasons, some clinical microbiology laboratories still employ outdated human blood from the hospital blood bank for preparation of blood agar. Human blood is an unacceptable source of erythrocytes for preparing blood agar. Beta hemolysis produced by Group A streptococci almost always is more complete and extensive on sheep blood as compared to human blood agar. Differentiation between beta- and alpha-hemolytic reactions, therefore, can be made with greater ease using sheep blood agar. Colonies of *Haemophilus hemolyticus,* a frequent component of the microbial flora of the oropharynx, especially in children, can produce beta hemolysis simulating or identical to that of Group A streptococci when it is grown on human blood agar. This gram negative coccobacillus does not produce beta hemolysis on sheep blood agar. Finally, sodium citrate is used as an anticoagulant by many hospital blood banks for collecting human blood from donors. The citrate ion can interfere with growth of Group A streptococci or the action of their hemolysins responsible for beta-hemolytic reactions on blood agar.

Incubation of Streaked Blood Agar Plates and Their Inspection

Blood agar plates carefully streaked to facilitate growth of isolated colonies on the surface of the agar and within its depths are incubated at 35°C for 12 to 18 hours. An environmental atmosphere of carbon dioxide accelerates growth and potentiates hemolytic reactions of most Group A strains, as well as other subclasses of streptococci and alpha-hemolytic streptococci. If a carbon dioxide incubator is not available, streak plates can be placed in a plastic bag which is then gassed with a filtered source of 5 per cent carbon dioxide in air, sealed, and placed in a conventional incubator. Alternatively, one can use a closed container such as an anaerobic jar with an atmosphere of 10 to 15 per cent carbon dioxide which is held at 35°C.

Inspection of the incubated plate by transmitted and reflected light is made with an eye for any evidence of beta hemolysis. Obvious beta hemolysis which is limited to areas of confluent growth on the plate usually means poor streaking. Growth from such areas must be restreaked onto a fresh blood agar plate in order to obtain isolated colonies. This causes a delay of almost 24 hours in the processing of the specimen.

Beta hemolysis around isolated colonies most often is confused with that produced by hemolytic staphylococci (see Chap. 37). These microorganisms can usually be differentiated by colony characteristics. Blood agar plates inoculated with throat swabs may reveal beta-hemolytic colonies which closely resemble Group A streptococci but are actually Group C or Group G streptococci (rarely Group D). This finding is not uncommon in material on swabs of the oropharyngeal flora of children. Close attention to colonial morphologic findings with respect to the average size of individual colonies and whether or not they have a distinct mucoid character is helpful in preliminary assessment of a beta-hemolytic colony. Occasionally, a typical dull *matt* colony indicative of Group A streptococci meets the experienced eye; such strains produce liberal amounts of M protein. Such strains are most apt to be seen in association with outbreaks of streptococcal infection within closed populations, i.e., military barracks, boarding schools, etc., because rapid serial passage of Group A streptococci in man as well as mice promotes synthesis of M protein. At some point, the one or two isolated colonies which are to be subjected to more detailed study usually are smeared and Gram stained to confirm that they consist of typical gram positive bacterial cocci.

Identification

There are several ways of determining whether a given beta-hemolytic colony on a blood agar plate is a Group A streptococcus. Each method has advantages and disadvantages; none are perfect. It is to be emphasized that the most accurate method is the Lancefield grouping technique. Availability and cost of requisite monospecific grouping sera, as well as time and expense in growing streptococcal populations of sufficient density to yield adequate amounts of group-specific carbohydrate when the microorganisms are extracted with a suitable reagent, restrict the routine use of Lancefield grouping in most laboratories. In any doubtful situation in which a given isolate must be definitively identified, the Lancefield method is the highest court of appeal. Presented below are the two most common methods which are used in a large number of different clinical microbiologic facilities.

Bacitracin Susceptibility

Growth of the majority of strains of Group A streptococci is inhibited by 0.02 unit of bacitracin, whereas that of other commonly encountered subclasses, i.e., Groups B, C, D, and G, is not. This property of Group A streptococci is the basis for their identification in most hospital microbiology laboratories.

A representative isolated hemolytic colony is taken from the blood agar plate and restreaked on fresh blood agar upon which is pressed a disc impregnated with 0.02 unit of bacitracin. From this point, the procedure is essentially as described elsewhere for conventional antibiotic susceptibility testing using the disc method (see Chap. 45). Two points in addition to those pertaining to disc susceptibility testing in general must be emphasized. First, the amount of antimicrobial agent in the bacitracin disc used for identification of Group A streptococci, i.e., the "A disc," is much less than that in discs routinely used for bacitracin susceptibility testing, i.e., 0.02 unit as opposed to 10.0 units for susceptibility tests. Using the wrong type of bacitracin disc could, therefore, result in a false positive reaction. Second, potency of A discs decreases with prolonged storage, even at refrigeration temperatures. Old A discs may not inhibit growth of classic Group A streptococci shown to be readily inhibited by fresh A discs.

Overall reproducibility of the bacitracin disc method of grouping streptococci is reasonably good. Close to 90 per cent of Group A streptococcal strains are inhibited; only 3 to 5 per cent of non–Group A strains are inhibited.

Immunofluorescence Microscopy

This method has been used most widely by municipal or state Public Health laboratories that handle large numbers of throat swabs mailed in by physicians in outlying areas. In this situation, time is of the essence in reporting the presence of Group A streptococci. A high proportion of Group A streptococcal cells have been shown to remain viable for up to 72 hours or even longer on Dacron fiber-tipped swabs mailed in moisture-impervious envelopes with added desiccant to retard drying of the swab. Upon receipt, the swabs are inoculated into broth which is then incubated at 37°C for four to six hours. The culture is then smeared on a slide and appropriately fixed and stained with a monospecific Group A carbohydrate antibody conjugated to fluorescein isothiocyanate. When viewed with a fluorescence microscope with suitable light source, exciter, and barrier filters, only Group A streptococci will be observed to fluoresce intensely.

The disadvantage of the immunofluorescence method, in addition to cost, is that it precludes the opportunity of examining a throat swab blood agar streak plate and gaining an idea of not only the general composition of the oropharyngeal flora but also the relative number of Group A streptococci on the original throat swab. The number of these bacteria as reflected by beta-hemolytic colonies on the streak plate can be a help in distinguishing between colonization of the oropharynx by Group A streptococci as opposed to clinically manifest streptococcal disease, i.e., tonsillitis-pharyngitis (see Chaps. 12 and 14).

References

Book

Wannamaker, L. W., and Matsen, J. M. (eds.): Streptococci and Streptococcal Diseases. Recognition, Understanding, and Management. New York, Academic Press, 1972.

Review Article

McCarty, M.: The streptococcal cell wall. Harvey Lect. *65:*73, 1971.

Original Articles

Ayoub, E. M., and Wannamaker, L. W.: Identification of group A streptococci. Evaluation of the use of the fluorescent antibody technique. J.A.M.A. *187:*908, 1964.

Braunstein, H., Tucker, E., and Gibson, B. C.: Infections caused by unusual beta hemolytic streptococci. Am. J. Pathol. *55:*424, 1971.

Eickhoff, T. C., Klein, J. O., Daly, A. L., Ingall, D., and Finland, M.: Neonatal sepsis and other infections due to group B beta-hemolytic streptococci. N. Engl. J. Med. *271:*1221, 1964.

Ellen, R. P., and Gibbons, R. J.: Parameters affecting the adherence and tissue tropisms of *Streptococcus pyogenes.* Infect. Immun. *9:*85, 1974.

Finegold, S. M., Smolens, B., Cohen, A. A., Hewitt, W. L., Miller, A. B., and Davis, A.: Necrotizing pneumonitis and empyema due to microaerophilic streptococci. N. Engl. J. Med. *273:*462, 1965.

Horn, K. A., Meyer, W. T., Wyrick, B. C., and Zimmerman, R. A.: Group B streptococcal neonatal infection. J.A.M.A. *230:*1165, 1974.

Kaplan, E. L., Ferrieri, P., and Wannamaker, L. W.: Comparison of the antibody response to streptococcal cellular and extracellular antigens in acute pharyngitis. J. Pediatr. *84:*21, 1974.

Maxted, W. R.: The use of bacitracin for identifying group A haemolytic streptococci. J. Clin. Pathol. *6:*224, 1953.

Mead, P. B., Ribble, J. C., and Dillon, T. F.: Group A streptococcal puerperal infection: Report of an epidemic. Obstet. Gynecol. *32:*460, 1968.

Pien, F. D., Thompson, R. L., and Martin, W. J.: Clinical and bacteriologic studies of anaerobic gram-positive cocci. Mayo Clin. Proc. *47:*251, 1972.

Stollerman, G. H.: The role of the selective throat culture for beta hemolytic streptococci in the diagnosis of acute pharyngitis. Am. J. Clin. Pathol. *37:*36, 1962.

Chapter 14

STREPTOCOCCAL PHARYNGITIS-TONSILLITIS

Introduction

Common Misconceptions

Group A beta-hemolytic streptococci are the most important cause of acute exudative pharyngitis-tonsillitis. There is only limited evidence that other streptococcal groups, e.g., B, C, and G, cause clinically manifest disease of the oropharynx. This is important to keep in mind, since these streptococcal groups not uncommonly are found in throat cultures of patients, especially children, with nonbacterial (viral) pharyngitis. Because each of these streptococcal groups may produce beta hemolysis on blood agar streak plates, they may be mistaken for Group A streptococci and therefore be the basis for initiating antimicrobial therapy when none is indicated. Virtually none of the other members of the normal microbial flora of the oropharynx have any capacity to induce clinically significant infections of the oropharynx. This means that a throat culture obtained from a patient with severe pharyngitis and which yields a very heavy growth of *Staphylococcus aureus* in no way indicates that the staphylococcus is responsible for the patient's illness. Although *Streptococcus pneumoniae* (pneumococcus) may be isolated in large numbers from patients with symptoms and objective evidence of pharyngitis, the bulk of evidence argues against these microorganisms having an etiologic role. Such pneumococci more often than not are nontypable or are shown to be one of the higher numbered serotypes and therefore are considered to be relatively nonpathogenic (see Chap. 20). *Haemophilus influenzae*, when isolated in appreciable numbers, may cause confusion, especially if the patient is a young child. However, just as for the pneumococcus, these isolates usually are nontypable or of a type distinct from *H. influenzae*, type b, and thus are viewed as having little or no capacity to produce disease (see Chap. 21).

Both physicians and patients have misconceptions concerning the diagnosis of streptococcal pharyngitis and its treatment. It is still not appreciated that streptococcal pharyngitis-tonsillitis *cannot* be diagnosed on the basis of clinical symptoms, physical signs, or routine laboratory tests such as total white blood cell count and differential. The key role of the throat culture for accurate recognition of streptococcal disease of the oropharynx cannot be overemphasized. The critical need for prompt recognition of Group A streptococci by means of a throat culture and the eradication of these microorganisms by appropriate antimicrobial therapy must be continually stressed by physicians in an attempt to prevent rheumatic fever and rheumatic heart disease.

Most patients and a fair proportion of physicians do not realize that even the most effective antimicrobial therapy directed against streptococcal pharyngitis-tonsillitis does not materially alter the natural course of the disease. Thus, it is *not* for symptomatic improvement but for prevention of rheumatic inflammation and suppurative complications that antimicrobial therapy is prescribed.

Spectrum of Clinical Disease

Rheumatic fever is a unique consequence of and a marker for recent, antecedent Group A streptococcal pharyngitis-tonsillitis (see Chap. 15). One can readily determine the spectrum of clinical manifestations characterizing streptococcal oropharyngeal infections through detailed health inventories of individual patients during the five- to six-week period preceding their attack of rheumatic fever. What emerges is a very variable clinical pattern. At one end of the spectrum are some patients who develop very severe, debilitating illness. At the other end of the spectrum is a larger proportion of patients who exhibit extremely mild or trivial clinical symptoms of infection or no symptoms at all. Thus, a major problem in detection of Group A streptococcal pharyngitis is education of patients so that they report promptly for a throat culture, regardless of the severity of their respiratory tract infection. This is particularly true for those persons already identified as being susceptible to rheumatic fever by virtue of their having had one or more attacks of the disease at some time in the past.

Three different studies bearing on these points are presented in Table 14–1. As many as one third of patients had no manifestations of illness whatsoever preceding their rheumatic illness. The precipitating streptococcal infection in these patients was subclinical in character; they had no reason to consult a physician. From one third to one half of the patients had upper respiratory tract symptoms or other evident illness which might have prompted physician consultation; however, for various reasons these patients did not see a physician. Finally, and of greater importance, rheumatic fever developed in one third to more than one half of the patients despite the fact that they saw a physician for antecedent upper respiratory tract disease or other complaints. In a high proportion of these patients (1) streptococcal infection was not considered or throat culturing was not done, (2) a correct diagnosis was made but incorrect antimicrobial therapy was prescribed, or

(3) everything was done correctly by the physician but the patient did not follow instructions and complete the prescribed course of antimicrobial therapy.

TABLE 14–1. Clinical Patterns of Antecedent Streptococcal Infections and Patient-Physician Factors in Occurrence of Initial Attacks of Rheumatic Fever*

| | | Did Not See MD (per cent) | | Saw MD (per cent) |
| | Number of | No | URT** or | URT or |
Study	Patients	symptoms	other symptoms	other symptoms
A	105	15.2	50.5	34.3
B	109	11.0	31.2	57.8
C	261	34.0	32.0	34.0

*Combined data from the following reports (see References): *Study A,* Czoniczer, Lees, and Massell, 1961; *Study B,* Grossman and Stamler, 1963; *Study C,* Gordis, Lilienfeld, and Rodriguez, 1969.
**Upper respiratory tract.

It is obvious from the data given in Table 14–1 that a sizable proportion of attacks of rheumatic fever could be prevented if patients could be better educated about seeking physician consultation, even for trivial respiratory tract complaints. It is also obvious that physicians need to adopt a more incisive and aggressive approach to management of respiratory disease, including careful instruction of patients about completing a full course of antimicrobial therapy prescribed for eradication of demonstrable Group A streptococci in the oropharynx.

Diagnosis

Clinical Features

Specific complaints and physical findings consistent with streptococcal pharyngitis-tonsillitis include an abrupt onset with nausea and vomiting (especially in children), a temperature above 102.5°F, and a very red, edematous, posterior pharynx, soft palate, and/or tonsils or tonsillar areas. Small, pinpoint, focal or confluent areas of yellow to gray exudate are often present over the tonsils in the early phases of the disease. There may be exquisite tenderness at the angle of the jaw due to acute submandibular cervical adenitis. Leukocytosis and an increase of circulating immature neutrophils may occur. Clinically, the important point is that any one or all of these features may be observed with any nonbacterial (viral) acute pharyngitis.

Several studies of the reliability of clinical diagnosis have shown that experienced physicians examining patients with a complaint of "sore throat" have only about a 50 per cent chance of correctly identifying those patients with Group A streptococcal disease as determined by the results of throat cultures and/or antibody assays. Physicians do somewhat better in identifying patients whom they believe do not have streptococcal infection as the basis for "sore throat," a correct diagnosis being made in about 70 per cent of such patients.

Throat Culture

A carefully collected throat swab which is properly streaked on a suitable blood agar plate constitutes the definitive method for recognition of streptococcal pharyngitis-tonsillitis. This is a sensitive, inexpensive, and relatively rapid diagnostic procedure. The throat culture has its greatest value in excluding streptococcal infection as a diagnostic possiblity. Within 24 hours it will enable a physician to identify the 90 to 95 per cent of adult patients who present with "sore throat" of nonstreptococcal etiology and who need no antimicrobial therapy (see Chaps. 12 and 13). Such patients will be recognized within 24 hours by the absence of colonies of bacteria in their throat swab blood agar streak plates giving a beta-hemolytic reaction.

If beta-hemolytic colonies are present, a representative colony should then be streaked onto a new blood agar plate and its susceptibility to bacitracin determined. This is a reliable screening method for identifying whether the hemolytic bacterial colony is a Group A streptococcus. Approximately 85 to 95 per cent of Group A streptococci are inhibited by the amount of bacitracin (0.02 to 0.04 units) incorporated into the standard "A" bacitracin disc manufactured for use in this fashion. Unfortunately, approximately 5 to 10 per cent of non-Group A streptococci are also susceptible to bacitracin. While the bacitracin disc method for identifying Group A streptococci does not have the precision of definitive Lancefield grouping by the precipitin method (see Chap. 13), it is a sufficiently reliable procedure to use for identifying Group A streptococci under most clinical microbiology laboratory circumstances.

The question frequently arises as to how one should interpret a very small number of beta-hemolytic colonies on a throat culture plate. What is the significance of only three or four discrete hemolytic Group A streptococcal colonies? Does this mean that the patient is merely a streptococcal carrier? Does it mean he should be treated for streptococcal disease? In many cases, the issue as to whether the patient is infected to a significant degree can be resolved only retrospectively by demonstrating a significant rise in antibodies that are reactive with one or more streptococcal antigenic constituents. However, retrospective information is useless in deciding how to manage this type of patient. The usual situation that causes confusion is the presence of only a few hemolytic colonies in the throat culture of a patient who quite clearly has a sore throat. It is the policy of most physicians to consider any Group A streptococci in the oropharynx as abnormal and to give the patient harboring such small numbers of streptococci eradicative antimicrobial therapy. This is especially true if the patient in question is known to have had rheumatic fever in the past.

Serologic Tests

There are a number of highly refined serologic tests available for detecting antibodies induced by Group A streptococcal infection (see Chap. 13). Indeed, in virtually no other infectious disease are as many definitive immunologic assays on hand for retrospectively documenting recent infection. In other words, if one wishes to employ several of these different assays for antibody production, it is possible to make a retrospective diagnosis of antecedent streptococcal infection in almost 99 per cent of patients.

The three procedures most widely employed in clinical laboratories for the serologic diagnosis of streptococcal infection are those which measure levels of antibody against streptolysin O, streptococcal hyaluronidase, and streptococcal DNAse B. The latter nuclease is antigenically specific for Group A streptococci. Using the anti-streptolysin O assay (ASO test), antibodies can be demonstrated in approximately 85 per cent of individuals within two to four weeks following an antecedent streptococcal infection. Using both the anti-streptolysin O and the anti-streptococcal hyaluronidase assays, antibody production can be demonstrated in approximately 95 per cent of patients. By including the anti-streptococcal DNAse B assay, a diagnostic rise in streptococcal antibody can be detected in nearly 100 per cent of patients.

Because of the retrospective nature of the antibody assays, detection of streptococcal immune responses are primarily useful in providing essential support for the diagnosis of acute rheumatic fever or in epidemiologic surveys. Indeed, the development of rheumatic fever is so closely linked to streptococcal infection that one important prerequisite for making the diagnosis is demonstration, by serologic means, of recent infection due to Group A streptococci (see Chap. 15).

Therapy

Rationale Underlying Treatment

There are two reasons for treating patients carrying Group A streptococci in their oropharynx or in whom the diagnosis of streptococcal pharyngitis-tonsillitis has been established. First and foremost is the desire to prevent an attack of rheumatic fever in patients known to have had rheumatic fever in the past. Recurrence of rheumatic fever is especially common among the latter group of patients. As many as 25 to 50 per cent of Group A streptococcal infections of the oropharynx in such individuals result in a recurrence of the disease (see Chap. 15). Second, eradicative therapy will prevent or decrease the likelihood of occurrence of suppurative complications, e.g., otitis media, mastoiditis, or peritonsillar abscess.

The administration of appropriate antimicrobial therapy does not significantly alter the clinical course of streptococcal pharyngitis-tonsillitis. Judging by such subjective criteria as pain or difficulty in swallowing, or such objective criteria as daily body temperature recordings and size of cervical lymph nodes, patients receiving penicillin in appropriate doses do not recover faster than nontreated control subjects. The practical extension of this observation which deserves reemphasis here is that the decision to institute antimicrobial therapy should in no way be based on a physician wanting to "make his patient feel better."

Since antimicrobial agents do not influence the clinical course of streptococcal disease, one must assume that host immunologic responses to the infecting streptococci play a major role in the development of the disease. Delayed-type hypersensitivity to streptococcal products appears to be especially important. In children less than two years of age, there may be very little or no fever and the throat may appear only slightly inflamed, or "injected," demonstrating no evidence of exudation. Despite these very mild manifestations, throat swabs may yield almost a pure culture of Group A streptococci. Data concerning the age-dependent incidence of delayed-type hypersensitivity to one important streptococcal antigen, viz., M protein, have been secured by Dr. Eugene Fox and his associates in connection with their work on streptococcal vaccines (see Chap. 15). Based on as yet unpublished data, acquisition of positive cutaneous reactions to purified M protein (1.0 μg test dose of type 12 material) is directly related to age as a consequence of increasing exposure to and infection by Group A streptococci. The findings are as follows: positive reactions occurred in only 10 per cent of children less than two years of age; one third of children three to six years of age gave positive reactions. More than one half of the reactions were positive by 7 to 10 years of age; two thirds were positive by 11 to 14 years, and positive reactions were recorded in three fourths of subjects aged 15 or older. Published data reveal that 75 per cent of 420 adults exhibited positive delayed-type cutaneous reactivity to type 12 M protein. A similar pattern of age-dependent cutaneous reactivity has been observed by other workers using other streptococcal antigens, e.g., Varidase, which is a commercial product containing streptodornase and streptokinase. In all likelihood, the miniature inflammatory response represented by the positive delayed-type skin reaction at the site of injected streptococcal antigen probably occurs on a larger scale in the oropharyngeal tissues of an individual with streptococcal pharyngitis-tonsillitis. Interaction of sensitized lymphocytes with M protein and other antigenic constituents elaborated and released by invading Group A strepto-cocci sets off a cascade of inflammatory events leading to erythema, edema, and cellular infiltration. It is this postulated sequence of events that many physicians believe accounts for the characteristic clinical picture of acute streptococcal oropharyngeal infections.

Eradicative Therapy

Penicillin. Definitive antimicrobial therapy for streptococcal pharyngitis-tonsillitis can be accomplished with several drugs. Penicillin is used most often. Benzathine penicillin, a long-acting form of the drug providing detectable levels of penicillin in the blood for about three weeks, is injected intramuscularly. It is the most effective therapy for streptococcal pharyngitis-tonsillitis, since it delivers an eradicative dose of penicillin with one injection and bypasses the uncertainty associated with oral penicillin and the problems of the patient's compliance. A single injection can be expected to eliminate streptococci from the oropharynx of 90 per cent of patients in a matter of 10 days.

The use of oral penicillin preparations is also effective but many patients do not complete the 10 days of penicillin therapy, which is mandatory for maximum eradication of the microorganisms.

Alternative Drugs. Alternative drugs to consider in patients allergic to penicillin include erythromycin and perhaps clindamycin. Many physicians prescribe tetracyclines. This practice must be condemned, since nearly 50 per cent of Group A streptococcal strains are highly resistant to this class of antimicrobial agent. In no way can tetracycline be considered a suitable drug for the treatment of streptococcal infection.

Another area of confusion concerns the use of sulfonamide derivatives. They *are* effective in preventing streptococci from colonizing the oropharynx and thereby *are* effective in prevention of rheumatic fever (see Chap. 15). They are *not* capable of eradicating streptococci already present in the oropharynx in numbers leading to clinical illness and *have no place* in the treatment of streptococcal pharyngitis-tonsillitis.

CASE PRESENTATION 1

A 23-year-old sixth grade school teacher saw her physician in early March because of a persistent sore throat and low-grade fever of approximately three days' duration. When her symptoms first began she had taken an oral tetracycline preparation which a neighbor had given to her. Physical examination revealed several discrete white to yellow-gray patches of exudate over both tonsillar areas. Marked point tenderness at the angle of the right jaw coincided with palpably enlarged submandibular cervical lymph nodes.

After a throat culture was obtained, the patient was given a prescription for an oral penicillin preparation, viz., phenoxymethyl penicillin. She was told that if she had streptococci in her throat culture she would be so notified and should then get the prescription filled and start penicillin therapy. Forty hours after this visit, the patient was contacted by telephone and told that a heavy growth of Group A hemolytic streptococcus was identified on the throat swab streak plate. Although the patient reported that her fever had subsided and that her sore throat was improved, she was strongly urged to take a full 10-day course of penicillin, at the end of which time she should report for a follow-up throat culture. The patient followed these instructions to the letter; her follow-up throat culture, taken 10 days after starting therapy, failed to reveal hemolytic streptococci.

There are several points about this case worth emphasizing. First, the patient is a school teacher and thus almost constantly exposed to young children of an age, i.e., 5 to 14 years, most prone to harbor Group A streptococci in their respiratory tract. Second, the time of year when the illness developed, viz., springtime, coincides with the peak occurrence of streptococcal oropharyngeal carriage and infection among susceptible children. Third, close questioning is often necessary to elicit a history of self-medication. In some instances, this may be a very important fact; e.g., it may help explain delay in isolation of a microorganism from culture material. Note that the neighbor had some of her oral tetracycline preparation "left over," thereby reinforcing the fact that a high percentage of patients do not consume all of an oral medication for the full period for which it was prescribed. While the physician who examined this patient found that there were clinical manifestations consistent with streptococcal disease of the oropharynx, certainly the exudative process was minimal and the pharynx was not classically "beefy red" as it is supposed to be. Perhaps the only hallmark of streptococcal pharyngitis-tonsillitis in this patient was the marked tenderness over the enlarged cervical lymph nodes beneath the right jaw. The way this physician handled this patient's problem is ideal. A throat culture was taken and the patient given a prescription to fill if the throat culture revealed streptococci. When streptococci were isolated and identified, the patient was instructed to take the eradicative 10-day course of penicillin therapy. Eradicative therapy was completed as shown by the fact that the follow-up throat culture was free of Group A streptococci.

CASE PRESENTATION 2

A 43-year-old mother, employed full time as an assembly plant worker, brought her 9-year-old daughter to a neighborhood Evening Clinic at 9 PM on April 16th. The mother had developed a "cold" during the preceding week. The cold was characterized initially by a watery nasal discharge, sneezing, and a "scratchy" throat. During the morning of April 15th, the daughter had complained of feeling chilly, vomited her breakfast, and complained of a severe sore throat and trouble in swallowing.

Physical examination of the mother revealed an oral temperature of 99°F, pulse rate of 82 per minute, and respirations 18 per minute. The nasal mucosa was noted to be slightly red and moderately edematous and covered with a yellowish mucoid secretion. The posterior pharynx was inflamed but free of exudate.

Physical examination of the daughter revealed a rectal temperature of 104°F, pulse rate of 110 per minute, and respirations 24 per minute. The child appeared acutely ill and quite toxic. The posterior pharynx, tonsils, and uvula were acutely inflamed, appearing bright red and edematous. Several discrete white to gray exudates were noted over each tonsillar area. The right tympanic membrane was dull and slightly erythematous.

Additional history elicited by a medical student who worked evenings in the Clinic revealed that there was no phone in the mother's home, she had two other younger children that were well and staying with a neighbor while she came to the Clinic, and that the mother's work schedule would not permit her and her daughter to return again for several days. The attending physician recommended that the mother and the daughter receive 1.2 million units and 600,000 units of intramuscular benzathine penicillin, respectively.

The mother, in all likelihood, was suffering from a rhinovirus infection of the upper respiratory tract, viz., a common cold. Her daughter, on the other hand, had several clinical features consistent with acute pharyngitis-tonsillitis due to Group A streptococci. Note the time of year, April, when streptococcal infections of the upper respiratory tract tend to be most prevalent. Also note that the daughter was of an age known to be highly susceptible to streptococcal infection of the oropharynx. It is also important to note that the 9-year-old daughter already had evidence of acute otitis media secondary to impaired drainage of secretions through the Eustachian tubes due to edema associated with the acutely inflamed posterior pharynx (see Chap. 12).

The attending physician correctly decided that any decision regarding antimicrobial therapy had to be made on the spot. Even if facilities for obtaining a throat culture had been available, there would have been no way to take advantage of the results of cultures if positive, e.g., by contacting the mother at a later date. The physician decided that the 9-year-old daughter most likely had acute streptococcal pharyngitis-tonsillitis, reflecting presence of a Group A hemolytic streptococcus in the family. He felt it best to give the child the most effective type of eradicative pencillin therapy, viz., benzathine penicillin. Even though he did not believe the mother was infected with Group A streptococci, he elected to treat her in a similar fashion, being aware of the uncertainty of clinical diagnosis of streptococcal disease involving the oropharynx. He also wanted to minimize the spread of the putative strain of streptococcus which the mother and/or daughter might harbor to other members of the family.

This case is a good example of one situation in which throat culturing and postponement of antimicrobial therapy are not in the best interests of patients. This one visit was the only opportunity the physician had to eradicate streptococci if they were present, and the decision quite correctly was made to do so without further delay.

CASE PRESENTATION 3

A 10-year-old boy was seen by an intern at 6 PM on July 2nd in the emergency clinic of a nearby University Medical Center because of fever of several hours' duration, headache, and sore throat. The temperature was 102.4°F orally. The posterior pharynx was intensely erythematous; the tonsils were swollen, red and partially covered with a skim milk-like exudate. The remainder of the physical examination was within normal limits. A throat culture was obtained. Aspirin, fluids, light diet, and bed rest were recommended to the parents as supportive therapy for the boy, and they were instructed to bring him back to the clinic for follow-up the next day.

On July 3rd, the patient was seen again and although he appeared to be less acutely ill, his temperature was 101.6°F and the tonsillar exudate was thicker, resembling cottage cheese in consistency. The original throat culture was reported to be free of any beta-hemolytic colonies on the blood agar streak plate. A second throat culture was taken at this time, and was subsequently found to be free of any Group A streptococci. In addition, because of the clinic director's interest in viral infections, throat and rectal swabbings for viral culture, together with an "acute phase" serum for base line serologic studies, were obtained.

The boy improved rapidly and felt clinically well by July 6th, at which time he returned to his normal activities. A "convalescent phase" serum was obtained from the patient three weeks later during a previously scheduled office visit for reimmunization of the patient with diphtheria and tetanus toxoid.

Subsequent laboratory studies revealed the following:

Viral cultures: Throat, adenovirus type 3; rectum, no virus isolated.

Serologic studies:

Antigen	Antibody Titer of Serums Collected July 3rd	July 24th
Streptolysin O	1/100	1/100
Adenovirus (group-soluble antigen)	< 1/4	1/16
Heterophil	< 1/56	< 1/56

This case is representative of the increasing tendency of patients to seek medical care for acute illnesses in emergency clinics in their geographic locality. It highlights the need for physicians who are part of the staff of such emergency clinics to be knowledgeable about the incisive approach to acute respiratory tract disease, since they are increasingly the ones initially consulted and responsible for decision making.

In many respects, the pattern of illness in this 10 year old boy could easily have been considered to be streptococcal in nature. The harried clinic staff could have simply decided to give the young patient a shot of penicillin and send him on his way. It is probable, however, that the intern who first saw the patient recognized the fact that summertime is not the time of year when Group A streptococcal respiratory tract disease is apt to be prevalent and that a virus would more likely be responsible for the illness in question. Therefore, supportive and symptomatic measures were employed, and the validity of this approach was indicated by each of two separate throat cultures failing to yield demonstrable Group A streptococci. One should note that the probably well-informed and cooperative parents did not demand that an antimicrobial agent be given and faithfully brought the patient back for follow-up visits.

Further evidence that the acute oropharyngeal infection was not streptococcal in nature was provided by the lack of any significant rise in anti–streptolysin O antibody titer (see Chap. 13). Proof that this young boy had sustained an intercurrent adenovirus infection, viz., isolation of type 3 adenovirus from the throat swab and a diagnostic, greater than four-fold rise in complement-fixing antibody to adenovirus group antigens (see Chaps. 11 and 18), was obtained through the luxury of special laboratory studies pertaining to viral infection.

It is interesting to note that the emergency clinic staff was aware of how often infectious mononucleosis can simulate streptococcal pharyngitis-tonsillitis, as evidenced by the request for a heterophil titer (see Chaps. 12 and 13).

Could this patient's illness initially have been thought to be diphtheria (see Chap. 17)? Why did the intern not request that a special culture be made for *Corynebacterium diphtheriae*? Why did he decide not to do a Schick test? Does the case abstract provide a clue or clues to these questions?

References

Book

Wannamaker, L. W., and Matsen, J. M. (eds.): Streptococci and Streptococcal Diseases. Recognition, Understanding, and Management. New York, Academic Press, 1972.

Original Articles

Breese, B. B., and Disney, F. A.: The accuracy of diagnosis of beta streptococcal infections on clinical grounds. J. Pediatr. *44:*670, 1954.

Brink, W. R., et al.: Effect of penicillin and aureomycin on natural course of streptococcal tonsillitis and pharyngitis. Am. J. Med. *10:*300, 1951.

Czoniczer, G., Lees, M., and Massell, B. F.: The need for improved recognition and treatment for the prevention of rheumatic fever. N. Engl. J. Med. *265:*951, 1961.

Denny, F. W., Wannamaker, L. W., and Hahn, E. O.: Comparative effects of penicillin, aureomycin and terramycin on streptococcal tonsillitis and pharyngitis. Pediatrics *11:*7, 1953.

Denny, F. W., Ayoub, E. M., Dillon, H. C., Jr., Disney, F. A., Kaplan, E. L., Moody, M. D., Paterson, P. Y., and Taranta, A.: Prevention of rheumatic fever (American Heart Association, Rheumatic Fever Committee). Circulation *43:*983, 1971.

Denny, F. W., Diehl, A. M., Jawetz, E., McCarty, M., Markowitz, M., Paterson, P. Y., Siegel, A. C., and Taranta, A.: House officer's knowledge of Group A streptococcal pharyngitis and its management. Am. J. Dis. Child. *124:*47, 1972.

Fox, E. N.: M proteins of Group A streptococci. Bacteriol. Rev. *38:*57, 1974.

Gordis, L., Lilienfeld, A., Rodriguez, R.: Studies in the epidemiology and preventability of rheumatic fever. III. An evaluation of the Maryland rheumatic fever registry. Publ. Health Reports *84:*333, 1969.

Grossman, B. J., and Stamler, J.: Potential preventability of first attacks of acute rheumatic fever in children. J.A.M.A. *183:*985, 1963.

Haverkorn, M. J., Valkenburg, H. A., and Goslings, W. R. O.: Streptococcal pharyngitis in the general population. I. A controlled study of streptococcal pharyngitis and its complications in the Netherlands. J. Infect. Dis. *124:*339, 1971.

James, W. E. S., Badger, G. F., and Dingle, J. H.: A study of illness in a group of Cleveland families. XIX. The epidemiology of the acquisition of Group A streptococci and of associated illnesses. N. Engl. J. Med. *262:*687, 1960.

Kuharic, H. A., Roberts, C. E., Jr., and Kirby, W. M. M.: Tetracycline resistance of Group A beta hemolytic streptococci. J.A.M.A. *174:*1779, 1960.

McCormack, R. G., Kaye, D., and Hook, E. W.: Resistance of Group A streptococci to tetracycline. N. Engl. J. Med. *267:*323, 1962.

Powers, G. F., and Boisvert, P. L.: Age as a factor in streptococcosis. J. Pediatr. *25:*481, 1944.

Siegel, A. C., Johnson, E. E., and Stollerman, G. H.: Controlled studies of streptococcal pharyngitis in a pediatric population. I. Factors related to attack rate of rheumatic fever. N. Engl. J. Med. *265:*559, 1961.

RHEUMATIC FEVER

Introduction

Rheumatic fever is an enigma. The specific event which initiates the disease is known, viz., antecedent Group A hemolytic streptococcal infection of the oropharynx. Since the medical field is armed with this fact and possesses a means of preventing recurrent streptococcal infections, rheumatic fever should be a preventable disease. However, even though we know what initiates the rheumatic process and what measures can prevent it, the specific events whereby the streptococcus causes rheumatic inflammation still remain unknown. Why must streptococci infect the upper respiratory tract passages in order to set the stage for rheumatic fever? Why must the streptococcus infect the oropharynx for at least eight days? Why is only a very small percentage of the general population susceptible to rheumatic fever? Why do the "target organs" bearing the brunt of inflammation, viz., the heart, nervous system, and joints, vary so much from one susceptible person to another?

Rheumatic fever may be defined as a nonsuppurative, poststreptococcal systemic inflammatory process primarily involving connective tissue with major clinical manifestations reflecting injury to the heart, joints, and central nervous system. The term *rheumatic fever*, although referring mainly to inflammation of the joints, i.e., the characteristic polyarthritis, also includes other organ system involvement. The terms *rheumatic carditis* and *chorea* refer specifically to involvement of the cardiovascular and nervous systems, respectively.

Rheumatic disease of the heart may involve primarily the pericardium, myocardium, or endocardium. Pericarditis and, to a lesser degree, myocarditis may be transitory processes and usually lead to no serious structural alterations. When rheumatic inflammation involves the endocardium, however, it exerts a continuing and scarring effect on this tissue, particularly the heart valves. This process leads to the characteristic changes of rheumatic heart disease.

Rheumatic inflammation of the myocardium involves the connective tissue elements rather than the myocardial fibers per se. The connective tissue injury may result in the formation of granuloma-like nodules called Aschoff bodies. The Aschoff body or nodule is traditionally considered to be the histopathologic hallmark of rheumatic carditis. While debate still goes on concerning the specificity of the Aschoff body and its morphogenesis, it is intimately intertwined with other stigmas of rheumatic heart disease and accepted as a valid signpost of rheumatic heart disease.

The most important aspect of the rheumatic process involves the endocardium, particularly where it is reflected upon itself to form the heart valves. It is the scarred and contracted malfunctioning heart valve which accounts for the clinical manifestations of rheumatic heart disease. It is the development of rheumatic valvulitis which especially marks Group A streptococcal pharyngitis-tonsillitis as a serious disease. The urgency in recognizing streptococcal infection of the oropharynx and promptly eradicating the infecting streptococcus from the upper respiratory tree is directly linked to prevention of irreversible rheumatic valvular disease.

The histopathologic as well as clinical features of rheumatic valvular inflammation are surprisingly nonspecific. The precise role of rheumatic inflammation as a cause of heart valve abnormalities, therefore, is difficult to determine. For example, atherosclerosis, especially of the aortic valve, may cause cardiodynamic changes simulating those of rheumatic aortic valve disease. There is some evidence that viruses may infect heart valves and cause malfunction similar to that resulting from rheumatic carditis. Most clinicians and pathologists agree that mitral stenosis, however, results solely from rheumatic inflammation. Any patient who has cardiodynamic evidence of mitral stenosis, with or without evidence of other valvular defects, can be considered to have rheumatic heart disease.

Interrelationships between Streptococcal Infection and Rheumatic Fever

Epidemiologic and Serologic Data

The following evidence clearly indicates that Group A streptococci are important in the etiology of rheumatic disease.

1. Close to two thirds of patients with either an initial or a recurrent attack of rheumatic fever give a history of a sore throat or some type of antecedent respiratory infection during the several weeks preceding onset of the rheumatic attack. The preceding respiratory infection may be extremely mild and be recalled by the patient only after close questioning (see Chap. 14). About one fifth of patients may still have Group A streptococci

readily demonstrable by throat culture when they consult a physician in the early phases of an attack of acute rheumatic fever.

2. Patients with acute rheumatic fever have elevated or rising titers of antibody to Group A streptococcal antigens which are indicative of relatively recent antecedent infection by this microorganism. As previously stated (see Chap. 13), a number of reliable tests for streptococcal antibodies are available which permit retrospective documentation of recent streptococcal infection in nearly 100 per cent of patients with acute rheumatic fever. Many clinicians would hold that such evidence of recent streptococcal infection is essential in making a firm diagnosis of rheumatic fever. The tests most often utilized are those which measure antibodies against streptolysin O, streptococcal hyaluronidase, and streptococcal DNAse B (see Chaps. 13 and 14).

3. Patients developing rheumatic fever respond to streptococcal infections with unusually high antibody responses compared to patients who demonstrate no propensity to develop rheumatic disease. They may be said to be "hyper-responders."

4. The peak age incidence of rheumatic disease parallels the peak age incidence of streptococcal infection. Maximum prevalence of both diseases is encountered in children between the ages of 5 and 14 years.

5. Antimicrobial therapy which eradicates the majority of colonizing streptococci from the upper respiratory tract prevents development of rheumatic fever. This point is especially important when dealing with patients known to be susceptible to the disease by virtue of having experienced an attack of the disease at some time in the past and who, on this basis, are candidates for a recurrent attack after each streptococcal infection of the oropharynx. Fortunately, there is at least a seven or eight day "grace period" between the time when the clinical manifestations of streptococcal pharyngitis-tonsillitis first appear and the time when appropriate antimicrobial therapy can be initiated and still be efficacious in prevention of rheumatic fever. It should be noted that it is not necessary to completely eradicate all of the streptococci infecting the oropharynx. Up to 10 per cent of throat cultures will still contain demonstrable streptococci in small numbers 10 days following initiation of a so-called eradicative course of penicillin therapy that is considered effective for rheumatic fever prophylaxis.

6. Long-term, continuous antimicrobial prophylaxis which prevents streptococcal infection will prevent recurrences of rheumatic fever in susceptible persons.

Antecedent Streptococcal Infection

Streptococcal infections causing acute rheumatic fever and carditis must involve the upper respiratory tract. Whether streptococcal respiratory tract infection is a prerequisite for chorea is less certain. Streptococcal infection of the skin does *not* appear to lead to rheumatic disease.

The virulence of the streptococcal strain infecting the upper respiratory tract, as expressed by the pattern of clinical disease, is an important factor in the incidence of rheumatic fever. From this it would follow that streptococcal strains causing especially severe pharyngitis-tonsillitis, i.e., high fever and marked exudation over the tonsils and severe edema-erythema of the pharynx, are more important in causing rheumatic fever than those strains associated with very mild or subclinical respiratory infections. Epidemiologic studies carried out during World War II at Warren Air Force Base in Wyoming showed that between 2 and 3 per cent of military recruits with severe exudative pharyngitis-tonsillitis could be expected to develop acute rheumatic fever. These were initial or first attacks of rheumatic disease for these men. In contrast, only 0.1 to 0.3 per cent of civilians with milder, often nonexudative, streptococcal oropharyngeal infections developed acute rheumatic fever. There is increasing evidence that specific Group A streptococcal serotypes are more virulent than others and have a greater propensity for causing exudative streptococcal pharyngitis and rheumatic inflammation. The virulence of these strains probably lies in their producing larger amounts of M protein. At least such strains are more apt to be typable and identified as a given M type than are those strains associated with mild, nonexudative streptococcal pharyngitis. These observations suggest that "rheumatogenic" serotypes of streptococci exist, analogous to "nephritogenic" serotypes of streptococci. While it is clear that a great number of different streptococcal serotypes can cause acute rheumatic fever, the majority of cases in a given locality appear to be associated with relatively few serotypes, i.e., perhaps no more than five to eight different serotypes. Such epidemiologic data are crucial in continuing efforts to develop an M protein streptococcal vaccine.

In summary, therefore, there are two types of streptococcal pharyngitis-tonsillitis with different risks of associated acute rheumatic fever. There is the classic exudative form of disease with a relatively high rate of rheumatic fever, viz., 2 to 3 per cent, especially likely to be observed in a fairly closed population living in close association with each other. This situation obtains among recent military recruits encountering virulent streptococci that are being rapidly disseminated within a military base. The same situation is found among large families crowded together in an urban setting and living under impoverished socioeconomic circumstances. In contrast, there is the less severe or nonexudative form of streptococcal pharyngitis which is far more common among "average" civilian populations and which is associated with a markedly lower risk of acute rheumatic fever.

Clinical Features

Age and Attack Rate

Rheumatic fever can occur at any age but is extremely uncommon in very young children less than two or three years of age or among individuals in the fifth decade of life or older. As already stated, peak incidence parallels that for streptococcal pharyngitis-tonsillitis, viz., 5 to 14 years of age. This age span corresponds to a time when children lacking immunity to Group A streptococcal infection are moving out of the relatively restricted home environment and, by virtue of school attendance and other associated activities, begin to intermingle with other individuals on an increasing scale. Through increasing contact with people they have a greater opportunity to become colonized by and develop infection from Group A streptococcal serotypes against which they have no protective M protein antibody (see Chap. 13).

Genetic and Environmental Factors

There is substantial evidence that chorea occurs with increased frequency among siblings as compared to unrelated individuals. More limited data suggest a relatively high degree of concordance of rheumatic fever and/or rheumatic carditis among identical twins. In all studies, however, it is difficult or impossible to dissociate the influence of gene effects from environmental determinants. For example, the socioeconomic status of young siblings and identical twins might dictate unusually close contact between familial members which, therefore, would favor person-to-person spread of streptococcal strains introduced into a family. This factor in turn would increase the frequency of recurrent streptococcal infections and enhance the likelihood of occurrence of rheumatic fever. Alternatively, serial passage of Group A streptococci within a family could be the result of basic host factors under genetic control which govern how susceptible the members of that family might be to colonization and infection by a given streptococcal serotype, e.g., the number of receptor sites on respiratory tract mucosa cells to which streptococci can bind or the capacity to elaborate and shed secretory IgA into the oropharyngeal secretions (see Chap. 13).

Latent Period

Two to four weeks usually elapse between the onset of clinically manifest streptococcal pharyngitis-tonsillitis and the initial signs of rheumatic inflammation. During the first seven to eight days of this latent period, i.e., during the first week of signs and symptoms of the streptococcal infection, appropriate antimicrobial therapy which reduces the number of streptococci within the upper respiratory tract will prevent rheumatic fever. It is important from the standpoint of pathogenesis to note that the latent period remains essentially the same for recurrent attacks of rheumatic fever in different individuals or even in the same patient. The fact that recurrent attacks of rheumatic fever are not characterized by any shortening of the latent period suggests that a "secondary" or "anamnestic" type of immune response equated with circulating antibody is not a major etiologic factor in development of the disease.

"Mimicry" of Rheumatic Fever

Most patients with rheumatic disease tend to exhibit a constellation of clinical signs which reflect inflammation of one organ system, viz., the joints, the cardiovascular system, or the central nervous system. Among persons suffering recurrent attacks of disease, the same constellation of clinical manifestations can be expected to occur as was associated with the initial attack. Patients who develop migratory polyarthritis during their first attack without any evidence of cardiac involvement show the same pattern of disease with each recurrent episode, i.e., joint inflammation unaccompanied by carditis. This propensity for the same constellation of clinical signs to be associated with recurrent attacks of the disease has been called the "mimicry" of rheumatic disease. Knowledge of the "mimicry" characteristic of rheumatic fever is important from the standpoint of prognosis in a given patient. It also must be considered in any discussion of pathogenetic mechanisms.

Mitral Stenosis

As already emphasized, this lesion is the only unique clinical and histopathologic "footprint" of the rheumatic process. Rheumatic carditis does cause mitral valve insufficiency and result in injury to and dysfunction of other heart valves, especially the aortic valve. From a diagnostic point of view, however, it is often difficult or impossible for a clinician to determine whether mitral insufficiency or other documented valvular malfunction has a rheumatic etiology. With the sole exception of mitral stenosis, virtually all other forms of rheumatic carditis, as well as all other manifestations of rheumatic inflammation involving other organ systems, can be simulated by a large number of other diseases of widely differing etiology. Furthermore, with the exception of rheumatic valvulitis, there are no permanent sequelae of rheumatic fever involving the joints, the central nervous system, or other noncardiac tissues. For all of these reasons, the physician focuses very specifically on mitral stenosis as one of the most important consequences of streptococcal respiratory tract infection.

Pathogenetic Considerations

Of several theories of pathogenesis in rheumatic fever, only two have sufficient supporting evidence to command serious attention. The first theory, which is accepted by the majority of clinicians, holds that rheumatic fever is a hypersensitivity or autoimmune disease caused by an antecedent streptococcal infection. Some of the reasons why this theory enjoys wide support are as follows: (1) the existence of a latent period between the onset of the preceding streptococcal infection and the development of rheumatic inflammation; (2) an exaggerated antibody response to streptococcal antigenic stimulation by persons developing rheumatic fever, in contrast to those who do not, and (3) cross-reactivity of the anti-streptococcal antibodies with mammalian cardiac myofibers and/or heart valves.

The second theory, which currently enjoys only minority support, holds that hypersensitivity induced by the streptococcus and which is inadvertently directed against host tissues does not play a significant role in the development of rheumatic fever per se. According to this theory, the tissue injury characterizing rheumatic inflammation results directly from cytotoxic constituents of Group A streptococci which impinge upon certain tissues of a susceptible host. As will be discussed later in this chapter, many of the features of the rheumatic process often cited in support of the disease having a hypersensitivity or autoimmune basis can be explained just as well in terms of cytotoxicity of streptococcal constituents.

Hypersensitivity or Autoimmunity

This theory is really concerned with rheumatic carditis. The main concept is that during the course of streptococcal infection, the patient makes an immune response against one or more streptococcal antigens which cross-reacts with his own heart valve or other autologous connective tissue "auto-antigens."

Concordant Evidence. Major points supporting the hypersensitivity theory, as presented in Table 15-1, can be summarized as follows:

Antigenic determinants are shared by Group A streptococci and mammalian cardiac myofibers and valve tissues. One cross-reactive system would appear to involve a constituent residing in the streptococcal cell membrane and/or cell wall and the sarcolemma membrane of heart myofibers. Another cross-reactive system consists of a streptococcal cell wall polysaccharide and a glycoprotein constituent of heart valve. This latter cross-reactive system is of special interest in the light of several studies indicating that patients who develop rheumatic heart disease but no other manifestations of rheumatic fever have very high, sustained levels of antibody against the Group A polysaccharide in streptococcal cell walls. This is the same polysaccharide which is the basis for the Lancefield grouping of streptococci.

Deposits of gamma globulin can be found in the myocardium and heart valves of patients who died of acute rheumatic carditis. It should be noted that little, if any, gamma globulin is demonstrable in association with the Aschoff body. This is true not only for Aschoff bodies in the hearts of patients that died of acute carditis but also for Aschoff bodies in atrial biopsies of patients with rheumatic heart disease who are undergoing open heart surgery. This seems odd in view of the fact that the Aschoff body is so widely accepted as the histopathologic hallmark of rheumatic heart disease.

Patients with rheumatic fever or carditis produce greater immunologic responses to streptococcal antigens during the course of their antecedent streptococcal infections than do other patients with seemingly comparable streptococcal infection but who do not develop rheumatic inflammation. One antibody elicitied by the streptococcus and reactive with heart tissue is found in especially high titer among patients developing acute rheumatic carditis. This antibody, demonstrated by direct or indirect immunofluorescence, reacts specifically with the subsarcolemma region of cardiac myofibers.

Discordant Evidence. It is just as important to highlight discordant evidence as concordant evidence in discussing any theory, and this side of the coin is also presented in Table 15-1.

As emphasized already, the streptococcus must infect the respiratory tract to cause rheumatic fever; yet circulating heart-reactive antibody also appears in patients who have streptococcal infections of the skin but who do

TABLE 15–1. Hypersensitivity-Autoimmune Pathogenetic
Theory of Rheumatic Carditis

Concordant Evidence	Discordant Evidence
Heart myofibers-valves and Group A streptococci share common antigens	Not all Group A streptococci share common antigens; heart muscle not primary site of injury
Immunoglobulin and complement deposits demonstrable in heart	Specificity of immunoglobulin not established; neither immunoglobulin nor complement in Aschoff body
Heart-reactive antibody in sera of rheumatic patients; highest titers associated with acute carditis	Antibody also associated with myocardial infarction, cardiotomy, and streptococcal skin infections

not develop rheumatic fever. In addition, patients who sustain heart injury, e.g., ischemic infarction, produce antibodies specifically reactive with myocardial fibers. For example, patients not uncommonly produce a specific heart-reactive antibody following open heart surgery. In some of these patients, pericardial inflammation and cardiac enlargement accompanied by fever and chest pain may occur, i.e., a syndrome called the post-cardiotomy syndrome. A very important finding still awaiting confirmation by other laboratories is that the cardiac myofiber antibody induced by cardiac injury, regardless of its cause, *does not* react with streptococcal cell membranes or cell walls. This antibody, in contrast to that induced by the streptococcus, is more of a true autoantibody since it seemingly is elicited by autologous heart tissue.

The immunologic specificity of the gamma globulin deposits found in patients that died of rheumatic carditis has yet to be defined. Before it can be accepted as heart-specific antibody fixed in situ to its "target antigen," additional studies are required. Can it be eluted or extracted and shown to bind specifically to sections of heart in vitro? More important, if injected into an experimental animal in reasonable amounts, will it bind to intact myocardium?

No animal model system is available which faithfully reproduces the histopathologic features of rheumatic inflammation or carditis. Repeated attempts by many investigators to produce experimental "allergic" carditis by injecting animals with heart extracts and/or streptococcal products combined with a variety of immunologic adjuvants have not been successful. This experience stands in contrast to the successful production of a large number of autoimmune or "allergic" experimental diseases of other organ systems induced at will in laboratory animals, e.g., disseminated encephalomyelitis, thyroiditis, and adrenalitis.

Cell-mediated immune responses, i.e., those responsible for delayed hypersensitivity, are believed to be of paramount importance in the pathogenesis of the experimental autoimmune diseases of animals. Presumably, such an immune response would be important in the development of rheumatic carditis in man if this disease has an autoimmune basis. There is no evidence, however, of cell-mediated or delayed hypersensitivity directed against heart antigens in patients with rheumatic carditis. In the few studies concerning this point, cultures of peripheral blood leukocytes of children or adults with acute, subacute, or inactive rheumatic carditis exhibited no evidence of in vitro lymphocyte proliferation when stimulated by heart extracts or purified myocardial fiber antigen. The peripheral blood leukocytes of such patients did exhibit lymphocyte proliferation after exposure to streptococcal cell walls, indicating that their cells had the capacity to express this in vitro correlate of cell-mediated immunity (or delayed-type hypersensitivity). By using a different in vitro correlate, viz., leukocyte migration inhibition, rheumatic fever patients, especially during the acute phases of their disease, can be shown to have a striking degree of reactivity to streptococcal cell membranes but not streptococcal cell walls.

Streptococcal Cytotoxicity

Group A streptococci produce a variety of extracellular products which exert injurious effects on mammaliam cells (see Chap. 13). Two of these products, viz., streptolysin O and streptolysin S, exert striking cytotoxicity when added to heart monolayer cultures. Certain constituents of streptococcal cell walls, e.g., the mucopeptide-polysaccharide complex, also are cytotoxic and can induce a variety of inflammatory responses when injected into experimental animals. Some of the histopathologic changes elicited in the heart by the mucopeptide-polysaccharide complex resemble the inflammatory reaction seen in rheumatic carditis.

It must be emphasized that the streptococcal cytotoxic theory becomes plausible only when the sequence of events leading to rheumatic carditis is considered in the following manner. It must be assumed that infection of the oropharynx provides a special environment essential for elaboration of relatively large amounts of "toxic" constituents by the infecting streptococci. This would explain why the streptococcus must infect the oropharynx and why the infection must span approximately 8 to 10 days before rheumatic fever occurs at a later date. Ten days would correspond to the period of time required for production, release, and dissemination of whatever amount of cytotoxic product is required to produce clinical manifestations of host tissue injury in patients with a propensity for developing rheumatic fever. Antimicrobial therapy, even when initiated as late as seven or eight days after the onset of streptococcal pharyngitis-tonsillitis, would prevent rheumatic fever by curtailing synthesis of the postulated cytotoxic products. Such products would then not accumulate in host target tissues, i.e., heart and joints, to a degree capable of causing injury recognized as rheumatic fever.

Mucopeptide-Polysaccharide Complex. Following injection of mice with this macromolecular streptococcal cell wall complex, tissue injury of the heart resembling the Aschoff nodule, as well as histopathologic changes in heart valves and synovial membranes simulating those of rheumatic inflammation, has been described. In addition, patients with rheumatic heart disease have a unique type of antibody response, viz., persistently elevated titers of antibody reactive with the Group A streptococcal cell wall polysaccharide. High-titer streptococcal polysaccharide antibody *does not* occur in patients who have rheumatic inflammation restricted to the joints or central nervous system. Thus, it seems to be uniquely associated with the development of rheumatic valvular disease. These findings are in need of additional confirmation because they represent one means for supporting a clinical diagnosis of rheumatic heart disease. They also may represent potentially important clues to the pathogenesis of rheumatic carditis.

Streptolysin O. This streptococcal hemolysin can irreversibly injure cultures of mammalian heart cells and induce inflammation of the synovium when injected in relatively large amounts into joint cavities of rabbits or other experimental animals. There is good evidence that its tissue-injuring and inflammation-provoking propensity lies in its capacity to labilize lysosomal membranes and cause release of a variety of proteolytic enzymes from lysosomal granules. Following streptococcal infection of the oropharynx, approximately 85 per cent of patients can be expected to have a demonstrable rise in titer of anti-streptolysin O antibody within approximately three to four weeks. In contrast, patients experiencing skin infections with streptococcal strains having the capacity to elaborate comparable amounts of streptolysin O produce little, if any, streptolysin O antibody (see Chap. 13). Recent studies have demonstrated that cholesterol or other sterols present in the skin can combine with streptolysin O and render this extracellular hemolysin relatively nonimmunogenic for rabbits. Conceivably, the cytotoxicity of the hemolysin might be similarly neutralized by combination with skin sterols. Should more evidence be mustered in the future to show that streptolysin O is an important factor in rheumatic fever, one might well have a rational explanation for why the disease follows streptococcal infections of the upper respiratory tract but is not observed in association with streptococcal infections of the skin. That is, streptolysin O would be "neutralized" when released by streptococci in the skin but not when shed by streptococci infecting the oropharynx.

At most, only 2 to 3 per cent of the general population has a predisposition to develop rheumatic fever. This segment of the population obviously differs in some way from the rest. Genetic factors might be important in several ways as follows.

1. Mucosal cells of the oropharynx of individuals predisposed to rheumatic fever might synthesize greater amounts of receptor material favoring specific attachment of Group A streptococci to oropharyngeal tissues (see Chap. 13). Alternatively, such individuals might have a deficiency in synthesis and/or shedding of secretory IgA within the upper respiratory tract, thereby facilitating colonization of the oropharynx by Group A streptococci and increasing the severity of streptococcal pharyngitis should it occur. In either case, the rheumatic individual would be more prone to develop streptococcal pharyngitis-tonsillitis, and infections in such individuals might well be associated with a greater output of streptococcal cytotoxic product.

2. Genetic factors might render specific target tissues of rheumatic individuals more permeable to circulating streptococcal cytotoxins or cell wall components. The individual who develops recurrent attacks of rheumatic polyarthritis may well possess synovial membranes which are more permeable to circulating cytotoxic products. Similarly, individuals who exhibit recurrent episodes of rheumatic carditis may have a permeability defect limited to the heart. In this manner, the "mimicry" of rheumatic fever would be easy to understand.

3. Genetic factors may govern the capacity of the host to elaborate enzymes which degrade streptococcal cytotoxic constituents which have been deposited in tissues. For example, the mucopeptide-polysaccharide complex does not exert cytotoxic effects until the polysaccharide moiety has been degraded sufficiently to expose toxic determinants associated with the mucopeptide moiety. Rheumatic fever patients might have an excessive capacity for degrading streptococcal Group A polysaccharides, thereby exposing mucopeptides in amounts sufficient to allow them to exert their tissue-injurious effects; or, alternatively, they may lack enzymes for degrading mucopeptide to a nontoxic state.

Treatment

The therapeutic approach to rheumatic fever consists mainly of relief of pain and other symptoms through suppression of inflammation. Since the 1930s, acetylsalicylic acid, i.e., aspirin, has proved to be a remarkably effective anti-inflammatory agent for controlling the acute manifestations of rheumatic fever, especially polyarthritis. Indeed, the capacity of aspirin to abolish pain and reduce swelling of acutely inflamed rheumatic joints in a matter of 24 hours or less serves as the basis of a therapeutic test to support the diagnosis of rheumatic fever in working through the differential diagnosis of polyarthritis.

During the 1950s, the newly discovered corticosteroids were generally believed to have anti-inflammatory activity surpassing that of aspirin and were widely used for management of rheumatic fever. A large, double-blind study finally showed that corticosteroids were no more effective than aspirin in the management of acute rheumatic polyarthritis. Furthermore, steroid therapy was associated with a higher incidence of undesirable side effects. It should be emphasized, however, that this study provided no data regarding the comparative efficacy of corticosteroids and aspirin in the treatment of other manifestations of rheumatic fever, specifically acute carditis. In patients with acute rheumatic carditis, especially in the face of developing heart failure, the anti-inflammatory action of corticosteroids is still considered advantageous by the majority of clinicians.

Prevention

Antimicrobial Agents

The Amercian Heart Association has published recommendations concerning rheumatic fever prophylaxis based on careful study and discussion of available data by members of its Committee on Prevention of Rheumatic Fever and Bacterial Endocarditis. Briefly stated, effective prevention of initial attacks of rheumatic fever, i.e., primary prevention, depends upon prompt recognition of and effective antimicrobial therapy for streptococcal infections. Therefore, rigorous use of throat cultures for *all* patients with upper respiratory tract complaints is called for. As already mentioned, however, a significant proportion of patients acquiring streptococcal pharyngitis experience either no symptoms or very trivial evidence of the disease (see Chap. 14). Such patients do not have any reason to seek medical attention, and there is no way of preventing their initial attacks of rheumatic fever.

The prevention of recurrences of rheumatic fever, i.e., secondary prevention, is more promising. Two methods have been found useful. Each method rests on two premises: (1) Group A streptococci are universally susceptible to a variety of antimicrobial agents, e.g., penicillin, and (2) if antimicrobial agents are used continuously or intermittently, they will prevent streptococcal infection and thereby prevent recurrences of rheumatic fever.

In the first method for prevention of recurrences of rheumatic fever, patients known to have already experienced an initial attack of rheumatic fever are placed on a regimen of daily penicillin administered orally once or twice a day. In patients with documented allergy to penicillin, one of the sulfonamide derivatives is employed as an alternative drug. This approach relies on low concentrations of the antimicrobial agent being excreted in the oropharyngeal secretions or reaching the superficial pharyngeal mucosa, thereby preventing colonization by Group A streptococci. Prophylaxis is maintained indefinitely or until the patient has reached an age when the risk of recurrent rheumatic fever begins to equal the risk of side reactions associated with long-term use of the ingested antimicrobial drug.

There are several limitations to this approach. A high percentage of patients find it difficult to continue daily oral prophylaxis for sustained periods of time. As the pain and fear provoked by the previous attack of rheumatic fever fades from their memory, the oral antimicrobial agent is ingested even more irregularly and finally discontinued. Compliance of patients regarding drug therapy is not merely a matter of intelligence or socioeconomic status. In a survey of college students, each of whom knew that he or she had a heart murmur signifying rheumatic heart disease, less than one fifth of the students were currently receiving any type of rheumatic fever prophylaxis despite the fact that such prophylactic measures had been strongly recommended and prescribed in the past. Another notable difficulty arises from the fact that, because sulfonamide derivatives are effective in preventing streptococcal infections, some physicians mistakenly believe they can be employed in the treatment of streptococcal pharyngitis-tonsillitis. Although sulfonamide derivatives are effective in preventing colonization of oropharyngeal tissues by streptococci, they unfortunately have very little capacity to eradicate colonies of these microorganisms already established in such tissues. Thus, they cannot be used for treatment of streptococcal disease.

The second method of antimicrobial prophylaxis assumes that streptococci may colonize oropharyngeal tissues from time to time but if eradicative antimicrobial therapy is started within a week or less following such colonization, rheumatic fever will be prevented. Patients on this prophylactic regimen receive monthly intramuscular injections of a long-acting preparation of penicillin, viz., benzathine penicillin G. Each dose is large enough to eradicate the majority of streptococcal microorganisms from the oropharynx should they be present. Significant penicillin blood levels persist for at least three weeks after each monthly injection of this form of penicillin. Thus, the streptococci have only a few days to colonize the oropharynx before the next monthly injection of penicillin is given and terminates the development of streptococcal infection before it gives rise to clinical manifestations.

There are several advantages of monthly benzathine penicillin as compared to daily oral penicillin prophylaxis. By clinical trial, it appears to be approximately 10 times more effective in preventing recurrent rheumatic fever than is either penicillin or sulfonamides by mouth. In addition, inspection of appointment records provides objective evidence as to which patients are not keeping their appointments, and special measures can be used to help them comply.

Some disadvantages of the monthly benzathine penicillin regimen also need to be mentioned. Most physicians worry about anaphylactic reactions to any drug that is administered parenterally. Anxiety concerning penicillin is especially common because it is an allergenic drug and is used on such a wide scale. Physicians prefer to prescribe oral penicillin on the premise that the risk of anaphylaxis is less. This is probably true, although it must be pointed out that in a sufficiently sensitized host one tablet of penicillin may induce an anaphylactic reaction. Some patients experience considerable pain at the site of injection of benzathine penicillin. This discomfort may cause them to break appointments, or they may want to switch over to an oral regimen. Furthermore, the necessity of coming to a physician's office for each monthly injection and then remaining for 20 or 30 minutes of observation can be a nuisance. Despite these drawbacks, the majority of patients can be convinced to accept intramuscular benzathine penicillin prophylaxis, especially if they are made aware of its greater efficacy. In view of the seriousness of recurrent rheumatic fever, particularly among patients already suffering from heart valve damage, physicians should strive to employ the most effective form of prophylaxis, viz., monthly injections of benzathine penicillin.

Patients with penicillin allergy, by necessity, cannot enjoy the benefits of benzathine penicillin prophylaxis. Since there are no data regarding rheumatic prophylaxis with antimicrobial agents other than sulfonamides, the only alternative for such patients is the oral sulfonamide regimen.

Streptococcal Vaccine

Theoretically, any one of the 50 or more antigenically distinct serotypes of Group A streptococci can cause rheumatic fever. However, epidemiologic studies indicate that a relatively small number of streptococcal serotypes, each elaborating a distinct M protein, cause a disproportionately large percentage of rheumatic attacks. These observations support the notion that "rheumatogenic" strains of Group A streptococci exist and are of special importance in rheumatic fever prophylaxis. Since immunity to Group A streptococcal infection appears to depend on immune responses against the M protein (see Chap. 13), considerable interest is directed towards developing vaccines consisting of the M proteins representing those serotypes most often implicated in causing rheumatic fever. The work has progressed slowly amid considerable technical handicaps and not a little concern over potential hazards. Methods for preparing M protein in an immunogenic form, relatively free of other biologically important streptococcal cell constituents, and in amounts large enough to use for vaccine development and production, represent major problems. Early trials of small amounts of vaccine induced low levels of M protein antibody and were associated with local or systemic hypersensitivity reactions. More progress has been made in recent years, and the results of trials with improved vaccines look encouraging.

References

Book

Markowitz, M., and Gordis, L.: Rheumatic Fever. Philadelphia, W. B. Saunders Co., 1972.

Symposium

Stetson, C. A.: The relation of antibody response to rheumatic fever. *In* McCarty, M. (ed.): Streptococcal Infections. New York, Columbia University Press, 1954.

Original Articles

Cromartie, W. J., and Craddock, J. G.: Rheumatic-like lesions in mice. Science *154:*285, 1966.

Denny, F. W., Ayoub, E. M., Dillon, H. C., Jr., Disney, F. A., Kaplan, E. L., Moody, M. D., Paterson, P. Y., and Taranta, A.: Prevention of rheumatic fever. Circulation *43:*983, 1971.

Dudding, B. A., and Ayoub, E. M.: Persistence of streptococcal group A antibody in patients with rheumatic valvular disease. J. Exp. Med. *128:*1081, 1968.

Fox, E. N., Waldman, R. H., Wittner, M. K., Mauceri, A. A., and Dorfman, A.: Protective study with a group A streptococcal M protein vaccine. Infectivity challenge of human volunteers. J. Clin. Invest. *52:*1885, 1973.

Ginsburg, I.: Mechanisms of cell and tissue injury induced by group A streptococci: Relation to poststreptococcal sequelae. J. Infect. Dis. *126:*294, 419, 1972.

Goldstein, W. J., Halpern, B., Parlebas, J., and Rebeyratte, P.: Isolation from heart valves of glycopeptides which share immunological properties with Streptococcus haemolyticus Group A polysaccharides. Nature *219:*866, 1968.

Gordis, L., and Markowitz, M.: Prevention of rheumatic fever revisited. Pediatr. Clin. North Am. *18:*1243, 1971.

Kaplan, E. L., Anthony, B. F., Chapman, S. S., Ayoub, E. M., and Wannamaker, L. W.: The influence of the site of infection on the immune response to Group A streptococci. J. Clin. Invest. *49:*1405, 1970.

Kaplan, M. H., Bolande, R., Rakita, L., and Blair, J.: Presence of bound immunoglobulins and complement in the myocardium in acute rheumatic fever. Association with cardiac failure. N. Engl. J. Med. *271:*637, 1964.

Kaplan, M. H., and Svec, K. H.: Immunologic relation of streptococcal and tissue antigens. III. Presence in human sera of streptococcal antibody cross-reactive with heart tissue. Association with streptococcal infection, rheumatic fever, and glomerulonephritis. J. Exp. Med. *119:*651, 1964.

McLaughlin, J. F., Paterson, P. Y., Hartz, R. S., and Embury, S. H.: Rheumatic carditis: in vitro responses of peripheral blood leukocytes to heart and streptococcal antigens. Arthritis Rheum. *15:*600, 1972.

Ohanian, S. H., Schwab, J. H., and Cromartie, W. J.: Relation of rheumatic-like cardiac lesions of the mouse to localization of group A streptococcal cell walls. J. Exp. Med. *129:*37, 1969.

Perry, L. W., Poitras, J. M., and Findlan, C.: Rheumatic fever and rheumatic heart disease among U. S. college freshman 1956–65. Prevalence and prophylaxis. Publ. Health Rep. *83:*919, 1968.

Rammelkamp, C. H., Jr.: The treatment and prevention of rheumatic fever. Pediatr. Clin. North Am. *2:*265, 1954.

Read, S. E., Fischetti, V. A., Utermohlen, V., Falk, R. E., and Zabriskie, J. B.: Cellular reactivity studies to streptococcal antigens. Migration inhibition studies in patients with streptococcal infections and rheumatic fever. J. Clin. Invest. *54:*439, 1974.

Schwab, J. H.: Analysis of the experimental lesion of connective tissue produced by a complex of C polysaccharide from group A streptococci. J. Exp. Med. *119:*401, 1964.

Siegel, A. C., Johnson, E. E., and Stollerman, G. H.: Controlled studies of streptococcal pharyngitis in a pediatric population. I. Factors related to the attack rate of rheumatic fever. N. Engl. J. Med. *265:*559, 1961.

Stollerman, G. H.: Factors determining the attack rate of rheumatic fever. J.A.M.A. *177:*823, 1961.

Stollerman, G. H.: Rheumatogenic and nephritogenic streptococci. Circulation *43:*915, 1971.

Wannamaker, L. W.: The chain that links the heart to the throat. Circulation *48:*9, 1973.

Wannamaker, L. W., and Ayoub, E. M.: Antibody titers in acute rheumatic fever. Circulation *21:*598, 1960.

Wood, H. F., Feinstein, A. R., Taranta, A., Epstein, J. A., and Simpson, R.: Rheumatic fever in children and adolescents. III. Comparative effectiveness of three prophylaxis regimens in preventing streptococcal infections and rheumatic recurrences. Ann. Intern. Med. *60* (suppl. 5):31, 1964.

Zabriskie, J. B.: Mimetic relationships between group A streptococci and mammalian tissues. Adv. Immunol. *7:*147, 1967.

Chapter 16

ACUTE GLOMERULONEPHRITIS: EPIDEMIOLOGIC, IMMUNOPATHOGENETIC, AND CLINICAL CONSIDERATIONS

Introduction: Biologic and Epidemiologic Contrasts Between Acute Glomerulonephritis and Acute Rheumatic Fever

Epidemiology

Both acute glomerulonephritis and acute rheumatic fever are remote nonsuppurative complications of Group A streptococcal infections. Several epidemiologic features of the two diseases depend on the epidemiology of streptococcal infections. However, many epidemiologic and biologic differences distinguish acute glomerulonephritis from acute rheumatic fever (see Table 16-1). These challenging differences demand explanations which very well might yield insight into the mechanisms of disease transmission and pathogenesis, and must be taken into account in designing prophylactic and therapeutic approaches.

Several epidemiologic differences between acute glomerulonephritis and acute rheumatic fever are of particular note. In contrast to acute rheumatic

TABLE 16-1. Biologic Difference Between Glomerulonephritis and
Rheumatic Fever

Biologic Feature	Glomerulonephritis	Rheumatic Fever
Geographical distribution	Uniform	More common in northern latitudes
Age	Any age	Rare in infancy
Familial factors	Family contacts	Familial tendency
Sex incidence	Males predominate	Equal
Preceding infection	Pharyngeal or skin	Pharyngeal only
Attack rate after streptococcal infection	Variable (to 28%)	Constant (3%)
Second attacks	Rare; may occur after skin infections	Common
Average latent period between infection and first attack	10 days	18 days
Latent period between infection and exacerbation	Shortened as compared to latent period in first attack	Same as latent period in first attack
Relation of degree of ASO* increase to incidence of first attacks	No relation	Incidence proportional to degree of ASO increase
Time of ASO increase in relation to onset of relapse	After	Before
Serum whole complement and C3	Decreased	Increased
M types of initiating Group A hemolytic streptococcus	Pharyngeal: 1, 4, 12, 18** Skin: 2, 31, 49, 52–55, 57, 60	Any pharyngeal type. Skin strains not rheumatogenic

*Anti–streptolysin O titer
**Limited evidence for 3, 6, 25

fever, in which the attack rate in well-defined streptococcal infections is fairly constant (3 per cent), the attack rate of acute glomerulonephritis has a range of 0 to 28 per cent. Some of this difference can be accounted for by the fact that acute rheumatic fever can follow pharyngeal infections with Group A streptococci of many M types, whereas only a few M types can precipitate acute glomerulonephritis.

The higher incidence of acute rheumatic fever in northern as compared to southern latitudes undoubtedly is related to the higher prevalence of streptococcal pharyngitis and upper respiratory infections in the northern latitudes. Streptococcal skin infections, which are more prevalent in warmer climates, are not rheumatogenic. Acute nephritis, however, can follow streptococcal infections of either the pharynx or skin. Thus, the higher prevalence of skin infections in the southern and tropical latitudes makes up for the lower prevalence of pharyngitis, resulting in a more even geographic distribution of acute glomerulonephritis as compared to acute rheumatic fever.

The reasons why acute glomerulonephritis but not rheumatic fever follows streptococcal skin infections are not clear. Nephritogenicity clearly can be a feature of both pharyngeal and skin strains of Group A streptococci. However, among "nephritogenic" streptococcal M types, only a few strains of a specific M type, such as type 12, may be nephritogenic. Thus, in sporadic type 12 streptococcal infections in northern latitudes, probably less than 1 per cent are followed by acute glomerulonephritis. On the other hand, during an epidemic of type 12 streptococcal pharyngitis in a military population, 11 per cent of these infections were followed by definite or probable acute glomerulonephritis. Several outbreaks of acute glomerulonephritis in families have involved 50 to 75 per cent of the siblings within periods of one to seven weeks. Such familial outbreaks of acute rheumatic fever have not been described, although a familial tendency has been documented. First attacks of acute rheumatic fever in different members of a family may occur years or even generations apart. The observation that acute glomerulonephritis occurs in infants may be related to streptococcal skin infections not uncommon in this age group. In contrast, streptococcal infections of the upper respiratory tract are unusual before the age of four years.

Infection with a particular M type of streptococcus results in a persistent protective immunity against the homologous organisms. Acute rheumatic fever can follow upper respiratory tract infections due to so many different M types of Group A streptococci that recurrences are not uncommon. In contrast, acute glomerulonephritis is precipitated by pharyngitis due to only a handful of M types (good evidence for 1, 4, and 12; limited evidence for 3, 6, and 25). Of these, type 12 has by far the widest distribution in the population. In view of the solid homologous immunity induced by type 12 infections and the unlikelihood of a subsequent infection by the less common nephritogenic types, second attacks are uncommon among patients whose initial episodes of acute glomerulonephritis have healed. For unknown reasons, exacerbations in chronic glomerulonephritis can follow infections due to any M type streptococcus, or even nonstreptococcal infections.

Second attacks of acute glomerulonephritis, although still not frequent, are more common in tropical or subtropical regions where epidemics of streptococcal skin infections may be associated with a number of different nephritogenic M types. Once a new streptococcal "skin" strain is introduced into a susceptible population, it may spread widely, thus setting the stage for second attacks of acute glomerulonephritis.

The basis for differences between acute glomerulonephritis and acute rheumatic fever that relate to other than epidemiologic factors is not well understood. The differences are striking, however, and emphasize that these two diseases have very different pathogenic mechanisms.

Biology

In most reported series of acute glomerulonephritis, males predominate by two to one, whereas acute rheumatic fever occurs with equal frequency in both sexes. Perhaps this incidence results from epidemiologic factors, such as greater exposure of school-age males to the minor trauma necessary to serve as a nidus for skin infection (see Chap. 36) or the concentration of young males in boarding schools or military camps where streptococcal infections are likely to become epidemic. However, this hypothesis is not well documented. Some unknown host factors may play equally essential roles in this difference in incidence.

No explanation is available for the shorter latent period (days between onset of infection and onset of sequelae) for acute glomerulonephritis as compared to acute rheumatic fever. The short latent period of one to three days for the exacerbation in chronic glomerulonephritis usually is considered to be evidence that poststreptococcal glomerulonephritis is related to an antigen-antibody reaction, since second episodes of serum sickness likewise exhibit a shortened latent period. In contrast, the latent period for recurrences of acute rheumatic fever remains the same as for that of the first attack.

One of the most striking differences between acute glomerulonephritis and acute rheumatic fever is the behavior of serum complement. Whole serum complement and C3 (see Chap. 3) are increased in acute rheumatic fever, as they are in other inflammatory conditions. In acute glomerulonephritis, however, whole serum complement, C3 and, properdin are reduced for the first two to six weeks, presumably reflecting some aspect of this condition's immunologic pathogenesis. General and local activation of the complement system by antigen-antibody complexes, circulating and deposited on glomerular capillary basement membrane, respectively, appears to play a role in the pathogenesis of acute glomerulonephritis but not acute rheumatic fever.

Acute glomerulonephritis and rheumatic fever very rarely occur in the same individual. When a patient with rheumatic heart disease has renal manifestations, subacute bacterial endocarditis should be suspected and sought.

Classification

Clinical

Acute glomerulonephritis can be overt or subclinical. Overt cases present little diagnostic difficulty. The acute nephritis syndrome is characterized by the abrupt onset of proteinuria, hematuria, edema of the face and legs, hypertension, and renal function impairment. Subclinical cases are detected by examination of the urine. Evidence should be sought for prior or current infection due to Group A streptococci or to certain other organisms (see below).

Poststreptococcal acute glomerulonephritis usually heals, especially in children. In some epidemics, healing rates have approached 100 per cent. However, the healing rate in sporadic instances of acute glomerulonephritis in the adult population is probably in the order of 85 to 90 per cent. The rate of progression of poststreptococcal chronic glomerulonephritis usually is quite slow, whether or not the patient suffers an exacerbation. Ten to thirty years may intervene before the endstage of chronic glomerulonephritis is reached. Rarely, the disease may follow a subacute course, reaching the terminal stage within a year or so. However, such a subacute course is more characteristic of other chronic glomerular diseases.

Pathologic

All glomeruli are diffusely involved in poststreptococcal acute glomerulonephritis. The glomerular lesions may be proliferative or exudative, or may present a combination of these two features (Fig. 16–1A). Proliferative changes may involve endothelial cells or the epithelial cells of Bowman's capsule, resulting in crescents. As the acute process subsides, hypercellularity usually is confined to the mesangial areas of the glomeruli. Lobular scars and adhesions between glomerular lobules and Bowman's capsule are monuments to prior exudative processes. On electron microscopy, subepithelial electron-dense deposits or humps are characteristic (Fig. 16–1B). By immunofluorescent histologic techniques, these deposits appear to contain immunoglobulin (IgG), C3 (a component of the complement system; see Chap. 3), and properdin (Fig. 16–1C). Fibrin or fibrin products localized in the glomeruli are responsible for proliferation of endothelial cells as well as the epithelial cells of Bowman's capsule, producing crescents (Fig. 16–1D).

Etiologic

A number of etiologies of acute glomerulonephritis are listed in Table 16–2. Most of these are related to glomerular deposits of circulating immune complexes. Group A streptococcal infection is by far the most common antecedent of acute glomerulonephritis. Acute focal or diffuse glomerular lesions may occur in the course of subacute bacterial endocarditis, usually due to *Streptococcus viridans* or Lancefield Group D enterococci. Bacteremia with *Staphylococcus epidermidis,* whether secondary to endocarditis or to infected prostheses such as ventricular-atrial shunts used to treat hydrocephalus, may be associated with acute glomerulonephritis. *Staphylococcus aureus* and pneumococcal pneumonia also have been reported as antecedents of acute glomerulonephritis, although concomitant streptococcal infection was excluded in only a handful of instances. The histopathology of the glomerular lesions in these circumstances is similar to that of poststreptococcal acute glomerulonephritis, although in subacute bacterial endocarditis, the lesions sometimes are distributed focally. The complement system is involved in the other conditions just discussed as it is in poststreptococcal acute glomerulonephritis.

Glomerulonephritis occurs in association with chronic quartan malaria, and in simian malaria. A variety of other infections from time to time have been implicated in the etiology of acute glomerulonephritis, usually on inadequate grounds. However, proteinuria and hematuria following infections of many types may be associated with glomerulitis. Other signs of acute glomerulonephritis, such as edema and hypertension, are rare in this

TABLE 16–2. Causes of Acute Glomerulonephritis

Group A streptococcal infections

Subacute bacterial endocarditis

Staphylococcal bacteremia – sustained (e.g., *Staphylococcus epidermidis*)

Pneumococcal lobar pneumonia

Quartan malaria

Viral infections

Miscellaneous infections – glomerulitis usually focal

Some tumors (especially lung carcinoma, Hodgkin's disease)

Systemic diseases
  Systemic lupus erythematosus
  Periarteritis nodosa
  Hypersensitivity angiitis

Idiopathic

condition. The urinary abnormalities in focal glomerulitis may reappear with recurrent infections.

Acute nephritis has been described in association with a number of different viral infections, including infectious mononucleosis, acute hepatitis (A and B), chicken pox, mumps, adenovirus 7, variola, varicella, and echovirus (type 9), and following vaccination. Deposits of immune globulins have been described in glomerular capillary basement membranes in association with some of these as well as other viral infections. In several viral infections in mice (e.g., lymphocytic choriomeningitis) and in Aleutian disease in mink, circulating antigen-antibody complexes are localized in glomeruli and are associated with glomerular lesions. However, in man, the cellular changes in glomeruli usually are not striking nor suggestive of the usual poststreptococcal alterations. An epidemic form of acute benign hemorrhagic nephritis has been described in association with nonstreptococcal pharyngitis, presumably of viral origin. The glomerular lesions were focal and usually very mild. Clinical recovery was the rule.

Finally, the acute nephritis syndrome may occur in the course of such systemic diseases as lupus erythematosus, periarteritis nodosa, or hypersensitivity angiitis.

Pathogenesis

Theories

Theories regarding the initiation of poststreptococcal acute glomerulonephritis are summarized in Table 16–3. The most likely mechanism is deposition of circulating antigen-antibody complexes on the glomerular

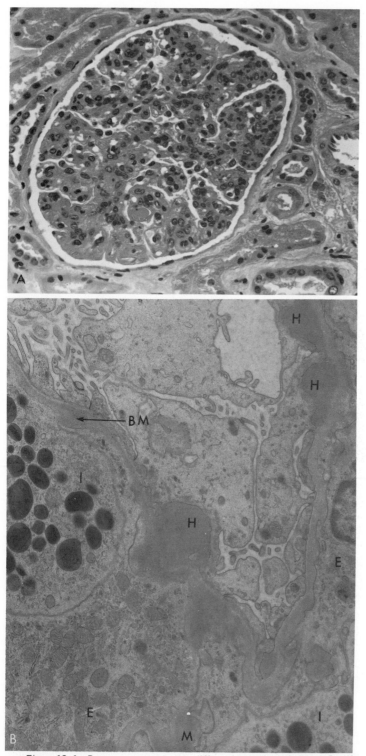

Figure 16-1. Poststreptococcal acute diffuse glomerulonephritis. *A,* Proliferation and exudation. Biopsy was obtained 30 days after onset of the condition. Hematoxylin and eosin stain. (X 147.) (From Jennings, R. B., and Earle, D. P.: *In* Becker, E. L. [ed.] : Structural Basis of Renal Diseases. New York, Harper and

(Figure 16-1 continued on opposite page.)

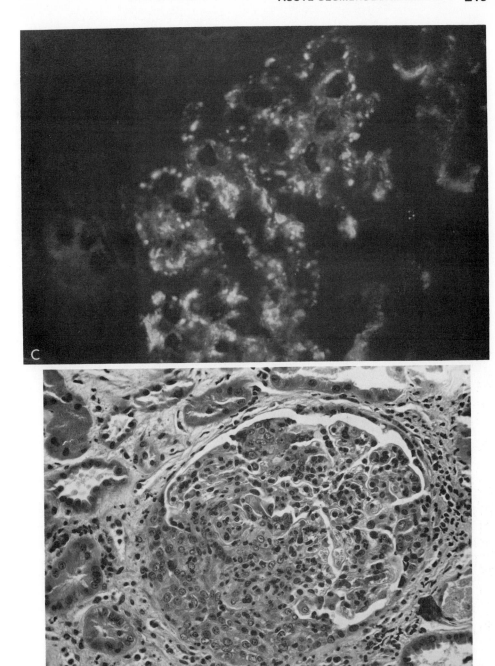

Figure 16–1 *(Continued).*

Row, 1968). *B,* Characteristic electron-dense subepithelial "humps." *BM* = basement membrane; *E* = endothelial cell; *H* = hump (immune deposit); *I* = inflammatory cell; *M* = basement membrane–like material (in mesangium). Electron microscopy. (X 12,000.) (From Jennings and Earle.)

C, Characteristic deposition of IgG in a granular pattern along the glomerular capillary basement membrane. Immunofluorescent anti-IgG stain. (X 25.) (Courtesy of Dr. Elizabeth V. Potter.) *D,* Crescent formation, characteristic of severe acute glomerulonephritis. Hematoxylin and eosin stain. (X 276.) (From Jennings and Earle.)

capillary basement membrane. This process is discussed at greater length below. Although the other three mechanisms are possible, and some evidence suggests that the theories of streptococcal products and streptococcal antigenic determinants (see below) should be kept in mind, none of these alone could satisfy all the known facts about the pathogenesis of poststreptococcal acute glomerulonephritis. A number of clinical and pathologic features of acute glomerulonephritis suggest that an immune response to Group A streptococcal infection plays a major role in its pathogenesis. The latent period of 5 to 28 days between Group A streptococcal infection and onset of acute glomerulonephritis and the early decrease in serum complement represent such evidence. Deposits of immune globulins and complement components on the glomerular capillary basement membranes, as demonstrated by electron microscopic and immunofluorescent histopathologic techniques, likewise support the immune pathogenetic hypothesis.

TABLE 16–3. Possible Initiating Mechanisms in Poststreptococcal
Acute Glomerulonephritis

Deposition of circulating antigen-antibody complexes on glomerular capillary basement membrane

Autoantibody formation following alteration of host protein or glomerular antigens by streptococcal products or antigens

Cross-reactive antigens between glomeruli and nephritogenic streptococci

Direct toxic effect of streptococcal toxins or products on glomerular basement membranes

The association of only a few M serotypes of Group A streptococci with acute glomerulonephritis suggests the possibility that nephritogenic strains produce some kind of toxic factor responsible for the lesion, or perhaps a factor that encourages localization of soluble complexes within the glomeruli.

Another rather remote pathogenetic possibility is a latent infection (e.g., L forms) that persists after subsidence of the initial streptococcal infection which in some way induces acute glomerulonephritis.

Streptococcal Products

Group A as well as other groups of streptococci produce a large number of antigenic extracellular products, most of which exhibit many different toxic effects in various tissues, as tested in vitro and in experimental animals. Many of these antigens induce serum antibodies which are useful in detecting streptococcal infections. However, only those effects which have some possible bearing on the pathogenesis of acute glomerulonephritis, or which involve the kidneys, are discussed here.

Large quantities of streptolysin S injected intravenously or intraperitoneally into mice cause necrosis of renal tubule cells. The amounts necessary for this effect are far in excess of the amount that could be formed by streptococcal infection of the pharynx, tonsils, or skin. Streptokinase has no direct effect on the kidneys but does activate conversion of plasminogen to plasmin which hydrolyzes various proteins, including fibrinogen or fibrin. It also activates complement components and generates permeability and chemotactic factors. All these activities could play a role in the pathogenesis of acute glomerulonephritis.

"Nephritogenic" streptococci have induced in rats tubular necrosis and sometimes glomerular lesions associated with proteinuria and hematuria. Similar lesions have also followed infections with non-nephritogenic streptococci. The tubular lesions, however, have little or no relationship to acute glomerulonephritis. Some of these experimental lesions resemble acute glomerulonephritis in man. A few studies have suggested the existence of a streptococcal extracellular nephrotoxin, but these results remain controversial at present. Intracellular nephrotoxins which induce acute glomerulonephritis in sensitized rabbits have been described but not yet confirmed.

Several streptococcal cell wall components such as the type specific M protein and hyaluronic acid play a role in the virulence of streptococci but apparently have no direct nephrotoxic effects.

Many streptococcal enzymes and other components or products are antigenic and thus could form circulating soluble complexes with their developing antibodies. These complexes could localize in the glomeruli and trigger the reactions which lead to acute glomerulonephritis. Unfortunately, unequivocal demonstrations of streptococcal antigens within the glomerular deposits of acute glomerulonephritis have been rare and often unconfirmed. Perhaps degraded streptococci or their cell wall components persisting within phagocytic leukocytes or mesangial cells could contribute to continuing tissue inflammation and antigenic responses.

Streptococcal Antigenic Determinants

Antigenic determinants common to both streptococci and mammalian tissue including the heart, skeletal muscles, and glomerular basement membranes have been demonstrated. Such cross-reactivity between components of nephritogenic streptococci and glomeruli has suggested the possiblity that the cross-reactive streptococcal antigen could induce nephrotoxic antibodies that react with glomerular basement membranes. This is an intriguing hypothesis, but if such a cross-reactive mechanism plays a role, it should be limited to nephritogenic strains of streptococci. This has not been demonstrated unequivocally. Another interesting hypothesis is that both immune complexes and cross-reactive immunity are involved in the pathogenesis of acute glomerulonephritis. Again, nephritogenic streptococci might somehow modify IgG in such a way that it develops the properties of immune complexes which initiate acute glomerulonephritis.

Recently, a possible role has been proposed for streptococcal plasma membrane components in initiating acute glomerulonephritis. Fluorescein-labeled IgG from sera of patients with acute glomerulonephritis localized in glomeruli of tissue obtained by biopsy in the early stages of acute glomerulonephritis. This staining property of IgG could be absorbed out by disrupted nephritogenic streptococci but not by non-nephritogenic strains. Further confirmation is needed.

Circulating Immune Complexes

Poststreptococcal acute glomerulonephritis and the glomerulonephritis of acute serum sickness in both man and experimental animals have many similarities, and both appear to represent "immune complex" disease. The latent period between infection, or injection of foreign protein, and the onset of acute glomerulonephritis is usually 7 to 14 days. Serum complement is reduced in acute glomerulonephritis and in serum sickness. Both glomerular lesions have similar characteristics on light microscopy, and on electron microscopy, these conditions exhibit characteristic electron-dense deposits (humps) on the epithelial side of the glomerular basement membranes. By immunofluorescent histopathologic techniques, the deposits contain IgG, C3, and properdin.

In the experimental model, a single intravenous injection of a large amount of a foreign protein (e.g., bovine serum albumin) in rabbits is followed in several days by specific antibody in the serum. Initially, high levels of antigen are still in the circulation, permitting formation of soluble antigen-antibody complexes. Most of the soluble complexes are taken up by the reticuloendothelial system, but some are deposited in the glomeruli over a period of several days, thus initiating acute glomerulonephritis in the animal host. As measurable antigen disappears from the circulation, serum C3 and properdin decreases while IgG, C3, and properdin are deposited in a granular pattern along the epithelial side of the glomerular capillary basement membranes.

Although the specific antigen in poststreptococcal acute glomerulonephritis has not been identified, its pathogenesis appears to be very similar to that of acute serum sickness in the rabbit (Fig. 16–2). Presumably, similar mechanisms are responsible for glomerular lesions in subacute bacterial endocarditis, staphylococcal bacteremia, pneumococcal pneumonia, and quartan malaria. The offending antigen has been eluted from kidneys of patients who died of glomerulonephritis due to the latter two conditions. Similarly, some viral infections may induce glomerulitis in the same fashion. Many instances of focal glomerulitis also appear to be based on soluble complex deposition. The considerable variations in the morphologic changes in the glomeruli could depend on such factors as species, amount of complex deposited, and different capacities of different complexes to initiate tissue reactions. Size of complexes does play a role in their localization. Small complexes which result from antigen excess are likely to remain in circulation, while precipitates formed in the zones of antibody equivalence or excess are rapidly taken up by phagocytic cells. The intermediate-size complexes (e.g., those with a sedimentation coefficient of 15S) formed in the presence of moderate antibody excess are soluble but still react with complement and can be deposited in vessel walls or glomeruli and thus induce inflammation.

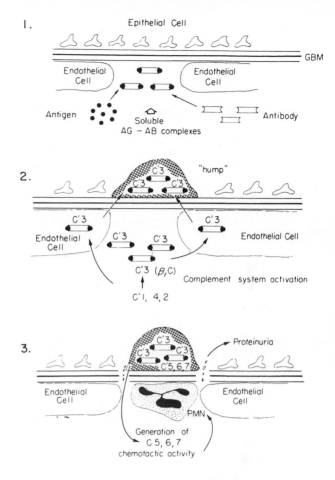

Figure 16–2. Diagrammatic representation of the development of glomerular injury by soluble antigen-antibody complexes. (From Fish, et al.: *In* Strauss, M. B., and Welt, L. G. (eds.): Diseases of the Kidney. 2nd ed. Boston, Little, Brown and Co., 1971.)

Mediators

Antigen-antibody complexes are responsible for the initiation of a number of secondary local mechanisms that contribute to the glomerular lesions. These include release of leukotaxines, and of anaphylatoxin and histamine that increase glomerular capillary and mesangial permeability and thus lead to further local trapping of immune complexes (Fig. 16–5). Furthermore, glomerular inflammatory changes result from proteolytic enzymes released by the leukocytes attracted to areas of antigen-antibody deposits. Antigen-antibody complexes may somehow trigger the coagulation process as well as activate the complement system. In any case, aggregation of platelets and deposition of fibrinogen, fibrin, and related products are common features of poststreptococcal acute glomerulonephritis. Without question, fibrin or fibrinogen ingested by phagocytic cells, both endothelial and epithelial, can result in cellular proliferation. Such proliferation causes

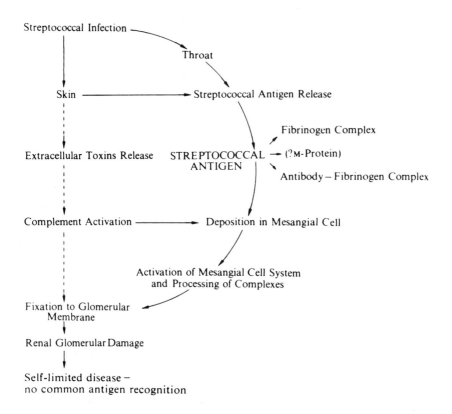

Figure 16–3. Proposed pathway of pathologic damage in acute poststreptococcal glomerulonephritis. (From Zabriskie, J. B., et al.: Streptococcus-related glomerulonephritis. Kidney Int. *3:*100, 1974.)

glomerular capillary obstruction and constriction of glomeruli within Bowman's space by crescent formation. These processes impair renal function.

When antigen fixes to antibody in vitro in the presence of fresh serum, a progressive and sequential activation of complement occurs as follows: C1, C4, C2, and then C3. Whole serum complement levels reflect the net effect of changes in these and sometimes other complement components. After C3 is activated, C5, C6, C7, C8, and C9 follow in line. A low molecular weight leukotactic agent is derived from activated C5. In experimental serum sickness nephritis in rabbits and in systemic lupus erythematosus nephritis in man, C1, C4, C2, and C3 are depressed. In contrast, in poststreptococcal acute glomerulonephritis and in chronic mesangiocapillary glomerulonephritis, C1, C4, and C2 are spared. Apparently C3 may be activated by an alternate pathway, which appears to involve properdin (see Chap. 3). The alternate pathway may be activated factors other than antigen-antibody complexes. On the other hand, complexes can activate both the classic and the alternate complement pathways.

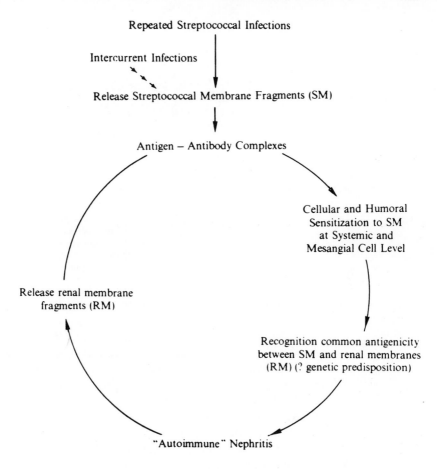

Figure 16–4. Proposed pathway of pathologic damage in progressive glomerulo-nephritis. (From Zabriskie, J. B., et al.: Streptococcus-related glomerulonephritis. Kidney Int. *3:*100, 1974.)

Diagnosis

Symptomatic acute glomerulonephritis is not a difficult diagnosis. Gross or microscopic hematuria, cylinduria, and proteinuria, with or without edema, circulatory congestion, hypertension, and impaired renal function suggest the diagnosis, especially if they develop one to three weeks after pharyngitis or in association with skin infections. Asymptomatic or "laboratory diagnosis" acute glomerulonephritis will be detected only if the clinician performs urinalyses at appropriate intervals after proven or suspected streptococcal infections, and in individuals exposed during epidemics or household outbreaks.

All of the signs and symptoms of glomerulonephritis may be associated with glomerular involvement in a number of systemic diseases; for example, subacute bacterial endocarditis, systemic lupus erythematosus, and peri-arteritis nodosa. Evidence for the associated systemic disease usually is readily detected by clinical examinations and appropriate tests.

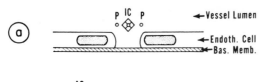

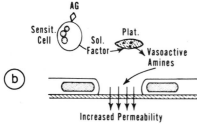

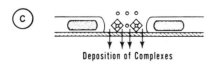

Figure 16–5. Theoretical summary of the mechanism responsible for the deposition of immune complexes from the circulation in acute immune complex disease. (From Cochrane, C. G.: *In* Proceedings of a Symposium on Immune Complexes and Disease. J. Exp. Med. *134:*75S, 1971.)

Serum complement determinations are helpful in the diagnosis of several glomerular diseases including poststreptococcal acute glomerulonephritis. Whole serum complement and C3 are depressed from the onset of acute glomerulonephritis and for the next two to six weeks. Sera for whole complement determinations must be promptly (within two hours) stored on dry ice. Such precautions are not necessary for C3, which is heat stable. C4 is not decreased in acute glomerulonephritis, but is in systemic lupus erythematosus and the nephritis associated with subacute bacterial endocarditis, thus serving as a useful differential feature.

Establishment of the streptococcal etiology of acute glomerulonephritis rests on both bacteriologic and immunologic studies. Recovery of a nephritogenic M type streptococcus on culture from a patient prior to or during the early phases of acute glomerulonephritis is fairly good evidence, but in view of the long latent period between infection and the onset of this condition, the offending organism already may have disappeared by the time the patient becomes symptomatic, especially in view of the widespread use of penicillin. Although penicillin may modify antibody response, 80 per cent of Group A streptococcal pharyngeal infections are followed by a significant increase in serum anti-streptolysin O titer. If another antibody such as antihyaluronidase is added, 90 per cent of the infections will be detected, while the further addition of antistreptokinase will increase the diagnosis rate to 95 per cent. Skin strains of streptococci only rarely induce an anti-streptolysin O response, probably because skin lipids inhibit streptolysin O. Therefore, an antihyaluronidase or antideoxyribonuclease should be utilized to detect streptococcal skin infection. Unless streptococcal antibody titers are definitely increased, serial observations are necessary.

M-type specific antibodies develop one to several months after streptococcal infections. However, this is rather late to be of practical clinical value.

Furthermore, measurement of serum M antibodies is difficult and performed only in research settings.

Treatment

Penicillin (or erythromycin for patients allergic to penicillin) is indicated in acute glomerulonephritis to eradicate the offending streptococci if still present. Treatment should be by injection of a long-acting penicillin (1,200,000 units benzathine penicillin) or should be continued for at least 10 days if the oral route (200,000 units penicillin G every six hours) is used. Although penicillin treatment is recommended since it will limit the spread of nephritogenic streptococci to other persons, it will not alter the outcome of already established acute glomerulonephritis. However, in periods of high incidence of streptococcal infections, temporary penicillin prophylaxis probably is worthwhile in the months immediately following the occurrence of acute glomerulonephritis to prevent a second attack or recurrence during convalescence that might lead to chronicity.

The immunologic pathogenesis of acute glomerulonephritis has suggested the use of steroids or other immunosuppressive therapy. However, since only rarely do patients with acute glomerulonephritis fail to recover and since even the severest instances may undergo spontaneous improvement, a very large prospective study will be necessary to establish the usefulness of such treatment. Careful observations of some patients with severe and progressive downhill courses suggest that large doses of steroids (60 to 80 mg prednisone or equivalent) daily in adults are worth further study. If steroids are used in patients with renal function impairment, the hazards of the catabolic effects of these drugs should be kept in mind.

The role of fibrin in experimental models of acute glomerulonephritis and its presence in glomeruli in patients with acute glomerulonephritis, have lead to trials with anticoagulant agents including heparin, Coumadin, and aspirin. In experimental models, promising results have been obtained, especially when treatment is instituted at the onset of the pathogenetic mechanism. However, clinical usefulness has not been demonstrated.

Prophylaxis

Except for temporary prophylaxis during early convalescence from poststreptococcal acute glomerulonephritis, long-term prophylaxis as practiced in rheumatic heart disease is not indicated for acute glomerulo-nephritis. Second attacks are very rare. Exacerbations occur in only 20 per cent of patients with poststreptococcal chronic glomerulonephritis, and when they do occur they rarely appear to result in more than transient renal function impairment. Thus, little would be gained by long-term prophylaxis.

In closed populations such as military camps, schools, and large family units, penicillin prophylaxis during periods when acute glomerulonephritis or nephritogenic streptococci have been detected probably is worthwhile.

CASE PRESENTATION 1

A 17-year-old high school student who had no prior known renal disease developed a sore throat and fever of 103°F on November 18. The fever and sore throat lasted for three days. On November 28, he developed hematuria, puffy eyelids, and swollen ankles. He went to a physician, who noted an inflamed pharynx, enlarged and reddened tonsils, and palpable cervical lymph nodes. The patient had pitting edema of his feet and pretibial areas and a blood pressure of 165/105 mm Hg; the urine contained 4+ protein, 20 to 30 erythrocytes and 25 to 30 leukocytes per high power field, some hyaline and granular casts, and one erythrocyte cast. The physician admitted the patient to a hospital where he made certain that laboratory investigations included throat culture, serum for anti-streptolysin O titer and beta 1C globulin (C3 component of the complement system), and evaluation of renal function. The patient was given bed rest and 1,200,000 units of procaine penicillin intramuscularly. The throat culture revealed Group A streptococci, the anti-streptolysin O titer was 166 units per ml, C3 was 53 mg per 100 ml (normal 110 to 160 mg per 100 ml), and the serum creatinine was 2.5 mg per 100 ml (normal < 1.5 mg per 100 ml).

The acute onset of the nephritic syndrome 10 days after a sore throat and fever, in a previously healthy young man, is the classic story of poststreptococcal acute glomerulonephritis. The leukocytes in the urine are not surprising in view of the glomerular exudative lesions characteristic of acute glomerulonephritis. The recovery of Group A hemolytic streptococci from the throat culture added weight to this diagnosis, especially when a streptococcal research laboratory several days later reported that the streptococci were M type 12. The initial anti-streptolysin O titer of 166 units per ml was borderline, but a repeat two weeks later was 500, a significant increase. The serum complement (C3) decrease provides further evidence in favor of acute glomerulonephritis. Because of the typical features and the probable favorable outcome, the attending physician elected not to obtain a confirmatory renal biopsy.

Penicillin therapy was given in order to prevent further spread of nephritogenic streptococci. The attending physician had no thought that this would alter the course of the already established disease in his patient. However, the patient had five younger siblings in his home. The physician obtained throat cultures and urine specimens from the siblings and both parents. Group A streptococci were found in the throat cultures from the mother and three siblings, two of whom had proteinuria and microscopic hematuria. Mild transient hypertension and ankle edema developed in one, while both had decreased serum C3.

The urine specimens in the original patient and the two siblings became normal within six weeks.

CASE PRESENTATION 2

A 26-year-old male civil engineer developed a severe sore throat and fever on February 27, 1964. This was treated with Achromycin. Eight days later, the urine became dark red, and the patient was admitted to a hospital. Aside from mild aching in the costovertebral angles, he had no other symptoms. The blood pressure was normal, edema was not present, but the urine had 3+ protein, innumerable erythrocytes, 200 to 300 leukocytes, and many erythrocyte casts. The blood urea nitrogen was increased to 84 mg per 100 ml. and the serum creatinine to 4.0 mg per 100 ml. Throat cultures did not yield Group A streptococci, but the anti-streptolysin O titer was 500 units per ml on admission, rising to 833 soon after; it subsequently fell to 62 three months later. Serum type specific M type 12 streptococcal antibodies appeared two months after the sore throat. The serum whole hemolytic complement was decreased to 26 units (normal 40 to 50 units) on admission but returned to normal within three weeks. The urine returned to normal color after eight days, but proteinuria 1 to 2+ and microscopic hematuria persisted. Renal function as reflected by the blood urea nitrogen and serum creatinine levels returned to normal in three weeks.

Although clinical history and laboratory observations associated with the acute episode described above strongly supported the diagnosis of post-streptococcal acute glomerulonephritis, several features of the patient's past history raised the possibility of an underlying chronic renal disease. Gross hematuria first occured at age 17 following an infection diagnosed as infectious mononucleosis. The patient became a member of the Naval Reserves, but after call to acitve duty at age 19, he was discharged because of abnormal urine. Gross hematuria again recurred transiently at age 24 at which time he was admitted to a Urology Service in a hosptial for evaluation. Except for persistent microscopic hematuria, the work-up, including cytoscopy, intravenous pyelogram, urine cultures, and renal function tests, all was normal.

The patient's 1964 hospital admission questioning revealed that his paternal grandfather also had had recurrent hematuria. Renal calculi were found at autopsy. A paternal cousin, while in the Army, had a kidney removed because of hematuria. Other details were not available. The patient's mother had been moderately deaf for many years following a series of serious otitis media infections. Audiometry on the mother revealed severe loss of air conduction hearing on the left, and the father had significant nerve conduction impairment for high frequencies bilaterally. The patient also had impairment of hearing for high frequencies but on the right only.

A renal biopsy was performed two weeks after onset of the gross hematuria. One glomerulus was hyalinized, and relatively fresh crescents were present in the remaining eight glomeruli. Thirty to fifty polymorphonuclear neutrophils were present in each glomerulus which were surrounded by extensive infiltrates of acute and chronic inflammatory cells. Erythrocyte casts were present in a number of tubules. The cortical architecture was disrupted by edema and interstitial fibrosis. The arterioles were normal. Electron microscopy demonstrated subepithelial deposits characteristic of poststreptococcal acute glomerulonephritis. Two subsequent biopsies revealed subsidence of the acute process. A biopsy obtained three months after onset revealed no inflammatory cells. Two of nine glomeruli were hyalinized, and the remaining had lobular scars and healed crescents. There were focal areas of interstitial fibrosis and tubular atrophy. The blood vessels again were normal.

The gross hematuria and transient impairment of renal function that followed an infection which proved serologically to be of Group A streptococcal origin, with subsequent demonstration of serum M type 12 antibodies and transient decrease in serum complement, made the diagnosis of poststreptococcal acute glomerulonephritis very likely. The crescents and glomerular exudation likewise were compatible with this diagnosis, and the glomerular subepithelial deposits seen on electron microscopy were characteristic. However, the prior history of recurrent hematuria and the hyalinized glomeruli and interstitial fibrosis on the first renal biopsy suggested underlying chronic renal disease. Working against the diagnosis of chronic glomerulonephritis with an exacerbation was the long latent period between infection and hematuria. The family history of hematuria and nerve deafness suggested familial nephritis (Alport's syndrome). However, the history of hematuria occurred in a grandfather who lived to be 86 and who had renal calculi at autopsy, and the patient's nerve deafness was confined to one side.

However, the subsequent course of events supported the diagnosis of Alport's syndrome. The patient's proteinuria gradually increased to the nephrotic range, and his renal function gradually declined to approximately one half of normal. He now had bilateral nerve deafness for high frequencies. A renal biopsy obtained nine years after his February, 1964, admission revealed that most glomeruli were normal but that a few had segmental hyalinization; several had periglomerular fibrosis in continuity with areas of intersititial fibrosis and infiltrations with chronic inflammatory cells. No deposits were noted on electron microscopy, although the glomerular capillary basement membranes were focally thickened. In 1967, the patient's then nine-year-old daughter developed abnormal urine and subsequently developed slowly progressive renal disease and nerve deafness.

CASE PRESENTATION 3

A 36-year-old housewife complained of progressive weakness for two months and malaise for one week. Upon careful questioning, she recalled confinement to bed for several weeks in her childhood because of joint pains. Subsequently, she enjoyed excellent health until her present illness. She appeared to be pale and had a temperature of 99.8°F orally. The heart had a grade 2/6 apical systolic murmer. The blood pressure was normal, and edema was absent. Two+ proteinuria, microscopic hematuria, and some hyaline and granular casts were present. The hemoglobin was 11 gm per 100 ml with normochromic erythrocytes but no reticulocytosis. The white blood cell count was 11,000 per cubic millimeter with 70 per cent polymorphonuclear leukocytes. The corrected erythrocyte sedimentation rate was 45 mm in one hour, the C-reactive protein was 4+, C3 was 60 mg per 100 ml, and the blood urea nitrogen was 65 mg per 100 ml.

The patient had neither petechiae nor clubbed fingers. The attending physician was not certain that he could palpate the spleen, but since he suspected subacute bacterial endocarditis, he ordered three consecutive blood cultures. These revealed *Streptococcus viridans* which proved to be only moderately sensitive to penicillin (1 unit per ml). Five million units penicillin

G were administered intramuscularly every six hours; probenecid, 0.5 gm orally, was given concurrently. The patient gradually improved and the blood cultures became sterile. The hemoglobin returned to normal, as did the white blood cell count, sedimentation rate, C-reactive protein, and C3. However, 1+ proteinuria persisted, and the blood urea nitrogen ranged between 70 and 80 mg per 100 ml.

This patient had some but not all the clinical features of subacute bacterial endocarditis. Despite prompt recognition of the disease almost as soon as the patient sought medical attention, and immediate institution of appropriate therapy which controlled the infection, renal function was already impaired and did not improve.

The attending physician was uncertain as to whether or not the patient had previous underlying chronic renal disease, nor was he certain about the prognosis. Therefore, he arranged for a renal biopsy after the patient had been in the hospital for three weeks and at a time when C3 was still decreased. A moderately severe diffuse proliferative and exudative glomerulo-nephritis was present. Some areas of focal necrosis and hyalinizing glomerular lobules, as well as adhesions between the glomerular tuft and Bowman's capsule, attested to permanent glomerular damage. A mild but definite early interstitial fibrosis was present. Electron microscopy revealed dense sub-epithelial deposits which, by immunofluorescent techniques, were shown to contain immunoglobulins and complement components, reflecting the immune-complex origin of the glomerulonephritis of subacute bacterial endocarditis. The glomerular lesions sometimes may be focally distributed.

Whether diffuse or focal, the glomerulonephritis of subacute bacterial endocarditis is rarely associated with gross hematuria, edema, or hyper-tension. Its onset is truly insidious. The physician must have a high index of suspicion and examine at least weekly the urine of patients with bacterial endocarditis.

References

Books

Becker, E. L. (ed.): Structural Basis of Renal Disease. New York, Hoeber Medical Division, Harper and Row, 1968.

Beeson, P. B., and McDermott, W. (eds.): Textbook of Medicine. 14th ed. Philadelphia, W. B. Saunders Co., 1975.

Harrison, T. R. (ed.): Principles of Internal Medicine. 7th ed. New York, McGraw-Hill Book Co., 1974.

Strauss, M. B., and Welt, L. G. (eds.): Diseases of the Kidney. 2nd ed. Boston, Little, Brown and Co., 1971.

Symposium Volumes

Becker, E. L. (ed.): Conference on Glomerulonephritis, New Heart Association, January 27, 1970. Bull. N. Y. Acad. Med. 46:747, 1970.

Kincaid-Smith, P., Matthew, T. H., and Becker, E. L. (eds.): Glomerulonephritis. A Symposium in Melbourne, Australia. New York, John Wiley & Sons, 1973.

Kunkel, H. G. (ed.): Proceedings of a Symposium on Immune Complexes and Disease. J. Exp. Med. *134:*Part 2, 1971.

Review Articles

Ginsberg, I.: Mechanisms of cell and tissue injury induced by Group A streptococci: relation to post-streptococcal sequelae. J. Infect. Dis. *126:*294, 419, 1972.

Granoff, A.: Kidney and viruses. *In* Rouiller, C., and Muller, A. F. (eds.): The Kidney. Vol. II. New York, Academic Press, 1969.

Merrill, J. P.: Glomerulonephritis. N. Engl. J. Med. *290:*257, 313, 374, 1974.

Original Articles

Bates, R. C., Jennings, R. B., and Earle, D. P.: Acute nephritis unrelated to Group A hemolytic streptococcal infection: Report of ten cases. Am. J. Med. *23:*510, 1957.

Dixon, F. J., Feldman, J. D., and Vasquez, J. J.: Experimental glomerulonephritis. The pathogenesis of a laboratory model resembling the spectrum of human glomerulonephritis. J. Exp. Med. *113:*889, 1961.

Earle, D. P., and Jennings, R. B.: Post-streptococcal glomerulonephritis. *In* Wolstenholme, G. E. W., and Cameron, M. P. (eds.): Ciba Foundation Symposium on Renal Biopsy. Boston, Little, Brown and Co., 1962.

Earle, D. P., and Seegal, D.: Natural history of glomerulonephritis. J. Chron. Dis. *5:*3, 1957.

Fish, A. J., Michael, A. F., Vernier, R. L., and Good, R. A.: Acute serum sickness nephritis in the rabbit: An immune deposit disease. Am. J. Pathol. *49:*997, 1966.

Herdson, P. B., Jennings, R. B., and Earle, D. P.: Glomerular fine structure in post-streptococcal acute glomerulonephritis. Arch. Pathol. *81:*117, 1966.

Jennings, R. B., and Earle, D. P.: Post-streptococcal glomerulonephritis: Histopathologic and clinical studies of the acute, subsiding acute and early chronic latent phases. J. Clin. Invest. *40:*1525, 1961.

Knicker, W. T., and Cochrane, C. G.: The localization of circulating immune complexes in experimental serum sickness: The role of vasoactive animes and hydrodynamic forces. J. Exp. Med. *127:*119, 1968.

Michael, A. F., Drummond, K. N., Good, R. A., and Vernier, R. L.: Acute post-streptococcal glomerulonephritis: Immune deposit disease. J. Clin. Invest. *45:*237, 1966.

Rammelkamp, C. H., Jr., and Weaver, R. S.: Acute glomerulonephritis: The significance of the variations in the incidence of the disease. J. Clin. Invest. *32:*345, 1953.

Vassali, P., and McCluskey, R. T.: The coagulation process and glomerular disease. Am. J. Med. *39:*179, 1965.

Zabriskie, J. B., Utermohlen, V., Read, S. A., and Fischetti, V. A.: Streptococcus-related glomerulonephritis. Kidney Int. *3:*100, 1974.

DIPHTHERIA

Introduction

Diphtheria is a prototype of bacterial diseases in which the major clinical manifestations result from the production by the invading bacterium of a poisonous extracellular substance that is called an exotoxin. A number of diseases fall into this category: tetanus, cholera, gas gangrene, botulism, and staphylococcal food poisoning. All of the microorganisms which cause the above diseases produce an exotoxin that is absorbed into the body from the site of infection, or from food upon which the bacterium has grown. In the latter case, the food is eaten, and the preformed toxin, ingested with the food, is absorbed from the intestinal tract (botulism, staphylococcal food poisoning). In some of these diseases, invasion and multiplication of the pathogen play an important part in the disease process, but the point to be emphasized is that, compared to the effects produced by the exotoxin, invasion and multiplication by themselves usually will produce only a mild, self-limited disease.

This is well illustrated by diphtheria in which pharyngeal disease produced by nontoxigenic *Corynebacterium diphtheriae* is mild, self-limited, and nonfatal. The nature and the manifestations of the "toxin" diseases mentioned above vary widely but, for the most part, the principles illustrated by the diphtheria model can apply equally well to the diagnosis, prevention, and treatment of the other diseases. More detailed consideration of some of the other diseases mentioned above is found in other chapters of this text.

Types of Disease

Diphtheria is caused by a gram positive pleomorphic bacillus called *Corynebacterium* (club-shaped bacterium) *diphtheriae.* More is said about the characteristics of this microorganism below. Two general types of diphtheria are recognized — pharyngeal and cutaneous.

The term *pharyngeal* is somewhat of a misnomer because diphtheritic infection can occur any place in the upper respiratory tract. It may on occasion extend into the lower respiratory tract. However, in most cases, the site of initial infection is the oropharynx. From this site the infection may spread to the posterior and anterior nares or the larynx and trachea. Generally, the greater the spread from the initial focus the greater the severity of the disease.

Corynebacterium diphtheriae is a normal inhabitant of the upper respiratory tract of human beings, and it is not found in the upper respiratory tract of lower animals nor does it produce disease in other species of animal. Therefore, although direct evidence is lacking, it is likely that *C. diphtheriae* cells have an affinity for the epithelial cells lining the upper respiratory tract of man which permits them to attach and colonize. Thus, colonization brought about by specific attachment to respiratory tract epithelium is probably the first step in the pathogenesis of pharyngeal diphtheria.

Only a small number of human beings who harbor *Corynebacterium diphtheriae* in their respiratory tracts will develop diphtheria. Whether disease occurs or not will depend upon the virulence (capacity to attach, multiply, and produce exotoxin) of the invading microorganism and the resistance of the host. The factor of greatest importance in deciding whether severe disease will occur is the capacity of a person whose upper respiratory tract is colonized by diphtheria bacilli to neutralize the action of the exotoxin. Diphtheria exotoxin is a protein and stimulates the production of antibody (antitoxin) which neutralizes the toxic acitivity. Because of subclinical infection during childhood, many adults who have never had clinically recognizable diphtheria will show protective levels of antitoxin in their serum. In addition, infants and children who have been adequately vaccinated will usually have protective levels of antitoxin. Persons with adequate circulating antitoxin may develop a mild pharyngitis due to attachment and multiplication of virulent diphtheria bacilli but they will not suffer from the effects of the exotoxin. Such so-called immune persons can, however, harbor virulent corynebacteria in the upper respiratory tract and therefore act as carriers and serve as sources of infection for less well-protected persons. Nonimmune (not enough antitoxin) persons may also harbor *C. diphtheriae* in the upper respiratory tract and serve as carriers and therefore sources of infection. These people, depending upon a number of poorly understood factors, either may or may not develop clinically evident disease.

The spread of *Corynebacterium diphtheriae* from person to person occurs mainly by droplet infection, although occasional accidental transmission by contaminated fomites cannot be ruled out. When diphtheria was very prevalent in the United States, transmission also occurred at times by means of contaminated milk or other food. These modes of transmission are presently uncommon.

Another and probably very important source of pharyngeal infection with *Corynebacterium diphtheriae* is infected cutaneous lesions. More is said about this below.

Pathogenesis

Clinical symptoms appear in susceptible persons in about two to five days following exposure and colonization. Because of the local multiplication and the production of exotoxin, the major clinical manifestation of diphtheria is pharyngitis, which varies in extent, depending upon the severity of the disease. In the highly susceptible person, the multiplication of the microorganisms and the production of toxin affect the mucous membrane so that serum exudes, cells infiltrate, and a typical adherent grayish pseudomembrane forms. This membrane consists of fibrin, bacteria, epithelial cells, infiltrating segmented neutrophils, and mononuclear cells. It is important to realize that toxin is not required for membrane formation, since persons infected with nontoxigenic strains may have typical-appearing membranes. Some patients may develop little or no membrane and show only mild signs of illness. Fever may not be high, 100 to 101°F, the pulse rate is not over 100 per minute, and, although the throat is sore, the discomfort frequently is not in proportion to the extent of the involvement or the amount of pseudomembrane which forms. Some difficulty may be encountered in swallowing, but the pain is not too severe. In severe cases, the membrane may extend inferiorly to the larynx or below, or superiorly into the nasopharynx, producing varying degrees of obstruction, and the person may appear acutely ill. Fever may rise to 103°F or more, and involvement of the regional lymph nodes may cause marked swelling and tenderness of the cervical lymph glands; when there is extensive involvement, the patient has the classic "bullneck" appearance. Laryngeal involvement may be so severe that respiratory obstruction may develop and emergency surgical intervention, i.e., tracheostomy, may be required to save the life of the patient. In diphtheria, a high fever and appreciable redness of the pharynx should always make one suspicious of a coexisting Group A streptococcal infection.

Regardless of the degree of pharyngeal involvement, it is of crucial importance to realize that infection due to fully virulent *Corynebacterium diphtheriae* results in formation of exotoxin which is absorbed through the mucous membranes into the general circulation. This toxin, by virtue of its effect on distant tissues and organs, is mainly responsible for the mortality associated with diphtheria. The two major actions of the toxin are on the heart and the peripheral nervous system, although other organs can also be affected. Unfortunately, the manifestations of myocarditis tend to occur late in the disease. The patient may appear to be recovering from the membranous pharyngitis only to develop a toxic myocarditis which may rapidly result in congestive heart failure. Depending upon various circumstances and treatment, the incidence of myocarditis can vary between 10 and 70 per cent of patients with diphtheria. Heart failure due to myocarditis is the most common cause of death following diphtheria. The heart failure is not very responsive to digitalis glycosides, since the cardiac myofibers are metabolically, as well as structurally, damaged by diphtheria toxin.

Neurologic complications also may appear as late as a month or six weeks after the onset of the infection. The incidence of neurologic complications may range from 2 to 75 per cent, depending upon the severity of the disease. The peripheral nerve involvement is manifested primarily as a motor defect. The severity may vary from a mild weakness to complete paralysis. The cranial nerves are usually affected first, and the most frequent symptoms are difficulty in swallowing and nasal regurgitation of fluid. Moreover, the voice may develop a nasal quality.

The involvement of the cranial nerves initially probably is due to the retrograde movement of the toxin along nerve fibers. Diphtheria causes demyelinization, hence the paralysis. Recovery from diphtheritic paralysis is the rule, since remyelinization will occur once the toxin has been catabolized.

Diphtheria toxin is a protein with a molecular weight of about 62,000 daltons which apparently consists of a single polypeptide chain. The diphtheria toxin molecule can be dissociated into two portions by the action of trypsin. One fraction (A) has a molecular weight of about 24,000 daltons, and fraction (B), a molecular weight of about 38,000 daltons. The toxicity apparently depends on a unique enzymatic activity associated with fraction A, but fraction A can reach the sensitive cell cytoplasm only when it is specifically associated with fraction B. After entering the cytoplasm of host cells, diphtheria toxin inhibits protein synthesis. Apparently, the toxin combines with nicotinamide adenine dinucleotide (NAD) to form a relatively dissociable complex. This toxin–nicotinamide adenine dinucleotide complex then reacts with transferase II to form an enzymatically inactive product that is but slightly dissociated. Thus, elongation of the peptide chains being synthesized in the cell is inhibited, and cell death eventually occurs.

One of the truly remarkable features of the production of toxin by *Corynebacterium diphtheriae* is that only those strains which have been lysogenized by a particular bacteriophage, called beta, will produce toxin. Strains of *C. diphtheriae* which do not produce toxin can be made toxin producers by exposing them to beta phage. Those cells which become lysogenized are then capable of producing toxin. Apparently, the gene which codes for the production of diphtheria toxin is part of the bacteriophage genome, and a culture of *C. diphtheriae* will produce diphtheria toxin only in the presence of this bacteriophage. The process of converting non–toxin-producing *C. diphtheriae* strains to toxin-producing strains by exposing them to beta phage is known as lysogenic conversion. To what extent this may occur naturally (e.g., in the upper respiratory tract of man) is not known.

It has long been recognized that *Corynebacterium diphtheriae* is capable of infecting other areas of the body; e.g., the conjunctiva, the umbilicus in the newborn, the penis after circumcision, the vagina, and even the cervix. Infection of skin wounds can also occur and has been noted to be particularly common in tropical climates. Until recently, infection of the skin with *C. diphtheriae* was thought to be quite rare in the United States. In the last few years, however, skin infections and in particular skin lesions produced by insect bites may commonly become infected with *C. diphtheriae* in people in the southern part of the United States. These cutaneous lesions may serve as an important reservoir of infection from which epidemics of pharyngeal diphtheria may arise. These lesions may also act as a source of micro-organisms which seed the upper respiratory tract and produce pharyngeal carriers. The epidemiologic importance of cutaneous infection is discussed in more detail below. It is important to mention here that diphtheritic infections of the skin or other organs in susceptible persons may show all of the toxic manifestations that occur after pharyngeal infection.

Diagnosis

In the United States today, the diagnosis of diphtheria is a difficult one for most physicians, pediatricians in particular, to entertain. The relative rarity of this disease at the present time in the United States and the frequency of Group A streptococcal infections and viral infections of the upper respiratory tract make diphtheria, in most cases, a remote possibility. The possibility of diphtheria should always be kept in mind, however, because failure to suspect it, should it be present, would result in delay of specific antitoxin therapy and fatal consequences for the patient. Diphtheria can occur in any community in the United States at any time and tends to appear in the form of abrupt small epidemics involving anywhere from six to several dozen people. The fatality rate is much higher among the first cases of diphtheria that occur during an epidemic owing to the facts that diphtheria usually is not suspected and treatment is delayed until there is laboratory confirmation. This delay of specific therapy may have serious consequences for the patient. Once the presence of diphtheria is recognized in a community, specific therapy may be given to patients sooner, hence the lower mortality rate in those who acquire the disease in the later stages of an epidemic.

Confirmation of the presence of pharyngeal diphtheria can be obtained only by isolation and identification of virulent toxin-producing *Corynebacterium diphtheriae* from the affected areas. In a case in which there is strong suspicion of diphtheria, antitoxin therapy should not be withheld until confirmation is obtained from the laboratory. Confirming the presence of typical-looking colonies of *C. diphtheriae* in culture may require one to four days, and several more days are needed to determine whether or not the isolated typical-looking bacterium actually produces exotoxin. Deferring treatment for this period might well have fatal consequences for the patient. Therefore, in the presence of a strong suspicion of diphtheria, material should be taken, using swabs, for culture and smears, and antitoxin should be administered immediately.

When diagnosing a possible case of diphtheria, it is helpful for the physician to keep in mind the following facts: diphtheria is more common in infants and children; severe disease occurs primarily in the nonvaccinated; diphtheria is more likely to occur in the fall months of the year, and it is more common in the southern and southeastern portions of the United States. Geographic distribution, however, may be misleading because diphtheria epidemics still occur in northern communities. The recent 1970 epidemic in Chicago (discussed later in this chapter) illustrates this point. Confirmation of diphtheritic infection in a patient can only be made by isolation and identification of virulent *Corynebacterium diphtheriae*. Material should be taken from the infected area in the pharynx with a cotton swab; the physician should be sure to collect material from, adjacent to, or even under the fibrinopurulent membrane if possible. This swab should then be used to inoculate suitable selective and differential media.

Traditionally, material removed by the swab for culture has been inoculated onto Loeffler's medium. This is a medium which consists of three parts of beef serum and one part of nutrient broth. It is solidified in the form of a slant in a tube by coagulating the serum with heat. Loeffler's medium is a rather deficient medium and does not sustain well the growth of many of the other fastidious bacteria which might produce disease in the upper respiratory tract. *Corynebacterium diphtheriae* appears to grow better on this medium that do streptococci, pneumococci, or neisseria. Therefore, smears prepared from bacterial growth on this medium after only 12 to 18 hours of incubation will not have a very heavy growth of contaminating micro-organism if *C. diphtheriae* is present. One of the benefits of this medium is that, since it is nutritionally poor, the pleomorphism of the bacterial cells is greater than that found when a more nutrient medium is used. In addition, the typical picture of club-shaped cells containing granules and cells arranged side by side in the characteristic palisade formation is more striking.

At the present time, however, Loeffler's medium is not regarded as the medium of choice for the isolation of *Corynebacterium diphtheriae*. A more nutrient medium containing whole blood to which has been added suitable concentrations of potassium tellurite is preferred. *C. diphtheriae* grows well on this medium and has the capacity to reduce the potassium tellurite to tellurium. The metal is deposited within the colonies and turns them black. Thus, the colonies suspected of being *C. diphtheriae* can easily be recognized. Other microorganisms, e.g., staphylococci, may at times also reduce potassium tellurite; however, confusion may be avoided by preparing a smear of a suspicious colony and staining it with a simple stain such as methylene blue which clearly brings out the pleomorphic appearance of *C. diphtheriae*. Thus, within 24 hours, tentative confirmation of the diagnosis of diphtheria can be made by detecting tellurite-positive colonies which show the typical pleomorphic morphology when stained with simple stains. However, definitive proof of the presence of virulent *C. diphtheriae* can be provided only by demonstrating that the isolated corynebacteria actually produce diphtheria toxin. This procedure, known as the "virulence test," is described below.

When the tellurite medium is inoculated, a sheep blood agar plate should be inoculated in a similar manner. This will permit the rapid detection of Group A streptococci. This is important not only because Group A streptococcal infections may clinically resemble diphtheria but also because Group A streptococci may sometimes coinfect diphtheritic lesions.

Some help can be obtained in the identification of *Corynebacterium diphtheriae* by noting the appearance of the tellurite-positive colonies. *C. diphtheriae* can be divided into three types — mitis, intermedius, and gravis — depending upon the appearance of the colonies. The mitis colonies are usually medium sized, smooth, and very black, with regular edges. The intermedius colonies are rather small, sometimes pinpoint colonies, and are also quite black. The gravis colonies, on the other hand, tend to be flatter and more gray than black and have irregular edges. Actually, these three forms represent the smooth to intermediate to rough transformations of

C. diphtheriae. They were originally described and given these names by British workers who isolated the three types from epidemic diphtheria in England and felt that there was an association between colony type and severity of the disease. The mitis type was associated more commonly with mild disease, the intermedius, with mild or severe disease, and the gravis type with severe diphtheria. It is now known that severe or mild diphtheria can be produced by any one of these three types, though there seems to be tendency for gravis strains to produce severe disease more frequently than the other two. There is no adequate explanation at the moment for the greater virulence of gravis types because it is known that all three types produce the same exotoxin and apparently do not differ greatly in their capacity to produce and excrete the toxin. *C. diphtheriae* can also be divided into types and groups by serologic reactions (agglutination) or by typing with bacteriophage. None of these methods has proved useful for the identification of *C. diphtheriae* in suspected cases of diphtheria, however.

As previously noted, the only way in which a suspected culture of *Corynebacterium diphtheriae* can be certified as being fully virulent is to determine by a virulence test whether the strain produces diphtheria toxin. There are a number of methods for determining this, either in vivo or in vitro, and the details of the techniques can be found in appropriate manuals. It is important here only to illustrate the principles involved; once these are grasped, the actual procedures become simple. The detection of the production of toxin by a culture of *C. diphtheriae* depends upon showing the capacity of diphtheria antitoxin to neutralize the toxic activity. To do this, two guinea pigs, for example, may be employed. One of these guinea pigs is given 500 units of antitoxin parenterally. An hour or two later, both guinea pigs are injected with a suspension of viable cells of the suspected culture of *C. diphtheriae*. If the culture produces diphtheria exotoxin, the guinea pig which did not receive the antitoxin will die in three to five days whereas the one which received the antitoxin will not. The same type of test can be performed in either rabbits or guinea pigs by injecting the viable *C. diphtheriae* cells intradermally into animals one or more of which have been given antitoxin. If the culture produces toxin, the animals which did not receive antitoxin will develop necrotic ulcerating dermal lesions. Lesions will not appear on the skin of the animals given antitoxin. If the culture does not produce diphtheria exotoxin, none of the animals, whether or not treated with antitoxin, will show dermal lesions.

Diphtheria toxin can be detected in vitro by incorporating antitoxin into a solid culture medium. The suspected culture is then plated out on this medium. If the culture produces exotoxin, a precipitate will form around the colonies on the plate that contain antitoxin whereas no such precipitate will be found around the colonies on the culture medium under similar conditions which do not contain antitoxin. There are a number of modifications of this technique.

The determination of whether or not *Corynebacterium diphtheriae* strains isolated from patients suspected of having diphtheria are toxigenic is important for several reasons. First, it provides confirmation, or lack of it, for the diagnosis of true diphtheria in a given patient. Secondly, the virulence test provides a differentiation between toxin-producing and non–toxin-producing strains of *C. diphtheriae*. This is of significance because it is clear that in diphtheria epidemics, a notable though small proportion of cases suspected of being diphtheria and showing evidence of pharyngeal infection may be caused by nontoxigenic diphtheria bacilli. In order to gain a better perspective of the disease, it is important to gather information on the incidence of disease due to nontoxigenic strains of *C. diphtheriae* and on the relationships between these strains and the toxin-producing ones.

It has already been noted that people can be carriers of *Corynebacterium diphtheriae*, which is found in either the upper respiratory tract or infected cutaneous lesions. It is frequently necessary, particularly during an epidemic, to determine not only which contacts of cases of diphtheria are carriers but also which ones carry toxigenic strains and which carry nontoxigenic strains of *C. diphtheriae*. If a person harbors only nontoxigenic strains, he cannot be regarded as much of a menace to the community; however, that person who harbors toxin-producing *C. diphtheriae* may be a potential source of severe disease. The results of the virulence test may determine whether or not carriers should be treated in an attempt to eliminate the bacteria they harbor. It should be routine to obtain material by swab from the pharynx of all members of the patient's family and from contacts of patients in order to identify who are carriers, and who, therefore, face a greater risk of contracting the disease.

Treatment

It is the primary aim of treatment in diphtheria to neutralize the toxin being produced by the microorganisms at the site of infection. The logic of this follows from the fact that the serious consequences of diphtheritic infection, excluding obstruction of the airway by pseudomembrane, come from the effects of diphtheria toxin. Therapy should be directed toward neutralization of toxin as soon as possible. Once toxin has entered susceptible cells, neutralization with antitoxin is impossible; therefore, if antitoxin therapy is delayed for a day or two, toxin may have entered cells in an amount sufficient to bring about a fatal outcome. This places a great burden upon a physician who first encounters a case of pharyngitis which might be diphtheria. If the physician, recognizing the possibility of diphtheria, gives antitoxin immediately, he may unnecessarily be administering a foreign serum to a human being and possibly inducing hypersensitivity to a foreign protein. Severe allergic reactions may be elicited in patients already hypersensitive to the foreign protein, or serum sickness may ensue. On the other hand, he may be preventing a serious outcome due to the toxic effects of diphtheria toxin. A physician cannot administer antitoxin to every patient with pharyngitis whom he encounters in his practice. Therefore, considerable clinical judgment is required. Help in this regard can be provided by a consideration of certain epidemiologic factors (see below).

If antitoxin is administered, the amounts given should be based upon the severity of the infection. For severe cases, it is usually recommended that 40,000 to 80,000 units be given intravenously; in moderately severe cases,

20,000 to 40,000 units. If there is uncertainty concerning the amount to be given, it is better to err on the side of giving too much rather than too little.

Antibiotic therapy should be used as a supplement but never as a substitute for specific antitoxin therapy. Antibiotic therapy as a supplement is aimed at reducing the microbial load at the focus of infection and reducing the amount of toxin being formed. It also serves to control any concomitant infection; for example, with beta-hemolytic streptococci. Such therapy also tends to decrease the length of the carrier state, which otherwise may persist for weeks following recovery from the disease. Although penicillin can be used, erythromycin appears to be the most effective drug for the treatment of carriers.

Epidemiology

A knowledge of the epidemiology of diphtheria not only aids the physician in suspecting diphtheria in a patient or in detecting the beginning of an epidemic but also provides insight into the reservoirs of infection and mode of spread. This knowledge then leads to the elaboration of methods of control or prevention of disease. Diphtheria is a disease which provides a good illustration of how such information has been used for the control of an epidemic infectious disease of the upper respiratory tract.

Mortality and Morbidity

Figure 17–1 shows the mortality and morbidity rates from diphtheria in the United States during the last 50 years, and Figure 17–2 shows the number of cases that occurred from 1958 to 1972. It can be seen that the incidence of the disease has markedly decreased. At present, there are seldom more than 100 or 200 cases of diphtheria per year in the United States.

In sharp contrast to the decrease in incidence, however, the graph shows that the mortality rate has not decreased, i.e., the proportion of deaths that occur in persons who contract the disease.

Age Distribution

Figure 17–3 demonstrates the distribution according to age. It is of significance that diphtheria is primarily a disease of infants and children. Shortly after birth and for a few weeks thereafter, infants are protected by antitoxin received from the mother by way of the placenta. As this protection wanes, susceptibility increases, as does the incidence of the disease. With increasing age, susceptibility decreases. This decrease in susceptibility may be due not only to vaccination but also to subclinical exposure to *Corynebacterium diphtheriae* and, presumably, to exposure to minute amounts of toxin; this gradually induces an active immunity.

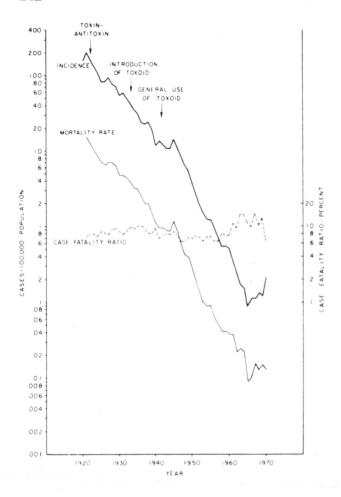

Figure 17-1. Diphtheria. Reported annual incidence, mortality rates, and case fatality ratio, United States, 1920 to 1970. (From Center for Disease Control, Morbidity and Mortality Weekly Report, No. 11, 1969–1970 Summary. December 31, 1971.)

Seasonal Distribution

Figure 17–4 shows the prevalence of diphtheria at different times during the year. In contrast to many upper respiratory diseases, the occurrence of diphtheria is greatest during the fall months. Classically, upper respiratory diseases usually have the highest incidence in the winter months. Diphtheria, however, can occur at any time of the year.

Geographic Distribution

Of particular importance is the geographic distribution (Fig. 17–5). The greatest incidence of diphtheria is in the southern and southeastern parts of the United States. A number of reasons can be given to account for this distribution. These areas of the country contain a large proportion of the

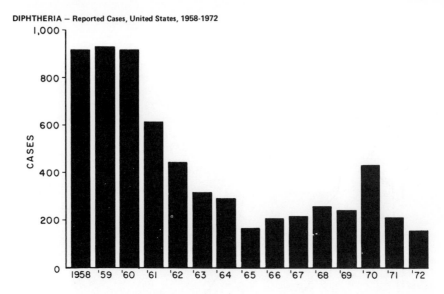

Figure 17–2. Diphtheria. Reported cases, United States, 1958 to 1972. (From Morbidity and Mortality Annual Supplement. Summary 1972. U. S. Department of Health, Education, and Welfare, Vol. 21, No. 53.)

people who do not have optimal living conditions. Crowding and lack of sanitation play a role in this situation because they promote the transmission of respiratory diseases. In addition, a great number of these people do not comprehend the need for vaccination. As a result, many of the children in these areas do not receive adequate vaccination. Currently, diphtheria is particularly prevalent among Mexican Americans living in the southern part of the United States. The somewhat warmer and more humid climate in the gulf States provides living conditions which promote the development of cutaneous diphtheria. Minor wounds and, in particular, insect bites traumatized by scratching can become infected from contact with playmates or from a pharyngeal carrier in the family. Infected cutaneous lesions may frequently follow an indolent course and remain open and discharge corynebacteria for long periods of time. These diphtheritic cutaneous lesions in turn can serve as a source for implantations of virulent corynebacteria in the pharynx of associates and family. There is a high correlation between the incidence of pharyngeal carriers of virulent *Corynebacterium diphtheriae* and the incidence of cutaneous lesions among these populations. Cutaneous lesions may be of greater importance in providing a persistent reservoir of diphtheritic infection in southern parts of the United States than are pharyngeal carriers.

Mode of Transmission

As has been previously noted, diphtheria is a disease which may be transmitted by droplet infection from active cases of the disease or from pharyngeal carriers. It also can be transmitted directly to susceptible persons

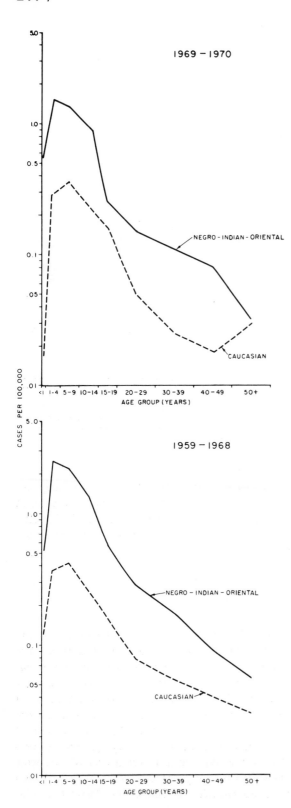

Figure 17–3. Average annual diphtheria attack rates, by age and racial groups, in the United States. (From Morbidity and Mortality Report No. 11. 1969–1970 Summary. U. S. Department of Health, Education, and Welfare, December 31, 1971.)

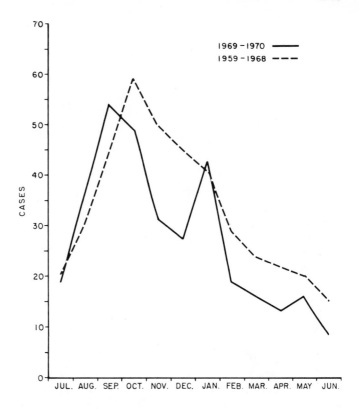

Figure 17-4. Average annual diphtheria cases, by month of onset, in the United States, 1969 to 1970 and 1959 to 1969. (From Morbidity and Mortality Report No. 11. 1969–1970 Summary. U. S. Department of Health, Education, and Welfare, December 31, 1971.)

from infected cutaneous lesions. Individuals with cutaneous lesions may also serve as a source of pharyngeal infection, and these carriers in turn may pass the infection to susceptible persons by droplet infection. Diphtheritic infection of susceptible persons by way of milk, other food, or by fomites is uncommon in the United States.

Nature of Outbreaks

Most cases of diphtheria in the United States at the present time occur in the form of small, or sometimes large, regional outbreaks. It is thus a true epidemic disease. The sources of many of these outbreaks are not known, but obviously certain conditions favoring spread must be present; i.e., a carrier of virulent corynebacteria, a supply of susceptible persons, and close association of persons. These epidemics occur primarily in the southern and southeastern parts of the United States for the reasons mentioned above. The pattern of appearance of diphtheria can be contrasted with that of epidemic cerebrospinal meningitis. In civilian populations, cases of meningococcal meningitis tend to be sporadic and separated from each other. There is no relationship between cases nor is there a recognizable common source of infection. This

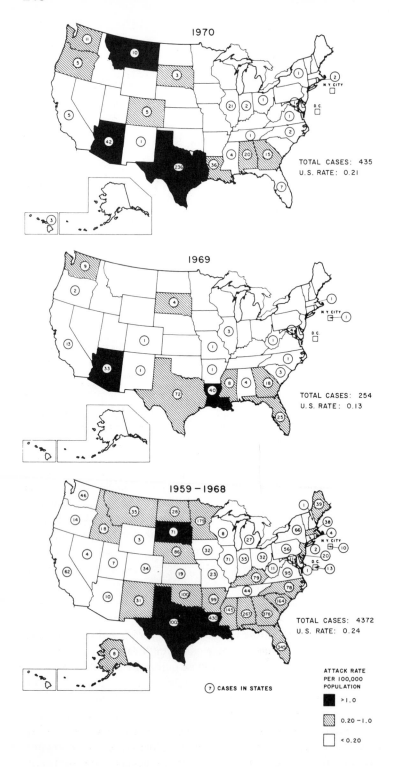

Figure 17–5. Reported diphtheria cases and annual attack rates by state in the United States. (From Morbidity and Mortality Report No. 11. 1969–1970 Summary. U. S. Department of Health, Education, and Welfare, December 31, 1971.)

can be accounted for by the fact that the carrier rate for virulent meningococci in the civilian population is much higher than the carrier rate for *Corynebacterium diphtheriae.* Meningococcal meningitis is really a disease of carriers because disease occurs only sporadically among a fairly large population of persons who harbor meningococci in the upper respiratory tract. On the other hand, the carrier rate for virulent *C. diphtheriae* in the general population is very low. Only when a carrier, or an individual with an unrecognized case of diphtheria, has contact with a population of susceptible persons will disease occur.

In epidemics of diphtheria, clinical disease occurs in both nonvaccinated susceptible persons and persons who have a history of some previous vaccination. Thus, vaccination does not necessarily prevent the development of infection and disease. This fact should be expected since it has already been noted that the diphtheria bacillus has the capacity to invade and multiply and bring about pseudomembrane formation independently of its capacity to produce exotoxin. Of particular importance, however, is the fact that mortality from the disease in epidemics is found almost exclusively in those persons who have not been vaccinated.

The explosiveness with which epidemic diphtherial disease can develop is well illustrated by the experience in Norway during the Second World War. In Norway, vaccination was not practiced, and thus a large pool of susceptible persons was built up. Prior to the German invasion, Norway had only about 50 cases of diphtheria a year, out of a total population of about 3 million. Within two years following the German invasion the number of cases of diphtheria had increased to approximately 50 thousand per year. The disruption of the economy and society brought about by the invasion may have played a role, but the presence of a large number of susceptible persons exposed to sources of infection, possibly brought in from Germany where the incidence of diphtheria had always been high, resulted in a rapid increase in the number of cases of the disease. Other European countries experienced some of the same problems with diphtheria during the early 1940s. Actually, diphtheria became the most prevalent infectious disease in Western Europe during World War II. Of interest is the fact that diphtheria also became the most common infectious disease among American troops in the European theater, even though many of these soldiers had been vaccinated. With this World War II experience to draw upon, one should not be too complacent about the low incidence of diphtheria in the United States today. A serious dislocation of the economy or society of the United States might well increase the problems with diphtheria as well as with other infectious diseases.

Prevention

Since diphtheria is a disease of the respiratory tract in which the major form of transmission is from person to person by droplet infection, there is no indirect way in which to control the spread of the disease. This situation stands in contrast to a disease such as typhoid fever, which is spread from person to person primarily by way of water and in which control is readily accomplished by purification of the drinking water supply. A disease that is transmitted from man to man or from animals to man by an insect vector can be prevented by elimination of the vector or eradication of the animal reservoir. No such methods exist for control of diseases of the respiratory tract. Physicans and public health workers have long realized that the only feasible way to control such a disease is to raise the level of resistance of the population at risk. Control of carriers and isolation or segregation of active cases of the respiratory disease offer partial solutions but are not sufficient in themselves.

The early discoveries that the severe manifestations of diphtheria come from the effects of diphtheria toxin and that toxin could be neutralized by antitoxin offered a logical procedure for reducing the prevalence of diphtheria. If toxin could be used to vaccinate susceptible persons, these individuals would produce antibody against toxin and if subsequently exposed to infection with virulent *Corynebacterium diphtheriae* would be immune since they would have antitoxin available to neutralize any toxin formed by the invading bacteria. This, at least, was the hope. Early attempts to immunize susceptible persons using toxin or toxin neutralized with antitoxin proved to be unfeasible because of the high incidence of morbidity due to the toxin. It was not until it was discovered that diphtheria toxin could be easily detoxified by exposing it to small amounts of formalin, without simultaneously affecting its antigenicity, did preparations become available that could safely be used for the immunization of susceptible infants, children, and adults. The best pediatric practice now requires vaccination of all infants and children against diphtheria, using diphtheria toxoid. Widespread use of the vaccination against diphtheria began about 1923, and there has since been a steady decline in the incidence of diphtheria until only 152 cases were reported in the whole United States in 1972.

It has been mentioned previously that some adults may produce enough antitoxin to be immune, presumably owing to subclinical exposure to *Corynebacterium diphtheriae*. These persons may also have developed a hypersensitivity either to toxin or other proteins found in *C. diphtheriae*. Persons who are hypersensitive to diphtheria toxin or other protein products of *C. diphtheriae* may develop serious local or systemic allergic reactions if given full vaccinating doses of diphtheria toxoid. Therefore, when the need arises to vaccinate adults, an attempt should be made to determine not only their immune status, which would indicate whether vaccination is really necessary, but also whether they are hypersensitive to the vaccine.

Fortunately, a test is available for this purpose. This is called the *Schick test* after Dr. Bela Schick, who devised the test. Essentially, this test consists of injecting a small amount of toxin (1/50 of a guinea pig minimal lethal dose) into the skin on the volar surface of one of the forearms of the person being tested. As a control, the same toxin preparation which has been heated to 70°C for at least 10 minutes to destroy toxicity should be injected into the skin on the volar surface of the other arm. This heated material will retain its capacity to elicit allergic reactions. A better control is to use the fluid toxoid vaccine preparation. This is usually diluted 1 to 10, and 0.1 ml is injected into the skin. The injection sites are inspected every day, and a recording is made of the degree of erythema, induration, and necrosis.

The interpretation of the results of the Schick test is difficult. The physician must keep in mind the fact that he is determining two things by this test: (1) the state of hypersensitivity to diphtheria toxin or other proteins of diphtheria cells, and (2) the presence of antitoxin and, therefore, information regarding the immunity of the person. If the person has sufficient circulating antitoxin to neutralize the Schick test toxic dose (immune) but happens to be sensitive to one or more antigens in the toxin preparation, he will show a reaction to both the toxoid (or the heated toxin control) and the toxin. However, these allergic reactions usually reach their peak at about 48 hours and then fade rapidly over the next one or two days. This is in marked contrast to a true positive Schick reaction which persists for many days. Such a result is known as a *pseudo-reaction.* If the person being tested does not have enough antitoxin in his serum to neutralize the Schick test dose but happens to be allergic to an antigen in the vaccine, he will exhibit reactions in both arms also; however, the reaction in the arm which receives the active toxin increases in size and does not reach a maximum until about five days later. Usually, this reaction eventually becomes necrotic, brown in color, and sloughs. The reaction in the arm which received the control injection almost completely subsides by day 5. Such a response is known as a *combined reaction.* A completely susceptible (no antitoxin) person who is not allergic will show a reaction only in the arm receiving the toxin. This is known as a *positive reaction,* whereas a person who is immune because of sufficient antitoxin but who is not allergic will not show a response in either arm. This person is regarded as being *immune.* The types of reactions which we have described are summarized in Table 17–1.

TABLE 17–1. Reactions to Schick Test*

	Skin Response				
	Toxin		Toxoid (or Heated Toxin)		
	36 hr	120 hr	36 hr	120 hr	Interpretation
Positive	−	+	−	−	Nonimmune; nonsensitive
Negative	−	−	−	−	Immune; nonsensitive
Pseudo	+	−	+	−	Immune; sensitive
Combined	+	+	+	−	Nonimmune; sensitive

*From Davis, B. D., et al.: Microbiology. 2nd ed. Hagerstown, Maryland, Harper and Row, 1973, p. 689.

Other types of reactions may sometimes be seen. Wheal and flare reactions which appear within a few minutes after injection can occur and may be due to reaginic antibody (IgE) produced by some people to toxin. The delayed allergic reactions are usually regarded as being true reactions of delayed hypersensitivity. However, one must always keep in mind the possibility that some of these may be Arthus type reactions due to interaction between toxin and antitoxin. Since even the most purified toxin is not completely free of contaminating material, it is difficult to be sure of the nature of the antigen responsible for all of the allergic reactions.

A person who is proved to be susceptible but allergic by the Schick test should be vaccinated with caution. Doses of the vaccine should be greatly reduced, and the number of injections increased. Such a person probably should be given another Schick test in about two weeks. A person who shows allergic reactions to the toxin preparations may well have his antitoxin level boosted sufficiently by the Schick test dose of toxin itself that a negative test will be obtained if he is retested two to three weeks later. Such a conversion would eliminate the necessity for a regular course of vaccination.

Diphtheria Outbreaks*

Chicago, Illinois

Between December 15, 1969 and February 8, 1970, 21 cases of diphtheria occurred in 12 unrelated households in the northwest part of the city, a low income, high population density area. There were two deaths yielding a case-fatality ratio of 9.5 per cent. The 12 household groups were 3/4 to 13 miles apart, the children of each of the 12 families attended different schools, and the family members had no contact with the other affected families through child care services, travel or holiday experience, or recreation or work experience. Nineteen of the patients had cultures positive for *Corynebacterium diphtheriae.* Fifteen isolates from patients in nine households were toxigenic *C. diphtheriae,* intermedius type. Toxigenic mitis types were cultured from three patients in two additional households and nontoxigenic mitis type from the sole patient in a different household. The lack of known epidemiologic association between the households suggests a multifocal origin.

Those patients with prior immunization tended to have mild or moderate disease while severe disease occurred only in unimmunized patients. Eleven of the 21 patients had mild illness at the time of diagnosis. Six patients had moderate disease, and the other four (including two fatal cases) were classified as severe.

Severe or moderately severe disease was reported early in the outbreak, while later the reported patients tended to have mild disease (Table 17–1). During a period of low awareness in Chicago, from January, 1957 to November, 1969, 45 cases of diphtheria were diagnosed with a case-fatality ratio of 29 per cent. During the 1969–1970 outbreak, the case-fatality ratio was 9.5 per cent, and both of the deaths occurred within the first month of the outbreak.

---

*The following discussions concerning diphtheria outbreaks in Illinois, Arizona, Oregon, and Texas are from the Center for Disease Control, United States Department of Health, Education, and Welfare.

TABLE 17-2. Diphtheria Cases by Week of Diagnosis, Clinical Severity, and Outcome, 1969-1970, Chicago, Cook County, Illinois*

Date of Diagnosis by Two-Week Periods Beginning	Clinical Severity			Fatal Outcome	Total Cases
	Mild	Moderate	Severe		
12/15/69	0	0	3	1	3
12/29/69	5	4	1	1	10
1/12/70	2	2	1	0	5
1/26/70	3	0	0	0	3
Total	10	6	5	2	21

*From Center for Disease Control, Report No. 11, 1969-1970 Summary, December 31, 1971.

In diphtheria outbreaks it has been a common experience that the index of clinical suspicion rises at a pace equal to the number of cases diagnosed and results in earlier diagnosis, earlier institution of treatment, and a lower case-fatality rate. In the Chicago outbreak, the first three cases diagnosed were severe (two were fatal) and the next 18 mild or moderate, suggesting that early in the outbreak only severe cases were recognized as diphtheria and that prior to the period of increased awareness milder cases may have existed, but were not diagnosed. For the United States a case-fatality ratio of about 10 per cent has been reported for each of the last 50 years. In outbreaks of diphtheria, however, case-fatality ratios of 5 per cent and less have been reported, in most instances decreasing as the outbreak progressed.

Arizona; New Mexico (Navajo Indian Reservation)

Between January 1 and October 7, 1973, 44 cases of diphtheria were reported on or near the Navajo Indian Reservation in Arizona and New Mexico (Fig. 17-6); 29 of the 44 cases occurred since August 1. Thirty-seven persons were hospitalized. Five patients had myocarditis and/or varying degrees of neurologic involvement, and two of these had respiratory arrests and required artificial ventilation. There were no deaths. Throat swabs from 28 of the 44 persons were positive for toxigenic Corynebacterium diphtheriae, biotype intermedius. From the same area, a total of 10 cases were reported in 1970, 30 cases in 1971, and 20 cases in 1972.

Of the 29 cases occurring since August 1, 1973, 22 were in females, and 24 were in persons 15 years of age or older (Table 17-3). Throat swabs from 118 contacts of 12 culture-proven cases were taken, and 18 were positive for toxigenic Corynebacterium diphtheriae, biotype intermedius (Table 17-4). Although the majority of cases were in persons 15 years of age or older, the carrier rates were highest in persons under 15 years.

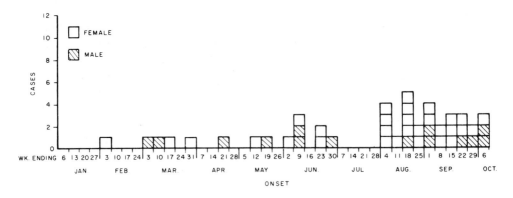

Figure 17–6. Forty-four diphtheria cases, by week of onset, Navajo Indian Reservation, January 1 to October 6, 1973. (From Morbidity and Mortality Weekly Report. U. S. Department of Health, Education, and Welfare, Vol. 22, No. 41.)

TABLE 17–3. Age and Sex Distribution for 29 Diphtheria Cases
Navajo Indian Reservation — August 1–October 7, 1973*

	Age Group (Years)			Total
	0–4	*5–14*	*15+*	
Male	1	1	5	7
Female	0	2	20	22
Total	1	3	25	29
Rate per 100,000	23	27	103	153

*From Center for Disease Control, Morbidity and Mortality Weekly Report, Vol. 22, No. 41, 1973.

TABLE 17–4. Age and Sex Distribution and Proportion of Persons Culture-Positive
for *C. diphtheriae* Among Contacts of 12 Culture-Proven Cases
Navajo Indian Reservation — 1973*

	Age Group (Years)			Total	Per Cent Positive
	0–4	*5–14*	*15+*		
Male	1/5**	6/21	3/28	10/50	20.0
Female	2/8	4/22	2/38	8/68	11.8
Total	3/13	10/43	5/66	18/118	15.3
Per cent positive	23.1	23.3	7.6	15.3	

*From Center for Disease Control, Morbidity and Mortality Weekly Report, Vol. 22, No. 41, 1973.
**Number positive/Number tested.

Epidemiologic investigation showed that five cases occurring before August 1 were in students at a single school, which accounted for almost half of the cases reported in the 5- to 14-year age group since January 1. In September a sixth case was reported in a teacher at the same school. The only other cases that could be linked epidemiologically were two cases in neighbors and two in a sister-in-law and a brother-in-law living in separate households.

Vaccination histories of injection dates from clinic and hospital records were available for 28 cases; 6 had been fully vaccinated, 14 had been incompletely vaccinated, and 8 had no history of vaccination.

Portland, Oregon

In April and May, 1970, three cases of diphtheria (one fatal) were reported from the Portland, Oregon, area. The first patient, a 59-year-old woman, had onset of illness on April 30. She had severe pharyngitis with membrane formation, fever, and respiratory distress, but no evidence of myocarditis or neuropathy. She was treated with 80,000 units of diphtheria antitoxin and underwent tracheostomy. She was also given erythromycin and recovered.

On May 11, a 64-year-old man with a history of hospitalization for chronic lung disease was again hospitalized after six days of an acute illness. He was resuscitated but died 18 hours later. At autopsy, a membrane was found in the trachea and the area near the carina, but no evidence of pharyngitis was found. A sputum culture obtained on admission grew toxigenic *Corynebacterium diphtheriae*.

On May 15 the third case was reported in a 56-year-old man with sore throat and fever of three days' duration. He had typical membranous pharyngitis which was confirmed by culture as toxigenic *Corynebacterium diphtheriae*. He was treated with antitoxin and penicillin and recovered.

Investigation determined that the only epidemiologic association common to the three patients was exposure to the skid row area of the city. The woman had been shopping in thrift shops in the area twice during the week prior to onset of illness. The two men lived in different hotels in the area but on opposite sides of the river. The patient who died had been out of the hospital for 15 days prior to his illness but had not left his hotel in the interim. Persons at both hotels were cultured, and nontoxigenic *Corynebacterium diphtheriae* was isolated from one asymptomatic person, the owner of one of the hotels.

The contacts of the woman patient were immunized, and an immunization program was begun in the skid row area. Twenty-three of 25 residents at one hotel and 22 of 30 residents at the second hotel were given boosters. Health department personnel also conducted immunization clinics in neighborhood gathering places (food lines, bars, and hotels).

San Antonio, Texas

From June, 1969, through December, 1970, 206 cases of diphtheria were reported from San Antonio, Bexar County, Texas. This total number of cases exceeded the number reported from this area over the preceding 20 years. There were three deaths, an overall case-fatality ratio of 1.5 per cent. One hundred and fifty-one (73 per cent) of the 206 cases were bacteriologically confirmed; the biotype of 92 isolates was determined: 61 per cent were intermedius, 18 per cent mitis, and 12 per cent gravis.

The number of cases per month rose from one in June, 1969, to 63 in August, 1970, when the epidemic peaked (Fig. 17–7). One hundred ninety-six of 206 cases occurred in 1970, and the attack rate for the city of San Antonio during 1970 was 25 per 100,000 population as compared to a rate of 0.21 per 100,000 for the United States. Within the city, the epidemic was centered in the lower socioeconomic areas, and the attack rate among Negroes was 45.6 per 100,000 population, among Spanish-Americans 48.6 per 100,000 population, compared with 3.8 per 100,000 population for others (Table 17–5).

In May, 1969, prior to the onset of the epidemic, an immunization survey in San Antonio showed that only 33 per cent of persons 5 to 14 years of age were adequately immunized (see Table 17–6), far below the 1969 national estimate of 62 per cent for persons aged 5 to 14 living in central cities in the United States. The highest age specific attack rates in San Antonio were 50.6 per 100,000 in the five to nine age group and 68.9 per 100,000 population in the 10 to 14 age group. The rates in these age groups exceeded those noted in all other major diphtheria outbreaks in the United States in recent years. Only one case was reported in an adult over age 50, and two cases in children less than one year of age. At the height of the epidemic in mid-August, 1970,

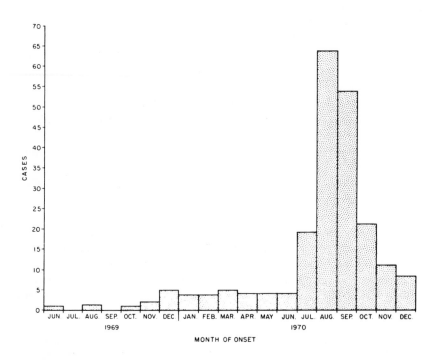

Figure 17–7. Diphtheria cases, by month of onset, San Antonio, Bexar County, Texas, 1969 to 1970. (From Morbidity and Mortality Report No. 11. 1969–1970 Summary. U. S. Department of Health, Education, and Welfare, December 31, 1971.)

TABLE 17–5. Diphtheria Attack Rate by Ethnic Group, San Antonio, Bexar County, Texas. June, 1969 to December, 1970*

Ethnic Group	Number of Cases	Attack Rate**
White, Spanish surname	156	48.6
Negro	25	45.6
White, Non-Spanish surname	15	3.8
ALL GROUPS	196	25.3

*From Center for Disease Control, Report No. 11, 1969–1970 Summary, December 31, 1971.
**Per 100,000 population based on projected total population for San Antonio, September, 1970, as per the Department of City Planning Statistical Guide, 1969 and the 1960 U. S. Census' distribution of the city's population by ethnic group.

mass immunization clinics were held and these were followed by neighborhood and school immunization clinics. During August and September, 1970, an estimated 452,000 vaccinations were administered; 15 per cent of these were boosters and the remainder constituted part of primary diphtheria immunization series. The monthly case rate gradually declined after October, 1970. In December, 1970, it was estimated that 74 per cent of children ages 5 to 14 in San Antonio were adequately immunized against diphtheria.

The immunization status was known for 182 of 196 cases with onset in 1970. Forty-six (23 per cent) were fully immunized and 136 (77 per cent) were inadequately immunized. Seventy-six per cent of the severe cases and all three of the fatalities occurred in inadequately immunized patients.

Certain segments of the United States population, predominantly those in the urban slums, remain inadequately immunized against diphtheria, and the danger of the occurrence of a large diphtheria outbreak is still present. San

TABLE 17–6. Per Cent of Population Fully Immunized Against Diphtheria by Age Group, and Socioeconomic Status, San Antonio, Bexar County, Texas, June, 1969 to December, 1970*

Age Group In Years	Socioeconomic Class			Total For City of San Antonio
	Lower	Middle	Upper	
1–4	60	58	85	67
5–14	28	24	49	33
15–39	24	23	35	27
40+	11	15	25	18

*From Center for Disease Control, Report No. 11, 1969–1970 Summary, December 31, 1971.

Antonio physicians were alert to the possibility of diphtheria because of the epidemic of 88 cases in Austin, Texas, from October, 1967, to April 1969. Although the estimated immunization level for San Antonio in May, 1969, was not sufficient to prevent the epidemic, the increased awareness of the disease probably led to earlier recognition and treatment during the epidemic and the low case-fatality ratio of 1.5 per cent.

References

Books

Davis, B. D., Dulbecco, R., Eisen, H. N., Ginsberg, H. S., Wood, W. B., and McCarty, M. (eds.): Microbiology. 2nd ed. Hagerstown, Maryland, Harper and Row, 1973.
Hoeprich, P. D. (ed.): Infectious Diseases. Hagerstown, Maryland, Harper and Row, 1972.

Original Articles

Belsey, M. A., Sinclair, M., Roder, M. R., et al.: Corynebacterium skin infections in Alabama and Louisiana. N. Engl. J. Med. *280:*135, 1969.
Boissard, J. M., and Fry, R. M.: Chronic nasal diphtheria carriers: Cure with sulphanilamide. Lancet *1:*610, 1942.
Brooks, G. F.: Recent trends in diphtheria in the United States. J. Infect. Dis. *120:*500, 1969.
Downes, J. J.: Primary diphtheritic otitis media. Arch. Otolaryngol. *70:*37, 1959.
Kallick, C. A., Brooks, G. F., Dover, A. S., Brown, M. C., and Brolnitsky, O.: A diphtheria outbreak in Chicago. Ill. Med. J. *12:*505, 1970.
Liebow, A. A., MacLean, J. H., Bumstead, J. M., and Welt, L. G.: Tropical ulcers and cutaneous diphtheria. Arch. Intern. Med. *78:*255, 1946.
Naiditch, M. J., and Bower, A. G.: Diphtheria. A study of 1433 cases observed during a 10-year period at the Los Angeles County Hospital. Am. J. Med. *17:*229, 1954.
San Antonio Metropolitan Health District, Bexar County, Texas, Immunization survey, May 1969, Appendix 4, Table 4, October 22, 1969.
Tasman A., and Lansberg, H. P.: Problems concerning the prophylaxis, pathogenesis, and therapy of diphtheria. Bull. WHO:939, 1957.
Zalma, V. M., Older, J. J., and Brooks, G. F.: The Austin, Texas diphtheria outbreak: Clinical and epidemiological aspects. J.A.M.A. *211:*2125, 1970.

Chapter 18

NONBACTERIAL UPPER RESPIRATORY TRACT DISEASE

Introduction

Nonbacterial infections of the upper respiratory tract are due to viruses and mycoplasma. These infectious agents are usually associated with mild localized illnesses which are accompanied by minor but discomforting constitutional symptoms. Typical diseases include rhinitis, pharyngitis, tonsillitis, laryngitis, and the common cold. Upper respiratory tract disease may also occur during the prodromal stage of more serious but less frequent constitutional illnesses such as measles or smallpox. The present discussion is concerned chiefly with those respiratory illnesses which are local rather than systemic in character.

Local upper respiratory tract infections cause morbidity at all age levels and are a source of great economic loss whether measured as lost wages, lost time, drug costs, or physicians' office visits. These illnesses are difficult to prevent and do not respond strikingly to medical treatment. Although for the most part, upper respiratory tract diseases are mild illnesses which lack the emotional overtones generally imparted to systemic diseases with high mortality rates, they are probably responsible for physiologic and immunologic stresses which acutely aggravate chronic diseases and may cause delayed effects which remain to be defined.

Nonbacterial agents that infect the upper respiratory tract are spread chiefly by airborne routes or by personal contact. Initial localization of these agents in the respiratory tract — a convenient portal of entry and exit — depends to a large extent on the particle size of the aerosol in which they are carried.

Large particles, usually greater than 5μ in diameters, are principally retained in the upper respiratory tract; smaller particles tend to be deposited in the lower respiratory passages. Following implantation on respiratory mucosa and penetration to mucosal cells, these infectious agents multiply locally and may subsequently spread to other portions of the body. (See Chap. 2.)

Normal respiratory tract infections are not, in general, precisely defined syndromes. They are better described as a set of disorders which chiefly affect nasopharyngeal tissues and present with a spectrum of clinical manifestations. As a rule, each illness is named after the anatomic site of maximal symptoms; e.g., an acute upper respiratory tract infection with mild sore throat, slight pain on swallowing, hoarseness, and fever would be called laryngitis. Moreover, each nonbacterial respiratory tract infectious agent has been associated with more than one clinical picture. Consequently, there is not a strict one-to-one correspondence between a particular clinical picture and a particular infectious agent (see Table 18–1).

TABLE 18-1. Spectrum of Illness by Some Respiratory Viruses*

	Cold	Febrile Cold	Influenza	Croup	Pneumonia	Bronchiolitis
Rhinovirus	++++	++				
Coxsackie A21	++++	+++	++			
Influenza A	+	++	++++	+++	++	+
Respiratory syncytial	++	++	+	+	+++	+++
Parainfluenza 3	++	++	+	+	++++	
Parainfluenza 1	++	++	+++	++++	+++	

*Modified from Tyrell, D. A. J.: Etiology of acute respiratory viral disease. *In* Conference on Newer Respiratory Disease Viruses. Am. Rev. Resp. Dis. Supplement, 1962.

Viral and mycoplasmal infections do not always result in overt clinical illnesses. Some resistance factors that determine susceptibility to these agents are known (see Chap. 4). Age, for example, is important because exposure to an increasing number of agents over a matter of time results in progressively broader immunity. Occupation is also important; e.g., housewives have more upper respiratory tract illness than their husbands because mothers usually have greater contact with their sick children than do fathers. Local barriers at respiratory mucosal surfaces include humoral factors such as mucoprotein nonspecific inhibitors, interferon, and specific immunoglobulins. Nonspecific factors that affect the physiologic state of respiratory membranes, e.g., humidity, smoke, and allergy, may affect the severity of upper respiratory tract disease.

Some Viruses and Mycoplasma Causing Upper Respiratory Tract Infections

A central fact to remember about upper respiratory tract infections is the great diversity of infectious agents which have been associated with illness. More than 50 per cent of the viruses which infect man (see Chap. 11) have been associated with upper respiratory tract infections. Two of six Mycoplasma species that infect man, *Mycoplasma pneumoniae* and *M. hominis,* also cause upper respiratory tract illnesses. A description of these agents involves examining a considerable portion of the area of human virology. Some appreciation of progress is gained by a more or less historic approach.

Influenza Viruses

The influenza viruses were the earliest viral agents associated with respiratory tract illnesses in man. Types A, B, and C influenza viruses belong to the orthomyxoviruses subgroup, i.e., the "true" myxoviruses. Orthomyxoviruses, which have a segmented genome, and paramyxoviruses, in which the genome is continuous, are subgroups of the myxovirus groups. The myxoviruses are so named because these viruses possess virus-specific neuraminidases which react with many mucoproteins containing an *N*-acetylneuraminic acid moiety.

Type A influenza virus, which was first isolated in England in 1933, is an important cause of upper respiratory tract disease, usually in association with yearly outbreaks of nonbacterial lower respiratory tract infection and the severe systemic syndrome called "la grippe" or "flu." *Type B* influenza viruses, which are antigenically distinct from type A and type C viruses, were first isolated in 1940 during an outbreak of pharyngitis in a boys' boarding school. Type B influenza causes outbreaks of respiratory disease with lower frequency than type A viruses and tends to cause a milder clinical illness than does type A virus. *Type C* influenza virus was first isolated in 1947. This agent causes mild respiratory tract disease in children and is not a major problem. Properties of influenza viruses and diseases associated with these agents are considered in greater detail in Chapter 22.

Adenoviruses

Adenoviruses are an important cause of nonbacterial pharyngitis, conjunctivitis, and respiratory tract disease. The earliest adenoviruses were isolated in 1953 directly from adenoidal tissue which was grown in tissue culture during studies of upper respiratory tract disease in children. When the adenoidal tissue or tonsil tissue was cultured, the cells appeared to proliferate well for three to seven weeks. Occasionally a few batches would show a typical cytopathic effect which was caused by a transmissible agent. Because of the tissues from which they were isolated, they were called *adenoidal* agents. Later, when similar viruses were isolated from adults and children with nonbacterial pharyngitis and epidemic forms of conjunctivitis, this group of agents was called the adenoidal-pharyngeal-conjunctival viruses, the A-P-C group.

Adenoviruses cause somewhat less that 10 per cent of all nonbacterial upper respiratory tract disease in civilian groups. Among military recruits, who live under somewhat crowded conditions, the proportion of adenovirus respiratory tract illnesses rises above 50 per cent. Recently, several adenoviruses have been associated with hemorrhagic cystitis of children.

Adenoviruses are nonenveloped DNA viruses (60 to 90 nm diameter) which show a high degree of symmetry in their structure. The viral capsid, or protein covering, has 20 triangular facets containing 252 capsomeres. There are 12 vertex capsomeres each consisting of a penton capsomere and a fiber projection. The remaining 240 nonvertex capsomeres make up faces and sides of the triangular facets (Fig. 18–1). Nonvertex capsomeres possess group-specific antigens which are common to all adenoviruses and type-specific antigens which identify the 33 human subtypes. The group antigen is recognized by the complement-fixation reaction, and individual serotypes are recognized by neutralization tests. Vertex-capsomeres and their fiber projection are chiefly concerned with attachment of virus to cells.

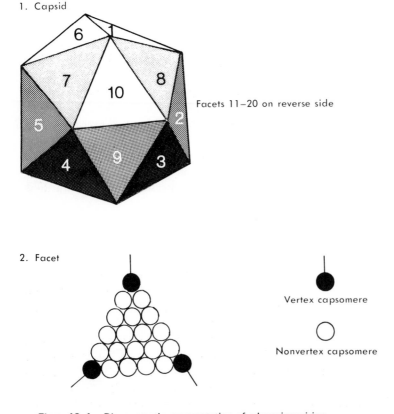

1. Capsid

Facets 11–20 on reverse side

2. Facet

Vertex capsomere

Nonvertex capsomere

Figure 18–1. Diagrammatic representation of adenovirus virion.

Most adenoviruses grow readily in tissue cultures and can be isolated without difficulty from throat swabs, conjunctival smears, and stools. The diagnosis of infection with adenovirus is made by viral isolation or by demonstrating a fourfold or greater increase in complement-fixation antibody titers between acute and convalescent antisera. Epidemiologic surveys show that types 1, 2, and 5 are important causes of upper respiratory tract disease in children; in addition, type 7 adenovirus causes severe pneumonia in children. Types 3, 4, 7, 14, and 21 are important causes of illness in military recruits.

The fact that some adenoviruses cause infection more frequently than others suggests that vaccines containing only a few of the many adenoviruses might be effective. Adenoviral vaccines made with killed virus were found to be effective against infection with homotypic viruses. However, studies in military groups showed that prevention of one type of adenoviral infection in a test population appeared to promote infection with a second adenovirus. For example, vaccination with type 4 adenoviral vaccine resulted in a decrease in type 4 infections but also an increase in the number of type 7 infections. This suggests that a polyvalent adenoviral vaccine might be more effective than a monovalent vaccine.

Further studies of adenoviral vaccines have been delayed, for the most part, by concern that batches of type 7 adenovirus which were grown in monkey kidney and intended as seed virus for vaccine preparation contained antigens of a simian virus that induced vacuolation of cells, SV40 virus. It was found that SV40 virus and hybrids of adenovirus with SV40 virus induced solid tumors in hamsters and malignant transformation of hamster cells and led to development of "T" or tumor antigens on the surface of the tumor cells. Subsequently, it was shown that adenoviruses types 3, 12, 18, and 31 also led to the development of tumors in baby hamsters. These animals developed type-specific neutralizing antibody against the infecting virus and also induced antibody against the T antigen. However, there is no direct evidence that SV40 virus or hybrids which may have inadvertently been injected cause tumors in man. Recently, the possibility that adenovirus might be a common cause of cancer was examined in a collaborative hospital study in which 197 cancer patients and 192 controls were examined for anti-T antibodies. The proportion showing such antibodies was the same in both groups.

Parainfluenza Viruses

Parainfluenza viruses are large (80 to 120 nm) RNA viruses which are classified among the paramyxoviruses. Four serotypes of parainfluenza virus infect man. The first, Sendai virus, the prototype parainfluenza type 1 virus, was isolated in mice that were inoculated with lung suspension from a case of pneumonia in a child and was initially called influenza D because it agglutinated chicken red blood cells. It now appears that the mice inoculated with the lung specimen had a latent infection with Sendai virus. Subsequently, several paramyxoviruses were found in man and also in cattle and monkeys. Types 1 and 2 parainfluenza viruses cause approximately one out of every three cases of croup in children one to four years of age, and type 3 virus is an infrequent cause of lower respiratory tract disease during the first year of life. Serologic surveys suggest that type 4 parainfluenza virus may be a common agent of respiratory tract infection in man, but its relation to human disease is not fully established.

Parainfluenza viruses cause recurrent illnesses in man. The initial illness in children which appears in the absence of antibody may be an upper respiratory tract infection with or without croup — or if more severe — bronchitis and pneumonia. Reinfection with the same type of parainfluenza virus can occur in the presence of circulating antibody, but the illness which results is less severe.

Recurrent parainfluenza viral infection in the adult usually causes mild respiratory illness. Occasionally, however, hoarseness — an adult equivalent of croup — is seen.

Parainfluenza viruses grow well in tissue culture. However, since they vary in their capacity to cause cytopathic changes, the presence of parainfluenza virus in tissue cultures is detected by placing fresh guinea pig cells in the culture tube and then rinsing the tubes with buffer. If parainfluenza virus infects the tissue culture, clusters of red cell adherence, called *hemadsorption,* are present (see Chap. 11). The reaction can be prevented by placing parainfluenza antiserum in the culture tube before adding red cells. Inhibition of hemadsorption is used to ascertain the serotype of an isolate.

Certain parainfluenza viruses, e.g., Sendai virus, can cause fusion of adjacent cells in tissue culture with production of syncytia. This property, which has been referred to earlier, appears to be independent of the ability of the virus to infect cells, since it is retained even after the virus is inactivated by ultraviolet light. This phenomenon has been employed as a possible means for recovery of latent viruses from tissues which may not be capable of supporting their growth. Apparently, virus which is latent within a non-permissive cell leaves its latency if the nonpermissive cell is fused with a cell which would support multiplication of the virus, i.e., a permissive cell (Fig. 18–2). Cell fusion was used recently for the isolation of polyoma-like virus from the brain of patients with multifocal leukoencephalopathy.

Another property of parainfluenza viruses is that they can establish a chronic noncytopathic infection in certain cells. The infected cells slowly release virus and can divide. The daughter cells also shed virus. The chronic infection apparently does not severely disrupt important cell biochemical mechanisms since the cells can be superinfected with other viruses, e.g., poliomyelitis virus. The implications of cell fusion and chronic infection by the parainfluenza viruses for potential human disease are still unexplored.

Respiratory Syncytial Viruses

In 1956, a new agent was isolated from pharyngeal secretions of a chimpanzee with an upper respiratory tract infection and from an animal caretaker responsible for the chimpanzee. This new agent, also a large RNA virus (80 to 120 nm), was serologically distinct from paramyxoviruses identified at that time. Because the agent also caused characteristic syncytial changes in tissue cultures, it was named *respiratory syncytial virus (RS).*

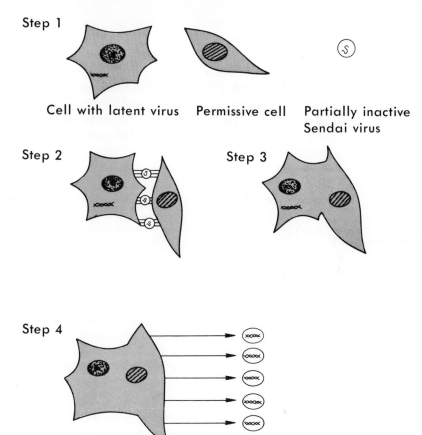

Figure 18–2. Schematic representation of cell fusion. *Step 1,* Mix components. *Step 2,* Agglutination of cells. *Step 3,* Fusion of cell walls. *Step 4,* Multiplication and release of latent virus from the hybrid.

This virus is an important cause of lower respiratory tract infections during the first six months of life. Reinfection occurs in older children and adults and causes less severe disease, affecting the upper respiratory tract. The lack of protection against reinfection by antibody seen in man has its laboratory counterpart and may be a model for other recurrent viral infection of man. Addition of respiratory syncytial virus antibody to cell cultures after inoculation with virus does not prevent formation of focal collections of infected cells and syncytia. This laboratory finding suggests that there is a cell-to-cell spread of the virus and accounts for spread of the virus in a partially immune host.

Inactivated viral vaccines prepared against this virus stimulate high levels of circulating antibody, and initially it was hoped that respiratory infections in infants could be prevented by vaccination. However, infants given these viral vaccines unexpectedly had more severe illnesses during subsequent outbreaks of respiratory syncytial virus than did unvaccinated controls. This adverse effect of vaccination of infants was attributed to a possible cellular reaction to antibody-virus complexes formed in vivo or to possible cellular hypersensitivity induced by the vaccine.

The reaction to respiratory syncytial viral vaccine is considered by many to be parallel to the reaction seen in children vaccinated with killed measles (rubeola) viral vaccine. Children inoculated with killed measles vaccine developed high titers of antimeasles antibody and experienced fewer cases of measles when exposed than did unvaccinated controls. After killed measles vaccine was released for general use and administered to large numbers of children, some recipients showed an unexpected effect. Following exposure to wild or "street" measles virus, measles infection occurred but demonstrated a modified illness which was associated with a peripheral rash. In the case of measles, the problem of immunization was solved by development of a live viral vaccine which does not induce the altered reactive state. A live vaccine for prevention of respiratory syncytial infection is not at hand.

Picornaviruses

The picornaviruses include two major subgroups: (1) rhinoviruses (15 to 30 nm), which grow best in tissue culture at 33°C, lose their infectivity when held one to three hours at a pH of 3 or lower, and (2) enteroviruses (30 to 50 nm), which grow well at 37°C and retain infectivity when kept at a pH of 3. These properties are believed to account for the facts that rhinoviruses are limited to nasal passages where low temperatures prevail and enteroviruses survive passage through the acidic environment of the stomach. Both groups are classed as nonenveloped RNA viruses.

The mid-1950s saw another major advance in the association of rhinoviruses with upper respiratory tract diseases. Serum neutralization methods have now identified 56 distinct serotypes of rhinoviruses that infect man, and more than 40 possibly unrelated strains remain to be classified, Rhinoviruses do not share a common antigen, and there seems to be little antigenic cross-reactivity between various serotypes. Each serotype induces homotypic antibody and probably prevents reinfection with the same serotype. However, there seems to be little protection against reinfection with another strain.

The clinical syndrome associated with the rhinoviruses is the "common cold." The benign nature of rhinoviral illnesses usually does not induce most physicians to attempt virologic studies in patients with this illness. The virus can be isolated from nasal and pharyngeal washings, and serologic and diagnostic procedures are available. Although rhinoviral vaccines are antigenic, the large number of serotypes suggests that vaccination is not the optimum of prevention.

The enterovirus group includes *coxsackieviruses, echoviruses* and *polioviruses.* Coxsackie- and echoviruses are not a major cause of upper respiratory tract disease but have been associated with mild respiratory illnesses, particularly in late summer and early fall.

The coxsackieviruses are named for the city of Coxsackie, New York where the prototype viruses were isolated in association with paralytic poliomyelitis. Coxsackieviruses are associated with several acute diseases, e.g., aseptic meningitis, pericarditis, myocarditis, and viral exanthema. Type A coxsackieviruses are associated with respiratory disease more commonly than are coxsackieviruses, type B.

Echoviruses (enteric cytopathic human orphan viruses) are known as "viruses in search of disease" because some are isolated with high frequency in the absence of clinical illness, i.e., in persons clinically well. They have been associated with mild febrile upper respiratory tract disease in children and rarely cause more severe respiratory tract illnesses. Like the coxsackieviruses, they are described chiefly for the sake of completeness.

Coronaviruses

The latest major group of viruses associated with upper respiratory tract disease was initially isolated in 1965 in Salisbury, England, and, in 1966, at the University of Chicago. The coronaviruses, so called because on electron microscopy they appear to be surrounded by a crown of projections with bulbous tips, are medium size (80 to 160 nm) enveloped RNA viruses. They are difficult to culture, usually requiring organ culture for isolation; e.g., human fetal tracheal organ cultures in which initial loss of ciliary motion and later destruction of tracheal lining cells indicated the presence of virus.

Corona viruses were found, in one study, to be a major cause of the common cold, particularly in adolescents and young adults. However, there is not sufficient information with which to adequately assess the relative importance of this group of agents in nonbacterial upper respiratory tract infections.

Mycoplasma Pneumoniae

Mycoplasma pneumoniae belongs to the genus Mycoplasma and is a nonviral, infectious agent considered to be the smallest free-living organism. It can be cultivated in cell-free media and responds to several antibiotics, e.g., erythromycin and tetracycline. *M. pneumoniae* is probably the only mycoplasma consistently shown to cause disease in man.

Mycoplasma pneumoniae is usually associated with lower respiratory tract illness but also causes pharyngitis, tracheobronchitis, and a form of infection of the tympanic membrane called bullous myringitis. *M. pneumoniae* pharyngitis may be indistinguishable from streptococcal pharyngitis and predominantly occurs in older children and young adults. Mycoplasmal infections have also been described in association with erythema multiforme (a skin disease), the Guillain-Barré syndrome (a neurologic illness), and other systemic illnesses that make up its protean manifestations.

A definite diagnosis is provided by isolation of *Mycoplasma pneumoniae,* but culture and identification of this agent usually require three to four weeks. Consequently, a serologic approach to diagnosis is recommended, usually by demonstrating high or increasing titers of cold agglutinins or complement-fixing antibodies. Cold agglutinin antibodies are directed against the large "I" antigens in the "I-i" red cell antigen system. The large I antigen, which is absent from fetal and cord red blood cells, is present on red cells of 97 per cent of adults. Cold agglutinin antibodies clump red cells strongly at 4°C and weakly at room temperature. High titers of cold agglutinins may be associated with a hemolytic process involving the patient's own red cells. In some patients, hemolysis may be so severe as to cause anemia. An earlier recommendation to remove serum from clotted blood before refrigeration is based on the possibility that the blood may contain cold agglutinins which would be absorbed from the serum unless previously separated from the red cells with which they react. Cold agglutinin antibodies are considered nonspecific because they do not react directly with intact *M. pneumoniae* and are not induced by injection of the agent.

On the other hand, complement-fixing antibodies are directed specifically against *Mycoplasma pneumoniae*. A serologic diagnosis depends on showing a fourfold or greater increase in titer between acute and convalescent serums. Not infrequently, serologic evidence is obtained also for a concurrent infection with one of the viruses described earlier in this chapter.

Prevention of Upper Respiratory Tract Infections

Vaccines prepared against the agents that cause respiratory illnesses, except for the influenza viruses, are still in the developmental stage.

Some problems related to these vaccines have already been described, but another consideration enters the picture; i.e., if it were possible to make a safe, effective vaccine for each virus, where should the effort be directed? This question arises because vaccination with vaccines prepared with each of the large number of viruses causing respiratory tract illnesses presents a logistic problem and an immunologic problem. The immunologic problem centers on a question concerning the ability of our immunologic system to respond to more than one antigen at a time. The logistic problem is concerned with how to prepare multivalent or multiantigenic vaccines which do not adversely affect the immunogenicity of any particular antigen.

One way to establish a developmental priority is to ascertain which agents cause the most disease. This question has been examined in several population groups and the results of such studies are in general agreement. The findings in a recently reported six-year study of the entire community of Tecumseh, Michigan, are shown in Table 18–2.

TABLE 18–2. Frequency of Infection with Respiratory Agents*

Agent	Frequency of Isolation	
	All Illnesses	Medical Consult
Rhinovirus	38.5	23.3
Parainfluenza	16.9	22.2
Group A streptococci	13.3	22.2
Influenza	11.9	15.0
Respiratory syncytial	5.9	5.6
Adenovirus	4.5	3.9
Enterovirus	4.3	3.3
Other	4.7	4.5

*From Monto, A. S., and Ullman, B. M.: Acute respiratory disease in an American community. The Tecumseh study. J.A.M.A. *227:*164, 1974.

The data describe the frequency with which agents isolated from patients who were ascertained to be ill caused acute respiratory tract illnesses.* Illness was uncovered by a continuing telephone survey, and specimens were collected within two days of onset by visiting either the home or the physician's office, if the patient sought medical attention. It was determined that if effective vaccines were available for more than 100 rhinoviruses and for 4 parainfluenza virus and 3 influenza virus types, it would be possible to prevent about two out of every three respiratory illnesses. This would mean that children less than five years of age would experience two instead of six respiratory tract infections per year, children from 5 to 14 years of age two instead of five infections per year, and adolescents and adults one instead of three per year.

Clearly, a major reason for the high frequency of upper respiratory tract illness, the apparent recurrence of respiratory disease, and the problems of preventing these illnesses is the large number of etiologic agents involved.

References

Books

Andrews, C., and Pereira, H. G.: Viruses of Vertebrates. 3rd ed. Baltimore, The Williams and Wilkins Co. 1972.

Bedson, S., Downie, A. W., MacCallum, F. O., and Stuart-Harris, C. H.: Virus and Rickettsial Diseases of Man. London, Edward Arnold Ltd., 1967.

Knight, V. (ed.): Viral and Mycoplasmal Infections of the Respiratory Tract. Philadelphia, Lea and Febiger, 1973.

Prier, J. E. (ed.): Basic Medical Virology. Baltimore, The Williams and Wilkins Co., 1966.

Original Articles

Chanock, R. M., Roizman, B., and Myers, R.: Recovery from infants with respiratory illness of virus related to chimpanzee coryzal agent (CCA): Isolation, properties and characterization. Am. J. Hyg. *66:*281, 1957.

Conference of Newer Respiratory Disease Viruses. Am. Rev. Resp. Dis. Supplement, 1962.

Denny, F. W., Clyde, W. A., Jr., and Glezen, W. P.: Mycoplasma pneumoniae disease: Clinical spectrum, pathophysiology, epidemiology and control. J. Infect. Dis. *123:*74, 1971.

Forsyth, B. R., Bloom, H. H., Johnson, K. M., and Chanock, R. M.: Patterns of illness in rhinovirus infections of military personnel. N. Engl. J. Med. *269:*602, 1963.

Francis, T., Jr.: Transmission of influenza by a filterable virus. Science *80:*457, 1934.

Glezen, W. P., and Denney, F. W.: Epidemiology of acute lower respiratory disease in children. N. Engl. J. Med. *288:*498, 1973.

Gwaltney, J. M., Jr., Hendley, J. O., Simon, G., and Jordan, W. S.: Rhinovirus infections in an industrial population. N. Engl. J. Med. *275:*1261, 1966.

Habel, K.: The nature of viruses and viral diseases. Med. Clin. North Am. *45:*1275, 1959.

McNamara, M. J., Pierce, W. E., Crawford, Y. E., and Miller, L. F.: Patterns of adenovirus infections in naval recruits. Am. Rev. Resp. Dis. *86:*485, 1962.

Monto, A. S., and Ullman, B. M.: Acute respiratory disease in an American community. The Tecumseh study. J.A.M.A. *227:*164, 1974.

Nichol, K. P., and Cherry, J. D.: Bacterial-viral interrelations in respiratory infections. N. Engl. J. Med. *277:*667, 1967.

---

*Thirty-seven per cent of these illnesses were due to lower respiratory tract infection.

Rowe, W. P., Huebner, R. J., Gilmore, L. K., Parrott, R. H., and Ward, T. G.: Isolation of cytopathogenic agent from human adenoids undergoing spontaneous degeneration in tissue culture. Proc. Soc. Exp. Biol. Med. *84:*570, 1973.

Tyrell, D. A. J.: Some recent trends in vaccination against respiratory viruses. Br. Med. Bull. *25:*165, 1969.

Tyrell, D. A. J.: Hunting common cold viruses by some new methods. J. Infect. Dis. *121:*561, 1970.

Valentine, R. C., and Pereira, H. G.: Antigens and structure of the adenovirus. J. Mol. Biol. *13:*13, 1965.

IV

LOWER
RESPIRATORY
TRACT
INFECTION

Chapter 19

LOWER RESPIRATORY TRACT INFECTION: GENERAL CONSIDERATIONS

Introduction

Nature of Lower Respiratory Tract Infections

Respiratory system infections are the most common of all infectious disorders (see Chap. 1). A significant proportion of all infectious respiratory tract disease is represented by acute infection of the lower respiratory tract, characterized by fever, a cough productive of increased or altered lower tract secretions, and chest pain associated with respiration.

In contrast to the upper respiratory system, lower respiratory tract infections often follow a life-threatening course. They can seriously compromise the terminal alveolar pulmonary airway system, especially in individuals with altered pulmonary function due to long-term cigarette smoking or chronic obstructive pulmonary disease, i.e., bronchitis and emphysema. When inflammation of the bronchial and alveolar spaces or the supporting interstitial tissue results in an abnormal density in the chest roentgenogram, it is called pneumonia. Progression of pneumonia, unchecked

271

by host immune defenses, inevitably compromises gas exchange across alveolar membranes and leads to ventilatory insufficiency. Insufficient oxygenation elicits a cascade of altered cardiopulmonary functions which collectively translate to appreciable morbidity and mortality. Primary pneumonia and especially secondary pneumonia, occurring as an intercurrent terminal event in patients with serious or fatal underlying diseases, are the major causes of death in the United States.

In further contrast to the upper respiratory tract, nearly 50 per cent of all lower respiratory tract infections have a bacterial origin. Relatively few species of bacteria account for the bulk of these infections. Virtually all of these bacterial species are susceptible to antimicrobial agents. It should be clear from the foregoing discussion that physicians must utilize an aggressive approach to the diagnosis and therapy of acute infections of the lower respiratory tract, especially in patients with pneumonia. By identifying and treating those pneumonias caused by microorganisms susceptible to antimicrobial drugs, morbidity and mortality can be diminished significantly.

The Lung as an "Extracorporeal" Organ

The lung and its secretions ordinarily are free of demonstrable microorganisms. The sterility of the pulmonary bed reflects the collective actions of natural and acquired host immune and other defense mechanisms, e.g., movement of the mucous sheet and beating of cilia (see Chaps. 2 and 3).

The pulmonary system is a direct anatomic extension of the upper respiratory tract. From birth on, the major branches of the lower respiratory tree are in potential direct communication with the microbial flora of the oropharynx and other regions of the upper respiratory tract. The pulmonary air conduit system also is perpetually exposed to the microbial-laden world in which we all live. In this sense, the lung, or at least a good portion of it, can be considered an "extracorporeal" organ system. Microorganisms in varying numbers, either within small droplets of respiratory secretions or rarely as free-suspended airborne individual infectious units, have ready access to the lower respiratory tract via the bronchi and smaller branches of the air conduit system. Approximately 80 per cent of the tidal air volume, with any infectious particles it may contain, impinges on the terminal airway system. Any disturbance in normal host defenses or inhalation of a critical number of pathogenic microorganisms can result in implantation, colonization, and infection of the trachea, major bronchi, or the terminal alveolar air system and its supporting interstitial tissue (see Chap. 2). Since every person has repetitive contact with infectious respiratory aerosols during his or her lifetime, it is remarkable that lower respiratory tract infectious disease does not occur more often.

Source and Transit of Microorganisms Reaching Lower Respiratory Tree

Microbes usually gain access to the lung by inhaled air, i.e., via an aerogenic pathway. Less commonly, they may reach the lung by means of the bloodstream. Recognition of whether pneumonia has resulted from infection via the aerogenic or hematogenous pathway can be helpful in diagnosis and management.

Aerogenic microorganisms are derived from two sources: (1) the normal microbial flora of the oropharynx and paranasal sinuses, and (2) aerosols created by coughing or sneezing by other individuals.

Transit of microorganisms via inhaled air to specific anatomic regions of the lower respiratory tract is a function of their size or the size of water or mucous droplets in which they are suspended (for a detailed discussion of this important principle, see Chap. 2). Infectious water droplets constituting respiratory tract aerosols are hygroscopic. Upon leaving the host and entering ambient air, the droplets immediately lose moisture and decrease in size. Inhaled by another individual in close proximity, the droplets quickly acquire moisture from the saturated air of the new host and increase in size to their original dimensions. In general, infectious particles with a diameter of 10 microns or greater are trapped in the upper respiratory tract passages and do not reach the tertiary bronchi, respiratory bronchioles, and alveolar air spaces. Particles ranging in size from 0.2 to 6 microns in diameter, especially those of 1 to 2 microns, are the ones which most readily gain access to the terminal alveolar airway system. Infectious units smaller than 0.2 micron usually stay suspended in the inhaled air and are then exhaled, posing little risk for the host.

The number of particles of different sizes in a representative sneeze and cough is depicted in Figure 19–1. The largest number of particles dispersed by either event produces a particle with a diameter approximately 2 microns or less that is capable of reaching the terminal bronchiolar-alveolar system of a new host. The number of water droplets in aerosols produced by sneezing and coughing can easily accommodate pathogenic microorganisms in numbers sufficient to initiate infection in a susceptible host. Studies such as that summarized in Figure 19–1 suggest that the time-honored practice of attempting to reduce the generation of infection-laden respiratory tract aerosols by covering the mouth and nose with a handkerchief, a hand or a mask, probably has some merit.

Prerequisites for Effective Management of Lower Respiratory Tract Infection

Three prerequisites must be met for optimal diagnosis and therapy of patients with lower respiratory tract infections. These are (1) a clinically useful system for classifying lower tract diseases, (2) guidelines for differentiating bacterial from nonbacterial types of infection, and (3) suitable methods for expeditiously securing and examining sputum and lower respiratory tract secretions.

A Meaningful Classification System. Many systems have been proposed, i.e., anatomic, etiologic, pathogenic, etc. Each has certain advantages. In order to be useful from a clinical standpoint, however, a classification system should be focused on specific microorganisms. Only by anticipating what specific microorganism is most likely responsible for pneumonia can the physician initiate efficacious antimicrobial therapy.

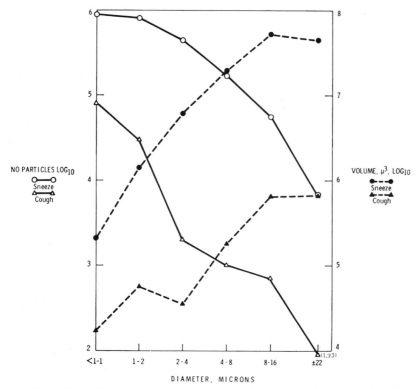

Figure 19–1. Distribution of particles by size in coughs and sneezes. (Data from Duguid, J. P.: The size and the duration of air-carriage of respiratory droplets and droplet-nuclei. J. Hyg. (Camb.) *44:*471, 1946; and Gerone, P. J., et al.: Assessment of experimental and natural viral aerosols. Bact. Rev. *30:*576, 1966. *In* Knight, V. (ed.): Viral and Mycoplasmal Infections of the Respiratory Tract. Philadelphia, Lea and Febiger, 1973.)

Differentiation of Bacterial from Nonbacterial Lower Respiratory Tract Disease. All thinking regarding initial management is based on this differentiation. The important decision of whether or not to employ antimicrobial therapy hinges on whether or not the clinician believes bacteria are causing the infection under consideration.

Proper Methods for Collecting and Examining Sputum and Lower Respiratory Tract Secretions. A Gram stain of sputum can supply objective data which are extremely valuable for clinical evaluation. Unfortunately, the methods often employed for securing and examining lower respiratory tract secretions are totally inadequate, and the data they yield can be seriously misleading. Reliance on such data can lead to faulty decision-making and suboptimal patient care.

Classification of Lower Respiratory Tract Infections

Each of several classification systems is briefly discussed below in terms of specific advantages each offers to the physician from the standpoint of clinical diagnosis and management.

Anatomic Classification

In this system of classification, lower respiratory tract infections are designated in terms of the specific anatomic sites initially involved, e.g., tracheitis, tracheobronchitis, bronchopneumonia, lobar pneumonia, or interstitial pneumonia. The term *pneumonitis* is a radiologic phrase; it has no place in a clinical vocabulary. One advantage of the anatomic classification system is the important distinction between inflammation primarily involving the alveolar spaces, i.e., lobar pneumonia, and inflammation of their supporting interstitium, i.e., interstitial pneumonia. This is an important distinction for the physician because completely different classes of microorganisms are etiologically associated with each type of infection and, consequently, each calls for materially different forms of therapy.

Pathogenetic Classification

This system of classification emphasizes how microorganisms gain access to lung tissue. Terminology is often confusing and deserves some explanation.

Primary infection or pneumonia denotes infection due to highly pathogenic microorganisms which reach the lower respiratory tract via the air passages, i.e., the aerogenic pathway, and initiate disease in an individual who does not have any underlying deficiency in the immunologic defense system.

Secondary infections or pneumonia are caused by less pathogenic microorganisms which induce lower respiratory tract disease largely because of some alteration in the patient's immune or natural defense mechanisms, e.g., occurrence of pneumonia in a pulmonary segment with impaired drainage of bronchial secretions secondary to obstruction of that segment by a carcinoma or an aspirated foreign body. As discussed in detail in Chapter 43, secondary pulmonary infections are often considered "opportunistic" in character; their causative microorganisms frequently are termed *opportunists*. A good example of an opportunistic infection in a compromised host is development of gram negative bacillary pneumonia in a patient on a respirator which has become heavily contaminated with *Pseudomonas sp.* owing to infrequent or improper sterilization. The respirator delivers aerosols heavily laden with the contaminating bacteria to the lower respiratory tract passages under pressure. Secondary pulmonary infections of this type are often referred to as "superinfections."

Hematogenous or *metastatic pulmonary infections* can result from microorganisms reaching the lung via the bloodstream. Pulmonary infections arising in this manner generally can be recognized from available clinical data, especially serial chest roentgenograms. The pulmonary densities are usually numerous and almost invariably involve both the right and left lungs. Early "highlights" signifying cavitation, if noted in association with some of the larger densities, are pathognomonic of abscess formation. Hematogenous pneumonia is indicative of bacteremia or showers of septic emboli secondary to a primary infection which is extrapulmonic in location, e.g., acute staphylococcal endocarditis involving the tricuspid valve in a mainlining heroin addict. Successful therapy must be directed at the extrapulmonic infection rather than the presenting pulmonary problem.

Finally, *aspiration pneumonia* resulting from inhalation of food, gastric contents, and upper respiratory tract bacteria and secretions is commonly encountered in chronic alcoholics or chronically ill patients being fed by gastric lavage. Aspiration of the foreign material disrupts normal host defense mechanisms, such as ciliary clearing of bronchi, and facilitates infection by the mixture of microorganisms swept along with the aspirated material. Any aspirated foreign body which causes obstruction, e.g., a peanut, also diminishes host defenses and potentiates infection in a similar fashion.

Etiologic Classification

The major advantage of this classification system is the emphasis which is placed on distinguishing bacterial from nonbacterial respiratory tract infections. Specific subdivisions of this classification include bacterial, mycoplasmal, rickettsial, viral, etc. These distinctions are important to the physician who must decide whether antimicrobial therapy is to be used and what drug should be selected. Correct decisions require thinking in terms of specific etiologic microorganisms, viz., *Streptococcus pneumoniae, Klebsiella pneumoniae, Staphylococcus aureus.*

Differentiation between Bacterial and Nonbacterial Lower Respiratory Tract Infections

General Aspects

A careful history identifying special features of the clinical setting, a thorough physical examination, and inspection of a Gram-stained sputum smear and chest roentgenogram provide the usual means for initial evaluation of the patient. Using the data from these sources, the clinician in most instances can reach a decision as to whether a patient has a bacterial or nonbacterial lower respiratory tract infection.

Expected clinical settings and specific etiologic agents and their relative frequency in relation to bacterial pneumonia are shown in Table 19–1. *Streptococcus pneumoniae* accounts for the large majority of cases and occurs in males or females of any age. Pneumonia due to *Klebsiella pneumoniae* and *Haemophilus influenzae* accounts for virtually all of the remaining cases, each occurring in a certain type of patient. Also included in Table 19–1 is an indication of the different type of antimicrobial therapy the physician utilizes in treating each of these major types of bacterial pneumonia. The fact that therapy does differ materially emphasizes the need for arriving at a diagnosis which is as specific as possible in terms of the causative microorganism.

From a practical standpoint, the first question the physician must answer is, Does the patient have pneumonia or not? In answering this question, the chest roentgenogram is indispensable in determining whether the patient has a

TABLE 19-1. Frequency and Clinical Settings of Major Types of Bacterial
Pneumonia and Indicated Antimicrobial Drug Therapy

Clinical Entity	Causative Microorganism	Per Cent of Cases	Clinical Setting	Indicated Antimicrobial Drug(s)
Pneumococcal lobar pneumonia	*Streptococcus pneumoniae*	⩾ 90	Males or females of any age; alcoholism often in history	Penicillin-class drug in low dosage
Klebsiella (Friedlander's) pneumonia	*Klebsiella pneumoniae* (Friedlander's bacillus)	1–5	Adult male; chronic alcoholic	Gentamicin or alternate aminoglycoside with or without chloramphenicol in usual dosage
"Flu" pneumonia	*Haemophilus influenzae,* type b	1–5	Child < 6 years; Adult > 60 years	Ampicillin in high dosage*

*With chloramphenicol initially until ampicillin-susceptibility of responsible strain of *Haemophilus influenzae* is determined (see Chaps. 21 and 33).

distinct lung infiltrate, i.e., whether pneumonia is present or not. At least two roentgenographic projections are used, viz., posteroanterior and lateral, as an aid in detecting small pulmonary densities which can be obscured by the heart or other anatomic structures.

If pneumonia is present, then the second question is, Does the pneumonia have a bacterial or nonbacterial origin? In answering this question, evaluation of all available data, especially the clinical setting, becomes crucial. Once having decided that bacterial pneumonia is the diagnosis, the clinician then must immediately decide whether the causative microorganism is *Streptococcus pneumoniae* or one of the less frequent bacterial etiologic agents (see Table 19–1). A carefully collected sputum specimen which is properly Gram stained can be of considerable help in arriving at this decision, which in turn will determine what type of antimicrobial therapy the physician should initiate.

Differential Diagnostic Features

Symptoms, signs, laboratory data, and chest roentgenographic findings most helpful in deciding on clinical grounds whether a patient with pneumonia has a bacterial or nonbacterial respiratory tract infection are listed in Table 19–2. Since *Streptococcus pneumoniae* accounts for at least 90 per cent of bacterial pneumonias, pneumococcal lobar pneumonia is used as the prototype bacterial disease. The features of pneumococcal pneumonia are compared with those of pneumonia caused by different viruses and by *Mycoplasma pneumoniae.*

TABLE 19-2. Differential Diagnostic Features of Bacterial Versus
Nonbacterial Pneumonia

Feature	Pneumococcal Lobar Pneumonia	Viral-Mycoplasmal Pneumonia
Onset[1]	Sudden	Gradual
Rigors[2]	Single chill	"Chilliness"
Facies[3]	"Toxic"	Well
Cough[4]	Productive	Paroxysmal; nonproductive
Sputum[5]	Purulent (bloody)	Mucoid
Herpes labialis[6]	Frequent	Rare
Temperature[7]	103°–104°F	< 103°F
Pleurisy[8]	Frequent	Rare
Consolidation[9]	Frequent	Rare
Gram stain (sputum)[10]	Neutrophils; cocci	Mononuclear cells; mixed flora
White blood cell and differential count[11]	> 15,000 Immature neutrophils	< 15,000 Normal
Chest x-ray[12]	Defined density	Nondefined infiltrate

1. Pneumococcal pneumonia usually begins suddenly, "with a bang." Its onset is often heralded by a hard, teeth clattering, shaking chill. The patient frequently can remember the exact time of day or night when he became abruptly ill. Close questioning often reveals that the patient had experienced a mild antecedent upper respiratory tract infection, e.g., a common cold, for several days. Nonbacterial pneumonia, in contrast, usually has a gradual onset, builds up slowly in crescendo fashion, and does not reach maximum intensity for several days.

2. Rigors are common in lobar pneumonia; a single shaking chill is the rule in pneumonia due to *Streptococcus pneumoniae.* Nonbacterial pneumonia, on the other hand, is rarely associated with a frank chill, although patients do complain of chilliness, i.e., difficulty in keeping sufficiently warm.

3. The patient with pneumococcal lobar pneumonia appears acutely ill and "toxic" from the very beginning of his illness. In contrast, patients with viral or mycoplasmal respiratory tract disease frequently appear well; only fever and a persistent cough serve as signs of illness. Progression of the interstitial inflammation, especially if it is widespread and causes ventilatory insufficiency, will render such patients just as "toxic" in appearance as those with acute pneumococcal pneumonia.

4. Pneumococcal pneumonia is accompanied by a cough productive of liberal amounts of sputum. In nonbacterial pneumonia, the cough is usually not productive and in cases in which it is, the secretions brought up have a mucoid white-yellowish cast.

5. The sputum produced in pneumococcal pneumonia has a dirty yellow or purulent character owing to its high content of segmented neutrophils. The purulent pulmonary secretions often contain blood or serosanguineous fluid which has entered acutely inflamed alveolar air spaces. In such instances, the sputum assumes a dark brown to purple hue, the so-called prune juice sputum considered typical for pneumococcal pneumonia. In contrast, the cough characteristic of viral or mycoplasmal pneumonia is usually persistent and troublesome but not productive of more than a small amount of mucoid or mucopurulent secretions. Long paroxysms of coughing are often triggered by deep breathing during examination of the chest and bring all efforts to continue the physical examination to a halt for several minutes.

6. On physical examination, herpes labialis (fever blisters) due to *Herpesvirus hominis* type 1 are frequent in pneumococcal lobar pneumonia; they are rare in viral or mycoplasmal pneumonia, despite

occasional temperature elevations equivalent to those accompanying bacterial pneumonia.

7. Body temperature usually exceeds 103°F and often spikes higher than 104°F in patients with pneumococcal pneumonia. A clinical rule of thumb, which still has merit, holds that in an adult patient an oral temperature greater than 104°F, especially if accompanied by a *single* rigor, can be considered diagnostic of acute pneumococcal lobar pneumonia until proved otherwise. Temperature spikes to above 104°F are often recorded in patients with acute pyelonephritis. However, the repetitive shaking chills which are so often associated with this infection provide a useful diagnostic clue in differentiating between acute pneumococcal pneumonia and acute pyelonephritis. Maximum temperatures in viral-mycoplasmal pneumonia usually do not exceed 103°F and sometimes stay well below this range.

8. Extension of pneumococcal pneumonia to the pleura is common and leads to complaints of pleurisy and physical evidence of pleural space inflammation, i.e., pleural friction rub or signs of fluid (transudate or exudate) in the costophrenic angle. Pleurisy and pleural fluid are exceedingly rare in nonbacterial pneumonias, since the inflammatory process only infrequently extends to and abuts on a pleural surface.

9. A flat percussion note and tubular breath sounds indicative of frank consolidation of lung tissue are to be expected in pneumococcal lobar pneumonia. These physical findings reflect inflammation and complete occlusion of the terminal bronchiolar and alveolar sac spaces by accumulating exudate. Pulmonary consolidation is rare in pneumonia of viral or mycoplasmal origin owing to the fact that these inflammatory processes are largely restricted to the interstitial tissues of the lung.

10. Additional differential aids are often derived from the initial laboratory and roentgenologic studies. Gram stains of smears of properly collected sputum from patients with pneumococcal pneumonia usually reveal an abundance of neutrophils and a distinct preponderance of gram positive coccal bacterial forms. Only occasional gram negative rods or cocci are observed. In nonbacterial pneumonia, the Gram-stained sputum smear usually reveals mononuclear inflammatory cells and a mixture of small numbers of different bacterial forms reflecting the normal oropharyngeal microbial flora.

11. In pneumococcal lobar pneumonia, the total peripheral blood leukocyte count is usually greater than 15,000 per cubic millimeter, with a sharp increase in the proportion of segmented neutrophils, many of which have an immature appearance. For reasons that are still unclear, severe leukopenia, with counts of less than 1000 per cubic millimeter, may be seen in bacterial pneumonia due to *Streptococcus pneumoniae* or *Klebsiella pneumoniae,* especially in patients with a history of chronic alcoholism. In contrast, in patients with nonbacterial pneumonia, the white blood cell count is most often only slightly elevated, i.e., less than 15,000 per cubic millimeter; the differential count is either normal or reflects an absolute or relative increase in the number of circulating small lymphocytes.

12. The chest roentgenogram usually reveals a sharply defined homogeneous pulmonary density in patients with pneumococcal pneumonia, since the inflammation is usually confined within normal anatomic boundaries of lung tissue to a segmental, lobar, or multilobar distribution. The density is often first evident emerging from the hilar region of the affected side and subsequently spreading into specific segments of a particular lobe. In contrast, the pulmonary density in nonbacterial pneumonia is often diffuse and poorly defined and has a moth-eaten appearance. The sharp anatomic boundaries so characteristic of pneumococcal pneumonia are absent. This is consistent with the fact that the interstitial tissue of the lung is the principal anatomic site of the inflammatory process.

Some appreciation of the specific microorganisms causing pneumonia among adult patients on a general medical service who have acute pneumonia can be gained by examining the data shown in Table 19–3. Two major points deserve emphasis: (1) in only one third of the patients could a specific etiologic agent be demonstrated, and (2) based on positive blood cultures, *Streptococcus pneumoniae* was the overwhelming single important cause of bacterial pneumonia. In this particular study (Table 19–3), if patients had been included from whom pneumococci had been isolated from the sputum or oropharyngeal cultures but not from the blood, another one third of the patients would have been considered to have had pneumococcal disease. This provides additional evidence for the important role of *S. pneumoniae* in the pathogenesis of pneumonia.

TABLE 19–3.   Relative Importance of Bacteria, Viruses and Mycoplasmas as Etiologic Factors in Pneumonia in 427 Adults*

Microorganism Isolated or Implicated	Per Cent of Cases Studied
Streptococcus pneumoniae	19.1
Staphylococcus aureus	0.7
Viruses (excluding herpesviruses)	15.2
Mycoplasma pneumoniae	4.0

*From Mufson, M. A., et al.: The role of viruses, mycoplasmas, and bacteria in acute pneumonia in civilian adults. Am. J. Epidemiol. *86:*526, 1967. Each patient was admitted to study with a diagnosis of pneumonia supported by an unequivocal pulmonary density in the initial chest roentgenogram.

Collection and Examination of Sputum, Lower Respiratory Tract Secretions, and Other Body Fluids

General concepts and specific guidelines concerning collection and microbiologic study of specimens pertaining to infections of the lower respiratory tract have been outlined in Chapter 10. The additional material included here relates specifically to problems concerning pneumonia that commonly arise in the clinical arena and which are the responsibility of the attending physician.

Sputum

Collection of sputum rarely receives the attention it deserves. An order for "sputum to lab for culture" may be written on the patient's chart, but whether a true sputum specimen is secured and transported promptly to the microbiology laboratory is quite another matter.

What actually happens in many instances is as follows: A sputum cup is placed by the patient's bed. The patient is told to provide sputum. No special instructions are given. The patient usually responds by coughing and spitting into the cup at intervals. What is produced may be mostly saliva heavily laden with oropharyngeal microorganisms, especially if the patient has a non-bacterial respiratory infection and a nonproductive cough. The expectorated secretions, together with their mixed microbial flora, usually are allowed to remain in the bedside cup for several hours before being taken to the clinical microbiology laboratory. During this period of time, various species of microorganisms, especially gram negative bacilli which normally inhabit the oropharynx in very small numbers, begin to replicate. These microbes may seriously hamper isolation and recognition of the more fastidious bacteria, e.g., *Streptococcus pneumoniae* or *Haemophilus influenzae,* for which purpose the sputum specimen was initially collected. What is often reported by the laboratory is a heavy growth of *Escherichia coli* or *Pseudomonas sp.* In most cases these microorganisms are not etiologically associated with the patient's illness; however, the unwary physician may believe that the heavy growth of bacteria indicates that they are responsible for the patient's disease. Acting on this assumption, he may order a change in antimicrobial therapy which will inhibit these gram negative microorganisms. By so doing, the patient may then receive an antimicrobial drug, e.g., gentamicin, which is far less effective than the antimicrobial agent initially prescribed, most likely a penicillin-class drug, or completely ineffective against pneumococci.

Sputum is a specific exudative product of the inflamed and injured respiratory tree. In response to injury, there is an outpouring of fluid, phagocytes, and blood into the tracheobronchial-alveolar airway. Accumulation of this exudate disrupts the normal ciliary action, leading to a cough reflex and forceful expulsion of the exudate up and through the oropharynx. It is only after the lower respiratory tract secretions have been so expelled that they can correctly be termed *sputum.*

Time is saved by giving the patient a brief idea of what sputum actually is and what he must do to produce some. With encouragement and coaching, the patient can usually draw a few deep breaths and give a few deep coughs sufficient to raise and expel material which quite clearly represents lower respiratory tract secretions or sputum. The sputum specimen can be caught on a wad of gauze sponge or folded tissue and then taken immediately to the laboratory, where it can be smeared, stained, and cultured as described in Chapter 10.

Aspiration of Lower Respiratory Tract Secretions

If a patient is too ill or too weak to cooperate in the collection of sputum, suitable material must then be collected by mechanical means. Many devices have been used at one time or another to aspirate lower respiratory tract secretions via the upper airway. With the exception of a triple-lumen bronchoscope, no device can be passed through the microbial-laden oropharynx for the purpose of aspirating lower respiratory tract secretions without considerable contamination of these secretions by upper respiratory tract microorganisms.

Translaryngeal aspiration has been used on an increasing scale to secure lower respiratory tract secretions uncontaminated by oropharyngeal microbes. Translaryngeal aspiration is not a new procedure, having been introduced many years ago by anesthesiologists as a convenient way for anesthetizing the larynx, trachea, and large bronchi, e.g., in preparation for bronchoscopy. This procedure has been discussed and illustrated in Chapter 10. Special emphasis is given here to the necessity that the needle puncture be made through the cricothyroid membrane (also called a ligament in some anatomy texts). The cricothyroid membrane lies within the larynx proper, as shown in Figure 19–2. Many physicians still refer to this procedure as transtracheal aspiration, which is incorrect terminology. Needle puncture of the trachea per se should be strenuously avoided if risk to the patient is to be minimized.

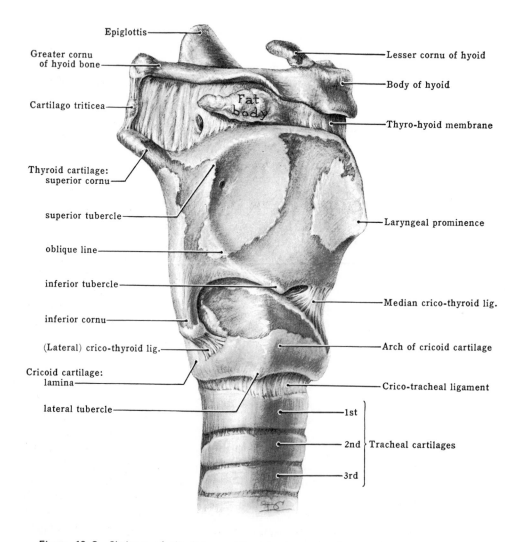

Figure 19–2. Skeleton of the larynx, side view. In performing translaryngeal aspiration, the site of the needle puncture is the median cricothyroid ligament. (From Grant, J. C. B.: Grant's Atlas of Anatomy. 6th ed. Baltimore, Williams & Wilkins Co., 1972. Copyright © 1972 The Williams & Wilkins Co. Reproduced by permission.

Blood

At least two blood cultures should be collected routinely as part of any febrile patient's work-up (described in Chap. 9). Up to one third of patients with pneumococcal pneumonia have *Streptococcus pneumoniae* demonstrable in their blood when admitted to the hospital. Positive blood cultures are the *only* definitive way of establishing an unequivocal diagnosis of pneumococcal lobar pneumonia because of the poor yield of typable pneumococci from sputa (see Chap. 10). The same also applies to pneumonia caused by *Klebsiella pneumoniae* or *Haemophilus influenzae*.

Pleural Fluid

If the physical examination and chest roentgenogram indicate presence of fluid in the costophrenic angle, diagnostic thoracentesis may yield material which is helpful for diagnosis. If microorganisms are seen in Gram-stained pleural fluid or grown from pleural fluid cultures, the patient has empyema by definition. *Empyema* is a rare complication of bacterial pneumonia and is usually seen only in patients who do not seek medical help until very late in the course of their illness.

Counterimmunoelectrophoresis

As mentioned in Chapters 9 and 10, enthusiasm has been rekindled over the feasibility of detecting specific microbial antigens in blood, urine, or other body fluids as a highly specific diagnostic test. The development of relatively inexpensive equipment for performing counterimmunoelectrophoresis and the availability of commercial antisera have allowed this procedure to be employed and evaluated in a number of infectious diseases, including pneumonia due to *Streptococcus pneumoniae* and *Klebsiella pneumoniae*. The initial results are encouraging and the speed of diagnosis is impressive, as illustrated by Case Presentation 2 in Chapter 21.

CASE PRESENTATION 1

A 23-year-old male was hospitalized in late December, 1971, because of increasing shortness of breath and development of a cough with blood-tinged sputum. Except for asthmatic attacks precipitated by various environmental allergies, he had always been in good health. One week before hospitalization, this patient had developed what he called "a cold," characterized by a mild sore throat and nonproductive cough, malaise, and a generalized dull headache. Three days prior to hospitalization, at 3:15 PM, the patient experienced a severe shaking chill which lasted approximately 15 minutes. Following the rigor, the cough became worse and more productive of sputum, which was frankly "bloody looking" a few hours before admission to the hospital.

Physical examination revealed a temperature of 103.8°F (orally), pulse 124 per minute, and blood pressure 112/70. Respirations were 36 per minute; each expiration was accompanied by an audible "grunt." The chest was hyperresonant to percussion and filled with inspiratory and expiratory wheezes. Fine crackling rales were heard on inspiration over the lower anterior chest just to the right of the sternum. A grade II/VI systolic ejection type murmur was clearly heard along the left sternal border.

Initial laboratory data included a total leukocyte count of 12,100 per cubic millimeter, with 71 per cent segmented neutrophils, 17 per cent band forms, 11 per cent lymphocytes, and 1 per cent eosinophils. Urine demonstrated a pH of 5.5 and gave a 1+ reaction for protein. A freshly collected sputum was Gram stained and revealed numerous erythrocytes, a considerable number of neutrophils, and a mixture of gram positive rods and cocci. Chest roentgenogram revealed a distinct infiltrate involving the right middle lobe (Figs. 19–3 and 19–4).

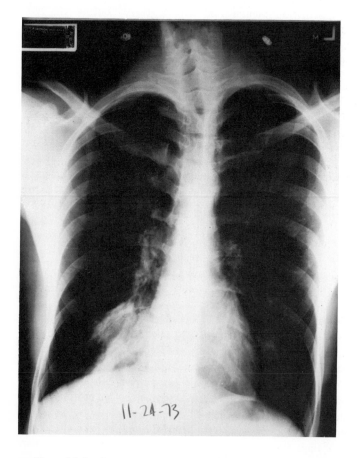

Figure 19–3. Posteroanterior chest roentgenogram of the patient discussed in Case Presentation 1. Note the fairly well-defined density in the lower right lung field. Without the right lateral roentgenographic projection (see Fig. 19–4), it would be impossible to know whether the pneumonic infiltrate occupies the right middle or right lower lobe of the lung.

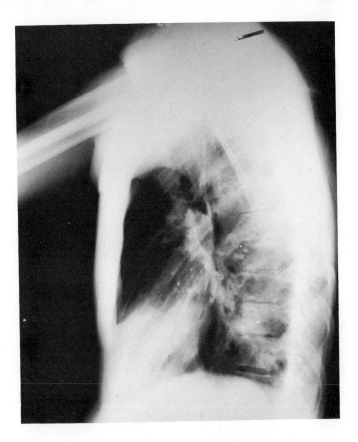

Figure 19-4. Right lateral chest roentgenogram of the patient discussed in Case Presentation 1. Although difficult to discern because of the cardiac shadow, the density noted in the right lung (Fig. 19-3) appears to be within the middle lobe and also the lower lobe of the right lung. The "stringy" densities confined to the hilar region are not uncommon in patients with bronchial asthma.

After drawing three blood cultures (from different sites) and learning that sputum had been inoculated onto appropriate bacteriologic culture media, the patient's physician ordered procaine penicillin, 600,000 units via the intramuscular route every six hours, aminophylline rectal suppositories, and intermittent positive pressure breathing treatments to relieve the bronchospasm and allow the patient to rest more comfortably.

The patient improved at a rapid rate, becoming afebrile on the fourth hospital day. At that time, the laboratory reported that two of the three blood cultures (the first two drawn) had yielded *Streptococcus pneumoniae*, which gave a quellung reaction with type 8 antiserum. Sputum culture, however, yielded only normal flora, including a few nontypable colonies of *S. pneumoniae*.

The features of the clinical setting — wintertime with its associated sharp increased incidence of respiratory diseases, the symptoms and physical findings, and chest roentgenographic evidence of a pulmonary infiltrative process — all point to acute pneumococcal lobar pneumonia. One wonders if the patient's asthmatic condition might have been a factor favoring infection of the lung. The history of a "cold" preceding onset of the acute illness is in accord with a high proportion of patients who experience some type of antecedent upper respiratory tract infection for several days before onset of bacterial pneumonia. Some investigators believe that the preceding upper respiratory tract symptoms result from an intercurrent viral infection which alters the host's immune defenses so as to allow pathogenic *Streptococcus pneumoniae* carried in the oropharynx to gain access to the lower respiratory tree. There are little data to support this notion. Many lines of evidence, however, indicate that the upper respiratory tract symptoms are not caused by *S. pneumoniae* per se (see also Chap. 12).

Note the dramatic sudden onset of symptoms of lower respiratory tract disease, i.e., a single rigor which is so characteristic of lobar pneumonia due to *Streptococcus pneumoniae*. Also note that in this patient herpes labialis (fever blisters) did not appear, and the recorded temperature did not exceed 104°F, as is so often the case.

A definitive diagnosis of pneumococcal pneumonia was possible because of the positive blood cultures. It is interesting that only the first two blood cultures yielded *Streptococcus pneumoniae*, emphasizing the fact that bacteremia associated with pneumonia due to this microorganism tends to be transitory. Indeed, had additional blood cultures been taken over a period as long as 24 hours before antimicrobial therapy was started and all cultures found to be positive for *S. pneumoniae*, the heart murmur would have been given much greater emphasis because of concern about acute pneumococcal bacterial endocarditis. Despite the positive blood cultures, neither the Gram stain of sputum nor the sputum culture provided any strong clue of *S. pneumoniae* infection. At least 50 per cent of sputum specimens cultured in the average hospital microbiology laboratory fail to yield *S. pneumoniae* in numbers consistent with their having an etiologic role in patients with pneumococcal pneumonia the diagnosis of which has been established by positive blood cultures (see Chap. 10). The nontypable pneumococci isolated from the sputum in this case undoubtedly represented relatively non-pathogenic *S. pneumoniae* which can be expected to be found in the normal oropharyngeal microbial flora of a high proportion of persons during the winter months.

CASE PRESENTATION 2

A 17-year-old healthy high school male noted fatigue and some generalized muscle aching on October 14, 1973. He awoke on the morning of October 15 feeling extremely chilly and suffering from a severe frontal headache. Shortly thereafter he became aware of fever, and his recorded oral body temperature was 102.6°F. Insidious onset of an increasingly troublesome, persistent, nonproductive cough, along with continued headache, remittent fever, and generalized muscle aching, was noted later during the day. On October 17, the patient complained of a severe left earache, and on October 18, primarily because of the continued earache and persistence of other symptoms he consulted a physician.

Physical examination revealed a temperature of 101°F and a pulse rate of 100 per minute; blood pressure was 124/76, and respirations were 24 per minute. The patient looked reasonably well but was obviously in pain because of the earache and the distressing and persistent cough which was productive of only a slight amount of mucoid sputum. The left tympanic membrane was diffusely erythematous; a small (1 to 3 mm) bleb was noted on the inferior portion of the inflamed drum. A single tender, enlarged, posterior cervical lymph node was palpable below the left ear lobe. Examination of the chest revealed crackling inspiratory rales over the right lower lungfield posteriorly.

Initial laboratory data included a hematocrit, total leukocyte count of 8000 cells per cubic millimeter and a urinalysis within normal limits. Chest roentgenogram, including posteroanterior and lateral views, showed a stringy, poorly delineated infiltrate in the most posterior and inferior segment of the right lower lobe (Figs. 19–5 and 19–6). Satisfactory sputum could not be obtained. After a throat culture was inoculated onto sheep blood agar, and

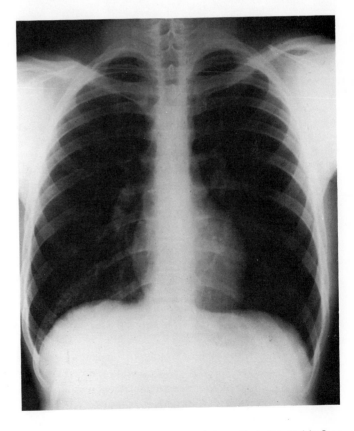

Figure 19–5. Posteroanterior chest roentgenogram of the patient discussed in Case Presentation 2. In addition to the increased hilar-bronchopulmonary markings consistent with a history of cigarette smoking, this film was interpreted to show a definite, poorly delineated and moth-eaten–like infiltrate in the very lower portion of the right lung field.

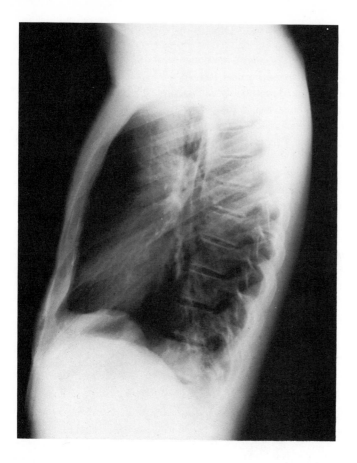

Figure 19–6. Right lateral roentgenographic projection of the patient discussed in Case Presentation 2. The moth-eaten appearance of the density occupying the most inferior segments of the right lower lobe is better visualized in this film.

two blood cultures were obtained, the patient was started on erythromycin stearate 0.5 gm four times a day. Subsequent serologic studies revealed serum collected on October 18 to have a complement-fixing antibody titer of 1:160 against *Mycoplasma pneumoniae*. Additional sera collected on October 19 and October 31 had titers of 1:320 and greater than 1:640, respectively.

The clinical setting of this illness — late fall rather than winter or spring season of the year; an adolescent, previously healthy patient; an insidious onset of an illness characterized primarily by nonproductive, persistent cough with headache and generalized muscle aching and moderate fever — is totally consistent with mycoplasmal disease. Occurrence of the earache probably was the most important symptom, suggesting to the physician that the patient might have pneumonia due to *Mycoplasma pneumoniae*. Up to one fourth of adolescent or college-age patients with established *M. pneumoniae* lower respiratory tract infections have the complaint of earache as part of their history. The basis for the earache is mycoplasmal infection of the tympanic membrane per se, i.e., myringitis. Sometimes one or more blebs filled with fluid may be present, as in Case Presentation 2, and shown to contain *M. pneumoniae,* thereby providing direct evidence for the mycoplasmal origin of the myringitis. Earache due to otitis media is uncommon in adolescence and adulthood since by this time the mass of lymphoid tissues surrounding the eustachian tube orifices has decreased in size and does not commonly enlarge and cause obstruction to drainage of middle ear secretions in association with acute respiratory tract infections.

The physical examination was not particularly revealing, with the exception of the evidence of left-sided tympanic membrane inflammation and associated adenopathy. Notable in this patient were the signs of inflammation in the right lower posterior lung. In many patients with mycoplasmal pneumonia, the examination of the chest may be completely unrevealing. Note also the persistent cough which did not produce enough secretions that could be termed *sputum.*

It is obvious from the way this patient was managed that the attending physician suspected pneumonia due to *Mycoplasma pneumoniae* from the outset and for this reason prescribed erythromycin. Serum was drawn at appropriate intervals to allow demonstration of a rising antibody titer specifically reactive with *M. pneumoniae.* Approximately 85 per cent of patients with mycoplasmal pneumonia have a diagnostic rise in this complement-fixing antibody immune response. Another serologic test which may be positive in this disease is a high titer of cold agglutinins or antibodies specifically reactive with a viridans streptococcus, designated Streptococcus MG.

Do you believe the patient responded promptly to the erythromycin therapy? What other evidence is there that the patient with mycoplasmal pneumonia does not exhibit prompt clearing of his Mycoplasma micro-organisms from the respiratory tract? Is this patient a communicable hazard in his school and family setting?

CASE PRESENTATION 3

A 39-year-old white female was brought to the hospital emergency room during the early evening of December 20, 1966 with a diagnosis of barbiturate intoxication. She had made two suicidal gestures during the previous year in association with marital and economic crises. An empty medicine vial marked sodium seconal had been found on her bedside table by the patient's friend, who had discovered the patient lying on the floor of her apartment bedroom in a totally unresponsive condition.

A brief examination made immediately upon admission to the hospital revealed the following: a rectal temperature of 96.8°F; blood pressure, 90/50; pulse rate, 82 per minute; and respirations (very shallow), 12 per minute. The pupils were equal, small, and sluggishly reactive to light. The patient appeared comatose, responding only slightly to deep pain. The neck was supple. Lung fields were clear to auscultation. The abdomen was soft. All deep tendon reflexes were present but markedly depressed. There was evidence of small amounts of dried vomitus on the patient's neck.

An endotracheal tube was immediately inserted, and the patient was placed on mechanical ventilation while intravenous fluids were started. Initial respiratory secretions periodically aspirated through the endotracheal tube were scanty and mucoid. A roentgenogram taken at the bedside four hours after hospitalization revealed a definite density in the middle and lower portions of the right lung fields. Reexamination of the chest at this time revealed unequivocal crackling rales over the right chest posteriorly. Secretions aspirated through the endotracheal tube now had a mucopurulent character, and Gram stained smear revealed some polymorphonuclear neutrophils and innumerable gram positive cocci, many of which were arranged in short chains and clusters. A very few gram negative cocci and rods were noted in occasional microscopic fields. At this time, the patient's total peripheral blood leukocyte count was found to be 18,000 per cubic millimeter. Upon reviewing the information in hand, the attending physician requested the house staff to secure two blood cultures in rapid succession, send the aspirated respiratory secretions to the laboratory for culture, and initiate intravenous nafcillin, 4 gm every six hours.

The clinical setting is classic: a patient known to be susceptible to depression with a history of attempted suicide in the past, all indications that her current comatose condition is due to an overdose of sodium seconal, and clinical and roentgenographic evidence of acute aspiration pneumonia secondary to emesis and inhalation of gastric and upper respiratory tract secretions. The Gram stain of the mucopurulent respiratory secretions pointed strongly to staphylococcal infection. The attending physician made the correct response by prescribing a penicillinase-resistant semisynthetic penicillin derivative, nafcillin, knowing that even in 1966 a fair proportion of patients outside hospitals harbor penicillinase-secreting and penicillinase-resistant staphylococci in their oropharynx or on their skin. He also undoubtedly knew that nafcillin would represent effective therapy for not only penicillin-susceptible staphylococci but also several other likely causes of aspiration pneumonia, viz., *Streptococcus pneumoniae*, microaerophilic streptococci, and at least a small proportion of strains of Bacteroides species.

Subsequently reported laboratory data revealed that the blood cultures remained sterile (very often the case in staphylococcal pneumonia acquired via the aerogenic as opposed to the hematogenous route) and that almost a pure culture of *Staphylococcus aureus* was obtained from the patient's lower respiratory tract secretions. This staphylococcal isolate was highly penicillin-resistant but was nafcillin-susceptible with minimal inhibitory concentrations for these two antimicrobial drugs of 62 μg per ml and 0.4 μg per ml, respectively.

References

Book

Knight, V. (ed.): Viral and Mycoplasmal Infections of the Respiratory Tract. Philadelphia, Lea and Febiger, 1973.

Original Articles

Austrian, R., and Gold, J.: Pneumococcal bacteremia with especial reference to bacteremic pneumococcal pneumonia. Ann. Intern. Med. *60:*759, 1964.

Bartlett, J. G., Gorbach, S. L., Thadepalli, H., and Finegold, S. M.: Bacteriology of empyema. Lancet *1:*338, 1974.

Bartlett, J. G., Gorbach, S. L., and Finegold, S. M.: The bacteriology of aspiration pneumonia. Am. J. Med. *56:*202, 1974.

Denny, F. W., Clyde, W. A., Jr., and Glezen, W. P.: Mycoplasma pneumoniae disease: clinical spectrum, pathophysiology, epidemiology, and control. J. Infect. Dis. *123:*74, 1971.

Dorff, G. J., Coonrod, J. D., and Rytel, M. W.: Detection by immunoelectrophoresis of antigen in sera of patients with pneumococcal bacteremia. Lancet *1:*578, 1971.

Glezen, W. P., Loda, F. A., Clyde, W. A., Jr., Senior, R. J., Sheaffer, C. I., Conley, W. G., and Denny, F. W.: Epidemiologic patterns of acute lower respiratory disease of children in a pediatric group practice. J. Pediatr. *78:*397, 1971.

Hahn, H. H., and Beaty, H. N.: Transtracheal aspiration in the evaluation of patients with pneumonia. Ann. Intern. Med. *72:*183, 1970.

Kalinske, R. W., Parker, R. H., Brandt, D., and Hoeprich, P. D.: Diagnostic usefulness and safety of transtracheal aspiration. N. Engl. J. Med. *276:*604, 1967.

Laurenzi, G. A., Potter, R. T., and Kass, E. H.: Bacteriologic flora of the lower respiratory tract. N. Engl. J. Med. *265:*1273, 1961.

Mays, B. B., Thomas, G. D., Leonard, J. S., Jr., Southern, P. M., Jr., Pierce, A. K., and Sanford, J. P.: Gram-negative bacillary necrotizing pneumonia: A bacteriologic correlation. J. Infect. Dis. *120:*687, 1969.

Merrill, C. W., Gwaltney, J. M., Jr., Hendley, J. O., and Sande, M. A.: Rapid identification of pneumococci. Gram stain vs. the Quellung reaction. N. Engl. J. Med. *288:*510, 1973.

Monto, A. S., and Ullman, B. M.: Acute respiratory illness in an American community. The Tecumseh study. J.A.M.A. *227:*164, 1974.

Mufson, M. A., Chang, V., Gill, V., Wood, S. C., Romansky, M. J., and Chanock, R. M.: The role of viruses, mycoplasmas and bacteria in acute pneumonia in civilian adults. Am. J. Epidemiol. *86:*526, 1967.

Chapter 20

STREPTOCOCCUS PNEUMONIAE (PNEUMOCOCCUS)

Introduction

The three microorganisms *Streptococcus pneumoniae, Haemophilus influenzae,* and *Klebsiella pneumoniae* are classic examples of true extracellular parasites. These microorganisms will not produce disease unless they are growing and multiplying outside of phagocytic cells because once they are phagocytosed by neutrophils and macrophages they are killed within a few minutes. All three commonly cause disease in man and, since they produce disease only when they are outside of phagocytic cells, they must possess some property which prevents phagocytosis. In the case of all three, this phagocytosis-resisting mechanism has been found to reside in a polysaccharide capsular material. This capsular material inhibits phagocytosis by preventing attachment of the bacteria to the cell membrane of phagocytic cells. Without this attachment, phagocytosis does not readily take place.

These three pathogenic bacteria have in common a number of other characteristics. All are normal inhabitants of the upper respiratory tract of man and produce disease under conditions in which host defense mechanisms have been weakened. These bacteria are morphologically and metabolically quite different; however, they produce similar types of disease, and the diseased host recovers only when antibody specific for the capsular polysaccharides is developed. This specific antibody combines with the capsular material on the bacterium and, together with complement, neutralizes the antiphagocytic activity of the capsular polysaccharide.

Streptococcus pneumoniae is a particularly good example of a facultative intracellular parasite which owes its pathogenicity solely to the antiphagocytic effect of the capsular material since, to the best of our knowledge, it produces no other substance capable of deleteriously affecting host defense mechanisms. However, the presence of these metabolizing and multiplying cells does initiate an inflammatory reaction which causes an outpouring of fibrin, white blood cells, and red blood cells.

Morphology

Characteristically, pneumococci appear as gram positive, lancet-shaped diplococci. The cells may occur in clumps and, not infrequently, they may form chains of varying lengths. Some strains are particularly prone to chain formation and may not be distinguished from other streptococci. Ordinarily, pneumococci cannot be differentiated from other gram positive cocci when specimens such as pus, sputum, spinal fluid, and other body tissues are stained by the Gram method. Furthermore, capsules cannot be seen when fresh material containing pneumococci is examined directly or when it is stained by Gram's method. The capsule can be demonstrated only by using special capsule stains or by taking advantage of the fact that the capsule swells and becomes visible when type-specific antiserum is added to the medium in which the pneumococci are suspended. This is known as the "quellung" (swelling) reaction. It is an effective and efficient method for the demonstration of capsules of *Streptococcus pneumoniae* but requires type-specific antiserum. At one time, hospital laboratories did serologic typing of all pneumococcal strains found in the sputum of patients with pneumonia so that the appropriate type-specific serum could be used for therapy. Currently, the effectivenss of penicillin therapy has made serologic typing, for the most part, unnecessary; therefore, supplies of antisera of each pneumococcal type are not readily available. Type-specific antibody also can be useful for the detection of antigen in body fluids by counterimmunoelectrophoresis.

Capsules can be detected by suspending pneumococci in methylene blue and then placing this suspension on a slide. A clear area around each diplococcus will be seen when examined under the microscope; this clear zone represents the capsule which has excluded the dye from that area.

Growth

Streptococcus pneumoniae requires an enriched medium for growth, and the colonies resemble those of other alpha-hemolytic streptococci. On blood agar plates, an alpha-hemolytic reaction is seen. If the amount of capsular polysaccharide produced is large, as in type 3 strains, the colonies may appear large and mucoid.

Metabolism

Pneumococci grow aerobically but are facultative anaerobes. They are classified with the lactic acid-producing bacteria because the major fermentative product is lactic acid. During fermentation, hydrogen peroxide accumulates and, since the pneumococci produce neither peroxidase nor catalase, viability becomes adversely affected in old cultures. Viability of the cells can be maintained by adding blood to the culture medium, since red cells contain adequate amounts of catalase.

Pneumococcal cells in broth cultures or in colonies on blood agar may die because of the activation of an endogenous autolytic enzyme. This enzyme is an L-alanine-muramyl amidase and is activated by a variety of surface active agents. This provides the basis for the *bile solubility test* which is used for the separation of pneumococci from the other streptococci. Practically, all other streptococci are bile insoluble since they do not possess this autolytic enzyme.

Pneumococci ferment a number of carbohydrates as do other strepto-cocci, but only the penumococcus will ferment inulin. Thus, a typical alpha-hemolytic streptococcus which is bile soluble and ferments inulin can be tentatively identified as *Streptococcus pneumoniae.*

Antigenic Components

The major antigenic component of the pneumococcus cell is the capsular polysaccharide. This determines the type specificity of the strain and over 80 distinct antigenic types have been found. There are cross-reactions between some types, and polysaccharides from some types cross-react with antibody to polysaccharides found in other alpha-hemolytic streptococci, in *Klebsiella pneumoniae,* and in some Salmonella species; the polysaccharide capsule of type 14 *Streptococcus pneumoniae* also will cross-react with antibody to type B human red blood cells. For a given type of pneumococcus, the size of the capsule seems to bear an important relation to pathogenicity. For example, there are mutants of type 3 pneumococcus which produce a capsule of small size. These are less virulent than type 3 strains which produce large amounts of capsular material. The intermediate mutants are more pathogenic than strains which produce no capsule. Conversely, the small capsule-producing strain of one type may be more virulent than a large capsule-producing strain of another type. The chemical composition of some of the type-specific pneumococcal polysaccharides has been determined; e.g., the capsule of type 3 cells is a polymer of cellobiuronic acid.

Other antigens are found in the cell walls of *Streptococcus pneumoniae.* Among these is the C substance, a polysaccharide antigen which is probably equivalent to the group-specific C substances found in the beta-hemolytic streptococci (see Chap. 13). The significance of this antigen is that it has the peculiar property of being able to combine with and precipitate a beta globulin that is found in the serum of persons who are suffering from inflammatory diseases. A precipitin test using the C substance has been developed and is used as a guide to determine the degree of activity of inflammatory diseases. The C reactive protein which is found in the serum of patients with these inflammatory diseases is not an antibody; rather, it is only one of several abnormal proteins that can be detected in the serum of patients during the acute phase of the inflammatory disease.

Protein antigens also are found in pneumococcal cells. An M antigen apparently equivalent to the M antigen found in the beta-hemolytic streptococci also is present (see Chap. 13). This antigen is not antiphagocytic, nor will it produce immunity to pneumococcal infections when used as a vaccine.

Pathogenesis

Streptococcus pneumoniae is the most common cause of pneumonia in man. Ninety per cent of all bacterial pneumonias are caused by this microorganism. Pneumococcal pneumonia is almost always caused by pneumococci found normally in the upper respiratory tract of the majority of persons. Epidemics of pneumococcal pneumonia have occurred in certain populations (see discussion of epidemiology later in this chapter) but they are rare. In the ordinary course of events, pneumococci found as inhabitants of the upper respiratory tract gain entrance to the alveoli of the lung and under appropriate circumstances will begin to grow and multiply and produce disease.

The normal human host is highly resistant to the induction of pneumonia by *Streptococcus pneumoniae*. Only when situations develop which lower host defense mechanisms will such disease occur. One of the most common predisposing factors is viral infection of the upper or lower respiratory tract. When penumococcus pneumonia occurs in otherwise healthy human beings, a history of a recent cold or of influenza can usually be obtained. Any impairment of the epiglottal reflex, the cough reflex, or the movement of the mucociliary stream also will predispose to pneumonia due to *S. pneumoniae*.

Pneumococcal lobar pneumonia is far more common among chronic alcoholics than any other class of human beings. Alcohol intoxication is known to interfere with the defense mechanisms just mentioned. The chronic alcoholic may also vomit while in a semicomatose state and is at much greater risk of aspirating gastric contents. Alcohol intoxication also has been shown to delay mobilization of segmented neutrophils as well as impair their migration into an area of inflammation.

Following entry of the microorganisms into the lower respiratory tract and its alveoli, there is an outpouring of edema fluid, and segmented neutrophils accumulate in enormous numbers. The infection spreads peripherally, with the pneumococci multiplying readily in the edema fluid. An entire lobe may be involved or frequently, more than one lobe.*

Unless prompt treatment is given, the pleura may be involved by direct extension with the development of pleurisy and possibly empyema.

The infection may spread to the lymphatics with involvement of the hilar lymph nodes. Pneumococci may be carried by way of the lymphatics to the bloodstream and then may spread by way of the blood, and metastatic lesions may develop in other tissues such as the meninges, heart valves, or joints.

Primary infection of the upper respiratory tract, including sinusitis, otitis media, and mastoiditis, may be caused by pneumococci. There may be direct extension to the meninges with subsequent meningitis.

---

*The student should review the evolution of the pulmonary lesion, from inception to final resolution, in his textbook of pathology.

In untreated pneumococcal pneumonia, approximately one third of patients will die, although the mortality rate varies depending upon the serologic type producing the disease. In the two thirds of patients who spontaneously get well, the recovery is exclusively due to the development of an immune response which produces enough antibody to neutralize polysaccharide capsular material. This in turn provides for opsonization of the invading bacteria before death occurs.

Even in patients adequately treated early in the disease with suitable antibiotics, final recovery, in large part, depends upon a similar adequate immune response.

Epidemiology

Although any type of pneumococcus may cause lobar pneumonia in man, pneumonia is caused more frequently by certain types. In the United States at the present time, the most commonly encountered pneumococcal types in adults are types 8, 4, 3, 1, 7, and 12, in that order. In children, types 19, 23, 14, 3, 6, and 1 are more frequently found. Type 3 pneumococcus is the most virulent and accounts for the highest mortality rate because it produces more capsular material.

Pneumococcal lobar pneumonia is a sporadic disease in that cases are scattered as to place, time, and person. The sporadic occurrence arises from the fact that pneumococcal pneumonia is essentially a disease of carriers. From 20 to 70 per cent of normal human beings carry pneumococci in their upper respiratory tracts. Pneumococcal lobar pneumonia will occur in a certain proportion of these persons when host resistance has been lowered by some environmental factor or by another disease. Viral upper and lower respiratory tract infections are especially prone to predispose to pneumococcal pneumonia.

In the Northern Hemisphere, occurrence of pneumonia shows a seasonal distribution comparable to that of other respiratory tract infections. The highest number of cases appear during the coldest months of the year. This has been attributed to the increased crowding of people into closed environments during the winter which favors the transmission of microorganisms from person to person. Outside environmental factors are more unfavorable and, probably most important, this is the time of highest incidence of viral respiratory tract infections. There is, therefore, an overall reduction in host resistance during the winter months as compared to the other seasons of the year.

The incidence of pneumococcal pneumonia is greatest in young children and infants under five years of age, and in old persons. After 50 years of age, the morbidity and mortality rates increase. This age distribution for pneumococcal pneumonia is similar to that of many other infectious diseases and probably reflects the lower capacity of the very young and the old to mount an effective immune response.

Epidemics of pneumococcal pneumonia also may occur. These are of two general types. In the first, there may be an unusually high incidence of pneumococcal pneumonia in fairly large population groups, and the cases are caused by a variety of pneumococcal types. This situation was encountered in some military installations during World War II. The rapid turnover of personnel causing a constant introduction of new susceptible people probably accounted for the high incidence in this instance. In addition, many factors, including antecedent upper respiratory tract viral infections, no doubt played a role. The parallel between this type of epidemic of pneumococcal lobar pneumonia and the epidemics of cerebrospinal meningitis which develop among new military recruits should be apparent. Both are diseases of carriers, and poorly understood factors which lower host resistance are considered to be responsible for the development of the unusual number of cases.

The second type of epidemic includes outbreaks which occur among the inmates of children's homes, orphanages, and hospitals for persons with mental diseases. In these epidemics, there is a marked increase in the number of cases of pneumococcal lobar pneumonia caused by a single type of pneumococcus. In addition to the factors existing in these institutions which may contribute to lowering of host resistance, the introduction of a particularly virulent type of pneumococcus may play a large role in the genesis of the epidemic. Here again there is a parallel with meningococcal meningitis in which the large epidemics and pandemics which occur every few years are primarily the result of the introduction into human populations of a meningococcal type of greater virulence (see Chap. 34).

Isolation and Identification

The diagnosis of bacterial pneumonia depends upon the isolation or identification of the microorganism from the patient suffering from the disease. Three types of clinical specimens are available as a source for culture of bacteria which may be causing pneumonia: (1) sputum coughed up by the patient, (2) aspirates from the pulmonary tree, and (3) blood. Pneumococci in a sample of sputum can be isolated by plating the material on blood agar and, following isolation, identifying the organism by its capacity to ferment inulin, the finding that it is bile soluble, and its sensitivity to optochin. The *Optochin test* (ethylhydrocupreine) is particularly useful in the clinical laboratory for identification of the organism because pneumococci are uniquely susceptible to this compound. The test can be conveniently performed by using a paper disc impregnated with the proper concentration of the drug and placing it on the blood agar plate inoculated with the strain to be identified. After incubation, if the organism is a pneumococcus, a clear zone will be noted around the disc where growth has been inhibited. Sometimes, an optochin disc can be placed on a blood agar plate which was initially streaked with a portion of the sputum sample. If the number of pneumococci present is large, evidence of lack of growth around the disc can be noted for a presumptive identification.

The usefulness of sputum as a source of material for isolation of pneumococci or of other bacteria causing pneumonia is affected by the fact that such specimens are always contaminated by the microflora normally found in the upper respiratory tract. It may be difficult to distinguish pneumococci from the numerous alpha-hemolytic streptococci which normally inhabit this region. Such sputum samples also may be contaminated with pneumococci normally resident in the upper respiratory tract, and conceivably a pneumococcus could be isolated which would have no relation to the underlying pulmonary disease (see Chap. 10).

When pneumococci in a sputum sample are numerous, direct identification can be made by applying the capsular swelling test, the quellung reaction. This test, however, demands the availability in suitable form of type-specific antisera for at least the most prevalent pneumococcal types.

The most suitable pulmonary aspirate is that which can be obtained by translaryngeal aspiration. Material obtained in this manner will be free of contamination with microorganisms from the upper respiratory tract (see Chap. 10).

Blood cultures constitute an important source of material for isolation of pneumococci. One third of patients with pneumococcal lobar pneumonia have detectable microorganisms in their blood at some time during their illness. When pneumococci are isolated from blood, they are found in pure culture and the final identification can be made much more easily.

Isolation of virulent pneumococci from sputum can be greatly facilitated by emulsifying some of the sputum in saline and injecting a small portion of this material intraperitoneally into one or more laboratory mice. Encapsulated pneumococci are highly virulent for the laboratory mouse and, since they are resistant to phagocytosis, will multiply in the peritoneal space; on the other hand, contaminating, nonencapsulated microorganisms of the normal flora will be phagocytized and killed. The mouse so inoculated will die of an overwhelming pneumococcal disease within 24 to 48 hours. Pneumococci can then be readily isolated from the blood of the mouse or can be directly visualized and typed by the quellung method, using peritoneal exudate as a source of encapsulated microorganisms. The problems associated with maintaining and working with an animal colony have prevented widespread use of this procedure in most clinical laboratories.

Prevention

The same problems are encountered in the prevention of pneumococcal pneumonia as are encountered in attempts to prevent any respiratory disease. There are no public health methods of sanitation which can be applied to the control of such a disease. The only recourse is to attempt to raise the level of immunity in the population at risk. This can be done artificially by vaccination. It has been known for many years that human beings can be vaccinated with small amounts of pneumococcal polysaccharide, and that sufficient antibody will be formed to provide immunity to pneumococcal disease. This immunity is type specific.

Since the advent of penicillin and the demonstration of its remarkable effectiveness in therapeutic use, the opinion has prevailed that pneumococcal disease is no longer a significant medical problem. Now it appears, however, that the use of penicillin, even though it has markedly reduced mortality from pneumococcal disease, has had little influence on the *incidence* of pneumococcal disease. Therefore, an interest has been revived in the vaccination with pneumococcal polysaccharides of people who are known to be at risk, i.e., elderly people, those with underlying predisposing pulmonary disease, and persons in certain institutions. The types of pneumococci that cause the majority of cases of pneumonia in human beings are known. Vaccines containing small amounts of polysaccharide capsular material of each of these types are now being tested in human volunteers. It is clear that when mixtures of from 6 to 18 different type-specific polysaccharides are injected into man, antibody will be produced against all or most of these. If this antibody response proves to be adequate for protection against the initiation of pneumococcal infection, vaccination may prove to be of great benefit to certain population groups.

References

Books

Beeson, P. B., and McDermott, W. (eds.): Textbook of Medicine, 14th ed. Philadelphia, W. B. Saunders Co., 1975.
Davis, B. D., Dulbecco, R., Eisen, H. N., Ginsberg, H. S., Wood, W. B., and McCarty, M. (eds.): Microbiology. 2nd ed. Hagerstown, Maryland, Harper and Row, 1973.
Hoeprich, P. D. (ed.): Infectious Diseases. Hagerstown, Maryland, Harper and Row, 1972.

Review Article

MacLeod, C. M.: Prevention of pneumococcal pneumonia by immunization with specific capsular polysaccharides. *In* Mudd, S. (ed.): Infectious Agents and Host Reactions. Philadelphia, W. B. Saunders Co., 1970.

Original Articles

Austrian, A., and Gold, J.: Pneumococcal bacteremia with special reference to bacteremic pneumococcal pneumonia. Ann. Intern. Med. *60:*759, 1964.
Toxicity of pneumococcal neuraminidase. Infect. Immun. *2:*115, 1970.

Chapter 21

HAEMOPHILUS INFLUENZAE AND KLEBSIELLA PNEUMONIAE

Introduction

Haemophilus influenzae and *Klebsiella pneumoniae*, although different in most respects, have certain features in common with *Streptococcus pneumoniae*. Both *K. pneumoniae* and *H. influenzae* are normal inhabitants of the upper respiratory tract of man and may produce both lower and upper respiratory tract disease similar to that produced by the pneumococcus. Both *K. pneumoniae* and *H. influenzae* share with *S. pneumoniae* the presence of a large polysaccharide capsule which protects them from phagocytosis and is largely responsible for their capacity to produce disease. *H. influenzae* and *K. pneumoniae*, next to *S. pneumoniae*, are the two most common encapsulated bacteria which produce infection of the upper and lower respiratory tract in human beings in the United States today.

Haemophilus Influenzae

Morphology

Haemophilus influenzae is a very small gram negative pleomorphic bacterium (rod). When the cells are young and growing under optimal conditions, they appear more like a coccobacillus than a true bacillus. In older cultures, or when growing under unfavorable conditions, the rods become elongated and frequently appear filamentous.

300

Growth

Haemophilus influenzae will grow in either the presence (aerobe) or absence (facultative anaerobe) of oxygen (air). This microorganism belongs to a group collectively referred to as the hemophilic bacteria. These microorganisms require enriched media for growth, and most must have available either one or both of two growth factors referred to as X and V. X factor has been identified as hematin, and V factor is found to be replaceable by NAD (nicotinamide-adenine dinucleotide, diphosphopyridine nucleotide), NADP (nicotinamide-adenine dinucleotide phosphate, triphosphopyridine nucleotide), or adenine nucleoside (see Table 21–1). V factor is heat labile and may be destroyed enzymatically by enzymes found in red blood cells. Therefore, for growth of *H. influenzae* it is better to use chocolate agar enriched with V factor rather than blood agar. Chocolate agar is blood agar which has been heated sufficiently to destroy red blood cells and inactivate the enzymes which might degrade the V factor.

TABLE 21–1. Differential Growth Characteristics of the
Haemophilus-Bordetella Group*

Species	Growth Factors		Hemolysis
	X	V	
Genus Haemophilus			
H. influenzae	+	+	−
H. parainfluenzae	−	+	−
H. aegypticus	+	+	−
H. ducreyi	+	−	+
H. suis	?	+	−
H. hemolyticus	+	+	+
Genus Bordetella			
B. pertussis	−	−	+
B. parapertussis	−	−	±
B. bronchiseptica	−	−	±

*From Davis, B. D., et al.: Microbiology. 2nd ed. Hagerstown, Maryland, Harper and Row, 1973.

Although *Haemophilus influenzae* requires both X and V factors for growth, not all of the species bacteria in the genus Haemophilus require these factors; some require only one. Table 21–1 lists the members of this genus, their requirements for X and V factors, and their capacity to produce hemolysis of red cells. The growth requirements as outlined in the table are useful for differentiating members of this group.

V factor required for growth by *Haemophilus influenzae* can also be furnished by other microorganisms. For example, colonies of staphylococci on chocolate agar may produce enough V factor to permit the growth of *H. influenzae* in the intermediate vicinity of the staphylococcal colony. This is known as the *satellite phenomenon* (Fig. 21–1). It is not known whether

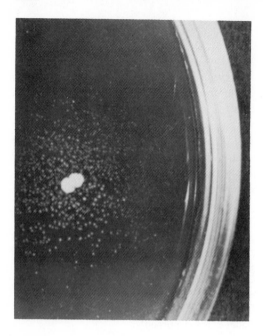

Figure 21–1. Satellite phenomenon. Colonies of *Haemophilus influenzae* growing only in vicinity of staphylococcal colonies on agar medium lacking V factor. The agar, which contained blood autoclaved to destroy the V factor, was uniformly seeded with a heavy inoculum of *H. influenzae* and a very light inoculum of *Staphylococcus aureus.* (From Davis, B. D., et al.: Microbiology. 2nd ed. Hagerstown, Maryland, Harper and Row, 1973.)

the production of V factor by other microorganisms, or by the host, may contribute to the growth of *H. influenzae* in vivo and therefore contribute to its pathogenicity.

Reference has already been made in Chapter 14 to practical problems arising from the fact that *Haemophilus hemolyticus* and staphylococci are common components of the normal oropharyngeal microbial flora, especially in children. In association with production of V factor by the staphylococci, *H. hemolyticus* colonies surrounded by areas of complete (beta-type) hemolysis may occur on blood agar plates streaked with throat swabs. These colonies may be mistaken for Group A streptococci. This problem can be avoided by using agar plates prepared from sheep blood rather than human blood, since the hemolysin produced by *H. hemolyticus* does not lyse sheep erythrocytes. A simple determination of the Gram reaction of any hemolytic colony suspected of being Group A streptococci on a throat swab streak plate also will help avert such cases of mistaken identity.

Antigenic Structure

The major antigenic component is the polysaccharide capsule. Six distinct antigenic types have been described and are labeled a, b, c, d, e, and f. *Haemophilus influenzae* can be typed by means of capsular swelling (Quellung) tests, using specific antiserum, or by other serologic tests. The capsular polysaccharide of *H. influenzae* type b, the type which most frequently causes diseases of humans, has been shown to be a polyribophosphate.

Other antigens are also present in *Haemophilus influenzae* cells. A protein M antigen is found to be present in all antigenic types and apparently is species specific. *H. influenzae,* as do most gram negative bacteria, also contains an endotoxin.

Immunologic relationships are found between some of the *Haemophilus influenzae* types and other bacteria. For example, type b cross-reacts with pneumococcus types 6, 15, 29, and 35; type c with pneumococcus type 11 and type a cross-reacts with pneumococcus type 6. Other cross-reactions have been noticed. For example, type b will cross-react with antigens found in *Staphylococcus aureus, Bacillus subtilis,* and some strains of *Escherichia coli.* The antigen in *E. coli* which cross-reacts with the *H. influenzae* polyribose phosphate capsule has been identified as a surface-stable, acidic capsular polysaccharide, the *E. coli* K antigen.

Pathogenesis

The pathogenesis of *Haemophilus influenzae* disease in some ways is similar to that of disease produced by *Streptococcus pneumoniae.* *H. influenzae* strains are normal inhabitants of the upper respiratory tract of a significant number of persons, and disease may result because of the absence in the serum of protective anticapsular antibody. Adults are infrequently infected since natural exposure to *H. influenzae* strains in the upper respiratory tract has led to the development of antibody following subclinical infection. Of the six antigenic types, by far the most pathogenic are those organisms constituting type b. Most of the disease seen in children is due to type b strains.

Disease in susceptible children probably starts as pharyngitis, and it may well be that there was some preceding viral infection that reduced resistance; this is similar to the clinical pattern found with *Streptococcus pneumoniae.* The upper respiratory tract may be involved, since sinusitis and, in some children, epiglottitis may occur. The latter infection can be severe and may lead to the rapid development of laryngeal obstruction (see Fig. 12–1). One of the characteristic clinical features of this disease is a cherry red, markedly edematous epiglottis. Prompt tracheotomy may be required to prevent asphyxia. *Haemophilus influenzae* pneumonia may also occur in children or adults, especially when resistance has been lowered by a preceding viral infection. The classic example of *H. influenzae* pneumonia following viral infection is provided by the occurrence of many cases of *H. influenzae* pneumonia during the 1918 influenza epidemic, which led to the erroneous conclusion that *H. influenzae* is the cause of influenza.

Bloodstream invasion is common, and one of the most frequently seen manifestations of *Haemophilus influenzae* infection is meningitis. Meningitis is almost invariably due to type b *H. influenzae,* and it may be fatal unless prompt diagnosis is made and adequate treatment given. If large numbers of microorganisms are present in cerebrospinal fluid, they can be typed and identified directly by the Quellung reaction.

It is probably safe to conclude that most if not all disease due to *Haemophilus influenzae* results from microorganisms harbored in the upper respiratory tract; however, in the case of type b, disease may on occasion be acquired from carriers of this organism. Disease due to *H. influenzae* usually occurs in infants and children who have not yet developed adequate protective antibodies as a result of subclinical infection.

Occasionally, pulmonary disease from *Haemophilus influenzae* is seen in adults. When this happens, it is usually associated with other factors, such as an antecedent viral infection, or other underlying pulmonary disease, e.g., chronic bronchitis, which modify animal host defense mechanisms for *H. influenzae* pneumonia.

It is of some interest that although *Haemophilus influenzae* is probably one of the most common causes of otitis media in children, most of the *H. influenzae* strains isolated from this condition are nontypable; i.e., they are not members of any one of the six antigenic types. Type b *H. influenzae* is responsible for only 5 to 10 per cent of the cases. The pathogenesis of otitis media caused by the nontypable *H. influenzae* strains is not clear.

Epidemiology

It has already been noted that *Haemophilus influenzae* is a normal inhabitant of the upper respiratory tract. One would expect, then, that meningitis and other infectious disease due to *H. influenzae* would occur sporadically, and this is the case. Epidemics of *H. influenzae* meningitis do not occur. As with meningitis caused by *Neisseria meningitidis*, *H. influenzae* meningitis is primarily a disease of carriers.

Certain racial differences in susceptibility to infection with *Haemophilus influenzae* have been noted. In certain southern states, the incidence of *H. influenzae* meningitis is four times as great in Negroes as in whites. This finding suggests that blacks may be genetically more susceptible to *H. influenzae*. However, in the northern city of Pittsburgh, there is no difference in the incidence of *H. influenzae* meningitis in blacks and whites. This suggests that rather than a genetic factor, the higher incidence may be a reflection of a lower socioeconomic status of blacks in the South which in some unknown way could reduce resistance to this microorganism.

Immunity

Immunity to infection with *Haemophilus influenzae* is directly related to age and is directly related to the amount of circulating bactericidal antibody found in the blood. Figure 21–2 shows the relationship of case incidence and age to the presence of circulating bactericidal antibody. As are many gram negative bacteria, *H. influenzae* is readily lysed by antibody and complement. This fact has provided over the years a convenient method of measuring immunity to *H. influenzae* infection. Whether or not antibody found in the

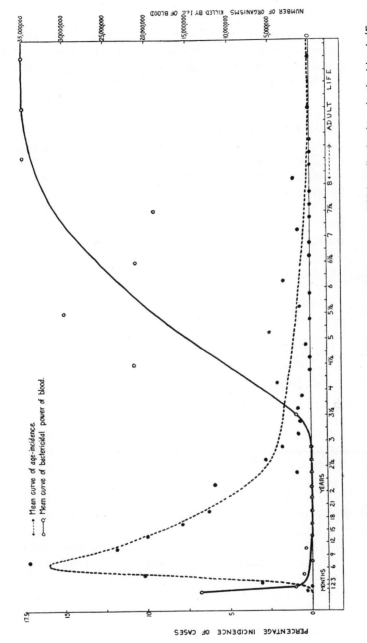

Figure 21-2. Relation of the age incidence of *H. influenzae* meningitis to bactericidal antibody titers in the blood. (From Fothergill, L. D., and Wright, J.: *J. Immunol. 24*:281, 1933.) © [1933] The Williams & Wilkins Co., Baltimore.

serum plays a role in prevention of infection in human beings is another matter. It is known that anticapsular polysaccharide antibody is protective and, since the major effect of this antibody is to promote phagocytosis through opsonization, opsonization and phagocytosis are probably the major immune factors and account for the protection of human beings against infection. Although the antibody can be readily demonstrated in vitro, it is not known whether bactericidal lysis actually takes place in vivo.

The increased immunity to *Haemophilus influenzae* infections which occurs with age should be accompanied by an increase in antibody to the polyribose phosphate capsular polysaccharide; this has been shown to be the case with type b *H. influenzae*. It has been assumed that the development of antibody with increase in age is due to subclinical exposure to *H. influenzae* types residing in the nasopharynx. Undoubtedly, this type of antigenic exposure is in part responsible. The demonstration that a variety of other bacteria, including strains of *Escherichia coli*, have antigens closely related to type-specific polysaccharide capsular antigens of *H. influenzae* types raises the possibility that some of the immunity which has developed may have come from exposure to these other microorganisms, many of which normally colonize the gut. The suggestion has been made that colonization of children with antigenically related *E. coli* strains might provide the antigenic stimulus needed to develop protective immunity to type b *H. influenzae*. Experimental studies in which rabbits have been colonized with specific *E. coli* indicate that protective immunity to type b *H. influenzae* can be developed in this manner. Whether or not immunization of this type would be a useful approach to the prevention of disease in human beings has yet to be determined.

Active immunization of infants and young children with the specific polyribophosphate which constitutes the capsule type b *Haemophilus influenzae* may also be feasible. It has been shown that single doses of 1 to 100 µg of polyribophosphate in adults and children are immunogenic and well tolerated. A single intramuscular dose of either 5 or 25 µg will produce anticapsular antibody rises in approximately 90 per cent of children to levels that exceed those found in presumably immune individuals.

Klebsiella Pneumoniae

Klebsiella pneumoniae, the third of our triumvirate of microorganisms which cause primary disease of the lower respiratory tract, is a small nonmotile gram negative bacillus which by Gram stain cannot be morphologically distinguished from other members of the Enterobacteriaceae. The major feature distinguishing this organism from other members of the Enterobacteriaceae is the presence of a large polysaccharide capsule. So much of this capsular material is produced on certain types of suitable solid culture media that the colonies are mucoid in appearance, and if touched with an inoculating wire, the sticky mucous-like material will adhere and can be drawn into long strands. Seventy-seven distinct antigenic types of polysaccharide have been identified to date. Strains of *K. pneumoniae* can be identified and typed by serologic means, including the capsular swelling test. *K. pneumoniae* is usually identified by the biochemical tests which are used to distinguish members of the Enterobacteriaceae (see Chap. 11).

The pathogenesis of pulmonary disease due to *Klebsiella pneumoniae* differs little from the pathogenesis of pulmonary disease caused by *Streptococcus pneumoniae*. Like *S. pneumoniae* and *Haemophilus influenzae*, *K. pneumoniae* is an inhabitant of the upper respiratory tract of from 1 to 6 per cent of normal human beings. It is also frequently found in the gastrointestinal tract. As does pneumonia due to *H. influenzae* and *S. pneumoniae*, that due to *K. pneumoniae* most frequently occurs in persons whose normal host resistance has been lowered in some manner. These include those suffering from some underlying systemic disease such as diabetes and those who may have underlying bronchopulmonary disease. Any illness which contributes to lowered resistance disposes to pneumonia due to *K. pneumoniae*. As does pneumococcal pneumonia, the disease occurs frequently in persons who are chronic alcoholics.

Although pneumonia due to *Klebsiella pneumoniae* is usually secondary, primary pneumonia can occur. From 0.5 to 5 per cent of all primary pneumonias are said to be due to *K. pneumoniae*.

Clinically, pneumonia caused by *Klebsiella pneumoniae* cannot be distinguished from that caused by *Streptococcus pneumoniae*. The presenting symptoms and the course of the pulmonary involvement are similar. In contrast to pneumonia caused by *S. pneumoniae*, disease due to *K. pneumoniae* usually shows a greater number of microorganisms in the areas of pulmonary consolidation. Unlike pneumococcal pneumonia, there also is a great deal of destruction of alveolar walls so that repair is by fibrosis. For this reason, pneumonia due to *K. pneumoniae* is a destructive disease, and abscess formation, often associated with bronchial obstruction, is common. The mortality rate ranges from 50 to over 90 per cent for untreated patients. Because of the rapid and excess amount of tissue destruction, early diagnosis and treatment are imperative.

Unlike *Streptococcus pneumoniae*, *Klebsiella pneumoniae* is resistant to penicillin. This emphasizes the need for early diagnosis and treatment with suitable microbial agents such as cephalothin or gentamicin. These are usually regarded as the preferred drugs but, in patients with serious disease or another underlying medical problem, two drugs may be necessary; e.g., cephalothin plus kanamycin or cephalothin plus gentamicin.

Procedures used for the diagnosis of any pneumonia should be instituted immediately so that recovery and identification of *Klebsiella pneumoniae* can be made as soon as possible. Gram stains of sputum, blood culture, induced sputum specimens, or possibly even translaryngeal aspiration are as appropriate here as in any pneumonia (see Chap. 11).

No specific methods of prevention are available. The large number of serologic types make vaccination impractical. In contrast to pneumonia produced by the pneumococcus, all *Klebsiella pneumoniae* types seem to be equally capable of causing serious disease.

In connection with this brief discussion of pneumonia caused by *Klebsiella pneumoniae*, it should be pointed out that a wide variety of other aerobic gram negative bacteria may cause pneumonia in man. These include *Escherichia coli, Serratia marcescens, Pseudomonas aeruginosa,* and Proteus species. These microorganisms are almost always encountered in hospitalized patients, and the pneumonia is frequently due to hospital-acquired microorganisms. Patients in hospitals who are receiving inhalation therapy for underlying pulmonary disease are particularly at risk, especially if they are also receiving antimicrobial therapy which can modify the flora of the upper respiratory tract. In the hospital setting, the number and proportion of gram negative bacteria found in the upper respiratory tract of patients may show a marked increase over that found in the general population. Pneumonia due to gram negative bacilli is found most frequently in those patients in whom a significant microbial flora consisting of gram negative bacilli has been established in the upper respiratory tract. In these patients, inappropriate therapy with antibiotics to which these microorganisms are resistant, such as penicillin, will significantly contribute to the building up of a gram negative bacillary upper respiratory microbial flora and predispose to further infection.

CASE PRESENTATION 1

A 75-year-old male, with a diagnosis of chronic obstructive pulmonary disease established 15 years previously by means of pulmonary function tests, was hospitalized because of "pneumonia" during the early morning hours of February 12, 1970. He had been in reasonably good health except for a chronic productive cough, dyspnea on exertion, and wheezing, all attributed to his underlying lung disorder and aggravated by his 60-year-old two-pack-a-day cigarette smoking habit. On February 10, the patient noted sore throat, an increase in cough with appearance of grossly purulent sputum, and marked shortness of breath. These symptoms, together with increasing right anterolateral chest pain intensified by respiratory movements, finally prompted hospitalization.

Physical examination revealed an acutely ill patient with labored respirations of 34 per minute, rectal and axillary temperatures ranging from 99.8° to 101.4°F, a pulse rate of 110 per minute, and a blood pressure of 166/90. Significant findings included a suggestive friction rub over the lower right lateral chest wall and coarse rhonchi, end-inspiratory crackling rales, and expiratory wheezes throughout both lung fields.

While waiting for an emergency chest roentgenogram to be taken, the attending physician prepared a Gram stain of freshly collected purulent sputum. The stained smear revealed innumerable neutrophils and a mixture of gram positive and gram negative bacteria, none of which predominated. Inspection of the chest roentgenogram showed a well-defined density in the right middle and lower lobes of the right lung, with evidence of fluid in the right pleural space. Other abnormalities consistent with chronic lung disease and believed to be unrelated to the patient's acute illness also were noted.

After two blood cultures were drawn in rapid succession at separate venipuncture sites and the sputum specimen had been inoculated onto appropriate media, the patient was started on moderately large doses of ampicillin by vein. Both the nurse in charge and the intern raised a question as to whether a respiratory ventilator should be ordered for the patient, but the attending physician indicated he did not wish this done. Two days later, when the patient had shown improvement in all spheres, both blood cultures and the sputum culture were reported to have yielded *Haemophilus influenzae,* type b.

The clinical setting for this case includes at least two factors which serve to diminish host defenses and predispose this patient to lower respiratory tract infection, viz., long-standing underlying lung disease and persistent inhalation of cigarette smoke. The patient's illness occurred at a time of year when infectious respiratory diseases of all kinds tend to attain peak incidence. The symptoms, physical findings, and chest roentgenogram collectively supported a presumptive diagnosis of acute bacterial lobar pneumonia. The Gram stained sputum smear also provided support for this diagnosis but did not offer any definite clues as to what specific microorganism was responsible for the patient's acute disease.

Two important facets of the clinical setting were responsible for the decision by the physician, who had a diagnosis of pneumonia due to *Haemophilus influenzae* specifically in mind, to initiate antimicrobial therapy with ampicillin. First, *H. influenzae* and *Streptococcus pneumoniae* are the two most common causes of acute exacerbations in patients with chronic obstructive pulmonary disease. While such exacerbations often reflect intercurrent infections limited to the tracheobronchial tree with little or no involvement of the lung parenchyma, pneumonia may develop. This is especially true when the acute exacerbations are due to strains of *H. influenzae* and *S. pneumoniae* representing serotypes clearly implicated in the pathogenesis of lobar pneumonia. Second, increasing evidence indicates that older persons and young children may be especially susceptible to disease caused by *H. influenzae*. Occurrence of such disease in older patients, despite demonstrable serum bactericidal antibody to *H. influenzae* type b laboratory strains, has been reported. This observation is at variance with the situation in children. It suggests that host immune responses other than the presence of type-specific bactericidal antibody may be important determinants in infections and disease due to *H. influenzae*. The question of subtypes or substrains of type b *H. influenzae* with subtle alterations in antigenic composition also can be raised.

Until very recently, the overwhelming majority of *Haemophilus influenzae* strains could be expected to exhibit greater in vitro susceptibility to ampicillin than to penicillin G. This is the basis for the widespread use of this extended spectrum penicillin-class antimicrobial drug in the therapy of disease due to *H. influenzae*. Since *Streptococcus pneumoniae* is invariably susceptible to ampicillin, this drug also can be used for the treatment of pneumococcal disease. Within the past year or so, however, disease caused by well-documented, ampicillin-resistant strains of *H. influenzae* has been reported from several quarters. Therefore, the spector of drug resistance once again presents a problem. Physicians must be ready to use alternate antimicrobial drugs should they have reason to believe a patient is infected with a strain of *H. influenzae* resistant to ampicillin.

CASE PRESENTATION 2

A 40-year-old male chronic alcoholic was hospitalized in January, 1969, with the complaint of left pleuritic chest pain of four days' duration accompanied by sweats, several hard "teeth clattering" rigors, a cough productive of "gray-black" sputum and mixed with fresh blood, and repeated emesis. The patient was known to the admitting room hospital staff because of previous hospitalizations for pneumonia and delirium tremens secondary to chronic and acute alcoholism.

The patient was tremulous and had a strong odor of liquor on his breath. He was tachypneic and appeared seriously ill. His blood pressure was 130/95 mm Hg; the pulse rate was 136 per minute; and respirations were 30 per minute. His oral temperature was 100.6°F, but when it was checked by a rectal thermometer it was found to be 103.8°F. Expansion of the left hemithorax on inspiration was impaired. Scattered rales were heard over the left posterolateral lung fields.

Initial laboratory studies revealed a white blood cell count of 6500 per cubic millimeter, with 50 per cent segmented neutrophils and 26 per cent band forms. Two separate Gram stained sputum specimens showed a striking predominance of gram negative bacilli. Several oil immersion fields contained only gram negative, rod-shaped microorganisms in large numbers. The chest roentgenogram showed a dense left lower lung infiltrate.

After securing two blood cultures and ascertaining that the sputum specimen was already inoculated onto suitable media, the attending physician ordered cephalothin and kanamycin. The presumptive diagnosis was acute pneumonia due to *Klebsiella pneumoniae.*

Approximately nine hours after hospitalization, the patient was evaluated by a consultant for infectious diseases, who drew additional blood for special testing. During the next 90 minutes, serum from this blood specimen was tested by means of counterimmunoelectrophoresis and found to give a single discrete precipitin line with type 1 monospecific *Klebsiella pneumoniae* antiserum as well as a polyvalent *K. pneumoniae* antiserum. No precipitin lines were observed with types 2 through 6 monospecific *K. pneumoniae* antisera or with various monospecific or polyvalent *Streptococcus pneumoniae* antisera. The infectious diseases consultant contacted the attending physician and informed him of finding *K. pneumoniae* type 1 antigen circulating in the blood of the patient, indicative of acute pneumonia due to type 1 *K. pneumoniae.* Thirty-six hours later, the hospital laboratory reported that the initial sputum specimen and both blood cultures had yielded *K. pneumoniae* which gave a quellung reaction with type 1 antisera only.

The clinical setting is prototypic for acute pneumonia due to *Klebsiella pneumoniae*; i.e., wintertime, a middle-aged chronic alcoholic male, and symptoms, physical findings, and a chest roentgenogram indicative of lobar pneumonia. Note that the patient had suffered a number of shaking chills instead of the single chill so commonly experienced with pneumonia due to *Streptococcus pneumoniae.* Although the patient's sputum contained a liberal amount of blood, it was not the so-called currant jelly sputum considered characteristic of *K. pneumoniae* pneumonia. The currant jelly designation reflects the extensive lung injury and considerable hemorrhage which may occur in *K. pneumoniae* infections of the lung, and the large amounts of viscous polysaccharide capsular material that are elaborated by the rapidly multiplying microorganisms, rendering the sputum almost mucilaginous in consistency and appearance.

The fact that the acute process involved the left lung of the patient helped exclude aspiration pneumonia, always a possibility in chronic alcoholics but which usually involves the right lung. The Gram stained sputum smear proved most helpful in considering the likelihood of pneumonia due to *Klebsiella pneumoniae.* The sputum smear, probably more than anything else in the initial evaluation, was the clue that led to starting antimicrobial therapy (cephalothin and kanamycin) effective against this specific microorganism.

The use of a relatively new diagnostic technique, counterimmunoelectrophoresis, illustrates the rewards that may accrue from searching for immunologically specific microbial antigens in blood and body fluids of patients (see Chap. 9). A specific diagnosis of pneumonia due to *Klebsiella pneumoniae* was in hand within 90 minutes after blood was drawn for testing by the infectious diseases consultant. The rapidity of this diagnostic procedure is invaluable for prompt recognition or differentiation of a number of acute, life-threatening, infectious problems, including pneumonia due to *K. pneumoniae,* in which highly selective antimicrobial therapy is required.

Two other points are worth noting in this case. First, oral temperatures are notoriously inaccurate in patients who are experiencing any respiratory distress and are unable to close their lips firmly around an oral thermometer. Second, the relatively low total leukocyte count of 6500 per cubic millimeter is not infrequent in pneumonia due to either *Streptococcus pneumoniae* or *Klebsiella pneumoniae.* Severe leukopenia, with total white cell counts as low as 700 to 800 per cubic millimeter, has occasionally been observed in patients. At the other end of the spectrum are some patients with extremely high total leukocyte counts, viz., 35,000 to 50,000 per cubic millimeter. Such leukocytosis probably reflects the propensity of *K. pneumoniae* to cause extensive destruction of lung tissue with complicating pulmonary abscess formation, an event which virtually never occurs in pneumonia due solely to *S. pneumoniae.*

References

Books

Beeson, P. B., and McDermott, W. (eds.): Textbook of Medicine. 14th ed. Philadelphia, W. B. Saunders Co., 1975.

Davis, B. D., Dulbecco, R., Eisen, H. N., Ginsberg, H. S., Wood, W. B., and McCarty, M.: Microbiology. 2nd ed. Hagerstown, Maryland, Harper and Row, 1973.

Hoeprich, P. D. (ed.): Infectious Diseases. Hagerstown, Maryland, Harper and Row, 1972.

Symposium Volume

Sell, H. E., and Karzon, D. T. (eds.): Haemophilus Influenzae. Nashville, Vanderbilt University Press, 1973.

Review Articles

Alford, R. H.: Transformation of human lymphocytes by a Haemophilus influenzae antigen. *In* Sell, H. E., and Karzon, D. T. (eds.): Haemophilus Influenzae. Nashville, Vanderbilt University Press, 1973.

Anderson, P., Johnston, R. B., Jr., and Smith, D. H.: Methodology in detection of human serum antibodies to Haemophilus influenzae, type b. *In* Sell, H. E., and Karzon, D. T. (eds.): Haemophilus Influenzae. Nashville, Vanderbilt University Press, 1973.

Argamman, M.: Serologic relationship between Haemophilus influenzae, type b, by capsular polysaccharide and polyribitol teichoic acids of gram-positive bacteria. *In* Sell, H. E., and Karzon, D. T. (eds.): Haemophilus Influenzae. Nashville, Vanderbilt University Press, 1973.

Feldman, R. A., Fraser, D. W., and Koehler, R. E.: Death certificates as a measure of Haemophilus influenzae meningitis mortality in the United States, 1962–1968. *In* Sell, H. E., and Karzon, D. T. (eds.): Haemophilus Influenzae. Nashville, Vanderbilt University Press, 1973.

Fine, D. P., Marney, S. R., Jr., Colley, D. G., and DesPrez, R. M.: Haemophilus influenzae decomplementation pattern in chelated and nonchelated serum. *In* Sell, H. E., and Karzon, D. T. (eds.): Haemophilus Influenzae. Nashville, Vanderbilt University Press, 1973.

Fraser, D. W., Darby, C. P., Koehler, R. E., Jacobs, C. F., and Feldman, R. A.: The epidemiology of Haemophilus influenzae meningitis. *In* Sell, H. E., and Karzon, D. T. (eds.): Haemophilus Influenzae. Nashville, Vanderbilt University Press, 1973.

Handzel, Z. T., Myerowitz, R. L., Schneerson, R., and Robbins, J. B.: Gastrointestinal colonization of neonatal rabbits with cross-reacting Escherichia coli: An approach to induction of immunity toward Haemophilus influenzae, type b. *In* Sell, H. E., and Karzon, D. T. (eds.): Haemophilus Influenzae. Nashville, Vanderbilt University Press, 1973.

Harding, A. L., Anderson, P., Howie, V. M., Ploussard, J. H., and Smith, D. H.: Haemophilus influenzae isolated from children with otitis media. *In* Sell, H. E., and Karzon, D. T. (eds.): Haemophilus influenzae. Nashville, Vanderbilt University Press, 1973.

Ingram, D. L., O'Reilly, R., Anderson, P., and Smith, D. H.: Detection of the capsular polysaccharide of Haemophilus influenzae, type b, in body fluids. *In* Sell, H. E., and Karzon, D. T. (eds.): Haemophilus Influenzae. Nashville, Vanderbilt University Press, 1973.

Johnston, R. B., Jr., Anderson, P., and Newman, S. L.: Opsonization and phagocytosis of Haemophilus influenzae, type b. *In* Sell, H. E., and Karzon, D. T. (eds.): Haemophilus Influenzae. Nashville, Vanderbilt University Press, 1973.

Michaels, R. H., and Schultz, W. F.: The frequency of Haemophilus influenzae infections: An analysis of racial and environmental factors. *In* Sell, H. E., and Karzon, D. T. (eds.): Haemophilus Influenzae. Nashville, Vanderbilt University Press, 1973.

Myerowitz, R. L., Handzel, Z. T., Schneerson, R., and Robbins, J. B.: Escherichia coli antigens cross-reactive with the capsular polysaccharides of Haemophilus influenzae, type b. *In* Sell, H. E., and Karzon, D. T. (eds.): Haemophilus Influenzae. Nashville, Vanderbilt University Press, 1973.

Norden, C. W., and Michaels, R. H.: Antibody production following Haemophilus influenzae meningitis. *In* Sell, H. E., and Karzon, D. T. (eds.): Haemophilus Influenzae. Nashville, Vanderbilt University Press, 1973.

Parke, J. C., Jr., Schneerson, R., and Robbins, J. B.: The attack rate, racial distribution, age incidence, and case fatality rate of Haemophilus influenzae, type b, meningitis in Mecklenburg County, North Carolina. *In* Sell, H. E., and Karzon, D. T. (eds.): Haemophilus Influenzae. Nashville, Vanderbilt University Press, 1973.

Peter, G., Anderson, P., and Smith, D. H.: Immunization of adults and children with polyribophosphate, the capsular antigen of Haemophilus influenzae, type b. *In* Sell, H. E., and Karzon, D. T. (eds.): Haemophilus Influenzae. Nashville, Vanderbilt University Press, 1973.

Robbins, J. B., Myerowitz, R. L., Schneerson, R., Whisnant, J. K., Gotschlich, E., and Liu, D. R.: Cross-reacting antigens of enteric bacteria as an antigenic source for "natural antibodies to bacteria causing meningitis." *In* Sell, H. E., and Karzon, D. T. (eds.): Haemophilus Influenzae. Nashville, Vanderbilt University Press, 1973.

Robbins, J. B., Parke, J. C., Jr., Schneerson, R., and Whisnant, J. K.: Quantitative measurement of "natural" and immunization-induced Haemophilus influenzae, type b, capsular polysaccharide antibodies. *In* Sell, H. E., and Karzon, D. T. (eds.): Haemophilus Influenzae. Nashville, Vanderbilt University Press, 1973.

Robinson, J. P., Sell, S. H., and Schuffman, S. S.: Electron microscopy studies of antibodies to Haemophilus influenzae, type b. *In* Sell, H. E., and Karzon, D. T. (eds.): Haemophilus Influenzae. Nashville, Vanderbilt University Press, 1973.

Schneerson, R., Robbins, J. B., and Parke, J. C., Jr.: Studies on Haemophilus influenzae, isolated from otitis media. *In* Sell, H. E., and Karzon, D. T. (eds.): Haemophilus Influenzae. Nashville, Vanderbilt University Press, 1973.

Sell, S. H., Turner, D. J., and Federspiel, C.: Natural infections with Haemophilus influenzae in children: Types identified. *In* Sell, H. E., and Karzon, D. T. (eds.): Haemophilus Influenzae. Nashville, Vanderbilt University Press, 1973.

Sell, S. H., Turner, D. J., Johnston, R. B., Jr., Federspiel, C. F., Zwaag, R. V., and Duke, L. J.: Natural infections with Haemophilus influenzae. II. Studies of serum antibody activity. *In* Sell, H. E., and Karzon, D. T. (eds.): Haemophilus Influenzae. Nashville, Vanderbilt University Press, 1973.

Sherwin, R. P., and Wilkins, J.: The ultrastructure of Haemophilus influenzae. *In* Sell, H. E., and Karzon, D. T. (eds.): Haemophilus Influenzae. Nashville, Vanderbilt University Press, 1973.

Smith, A. L., Averill, D. R., Moxon, E. R., Weller, P. F., Marino, J., and Smith, D. H.: Haemophilus influenzae, type b. *In* Sell, H. E., and Karzon, D. T. (eds.): Haemophilus Influenzae. Nashville, Vanderbilt University Press, 1973.

Smith, D. H., Hann, S., Howie, V. M., Ploussard, J. H., Harding, A. L., and Anderson, P.: Studies of the prevalence of antibodies to Haemophilus influenzae, type b. *In* Sell, H. E., and Karzon, D. T. (eds.): Haemophilus Influenzae. Nashville, Vanderbilt University Press, 1973.

Whisnant, J. K., Rogentine, G. N., and Robbins, J. B.: Studies on mechanism of susceptibility to Haemophilus influenzae, type b, disease: Relationship of erythrocytes and histocompatibility antigens with Haemophilus influenzae, type b, meningitis and epiglottitis. *In* Sell, H. E., and Karzon, D. T. (eds.): Haemophilus Influenzae. Nashville, Vanderbilt University Press, 1973.

Original Articles

Anderson, P., Johnston, R. B., Jr., and Smith, D. H.: Human serum activities against Haemophilus influenzae, type b. J. Clin. Invest. *51:*31, 1972.

Anderson, P., Peter, G., Johnston, R. B., Jr., Wetterlow, L. W., and Smith, D. H.: Immunization of humans with polyribophosphate, the capsular antigen of Haemophilus influenzae, type b. J. Clin. Invest. *51:*39, 1972.

Bradshaw, W., Schneerson, R., Parke, J. C., Jr., and Robbins, J. B.: Bacterial antigens cross-reactive with the capsular polysaccharide of Haemophilus influenzae, type b. Lancet *1:*1095, 1971.

Michaels, R. H.: Increase in influenzal meningitis. N. Engl. J. Med. *285:*666, 1974.

Norden, C. W., Callerame, M. L., and Baum, J.: Haemophilus influenzae meningitis in an adult: antibody and immunoglobulins. N. Engl. J. Med. *282:*190, 1970.

Schiffer, M. S., MacLowry, J., Schneerson, R., and Robbins, J. B.: Clinical, bacteriological, and immunological characterization of ampicillin-resistant Haemophilus influenzae type b. Lancet *1:*257, 1974.

Schneerson, R., Bradshaw, M., Whisnant, J. K., Myerowitz, R. L., Parke, J. C., Jr., and Robbins, J. B.: An Escherichia coli antigen cross-reactive with the capsular polysaccharide of Haemophilus influenzae, type b: Occurrence among known serotypes, and immunochemical and biologic properties of E. coli antisera to H. influenzae, type b. J. Immunol. *108:*1551, 1972.

Schneerson, R., Rodrigues, L. P., Parke, J. C., Jr., and Robbins, J. B.: Immunity to disease caused by Haemophilus influenzae, type b. J. Immunol. *107:*1081, 1971.

Sell, S. H.: The clinical importance of Haemophilus influenzae infections in children. Pediatr. Clin. North Am. *17:*415, 1970.

Chapter 22

INFLUENZA

Introduction

Influenza is an epidemic disease which spreads rapidly through a community and causes an acute febrile illness which is disabling but not usually fatal. Influenza most often occurs as a sudden, brief, winter outbreak, with greatest severity in the very young and in adults who have reduced chronic cardiopulmonary reserve. Periodically, the disease occurs in pandemic form and is then associated with an alarming increase in deaths due to pneumonia. For example, more than 15 million deaths occurred throughout the world in the pandemic of 1917 to 1918. A major concern of physicians is that influenza may return in that dreadful form.

The influenza viruses are divided on the basis of their distinctive antigenic characteristics into three major types: A, B, and C. There are no cross-reacting antigens between the three groups. The focus of this discussion is on type A influenza viruses which were first isolated in 1933 and were among the earliest human viruses shown to cause disease in man. Type A influenza viruses are usually considered the prototype for the myxoviruses.

The Virus

Gross Structure

Influenza type A viruses are pleomorphic, varying from spherical to filamentous forms. The spherical particles, which are 80 to 100 μ in diameter, are covered with several thousand projections — or "spikes" — which arise from the viral envelope. The envelope is a protein and lipid structure which releases viral nucleocapsid when treated with ether and detergent (see Fig. 22–1).

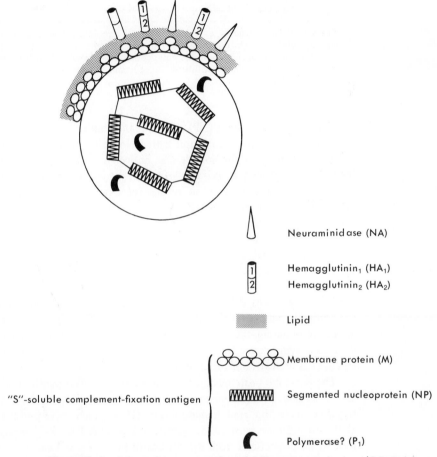

Figure 22–1. Schematic representation of influenza type A virus. (Adapted from Schulze, I. T.: The structure of influenza. II. A model based on the morphology and composition of subviral particles. Virology *47*:181, 1972.)

Structural Proteins

The RNA (ribonucleic acid) of influenza virus consists of five or more pieces of single-stranded RNA rather than one RNA molecule as found in other viruses. Biophysical and immunologic studies identify seven structural polypeptides in influenza type A viruses (see Table 22–1).

TABLE 22–1. Structural Polypeptides of Type A Influenza Virus

Structural Unit	Designation*	Molecular Weight (Daltons)
DNA-dependent RNA polymerase	P_1	81000–94000
Unknown	P_2	81000–94000
Nucleocapsid subunit	NP	53000–60000
Neuraminidase	NA	55000–70000
Hemagglutinin	HA_1	23000–30000
Hemagglutinin	HA_2	50000–60000
Membrane protein of envelope	M	21000–27000

*Polypeptides designated as P_1, P_2, and NP are internal or capsid proteins and ribonucleoprotein which constitute 1, 2, and 26 per cent, respectively, of the polypeptide content of the virion; the polypeptides designated as NA, HA_1, HA_2, and M are envelope proteins and constitute 6, 20, 12, and 33 per cent, respectively, of the virion polypeptides.

The ribonucleoprotein (NP) antigen is the major constituent of the capsid and is present in close association with RNA in the intact virion. It is also a major component of the soluble "S" antigen used for complement-fixation tests. The S antigen is extracted from infected tissues and is freed from hemagglutinating activity by adsorbing the extract with chicken red blood cells. The capsid antigens NP, P_1, and P_2 are type-specific and form the basis for classifying influenza viruses into types A, B, and C. The capsid polypeptides also seem to be invariant among strains of virus of the same type. The internal antigens are intimately concerned in the biochemical events of viral replication. However, it is not known whether the internal antigens are associated with immediate causes of cellular injury. In addition, the capsid antigens can be identified by their reaction with their specific antibodies in immunodiffusion in agar gel. The detection of antibody to S antigen containing the capsid proteins by complement-fixation tests is of diagnostic significance, since high titers of complement-fixation antibody are regarded as indicative of recent infection.

The envelope proteins consist of three surface glycopeptides, HA_1, HA_2, and NA, and a single nonglycosylated core protein, M. HA_1 and HA_2 together make the viral hemagglutinin (HA) which is responsible for the ability of influenza viruses to agglutinate red cells. The viral hemagglutinin is located on projections from the surface of the virion and enables the virus to adsorb to the walls of susceptible cells with high specificity. Destruction of viral hemagglutinin or inhibition of its activity by specific hemagglutination-inhibition (HI) antibody or certain glycoprotein nonspecific inhibitors of viral hemagglutinin interferes with the ability of the virus to infect susceptible cells. Antigenic differences between viral hemagglutinins from influenza viruses within the same type form the antigenic basis for classification of the viruses into families within the type. The other major surface antigen is the neuraminidase (NA). This glycoprotein exerts its enzymatic action on receptors which are located on susceptible cells and, by releasing *N*-acetyl-neuraminic acid (NANA), enables the virus to come off the cell surface. The action of neuraminidase in vitro on glycoproteins with the release of *N*-acetylneuraminic acid is the basis for a means of quantitatively estimating the amount of enzyme activity in a viral suspension. Destruction of neuraminidase by heat or pronase does not prevent adsorption to the surface of susceptible cells but does interfere with the elution of virus from the cell. Neuraminidase, like viral hemagglutinin, is also strain specific and is an additional means for classifying the viruses into families.

The remaining structural protein is the core protein, M, which apparently forms the backbone for the viral envelope. It is not glycosylated and is closely associated with the lipid matrix which makes up approximately 15 per cent of the mass of the virus. Persons with naturally occurring influenzal infection apparently develop antibody to M, but its relevance to immunity or pathogenesis is unknown.

The viral hemagglutinin and neuraminidase polypeptides of type A influenza viruses periodically undergo major antigenic shifts which are associated with the appearance of a new family of viruses. Four families of type A influenza viruses have been identified since isolation of the first influenza virus in 1933. The method for designating the viral hemagglutinin and neuraminidase antigens of the various families and their interval of prevalence are shown in Table 22–2.

TABLE 22–2. Surface Antigens of Type A Influenza Viruses

Family	Surface Antigen*		Dates
A_0	H_0	N_1	1933–1946
A_1	H_1	N_1	1947–1957
A_2	H_2	N_2	1957–1968
(A_3)**	H_3	(N_3)**	1968–present

*H_X: The hemagglutinin (HA).
N_X: The neuraminidase (NA).
**Hypothetical, as yet not found in nature.

Each influenza viral isolate is identified by a standard form of nomenclature which describes (1) type and family, (2) place of isolation and identifying number, (3) year of isolation, and (4) surface antigens. Thus, a strain of A_2 virus which was isolated in the Clinical Virology Laboratory, Northwestern Memorial Hospital, from a throat swab of patient number 1404 is designated as

$$A_2/NUMS\ 1404/1971\ (H_3N_2)$$

Genetics

The major phenotypic surface changes associated with epidemic spread of influenza are considered to reflect marked genetic lability or "plasticity" which probably is a consequence of their segmented RNA. The mechanism by which these changes occur may be a form of genetic recombination. This possibility is suggested by laboratory experiments which demonstrated that (1) certain traits, e.g., growth characteristics and surface antigens, can be transferred between strains belonging to different influenza virus families and (2) the hybrids breed true.

Proponents of a recombination hypothesis suggest that new families of type A viruses for man might occur by an interchange of genetic material between human influenza viruses and influenza viruses from animal reservoirs. Recently, Webster et al showed hybridization of human and swine influenza viruses. They infected one pig with a swine-adapted Hong Kong (HK) influenza virus and another pig with a swine influenza virus. Both animals were housed with four uninfected pigs from which they later isolated the original two strains of virus plus two hybrid strains with characteristics shown in Figure 22–2. Presumably, hybrids which possess new surface antigen are able to spread because man lacks protective antibody.

If pandemic spread of type A influenza is associated with major antigenic shifts in the virus, the interpandemic interval is characterized by less sudden antigenic changes, i.e., an interval of antigenic drift. During the inter-epidemic interval, there is a perceptible change in the antigenicity of the prevalent strains of virus such that younger strains in a family of influenza virus can be distinguished from the older ones. The nature of antigenic drift is characteristic: new strains react strongly with homologous antisera but do not react well with antisera against older strains. In contrast, older strains react almost as well with antisera against the new strains as they do with homologous antisera. This serologic interrelationship between the older and newer strains of virus and their antiserums is referred to as a one-way cross. Antigenic drift is almost certainly due to selection pressures exerted by antibody, and laboratory models in which influenza virus is grown in partially immune animals also reproduce the phenomenon of one-way antigenic crossing.

Inocula

a. Hong Kong (HK) Virus

    $HA_{(HK)}$ $NA_{(HK)}$

b. Swine (SW) Virus

    $HA_{(SW)}$ $NA_{(SW)}$

Recovered

a. Hong Kong Virus

    $HA_{(HK)}$ $NA_{(HK)}$

b. Swine Virus

    $HA_{(SW)}$ $NA_{(SW)}$

c. Hybrid Virus No. 1

    $HA_{(HK)}$ $NA_{(SW)}$

d. Hybrid Virus No. 2

    $HA_{(SW)}$ $NA_{(HK)}$

Figure 22-2. Hybridization of human and swine influenza viruses.

Proponents of the antigenic drift hypothesis suggest that the antibody responses of man to past and recent influenza virus force the emergence of new antigenic characteristics.

Biologic Activity

Influenza virus is transmitted from man to man as an airborne infection, and its localization in the respiratory tract depends largely on the size of the particles of droplets containing virus that are inhaled. Aerosol droplets created by sneezing and coughing contain a proportion of droplets in the 1.5 μ range. When inhaled, approximately one third of droplets in that size range are retained in the nose and almost two thirds are retained in the lower respiratory tract. If the aerosol arises from a person shedding influenza virus and the 1.5 μ droplets contain approximately 10 viral particles, there is an even chance that infection will occur (see Chap. 2).

In addition to the protective action of cilia on respiratory tract epithelium, mucoproteins covering the mucosa also serve to trap the virus. Some mucoproteins can neutralize viral infectivity in vitro and probably compete in vivo with receptors on epithelial cells for the virus. Attachment of the virus to nasal and bronchial epithelial cells is through the viral hemagglutinin antigen, and specific immunoglobulins against the viral hemagglutinin antigen can prevent infection. The relative importance of serum IgG or IgA on the nasal mucosa in protection is not clear at present.

Once the virus infects the cell, production of new virus begins in a few hours. Replicative events in influenza viral infection appear to be unique in that viral RNA is produced in the cell nucleus, while at the same time surface antigens for the virus appear at the cell membrane. New virus is apparently assembled at the cell surface and is released from the cell by the action of viral neuraminidase. The neuraminidase apparently is also responsible, in part, for lytic effects of influenza virus on cells.

Intranasal inoculation of high titer influenza virus produces pneumonia in mice. This phenomenon is independent of viral production in the lung of the mouse and is considered to be due to a viral toxin which has yet to be isolated. Influenza virus also induces fever when injected intravenously into rabbits. However, the pyrogenic effect is not as prompt nor as strong as that obtained with salmonella lipopolysaccharide endotoxin. The viral pyrogen is associated with the viral particle and is not due to contaminating materials.

Clinical Influenza

Uncomplicated Influenza

The uncomplicated form of influenza is usually a systemic illness with few localizing symptoms other than a severe retro-orbital headache. In some outbreaks, however, influenza may cause widespread pharyngitis and laryngitis which cannot be associated with a bacterial cause. The clinical picture of influenza during epidemics is characteristic; however, between epidemics, this disease usually cannot be distinguished from illness due to other respiratory tract infections.

Onset. During an epidemic period, uncomplicated influenza can frequently be diagnosed on the basis of the clinical history alone. Illness generally begins abruptly two to three days after exposure, and it is not uncommon for a patient to know the day and hour at which he became aware of the disease. The onset may consist of malaise, chilliness, and shivering, followed soon by headache, fever, lassitude, and diffuse myalgia. It is not unusual for a patient who went to work feeling well in the morning to have onset of influenza in the afternoon and be prostrated in bed by early evening with a temperature of 102°F. There are few characteristic signs of influenza. On physical examination, the patient may have a flushed face and show a slight to moderate degree of inflammation of the conjunctivae and pharynx.

Course. The period of acute illness with fever and prostration lasts three to five days. During that time, nasal obstruction, a "scratchy" sore throat, and a dry cough are common. Following the acute illness, defervescence of fever and a diminution of the principal symptoms occur in one or two days. Although the patient then feels much better, he experiences residual weakness and easy fatigability for more than a week. Many patients overestimate their capacity for physical activity following influenza and attempt to return to a normal schedule without adequate convalescence.

The factors responsible for recovery from acute influenza are not well understood. Release of interferon and production of antiviral antibody are probably major factors. Studies in mice treated with antilymphocyte sera or exposed to ionizing radiation suggest that cellular immune mechanisms have little, if any, role in recovery from influenza. Recovery from infection results in increased resistance to reinfection by homologous virus, but may not give much protection against viruses with different antigenic characteristics. Consequently, second attacks may occur in some future epidemic.

Bronchopulmonary Influenza

Tracheobronchitis. The clinical syndrome of influenza may be accompanied by signs of lower respiratory tract involvement without associated x-ray findings in more severe cases. Cough is usually more severe than in the uncomplicated form of influenza and is associated with production of blood-tinged sputum. Dyspnea and pleuritic chest pain may be additional complaints. Crepitant and musical inspiratory rales are found bilaterally, but no signs of consolidation appear. A Gram stain of the sputum shows few bacteria or cells. Patients with this form may be ill as long as three weeks, and antimicrobial therapy is not needed. This variant occurs in normal persons as well as in those with organic heart disease, and the prognosis is good.

Primary Viral Pneumonia. Primary influenza viral pneumonia usually occurs in middle-aged and older patients with chronic pulmonary disease or organic heart disease such as rheumatic heart disease with mitral stenosis, myocardial infarction, and advanced arteriosclerotic heart disease. The onset may be typical of severe uncomplicated influenza, but over the next 24 hours the patient experiences increasing respiratory distress and the cough soon becomes productive of a frothy, blood-tinged sputum. On physical examination, the patient appears seriously ill and extremely dyspneic, and shows moderate to deep cyanosis. The temperature is high, usually 102°F or above. Pulmonary findings are diffuse, with no signs of local consolidation. The patient may have fine, inspiratory rales and wheezes with a prolonged expiratory phase. Signs of congestive heart failure are usually not found.

X-ray findings suggest pulmonary edema or resemble an interstitial pneumonia fanning from the perihilar area toward the periphery. There may be a leukocytosis of 13,000 to 20,000 white cells consisting of a high percentage of polymorphonuclear cells with many immature band forms. In some patients, the sedimentation rate may be in the normal range. A Gram stain of the sputum shows few bacteria or polymorphonucelar cells, and sputum cultures may yield colonies which are representative of oropharyngeal bacterial flora.

The course of the interstitial viral pneumonia is rapid, and the prognosis is poor. A 36-hour interval from onset to hospitalization is not unusual. As air exchange becomes more difficult, dyspnea and cyanosis increase, and breath sounds are less readily heard. Arterial oxygen saturation is low and is not easily corrected. Progressive respiratory acidosis with an increased partial pressure of CO_2 and a fall in arterial pH has been described in some patients.

Patients with primary influenza viral pneumonia fail to respond to antimicrobial therapy, and steroids have not been found to have significant effect. Terminally, there may be a marked suppression of breath sounds, sticky inspiratory rales, and coarse bubbling rales during a prolonged expiratory phase. The patient shows rapid, gasping respirations, is deeply cyanotic, and may be agitated. Death is due to anoxia. A representative case is presented at the end of this chapter.

Bacterial Complications

Postinfluenzal Pneumonia. Bacterial pneumonia is probably the most common complication of influenza and occurs both in patients who otherwise seem healthy and in people with underlying disease. The usual history is that of influenza followed by one to seven days of definite improvement which is interrupted by a sudden reappearance of chills, fever, and pleuritic chest pain. A cough which is productive of bloody or rusty sputum is also seen. Patients again become acutely ill and have a high fever. On physical examination, there are classic signs of pulmonary consolidation, and the x-rays show dense, well-localized infiltrates, usually with lobar or lobular localization. Most patients have a leukocytosis with a predominance of polymorphonuclear cells and an increase in band forms. The erythrocyte sedimentation rate is usually increased. A Gram stain of the sputum shows many polymorphonuclear cells and bacteria, most commonly gram positive cocci. Influenza virus is usually not isolated from throat swabs or from sputum obtained at this stage, but high complement-fixation titers against S antigen may provide evidence of the antecedent influenzal infection.

Streptococcus pneumoniae is the bacterial agent most frequently found in postinfluenzal pneumonia, which probably reflects the fact that it is also the most common agent seen in noninfluenzal periods. However, *Staphylococcus aureus* is a common bacterial isolate from fatal cases of pneumonia associated with influenza. Since staphylococcal pneumonia can proceed rapidly to a fatal outcome, and because 50 per cent or more of staphylococcal isolates from patients admitted with infections acquired outside of the hospital are resistant to penicillin G, the initial therapy of postinfluenzal pneumonia, before the causative agent has been identified, should be with a semisynthetic penicillinase-resistant penicillin derivative directed against the staphylococcus. This therapy also has antipneumococcal action. Several authors claim that the response of patients with postinfluenzal pneumonia to antimicrobial therapy does not differ from that of patients with pneumonia during the interepidemic period and, on the whole, the mortality rate from postinfluenzal pneumonia is low.

Combined Viral and Bacterial Pneumonia. Bacterial infection may complicate primary viral interstitial pneumonia, resulting in an even more stormy course and worsening of an already poor prognosis. Instead of a frothy, blood-tinged sputum, there may be a tenacious, purulent material which shows a large number of bacteria on Gram stain. The patient with this condition appears seriously ill early in the course of the illness, and cyanosis may develop in less than 36 hours. Physical signs of consolidation in one or more lobes, in addition to the evidence for diffuse pulmonary disease in other portions of the lungs, are seen. X-rays show both lobar consolidation and perihilar infiltrates. There is most usually a leukocytosis; leukopenia should be regarded as a poor prognostic sign. Virus can usually be recovered at this early stage. Antimicrobial therapy directed against the bacterial infection should be started directly, but the response is usually disappointing and unpredictable. Apparently, death is due to the viral component of the disease even though the bacterial component seems controlled.

Other Complications

The importance of other complications of influenza is difficult to evaluate because they have been inadequately studied and their relation to influenza is uncertain. The severity of the prostration and the vasomotor instability that follows influenza suggested to some investigators that influenza has serious cardiovascular effects. So far, the only specific supportive evidence for myocardial damage is reversible T-wave changes which appear in precordial leads during the acute episode and are considered as a nonspecific evidence of injury. Neurologic complications, especially encephalitis, have also been described, but these have been infrequent. Even when delirium, convulsions, and coma have occurred, influenza virus has not been isolated from cerebrospinal fluid. Hypersensitivity and serum sickness–like and immune complex complications are rare: This may be due to the fact that the viremia which occurs at the height of viral growth is transient and probably ends before circulating antibody appears. Moreover, during viremia, virus adsorbs rapidly to white cells, and probably also to red cells, and in doing so may circumvent the customary pathways for depositing of antigen-antibody complexes.

Diagnostic Procedures

The clinical diagnosis of influenzal infection can usually be confirmed in the laboratory by viral isolation or appropriate serologic studies.

Viral Isolation

Viral isolation is accomplished by inoculating nasal swabs, throat swabs, or sputum into embryonated chicken eggs or onto monolayer Rhesus monkey kidney tissue cultures. Usually from two to four days are required for initial isolation of virus in eggs. Identification procedures generally require an additional two to three days. Isolation and identification in cell culture take approximately the same time. Both methods are commonly used at the beginning of an outbreak until the most appropriate method of isolating and identifying the prevalent strain can be ascertained. Sputum, throat gargles, and nasopharyngeal swabs offer adequate clinical materials, provided they are obtained during the first three, or occasionally four, days of illness. Usually, by the time the virus is identified, the patient with uncomplicated influenza has reached the stage of convalescence. In the complicated form of influenza, recovery of virus may be the only real evidence of the primary disease. The information is important, since it may explain a lack of response to antimicrobial therapy in certain patients with pneumonia.

Serologic Diagnosis

Patients who have recovered from influenzal illness generally possess several antibodies which demonstrate that they have made an immune response to some of the structural polypeptides. Immune response to viral hemagglutinin and neuraminidase antigens can be demonstrated in vitro by hemagglutination-inhibition and enzyme-inhibition (EI) antibodies, respectively. Immunoglobulins against NP, M, and possibly P_1 and P_2 are probably detected as part of the serum complement-fixation activity directed against S antigens, but reactions between the individual internal polypeptides and their specific antibodies have not been reported. There is general agreement that serologic diagnosis of influenza type A is most readily obtained by complement-fixation with the soluble or S antigen which is common to all type A viruses, since infection with new strains of influenza can be detected as well as can that of older strains. Diagnosis depends on demonstrating a fourfold increase in complement-fixing antibody titers or hemagglutinin-inhibiting antibody titers between acute serum taken as early as possible in the course of infection and convalescent serum taken after defervescence of symptoms.

Complement-fixing antibody to the S antigen can appear as early as nine days after infection and thus is a good indicator of infection. High titers of complement-fixing antibodies to the S antigen appear only as a result of infection and are not stimulated by presently acceptable influenza vaccines which are made with killed virus. Therefore, a complement-fixation titer of 1:80 or higher in a single serum taken early in convalescence can be accepted as presumptive evidence of influenzal infection (useful information in complicated cases of influenzal infection). A second blood sample obtained 7 to 10 days after the first should be tested to confirm the diagnosis.

Diagnosis of influenza by the hemagglutination-inhibition method always requires at least a fourfold increase in hemagglutination-inhibition titer between serum obtained in acute and convalescent stages of the illness. Infection cannot be diagnosed on the basis of results with a single serum sample, since hemagglutinin-inhibiting antibodies can be present as a result of previous infection or vaccination. Moreover, human sera usually contain mucoprotein nonspecific inhibitors of viral hemagglutination which must be removed before the sera are tested to ensure that hemagglutination-inhibition activity is due to antibody. There are two other major reasons why the hemagglutination-inhibition test is not the most efficient clinical laboratory procedure for diagnosis of influenzal infections. The hemagglutination-inhibition test easily distinguishes between various families of influenza viruses, i.e., A_0, A_1, and A_2 families, because it tests for differences between surface antigens. The high degree of specificity is a disadvantage in the clinical laboratory because it would be necessary to test each serum with many strains of virus just to be certain of testing with the one strain that contained the antigens which were homologous to the virus which caused the patient's illness. In addition, if the patient had been infected by a virus with new surface antigens which were not present in laboratory strains, antibody against the new virus would go undetected. Moreover, hemagglutination-inhibition tests require chicken red cells, which are not useful in tests for many other viruses and are not readily available at all laboratories.

The complement-fixation test with the soluble S ribonucleoprotein antigen is preferred because (1) it does not have the disadvantage of being strain-specific, and (2) the methodology and test components are applicable for testing for antibodies against a number of viruses. The S antigen (soluble nucleoprotein antigen) is obtained from the chorioallantoic membranes of embryonated eggs which were infected with one of the group A influenza viruses. Fluids extracted from infected membranes contain influenza virions as well as the S antigen. Preparations of S antigen used in the diagnostic laboratory are first treated with chicken red cells so as to adsorb the viral particle. The red cells are separated from the extracts by centrifugation, taking along the unwanted viral particles. Consequently, the S antigen preparations do not agglutinate chicken red cells and probably do not contain much surface antigen. The S antigen of one group A influenza virus family is antigenically similar to that from other group A viruses; i.e., antisera which react with S antigen from one family of influenza virus will react also with S antigen from other group A viruses. This is an advantage in the clinical laboratory since serums must be tested against a single S antigen for serologic diagnosis of influenza. Moreover, complement-fixing titer of 1:80 or higher in a single serum is evidence for a presumptive diagnosis of recent influenzal infection.

The ability of the S antigen of influenza type A viruses to react in the complement-fixation test with analogous antibody against all type A viruses means that one antigen can be used to test for infection with type A influenza. The broadness of reactivity of the S antigen of influenza should recall the nature of the complement-fixing antigen with adenoviruses (see Chap. 18). In the adenoviral system, one complement-fixing antigen can be used to detect antibody against 33 strains of adenovirus. If the complement-fixation test were not used for diagnosis of adenoviral infections, it would be necessary to perform neutralization tests with many strains of the virus in order to make a diagnosis.

Prevention

Vaccination

Vaccination and previous infection actively immunize against reinfection by influenza viruses with homologous or closely related surface antigens. The marked genotypic and phenotypic lability of influenza type A viruses has important clinical implications. For example, vaccination with an A_2 immunogen which contains H_2 and N_2 surface antigens increases the resistance of the vaccine recipient to infection with other A_2 influenza viruses. However, because A_2 viruses undergo antigenic drift from year to year, the strength of the immunity stimulated by the vaccine depends not only on the intensity of the response to the vaccine but also on the extent to which the A_2 immunogen cross-reacts with the new challenge A_2 virus which may be in circulation. Vaccination with an A_2 virus would not be expected to protect against infection with an influenza virus of a markedly different genotype which might arise because of an antigenic shift.

Killed influenza virus vaccines have reduced the incidence of influenza virus infections by 80 per cent or better. Vaccination with influenza virus vaccines does not provide protection against other viruses which can also cause influenza-like respiratory syndromes. Since several agents other than influenza may also be present in a community at the same time, the effect of influenza virus vaccination may be unrecognized without special studies to identify the cause of individual illnesses. Vaccination should be done at least three to four weeks before exposure to infection. Yearly or biennial vaccination is usually required with killed vaccine since protection does not persist indefinitely.

Procedures and indications for use of influenza vaccine appear yearly in a weekly publication of the United States Public Health Service called Morbidity and Mortality Weekly Report. Annual vaccination is recommended for (1) persons with chronic cardiorespiratory diseases, e.g., rheumatic valvular heart disease, emphysema, etc, (2) persons with chronic metabolic diseases, e.g., diabetes mellitus, and (3) older patients. Vaccination is also recommended for individuals who provide essential community services, because severe outbreaks can become so widespread as to disrupt and immobilize our complex society. Vaccination schedules should be completed by mid-November. United States Public Health Service recommendations should be ascertained yearly, since they are frequently changed according to anticipated variations in the status of influenza in the country.

Effective use of influenza virus vaccines depends directly on incorporating hemagglutinating and neuraminidase surface antigens which are either homologous to or cross-react strongly with the prevalent strain of virus. If influenza viruses exhibited the same stable genetic properties seen with many other viruses, the preparation and use of influenza vaccines would probably present fewer problems. Strenuous efforts are being made by the World Health Organization to monitor the antigenic properties of influenza viruses throughout the world. When new antigens are seen, they are compared to prevalent antigens and, if found to be markedly different, lead to incorporating the new virus into vaccines. The lead time for vaccine production is only a few months; previously, the lapsed time between identification of a new virus and its incorporation into vaccines resulted in a considerable delay in preparing new vaccines. Use of genetic recombination procedures for transferring new antigens to older viral strains which are presently used in vaccine production should shorten the interval between discovery of a new antigen and its eventual incorporation into new vaccines.

Chemoprophylaxis

Amantadine hydrochloride protects against infection with A_2 influenza viruses. In patients in whom protection is not complete, amantadine ingestion results in lesser symptoms and a reduced antibody response. Amantadine is a primary amine of a distinctive saturated ringed hydrocarbon. It is distributed to most tissues and is excreted unchanged with a half-life of 20 to 40 hours. It is administered in doses of 100 to 200 mg per day and can be given for several months without serious reactions. When given at doses of 200 to 300 mg daily, it may cause such side effects as drowsiness or sleepiness, or, in contrast, it may produce psychoenergizer effects such as those seen with amphetamines. Since amantadine is excreted almost exclusively through the kidneys, the drug is contraindicated in patients with impaired renal function, at least until additional knowledge of dose-effect relations is gained.

To be effective, amantadine must be given during the epidemic period, and it does not have persisting effects. It protects against A_2 influenza but not against type B influenza. Its mode of action is thought to be the prevention of penetration of infected cells. It augments the protective effect obtained with vaccination. At present, the greatest use of amantadine is prevention of A_2 influenza when there is reason to suspect that insufficient time remains to obtain a response to vaccination. The optimal approach in the face of an epidemic may be to vaccinate and then start amantadine chemoprophylaxis. In addition, preliminary observations suggest that amantadine can shorten the course of uncomplicated influenza if given early in the course of the illness. Thus, amantadine may be the first practical specific chemotherapeutic antiviral agent.

CASE PRESENTATION

Mr. F., 63 years old, was a heavy set, barrel-chested, slightly obese man. He was too short of breath to talk and the medical history was obtained from his wife.

The onset of the patient's illness occurred seven days before admission, with fever up to 100°F, generalized myalgia, and a moderately severe, nonproductive cough which was not accompanied by chest pain. His wife had had a respiratory infection the previous week and she assumed that her husband contracted her illness. Over the next several days, Mr. F.'s fever rose and his cough became more severe. Four days before admission, his temperature rose to 103°F. On the day of admission, his cough was persistent and was accompanied by blood-tinged frothy white sputum.

The patient had a myocardial infarct fourteen years earlier and apparently had been experiencing a progressive decrease in his physical and intellectual abilities over the past several years.

His pulse was 110 and regular, respiration 30 but labored, blood pressure 110/70, and rectal temperature was 104°F. He was cyanotic, and his neck veins were distended, especially during expiration. Moist crepitant rales were heard posteriorly below both scapulas. His heart was not enlarged by percussion. No murmurs nor any focal neurologic signs were noted.

Chest roentgenogram showed bilateral densities in the left lower and right upper lobes and 15 per cent cardiomegaly.

An electrocardiogram was made, and no acute changes from previous tracings were seen.

The laboratory found a hematocrit of 55 per cent; hemoglobin was 18 gm per 100 ml; and the white blood cell count was 5000, with 80 per cent neutrophils. The blood urea nitrogen was 37 mg per 100 ml. Blood gases showed pO_2, 38 mm; pCO_2, 21.5 mm; pH, 7.54; and O_2 saturation, 80 per cent.

The patient was initially treated with penicillin G administered intravenously (10×10^6 units per day) and then switched to cephalothin (6 gm per day). He was placed on oxygen by mask at a flow of 10 liters per minute. Subsequent blood gases showed pO_2, 50 mm; pCO_2, 27 mm; pH, 7.51; and O_2 saturation, 88 per cent.

A translaryngeal aspiration was done to obtain material for culture. Type A_2 influenza virus was recovered from the aspirate, but no bacteria were demonstrated.

The patient did not respond to these measures and died on the second hospital day.

This case history typifies the rapidly fatal disease caused by viral pneumonia in a patient with reduced cardiopulmonary reserve. The severe nonproductive cough suggests that the patient had a severe tracheitis before the onset of pneumonia. The cough associated with nonbacterial pneumonia is described as nonproductive, persistent, and sometimes paroxysmal, and usually is not associated with chest pain. The patient often is not able to limit coughing. Influenza is generally not accompanied by cough unless it is complicated by tracheitis or pneumonitis.

The past history of myocardial infarct and physical evidence of barrel-chestedness suggested impairment of the respiratory system and portended a poor prognosis.

Influenza viral pneumonia can simulate pulmonary edema by placing additional stress on a cardiovascular system which is already compromised thus precipitating cardiac decompensation. The differentiation between viral pneumonia and pulmonary edema is not easily made by either physical examination or x-ray in some cases, and treatment for a failing heart should be initiated. While a density in the chest roentgenogram suggests bacterial pneumonia, primary viral pneumonia may also cause lobar consolidation. In bacterial pneumonia, the physical examination and x-ray examination show abnormality in the same region of the thorax. In viral pneumonia, x-ray and physical examination may be temporally and spatially disparate.

Hypoxia and cyanosis occur as a result of interstitial infiltration of lung parenchyma and reduced diffusion of oxygen across the alveolar-capillary barrier. Since CO_2 is more diffusible, it crosses the barrier more readily and in this patient was decreased by the hypernea. In later stages or when secondary infection produces infiltration of alveoli, some shunting may be seen.

The patient was switched from penicillin to cephalothin in order to treat a possible staphylococcal pneumonia secondary to the viral pneumonitis. If staphylococci were present, therapy would preferably be with nafcillin, which has a more sharply defined bacterial spectrum than cephalothin and is specifically indicated for penicillinase-resistant cocci in patients who can tolerate this antimicrobial agent. The subsequent failure to culture pathogens from the translaryngeal aspirate in no way can be ascribed to the brief period of administration of an antimicrobial prior to collecting the translaryngeal aspirate.

Autopsy findings verified the diagnosis of viral pneumonia and in addition showed arteriosclerotic heart disease, left ventricular enlargement, and evidence of old myocardial infarcts.

Immunization against influenza virus is recommended for patients with a history of previous myocardial infarct as well as for those with altered pulmonary function. This patient had not been immunized.

References

Books

Bedson, S., Downie, A. W., MacCallum, F. O., and Stuart-Harris, C. H.: Virus and Rickettsial Diseases of Man. London, Edward Arnold Ltd., 1967.
Francis, T., Jr.: Serological variation in the viruses. In Burnet, F. M., and Stanley, W. M. (eds.): Viruses: Biochemical, Biological and Biophysical Properties. New York, Academic Press, 1959.
Hoyle, L.: The Influenza Viruses. New York, Springer-Verlag, Inc., 1968.
Knight, V. (ed.): Viral and Mycoplasmal Infections of the Respiratory Tract. Philadelphia, Lea and Febiger, 1973.

Original Articles

Choppin, P. W., and Pons, M. W.: The RNAs of infective and incomplete influenza viruses grown in MDBK and HeLa Cells. Virology *42:*603, 1970.

Francis, T., Jr.: Influenza: New acquaintance. Ann. Intern. Med. *39:*203, 1953.

Francis, T., Jr.: Influenza. Med. Clin. North Am. *45:*1275, 1959.

Hoyle, L., Horne, R. W., and Waterson, A. P.: The structure and composition of the myxoviruses. II. Components released from the influenza virus particle by ether. Virology *13:*448, 1961.

International Conference on Hong Kong Influenza. Bull. WHO *41:*335–748, 1969.

Louria, D. B., Blumenfeld, H. L., Ellis, J. T., Kilbourne, E. D., and Rogers, D. E.: Studies on influenza in the pandemic of 1957–1958. II. Pulmonary complications of influenza. J. Clin. Invest. *38:*213, 1959.

Schulman, J. L., and Kilbourne, E. D.: Independent variation in the nature of hemagglutinin and neuraminidase antigens of influenza virus: Distinctiveness of hemagglutinin antigen of Hong Kong, 68 Virus. Proc. Nat. Acad. Sci. *63:*326, 1969.

Webster, R. G., Campbell R. H., and Granoff, A.: The "in vivo" production of "new" influenza viruses. III. Isolation of recombinant influenza viruses under simulated conditions of natural transmission. Virology *51:*149, 1973.

Chapter 23

GENERAL CHARACTERISTICS OF MYCOBACTERIA

Introduction

The mycobacterioses constitute a large group of diseases of man and lower animals which are caused by members of the family Mycobacteriaciae. In man, these diseases range from the superficial self-limited infections of the skin caused by *Mycobacterium marinum,* to tuberculosis, a disease (the white plague) which decimated human populations in the Western nations until very recent times. At present, tuberculosis is a major infectious disease problem in the developing countries. In lower animals, tuberculosis of cattle and Johne's disease in cattle have posed serious problems which have only recently been surmounted in the Western world. There are also mycobacteria which produce disease in fowl, rodents, reptiles, and fish.

Classification of Mycobacteria

Although the mycobacteria can be separated into species on the basis of a variety of morphologic, biochemical, and antigenic characteristics, the really meaningful classification for the student of medicine is the one based upon the capacity of these microorganisms to produce disease.

Obligate Intracellular Parasites

This group includes *Mycobacterium leprae,* the causative agent of the disease leprosy (Hansen's disease), and *Mycobacterium lepraemurium,* the causative agent of rat leprosy. The outstanding feature of these mycobacteria is that they cannot be cultivated upon artificial media. *M. leprae* grows only in man and, to a limited extent, after inoculation into the footpad of the mouse. *M. lepraemurium* grows only in rodents and within macrophages in tissue culture. There are other mycobacteria which are obligate intracellular parasites and which produce disease in lower animals. However, these diseases of lower animals are of little importance to man except as experimental models for the study of leprosy; e.g., rat leprosy has been used extensively for this purpose.

Facultative Intracellular Parasites

Most of the pathogenic mycobacteria fall into this group. The principal cell which serves as the host for the mycobacteria of this class is the large mononuclear phagocyte called the *macrophage.* Therefore, at least in the initial stages of most mycobacterial infections, these microorganisms act essentially as parasites of the mononuclear phagocytic system. The most important members of this class of mycobacterial parasite are listed in Table 23–1.

TABLE 23–1. Mycobacterial Facultative Intracellular Parasites

Microorganism	Disease Produced
Mycobacterium tuberculosis	Tuberculosis in man
Mycobacterium bovis	Tuberculosis in cattle and man
Mycobacterium avium	Tuberculosis in fowl and man
Mycobacterium marinum (balnei)	Tuberculosis in fish and cutaneous lesions in man
Mycobacterium ulcerans	Superficial and deep ulcerations in the skin of man
Mycobacterium kansasii	Tuberculosis-like disease in man
Mycobacterium intracellulare	Tuberculosis-like disease in man
Mycobacterium scrofulaceum	Lymph node infection (scrofula)
Mycobacterium fortuitum	Various types of disease in man and lower animals

Other mycobacteria (atypical, unclassified, anonymous)
  A variety of strains and species many of which occasionally are associated with disease in man. These are discussed in Chapter 24.

Saprophytes

Saprophytes consist of a large number of species which are widely distributed in nature. They are found in soil and water, and at times as normal inhabitants of the skin, genital tract, or upper respiratory tract of man, where they may be mistaken for virulent tubercle bacilli. These mycobacteria, by definition, do not cause disease in man. A few of the more commonly recognized species are *Mycobacterium smegmatis,* found on the skin and in the smegma of man; *Mycobacterium phlei,* found in soil;

Mycobacterium butyricum, found in butter; and *Mycobacterium gordonae,* found in water supplies, including frequently tap water and water-distilling apparatus.

Medically Important Characteristics of Mycobacteria

The mycobacteria are slender, rod-shaped microorganisms which have a number of characteristics distinguishing them from other bacteria. Certain characteristics, however, are of particular importance because they have a relationship to the capacity of these bacteria to produce disease, to the pathology of the disease process, to the ability of infected hosts to control or eliminate infection due to mycobacteria, and to the diagnosis and treatment of mycobacterial disease. These characteristics are listed below. The more precise significance of these characteristics is discussed in subsequent chapters. Certain other characteristics of mycobacteria which are of importance for the identification of species are found in the next chapter in the section headed Diagnosis and also in Table 24–1.

1. The mycobacteria are acid-fast; i.e., they cannot readily be stained by the usual aniline dyes but, when once stained by the use of special procedures, cannot easily be decolorized even when strong decolorizing agents, such as acid-alcohol, are used.

2. The mycobacteria contain a much higher proportion of lipid material than do most bacteria; as much as 60 per cent of the dry weight of the cell may be composed of high molecular weight fatty acids and waxes. Most of these are found in or upon the cell wall. Therefore, these cells are very hydrophobic and they will not grow diffusely in liquid media unless surface active agents are present. In the absence of surface active agents, they adhere tightly to each other and form clumps of cells which are very difficult to disperse.

3. In part because of the high lipid content, the mycobacteria are appreciably more resistant than other pathogenic bacteria to the deleterious action of acids, alkalis, many germicides, and most antibiotics.

4. The pathogenic mycobacteria are strict aerobes.

5. Mycobacteria multiply much more slowly than most of the common pathogenic bacteria. Some saprophytic species have generation times of from four to six hours; at the other extreme is *Mycobacterium leprae* which, in the mouse footpad, has a generation time of about 12 days. *Mycobacterium tuberculosis,* the species which most commonly produces disease in man, has a generation time in vitro of from 10 to 20 hours, depending upon the nature of the culture medium.

6. Some pathogenic species, e.g., *Mycobacterium marinum* and *Mycobacterium ulcerans,* have low optimal growth temperatures and will not grow at all above 33°C. *Mycobacterium avium* grows best at temperatures of 42 to 45°C.

7. Mycobacteria are potent inducers of granuloma formation; i.e., in animal hosts they stimulate the proliferation and accumulation of mono-nuclear phagocytes (macrophages). In fact, the nodular lesion from which the

disease tuberculosis gets its name is composed principally of macrophages. The component of the mycobacterial cell which seems to be primarily responsible for inducing the granulomatous response is the *cord factor,* (trehalose, 6,6'dimycolate). This substance, found in the cell surface, was formerly thought to be responsible for the manner in which virulent mycobacteria adhere to one another and grow in cords.

8. Macrophages which have been exposed to, and have ingested, mycobacterial cells become greatly activated; i.e., they become more phagocytic and more motile, metabolic activity increases, and many lysosomes containing a variety of hydrolytic enzymes are produced.

9. Mycobacterial cells are potent adjuvants since, when injected together with antigens, they stimulate the production of antibody to the antigen. In particular, mycobacterial cells markedly promote the development of delayed hypersensitivity to protein antigens. For example, rabbits which, when injected with bovine serum albumin alone, will only respond by forming antibody will, when injected with bovine serum albumin and mycobacterial cells, also develop delayed hypersensitivity to bovine serum albumin.

10. Many pathogenic mycobacteria are uniquely susceptible to the two antimicrobial agents isoniazid and para-aminosalicylic acid.

Nature of Virulence of Mycobacteria

No virulence factors are produced by pathogenic mycobacteria. Endotoxins, exotoxins, extracellular enzymes, hemolysins, leukocidins, etc., have not been detected. No capsular material which might interfere with phagocytosis is present. In fact, mycobacteria are very readily phagocytosed by both segmented neutrophils and by macrophages even in the absence of opsonin. The high lipid content of the mycobacterial cell wall apparently has a great affinity for the lipid rich macrophage cell membrane because mycobacteria readily attach to the surface of these phagocytic cells and are rapidly ingested. Cord factor, mentioned above, when extracted from virulent mycobacterial cells and injected into mice in sufficient quantity, does produce toxic effects. A role for this substance in virulence, however, is doubtful, since it is also produced by nonpathogenic mycobacteria. In addition, enormous numbers of virulent mycobacterial cells can be injected into mice (2 to 3 $\times$ 10^8 cells) without producing severe adverse reactions. These animals will, of course, develop an overwhelming tuberculous infection and eventually die, but signs of toxicity in the first few days are usually minimal.

As far as can be determined, then, the disease-producing power of virulent mycobacteria resides solely in their capacity to multiply within phagocytic cells of the mononuclear phagocytic system. This capacity to multiply within host cells depends upon two factors: (1) the adequacy of the intracellular nutritional environment, and (2) the ability of the mycobacterial cell to withstand the antimicrobial armamentarium of the phagocytic cell. We have already pointed out that mycobacteria are far more resistant than most bacteria to a variety of chemical agents. The capacity to resist digestion and degradation within phagocytes undoubtedly is related in part to this generally greater tolerance to lethal agents. It is of interest to note, also, that virulent mycobacteria are good catalase producers, and when mutants such as isoniazid-resistant cells, which are poor catalase producers, appear, they are much less virulent. This suggests that the myeloperoxidase system is ineffective against drug-sensitive virulent mycobacteria. This is not the only factor, however, since there are strains of mycobacteria that are good catalase producers which, nevertheless, are not capable of producing disease. The activated macrophage is slightly more capable of coping with virulent mycobacteria, but it is not until acquired immunity develops that the body can mount a really efficient antimycobacterial defense.

Although we have little information on the specific factors responsible for the virulence of mycobacteria, there is one factor that is well defined and that is body temperature. As mentioned before, certain mycobacteria will not grow at temperatures above 33°C. These mycobacteria, *Mycobacterium ulcerans,* and *Mycobacterium marinum,* when infecting man will produce lesions only where the body temperature is low, i.e., the skin. If cultures of *M. ulcerans,* for example, are injected intravenously into mice, disease will develop, but the lesions will appear only where the body temperature is lower, i.e., skin, ears, tail, feet, etc. The viscera are not affected. Leprosy is a disease in which infection occurs only in the colder tissues of the body, i.e., the skin, peripheral nerves, nasal mucous membranes, etc. This observation, together with the fact that visceral lesions seldom occur, leads most leprologists to believe that *Mycobacterium leprae* also has a low optimal growth temperature.

Mycobacteria vary widely in their capacity to produce disease in different species of animals. Some, such as *Mycobacterium tuberculosis* and *Mycobacterium bovis,* will produce disease when injected into a wide range of mammalian hosts, even though these microorganisms, for the most part, produce natural disease in man and cattle, respectively; other species of mycobacteria will produce disease in one host only.

Finally, considerable differences in susceptibility to infection occur between different strains or races of animals. For example, it is well recognized that the colored races of human beings are more susceptible to tuberculous infection than is the white race.

References

Books

Davis, B. D., Dulbecco, R., Eisen, H. N., Ginsberg, H. S., and Wood, W. B., Jr.: Microbiology. 2nd ed. Hagerstown, Maryland, Harper and Row, 1973.

Smith, D., Conant, N. F., and Willett, H. P.: Zinsser Microbiology. 14th ed. New York, Appleton-Century-Crofts, 1968, pp. 520, 531, 564.

Sommers, H. B., and Russell, J. P.: Manual for the Clinically Significant Mycobacteria. Their Recognition and Identification. Commission on Continuing Education Council on Microbiology. American Society of Clinical Pathologists, 1967.

TUBERCULOSIS

Tuberculosis by definition is a chronic infectious disease of long duration in human beings which is caused by *Mycobacterium tuberculosis.* This definition is now too restrictive because we know that *Mycobacterium bovis, Mycobacterium avium, Mycobacterium kansasii,* and *Mycobacterium intracellulare* all may produce a pulmonary disease picture in man which is indistinguishable from that caused by *M. tuberculosis* (see Chap. 25). Certain types of disease caused by *M. tuberculosis* (e.g., infection of the skin and the lymph glands) can also be produced by other microorganisms such as *Mycobacterium marinum, Mycobacterium ulcerans,* and *Mycobacterium scrofulaceum* (see Chap. 25). However, the discussion which follows in this chapter refers only to *M. tuberculosis* and to the host response to this microorganism, unless other mycobacteria are specifically mentioned.

Transmission and Reservoir of Infection

Tuberculosis is primarily a disease of man. The major reservoir of infection is man and the disease is transmitted from man to man principally by droplet-nuclei which form when infectious material is discharged into the air by coughing. The portal of entry for the infection is usually the lower respiratory tract, and the major site of initial infection, therefore, is the lung. With the development of pulmonary disease and particularly with the formation of cavities, large numbers of virulent tubercle bacilli may be excreted. The transmission of the disease, then, is from an individual with an active case to susceptible persons by infected droplet-nuclei. Indirect transmission can occur from contaminated objects (fomites) handled by both diseased persons and susceptible persons, but this form of transmission is relatively uncommon. Any other conditions which create aerosols, and therefore infected droplet-nuclei containing virulent tubercle bacilli, can also serve as modes of transmission. For example, a person suffering from renal tuberculosis may excrete large numbers of tubercle bacilli in the urine;

aerosols and droplet-nuclei can be created when such a person urinates and flushes the toilet.

Infection with virulent tubercle bacilli can also take place through the skin. This is called *inoculation tuberculosis* and rarely occurs under natural conditions but is not infrequently seen in pathologists, medical students, and laboratory workers as a result of handling infectious materials.

Tuberculosis also can be acquired by way of the gastrointestinal tract. This is the principal way in which infection with *Mycobacterium bovis* occurs. This microorganism may be excreted in large numbers in the milk of infected cows. Ingestion by human beings of such milk may result in extensive tuberculous disease. In some areas of the world, this is still a major source of infection. In the United States, control of tuberculosis in cattle and the pasteurization of milk have virtually eliminated tuberculosis in man caused by *M. bovis.*

Although man is the major reservoir of infection for *Mycobacterium tuberculosis,* other reservoirs of infection may be established under special circumstances. For example, monkeys, cattle, dogs, and even cats can become infected if they are exposed to a master who has active pulmonary tuberculosis. Such animals, if they develop active disease, can serve as reservoirs of infection and transmit the disease to susceptible human beings with whom they may come into close contact.

Pathogenesis

Since infection usually takes place by way of the lower respiratory tract, the lung is the first organ involved and it is here that the initial major manifestations of disease occur. *Mycobacterium tuberculosis* can produce infection and disease in almost every tissue and organ in the body, but such disease is usually the result of dissemination from an initial pulmonary focus. There is evidence which suggests that the prediliction of *M. tuberculosis* for pulmonary tissue is directly related to its requirement for molecular oxygen for growth. Although, as mentioned before, infection and multiplication of the microorganisms will take place in other tissues, they proceed most rapidly in the lung. Therefore, the sequence of events which follow infection of the lung with *M. tuberculosis* can be used as an example of what may occur following infection of any organ or tissue.

In observing the progress of tuberculous infection, it is important to differentiate between that which occurs following infection of a person who has had no previous experience with *Mycobacterium tuberculosis* and that which occurs in a person who has previously been infected. In the former instance, there develops what we call primary infection or primary disease. In primary infection, one or more mycobacterial cells lodge within an alveolus where they are rapidly phagocytosed, most likely by alveolar macrophages. Because of their resistance to destruction, these virulent mycobacteria multiply within these macrophages almost as rapidly as they do in an artificial culture medium (Figs. 24–1 to 24–4). However, since the maximum rate of multiplication is still slow, the increase in numbers of virulent tubercle bacilli will be slow. Therefore, the appearance of symptoms or pathologic condition

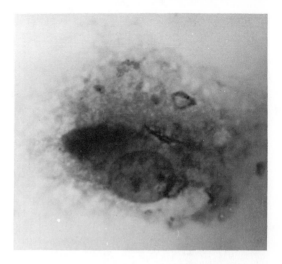

Figure 24-1. Peritoneal macrophage in tissue culture containing small clump of tubercle bacilli.

due to the infection may require several weeks. When the number of tubercle bacilli becomes significant, an inflammatory cellular exudate appears. Therefore, primary tuberculous infection is characterized by being pneumonic.

In spite of the cellular reaction, there is little resistance to the multiplication of the tubercle bacilli, and soon after infection, dissemination from this focus occurs. This dissemination is primarily by way of the lymphatics, and there is early extensive involvement of the regional (hilar) lymph nodes. At the same time, there is spillover from the lymphatics into the bloodstream with a seeding of virulent tubercle bacilli in all of the organs and tissues of the body. In a small proportion of persons thus affected, this process advances until widespread tuberculous disease, and possibly death,

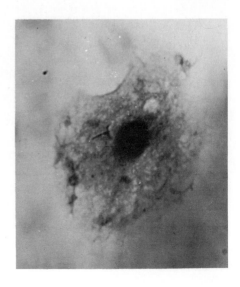

Figure 24-2. Peritoneal macrophage in tissue culture containing two tubercle bacilli.

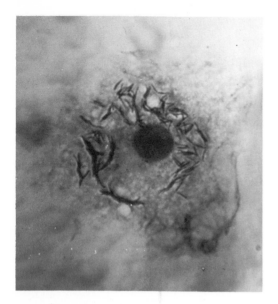

Figure 24–3. Peritoneal macrophage in tissue culture containing numerous tubercle bacilli. Note the alignment of the tubercle bacilli in the clumps as "cords."

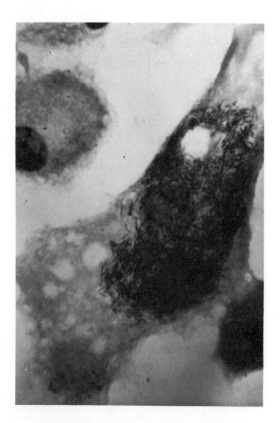

Figure 24–4. Peritoneal macrophage in tissue culture containing enormous numbers of tubercle bacilli.

occurs, provided treatment is not given. In the majority of such persons, however, after a period of a few weeks the following dramatic changes are seen. The rate of multiplication markedly decreases, the pneumonic process resolves, and the dissemination of tubercle bacilli to other organs ceases. The same changes also occur in all other tissues where tubercle bacilli may reside. Resolution of the disease process may proceed to a point such that, in many people so infected, little or no residue of the infection remains. In some, particularly in infants and children, all that may remain may be a Ghon complex; that is, a small calcified nodule in the lung and enlarged hilar lymph nodes.

Coincident with the changes described above, two immunologic manifestations appear. First, the affected individual becomes tuberculin positive. In other words, he shows reactions of delayed hypersensitivity to certain low molecular weight proteins or polypeptides which are found in the tubercle bacillus. We have already noted that mycobacteria markedly promote induction of delayed hypersensitivity to other proteins so it is no wonder that they exert the same effect for their own protein constituents. Secondly, the macrophages within which the tubercle bacilli previously were able to multiply so readily now have acquired the ability to markedly inhibit the multiplication of virulent tubercle bacilli. Therefore, since the tubercle bacilli are now unable to grow within these cells, the disease process is arrested and, with time, many of the virulent cells are destroyed. In other words, the diseased person has now become immunized as a consequence of the reaction of his immunologic system to the infection. This type of immunity is known as *acquired cellular immunity.*

It is of critical importance at this point to examine the relationship between tuberculin hypersensitivity and acquired cellular immunity. Tuberculin hypersensitivity is a specific immunologic response to tuberculoprotein or polypeptide. This hypersensitivity does not involve circulating antibody, cannot be passively transferred by serum, but can be passively transferred using lymphocytes obtained from tuberculin-sensitivie animals. Such lymphocytes in the presence of tuberculoprotein apparently elaborate a substance or substances (lymphotoxin) which destroy tissue cells and may be responsible for the destructive inflammatory reaction. On the other hand, the acquired cellular immunity to infection manifests itself as the intracellular inhibition of multiplication of virulent tubercle bacilli; it also cannot be transferred with serum (i.e., circulating antibodies are not involved), and there is evidence that it can be transferred with lymphocytes. Thus, there are some parallels between these two phenomena, and, because of these parallels, the majority of investigators and physicians take the position that tuberculin hypersensitivity is responsible for acquired cellular immunity. This appears reasonable when one realizes that when a tuberculin reaction occurs, macrophages accumulate and become activated. Therefore, they are better able to prevent the multiplication of virulent tubercle bacilli. This explanation requires that immunity to tuberculosis be specifically engendered (since the tuberculin reaction is specific for tuberculoprotein) but that the immune process itself (the inhibition of multiplication of virulent tubercle bacilli) be nonspecific because it depends only on macrophage activation, and activated macrophages are more capable of handling all species bacteria.

There are a number of findings, however, which make it difficult to accept this relationship between tuberculin hypersensitivity and immunity to tuberculosis. In the first place, animals can be rendered highly tuberculin sensitive by injecting them with Wax D and tuberculoprotein, both extracted from tubercle bacilli. These animals, however, do not show any increased resistance to infection over animals which have not been rendered tuberculin sensitive. Secondly, certain RNA protein complexes can be isolated from mycobacterial cells which will induce high degrees of increased resistance to infection with tuberculosis but which do not induce any detectable tuberculin hypersensitivity. Finally, there is strong evidence which indicates that there is a specific element in the acquired immune state in tuberculosis. For example, animals immunized with a mycobacterial RNA protein complex do not show any increased resistance to infection with other facultative intracellular parasites. Since these two phenomena, tuberculin hypersensitivity and acquired cellular immunity, can be dissociated, and since there is a specific element in resistance to tuberculosis, it would appear more reasonable to take the position that tuberculin hypersensitivity is not responsible for acquired immunity. It is more likely that, while macrophage activation, regardless of how it occurs, may play a role in resistance to tuberculous infection, this role is a minor one compared to the specific resistance which develops and which recently has been shown to be lymphocyte mediated.

In fact, it has been shown that splenic lymphocytes obtained from animals immunized with viable attenuated mycobacterial cells, or with RNA protein complexes obtained from these cells, will, when specifically stimulated, release a soluble substance which will cause inhibition of multiplication of virulent tubercle bacilli within macrophages in tissue culture. There are two possible mechanisms whereby this soluble substance might adversely affect the intracellular virulent bacilli: (1) This soluble substance might activate the macrophage to make it more capable of coping with the virulent cells; the macrophage would be the effector cell, and the lymphocyte the affector cell. (2) This soluble lymphocyte product might enter the macrophage and affect the tubercle bacilli directly. At the moment we have no information which permits us to decide which mechanism is operating.

Another reason for being skeptical of the role of tuberculin hypersensitivity in immunity to tuberculosis is the fact that tuberculin hypersensitivity is largely responsible for the destructive lesions, i.e., necrosis and cavity formation, which occur in tuberculous disease. This can be well illustrated by looking at the sequence of events in so-called secondary, or reinfection, tuberculosis (sometimes called *adult tuberculosis*).

We have seen that primary tuberculosis is the disease which occurs in persons who have never been exposed to tubercle bacilli and, therefore, are not tuberculin sensitive, nor do they have any acquired cellular immunity to infection. Until tuberculin hypersensitivity and acquired immunity develop, primary tuberculosis is for the most part a nondestructive disease process with rapid dissemination of the infecting microorganisms. On the other hand, reinfection tuberculosis is a disease which occurs in the presence of tuberculin hypersensitivity and in spite of the presence of acquired cellular immunity. Secondary tuberculosis may occur as a result of recrudescence of an old infection (endogenous) or by reinfection from an active case (exogenous). Regardless of source, the initial lesion is characterized by necrosis and by being circumscribed (localized). The necrosis is the result of the destructive nature of the inflammatory reaction of tuberculin hypersensitivity. The lesion is circumscribed and localized because of cellular immunity, which, operating in all of the adjacent tissues and within the lymphatic system that drains the lesion, prevents multiplication of tubercle bacilli and spread of the disease. Initially, the tubercle bacilli multiplies only in or near the necrotic area where cellular immunity has been reduced or abolished. The disease may progress, however, by extension as adjacent tissues develop necrosis as a consequence of allergic inflammation. In the lung, spread may also occur when a bronchus is eroded and infected material enters (bronchogenic spread), or spread may occur via the bloodstream if a blood vessel is eroded (hematogenous spread).

The reasons for the local breakdown of resistance which leads to a necrotic focus and disease are not well known. It is known that any factor, e.g., age, degenerative disease, immunosuppressive therapy, etc., which lowers resistance to infection will promote the development of tuberculous disease in previously infected people. Therefore, there must be a breakdown in cellular immunity which permits growth of the tubercle bacilli to the point where enough tuberculoprotein is produced to elicit a local necrotizing allergic reaction. Since necrosis is the outstanding feature of secondary, adult, or reinfection tuberculosis, the resolution of the disease process becomes far more difficult than is the resolution of a primary infection, which frequently is overcome by the acquired cellular immunity before the allergic state develops to the point where extensive necrosis occurs.

To recapitulate, primary tuberculous disease occurs in the nonimmune, nonallergic host and is characterized by rapid multiplication of tubercle bacilli and wide dissemination by way of the lymphatics and bloodstream of virulent organisms without extensive necrosis. Reinfection tuberculosis, on the other hand, is characterized by its initial localization, the early appearance of necrosis, and the lack of early general dissemination of the infecting microorganism. The disease progresses by local extension unless a bronchus or blood vessel is eroded, in which case infected material can be transported to other parts of the body. Thus, the major features of tuberculous disease can readily be explained on the basis of the relative participation of tuberculin hypersensitivity and acquired cellular immunity.

It is important to realize that tubercle bacilli may remain viable but dormant within the tissues of human beings for many months, or years, or even a lifetime. This follows from the fact that the acquired immune response inhibits the multiplication of tubercle bacilli but apparently does not confer upon the cells the capability to destroy all of the tubercle bacilli. Therefore, tubercle bacilli within macrophages located in a small tubercle in a lymph node, for example, or in the lung, may be held in check for long periods but are perfectly capable of again beginning to metabolize and divide if local resistance is lowered. Evidence for this type of infection is provided by the fact that tuberculin hypersensitivity persists in many persons for years following a primary infection even though all signs of tuberculous disease have disappeared. We must differentiate between tuberculous infection, which can be defined as the presence of viable and frequently nonmultiplying virulent tubercle bacilli within the cells or tissues of a host, and tuberculous disease due to viable multiplying tubercle bacilli within cells or tissues or necrotic foci which produce overt manifestations of disease. As we will see in Chapter 25, mycobacterial infection in humans is far more common than tuberculous disease.

Isolation and Identification

The diagnosis of active tuberculosis can only be made with certainty by showing that viable virulent tubercle bacilli are associated with a lesion or an affected organ. This association, in turn, can only be revealed by the isolation of virulent tubercle bacilli from the lesion or the affected organ. Tuberculosis usually is a pulmonary infection; therefore, sputum is the specimen most commonly examined for the presence of tubercle bacilli. However, other materials, such as urine, spinal fluid, or tissue biopsy specimens, may need to be examined.

The technical details involved in the isolation and identification of *Mycobacterium tuberculosis* from sputum or other material are not given here since they can be readily found in any standard textbook of microbiology or clinical pathology. Instead, emphasis is placed upon the obtaining of a suitable specimen for bacteriologic examination. This is of particular importance in the case of sputum samples, since sputum is always contaminated with microorganisms from the oral cavity. In the laboratory, such contaminated specimens must be decontaminated and then inoculated upon media selective for the growth of mycobacteria. In the decontamination process, advantage is taken of the fact that tubercle bacilli are much more resistant to deleterious agents such as acids and alkali than are most other bacteria. Treatment of the sputum sample with alkali, for example, markedly reduces the nonmycobacterial microbial population without seriously affecting the tubercle bacilli. Not all of the contaminating bacteria are killed in this manner, however; therefore, the treated sputum specimens should be inoculated upon a medium containing an inhibitory dye such as malachite green. Although growth of the mycobacteria will be retarded somewhat, the growth of a wide variety of other bacteria will be inhibited almost completely.

It follows that a sputum specimen which contains the fewest contaminating microorganisms is the best material for the isolation of *Mycobacterium tuberculosis*. Therefore, the collection of 24-hour sputum specimens, as is commonly done, is not always an appropriate procedure. These specimens, many of which are kept at room temperature for hours, will have a heavy growth of oral bacteria, and the decontaminating procedures used in the laboratory may not be adequate to dispose of them. The preferred procedure is to nebulize the patient early in the morning in order to take advantage of the presence of overnight pooled bronchial secretions. These specimens should then immediately be taken to the microbiology laboratory for prompt processing and inoculation upon suitable media. It is important not to use propylene glycol in the nebulizer, for this substance may inhibit the growth of, or even kill, tubercle bacilli.

Gastric contents are sometimes aspirated in order to obtain material from which tubercle bacilli may be isolated. Since bronchial secretions are automatically swallowed, the stomach may become a repository for virulent tubercle bacilli in patients suffering from pulmonary tuberculosis. Gastric aspiration should be avoided unless absolutely necessary because such specimens are frequently contaminated with saprophytic mycobacteria which, as has already been seen, may be found in water and soil and therefore be ingested with food. The presence of such saprophytic mycobacteria makes the isolation and identification of virulent tubercle bacilli more difficult. However, at times, gastric aspiration may be necessary in children and adults from whom bronchial secretions, for one reason or another, may not readily be obtained.

It is important to recognize that several specimens, not less than three and preferably not more than six, of sputum, urine, etc., should be collected from each patient with suspected tuberculosis. This is essential because the number of tubercle bacilli excreted may be small, and in many cases not every sample collected will contain tubercle bacilli. This is due to the fact that there may be only occasional release of tubercle bacilli from subepithelial bronchial abscesses. Single, early morning urine specimens are better than specimens collected over a 24-hour period for the same reasons noted above for the collection of sputum.

Owing to the slow multiplication rate of virulent tubercle bacilli, growth will not be detected on a medium inoculated with material containing tubercle bacilli in most cases for three to six weeks. In some cases, two to three months may be required for growth to appear. When large numbers of tubercle bacilli are present, e.g., in a sputum sample, growth will be evident in a shorter time than when specimens are inoculated which contain very few tubercle bacilli. Therefore, the result of the microbiologic examination of sputum samples is not rapidly forthcoming.

Once growth has appeared, *Mycobacterium tuberculosis* can be identified by virulence for animals, or by certain chemical tests.

Microscopic examination of sputum specimens is also frequently employed. The advantage of this procedure is the fact that mycobacteria are acid fast and are revealed as red, rodlike organisms against a blue background in the material placed upon the microscopic slide. Unfortunately, acid-fast staining does not distinguish virulent tubercle bacilli from contaminating saprophytic bacteria or from atypical mycobacteria. Therefore, the presence of acid-fast bacteria in the sputum specimen from a person suspected of having tuberculosis does not provide a definitive diagnosis. The presence of large numbers of acid-fast rods in the sputum of a patient with gross manifestations of pulmonary involvement may be suggestive but must be confirmed by isolation and identification of virulent tubercle bacilli. One exception to this rule, however, should be noted. In certain underdeveloped areas of the world, active pulmonary tuberculosis is common and laboratory facilities which can be used for the isolation and identification of myco-bacteria are almost nonexistent. In such areas, the finding of numerous acid-fast rods in sputum samples by the Ziehl-Neelsen technique can be considered sufficient evidence for the presence of active pulmonary tuberculosis and justifies the initiation of treatment with antituberculous drugs. The effect of chemotherapy on the course of the disease in such cases can also be determined by the use of the acid-fast stain. Of course, such an assumption cannot be made in the United States, where tuberculous disease, relatively speaking, is uncommon and where adequate facilities can be found for the isolation and identification of the offending microorganisms. Furthermore, the isolation of tubercle bacilli by culture upon a suitable medium is a far more sensitive and reliable method than the demonstration of acid-fast microorganisms by smear and staining.

In past years, frequent use was made of the fact that guinea pigs are very susceptible to infection with *Mycobacterium tuberculosis*. These animals could be injected with small amounts of sputum homogenate and, if sufficient numbers of tubercle bacilli were present, characteristic tuberculous disease would develop in the animal. This procedure for isolation and identification of tubercle bacilli is no longer appropriate because (1) this is not as sensitive a method for the detection of tubercle bacilli as is cultivation upon an artificial medium, (2) a number of mycobacteria which may produce pulmonary tuberculosis in man do not produce disease in guinea pigs.

Tuberculin Test

It has already been noted that persons who develop tuberculous disease or become infected with tubercle bacilli demonstrate delayed-type hypersensitivity to certain low molecular weight proteins or polypeptides of the tubercle bacillus. This hypersensitivity, when detected, can serve as an indication of the presence of tuberculous disease or infection. Such hypersensitivity can readily be detected by introducing small amounts of tuberculoprotein (tuberculin) into the skin; then, if hypersensitivity is present, a delayed inflammatory and indurated reaction will occur at the site of the injection. This procedure is feasible and practical and is known as the tuberculin test. There are two major types of tuberculin, one, called old tuberculin (OT), was introduced by Robert Koch many years ago and consists essentially of a concentrate of a culture medium upon which tubercle bacilli have grown. The material is concentrated by evaporating the fluid by boiling. Old tuberculin, however, contains many impurities and is difficult to standardize. It is not used very much today. The other material, purified protein derivative (PPD), is prepared from culture filtrates of tubercle bacilli by ammonium sulfate precipitation. Purified protein derivative is much purer, is easier to standardize, and gives fewer nonspecific reactions. However, it should not be regarded as being totally pure, since preparations contain a heterogeneous population of protein and polypeptide molecules and also may contain polysaccharides derived from the tubercle bacillus.

In order that comparable reactions may be obtained when different batches of purified protein derivative are used in different areas of the world, it must be standardized. A standard purified protein derivative is maintained by the World Health Organization against which the potency of other preparations may be measured. This standard PPD has been arbitrarily designated as containing 50,000 units per milligram. Other purified protein derivatives can then be compared with the standard by appropriate skin tests in human beings or infected guinea pigs.

When tuberculin testing human beings who may have tuberculous disease, care must be taken not to introduce too much tuberculin into the skin, since severe and damaging local and systemic reactions may occur. The whole forearm may become swollen, red, and tender. The axillary lymph nodes may become enlarged and tender, and fever with a temperature as high as 104°F may occur. The site of the injection of tuberculin becomes necrotic and eventually sloughs. With the fever, the patient experiences considerable malaise and may be prostrated for several days. In addition, complications such as pleural effusion or monoarticular joint effusions may occur.

Three dosages of purified protein derivative are generally recognized as being suitable. These are (1) first strength PPD, which consists of 0.00002 mg (1 tuberculin unit), (2) intermediate strength PPD, which contains 0.0001 mg (5 tuberculin units), and (3) second strength PPD, which contains 0.005 mg (250 tuberculin units). (See Table 24–1.) When testing persons strongly suspected of having active tuberculosis, the first strength purified protein derivative is the dosage of choice; certainly no dosage higher than the intermediate strength should be used. When making tuberculin surveys in healthy people to determine the presence of tuberculous infection, the intermediate strength is the dosage of choice. The second strength purified protein derivative should be used only in persons who are negative to the intermediate strength test dose, and therefore is of value only for the detection of rather low levels of hypersensitivity to tuberculoprotein. In Table 24–1, the various doses of old tuberculin and purified protein derivative are summarized and their relationship to each other given.

TABLE 24-1. Comparable Doses of Old Tuberculin (OT) and Purified Protein Derivative (PPD)*

Dilution of OT	Tuberculin Injected (MG)**	PPD Injected (MG)†	Tuberculin Units (TU)	Strength
1:100,000	0.001		0.1	
1:10,000	0.01	.00002	1.0	First
1:2,000	0.05	.0001	5.0	Intermediate
1:1,000	0.1		10.0	
1:100	1.0	.005	250.0	Second

*From Smith, D. T., et al. (eds.): Zinsser Microbiology. 14th ed. New York, Appleton-Century-Crofts, 1968, p. 541.
**Based on 1 ml of concentrated OT = 1000 mg.
†Based on milligrams of protein.

A variety of techniques can be employed to introduce either old tuberculin or purified protein derivative into the skin of human beings. These include the following:

1. The Mantoux test procedure, in which the desired amount of purified protein derivative or old tuberculin is injected directly into the skin in a volume of 0.1 ml.

2. The Vollmer patch test, in which tuberculin is merely placed on a piece of gauze which is held in contact with the skin by a strip of adhesive.

3. The tine test, in which old tuberculin is dried upon the points of several small tines and punctures are made in the skin so that small amounts of tuberculin are introduced.

All of these procedures have a certain usefulness, but by far the best is the Mantoux procedure since it permits the introduction directly into the skin of a standard volume and amount of tuberculin. More reliable and reproducible skin test reactions are obtained by this procedure than by any of the others. The Vollmer patch test, for instance, is sometimes particularly useful when tuberculin testing infants and children, in whom performing skin tests may be difficult, and the tine test provides a rapid and easy procedure for skin testing large population groups. It is sometimes worthwhile to sacrifice some sensitivity for the number of skin tests that can be done. When testing individual patients, however, the Mantoux test is the only acceptable procedure.

After the Mantoux test has been performed by the intradermal injection of 0.1 ml of diluent containing the desired amount of purified protein derivative, the ensuing reactions must be read and interpreted with care. The major reaction which occurs is one of delayed hypersensitivity; therefore, the inflammatory reaction becomes visible only after a matter of hours and reaches a peak at 48 to 72 hours. This reaction in human beings is characteristically erythematous and indurated. The area of induration should be outlined, and the diameter of the induration measured. Some clinicians measure the erythema because there usually is a direct relationship between the amount of erythema and the amount of induration. However, since this correlation is not absolute, the amount of induration should be recorded either in terms of the diameter of the induration in millimeters or by calculation of the area of induration. Arthus reactions, probably due to antibody specific for the polysaccharides found in tuberculin preparations, may be seen which appear earlier and reach a peak at about 24 hours and frequently are nearly gone at 48 hours. These reactions are inflammatory and edematous and therefore soft to the touch. These are not regarded as true tuberculin reactions. In addition, atypical wheal-flare reactions may occasionally occur. These subside rapidly and are not confused with a true tuberculin reaction. Rarely, persons who show no reaction whatsoever within 72 hours may develop, in approximately 7 to 10 days, an erythematous reaction at the site of the injection of tuberculin. This undoubtedly represents an Arthus-type reaction which develops because antibodies are produced to some ingredient of the purified protein derivative which reaches a level such that when it combines with antigen that is retained at the injection site produces an inflammatory reaction. This type of reaction should never be regarded as evidence of tuberculous infection or disease.

Since nonspecific reactions do occur, either due to the trauma of the injection or because of sensitization by infection with mycobacteria other than tubercle bacilli, small indurative or erythematous tuberculin reactions are not regarded as positive. Different workers use different criteria. Some maintain that no reaction under 10 mm in diameter is positive, whereas others set the limit at 5 or 6 mm. Most commonly, the dividing line is set at

10 mm. In other words, to be truly positive a tuberculin reaction following the intradermal injection of purified protein derivative should be 10 mm or more in diameter. The size of the tuberculin reaction to a given dose of purified protein derivative is a rough indication of the degree of sensitivity. A person showing a reaction over 15 mm has a substantially greater degree of hypersensitivity to tuberculin than the person who shows a reaction of less than 15 mm (see Table 24–2). A person who reacts negatively to first strength and intermediate strength but who shows a positive reaction to second strength probably has never been infected with *Mycobacterium tuberculosis* but has been infected with one or more atypical mycobacteria. In addition, reactions of less than 10 mm of induration to either first or intermediate strength purified protein derivative probably represent, in most cases, infection with one or more atypical mycobacteria. Positive reactions in adults to first strength or intermediate strength purified protein derivative in the absence of any other signs or symptoms of what might be tuberculous disease are regarded as indications of infection with *M. tuberculosis* but cannot be regarded as an indication of tuberculous disease. On the other hand, strong reactions in adults to first strength or intermediate strength purified protein derivative in the presence of evidence of pulmonary involvement strongly suggest but do not prove the presence of tuberculous disease. Infants and young children who have not lived long enough to become infected with other mycobacteria and who have had no time to control an active tuberculous infection and set up a dormant infection, but who show strong reactions to first or intermediate strength purified protein derivative, are regarded as probably having an active tuberculous process.

Reactions to purified protein derivative also have some prognostic significance because the incidence of active tuberculous disease is significantly higher in those persons who have reactions greater than 15 mm in diameter. These large reactions indicate a high degree of tuberculin hypersensitivity which in turn, probably reflects some, possibly microscopic, active disease. Therefore, a high degree of tuberculin sensitivity is associated with less immunity, and progressive disease is more probable. On the other hand, small reactions or a reaction to the second strength purified protein derivative only, represent little or no mycobacterial activity because of a high degree of acquired immunity (see Table 24–2).

Positive tuberculin reactions must be interpreted with caution for another reason. In view of the widespread use of BCG (bacille Calmette Guérin) vaccine in other parts of the world (see Prevention, below), tuberculin hypersensitivity may exist in people so vaccinated. Therefore, BCG vaccination may be the cause of tuberculin hypersensitivity in foreigners resident in the United States.

Perhaps the greatest value of tuberculin testing resides in its negative implications. A properly executed negative tuberculin test, even in the face of pulmonary disease, constitutes strong evidence against the presence of active tuberculous disease in the majority of cases. Two points deserve emphasis in considering negative tuberculin tests. First, a dilute purified protein derivative solution may lose potency rapidly due to adsorption of purified protein derivative to the glass surface of the vial or syringe within which it is contained. This can be prevented by dissolving the purified protein derivative

TABLE 24-2. Definite Cases of Tuberculosis, According to the Interval Between Entry and the Earliest Radiographic or Clinical Manifestation (the Starting Point) of the Illness*

Total Group	Number of Participants	Starting Period of Intensive Follow-up (to September, 1960)						
		Cases of Tuberculosis			Annual Incidence per 1,000 Participants			
		Starting Within 2½ Years of Entry	Starting Between 2½ and 5 Years After Entry	Starting Between 7½ and 10 Years After Entry	0-2 Years	2-5 Years	5-7 Years	7-10 Years
Negative unvaccinated	12,867	68	91	14	2.11	2.83	1.34	0.85
Negative BCG-vaccinated	13,598	14	14	7	0.41	0.41	0.38	0.40
Positive Induration 15 mm or more in diameter	6,866	63	31	7	3.67	1.81	0.99	0.79
Induration 5–14 mm in diameter	8,838	17	19	7	0.77	0.86	0.54	0.62
Positive only to 100 TU	6,253	12	19	5	0.77	1.22	0.58	0.62
All groups	54,239	181	179	44	—	—	—	—

*From Third Report to the Medical Research Council: B. C. G. and Vole bacillus vaccines in the prevention of tuberculosis in adolescence and early adult life. Br. Med. J. 1:973, 1963.

in a solution containing a small amount of an anti-absorbent such as Tween-80. All available purified protein derivative products are now prepared in this fashion.

Increasing evidence suggests that patients with active tuberculosis may exhibit two patterns of altered delayed hypersensitivity responses. Occasionally, a patient will appear to be completely anergic, giving negative skin test responses to purified protein derivative as well as other skin test antigens (mumps, trichophyton, streptococcal streptokinase-streptodornase, and monilia) routinely employed to assess overall cutaneous reactivity of the delayed type. More commonly, patients will exhibit a negative tuberculin test while simultaneously giving positive responses to one or more of the other test reagents. While both cutaneous anergy and specific purified protein derivative–negativity are known to be associated with far advanced tuberculosis, especially the miliary form of the disease, both types of altered cutaneous reactivity may be observed in patients with active disease confined to one pulmonary segment or lobe. Furthermore, these patients do not appear seriously ill by the usual clinical criteria. After instituting effective antituberculous therapy, positive responses to purified protein derivative or other test antigens in those subjects with anergy can be anticipated to occur within two to four weeks. The occurrence of purified protein derivative–positivity may antedate isolation of *Mycobacterium tuberculosis* from sputum or other specimens and provide welcome indirect support, especially in patients with negative acid-fast smears, for the clinical diagnosis of active tuberculosis.

Prevention

Tuberculosis is transmitted from a person with active pulmonary disease to a susceptible person who inhales infected droplet-nuclei generated from the bronchial secretions of the diseased person. The basic principle involved in the prevention of tuberculosis, therefore, revolves around procedures which prevent contact between susceptible persons and the diseased carrier. Since tuberculosis develops slowly, a person may be excreting tubercle bacilli long before he is aware that he is ill. Therefore, the prevention of spread of tuberculosis depends upon the early detection of pulmonary disease, the isolation of the diseased person, and finally the treatment of the diseased person to the point where he is no longer excreting tubercle bacilli. In the twentieth century, intensive efforts have been made to control tuberculosis by these means. In addition to the cases of tuberculosis that have been found in persons examined by physicians because of some other illness, mass x-ray screening programs have been conducted in order to detect persons with pulmonary pathologic findings. Such individuals have then been checked to determine whether they have tuberculosis. When active cases are discovered in this manner, the family and contacts of the patient are examined in order to reveal possible sources for the infection and to determine whether the patient has infected others. In this way, many cases of tuberculosis have been located. These diseased persons are then intensively treated with chemotherapeutic agents to render them noninfectious. Today, this treatment can frequently be accomplished without confining the patient to a hospital or sanitorium.

In many communities, tuberculin testing surveys of populations, particularly school children, are conducted regularly. Those found to be tuberculin positive to the intermediate strength purified protein derivative are then examined by x-ray for the presence of pulmonary disease; if found, the contacts are investigated to reveal possible sources of infection. Intensive applications of these procedures for the detection, isolation, and treatment of tuberculosis in the United States and other countries in the western world has resulted in a steady drop in the incidence, prevalence and mortality from tuberculosis. There is little doubt that the complete application of these procedures to an entire population would result in the reduction of tuberculosis in human beings to an insignificant level.

The preventive programs described above, however, are enormously expensive, and it is impossible to obtain the full cooperation of every person. Although tuberculosis in the United States has been reduced to a very low level in most rural areas, there still remain large endemic foci in certain population groups found in our large cities. As might be expected from the mode of transmission, most cases of tuberculosis are found in those areas of our cities where there is overpopulation, overcrowding, and lower standards of personal hygiene and sanitation.

The application of the above-mentioned methods for the prevention of tuberculosis is also difficult if not impossible in many of the underdeveloped areas of the world. In primitive cultures with a low level of education, lack of sanitation, and crowding, tuberculosis is a major problem. Facilities for the detection of tuberculosis and the isolation and treatment of cases do not exist, nor is there money available to provide them. In addition, the low level of education and understanding limits the degree of cooperation necessary from a large portion of the population. Therefore, other means for the control of tuberculosis in such population groups must be found.

Fortunately, another approach to this problem is available. It is well recognized that if the level of resistance of a population to an infectious disease can be increased and maintained to the point where the number of the susceptible persons is reduced to a small proportion of the population, the disease cannot maintain itself readily and may eventually disappear. This end has been realized in certain parts of the world as the result of vaccination against such diseases as diphtheria and smallpox. A potent vaccine against tuberculosis could be expected to reduce markedly the incidence of tuberculosis in susceptible persons, even though there are factors which make the elimination of this disease by vaccination very improbable. Such a vaccine would also be of particular usefulness in areas where the conventional procedures of detection, isolation, and treatment of cases cannot be applied. Such a vaccine is available in the form of BCG (bacille Calmette Guérin). BCG is an attenuated mutant of a virulent strain of *Mycobacterium bovis* developed by the French scientists Calmette and Guérin in the early years of the twentieth century. The vaccine, which consists of living cells of this attenuated strain, when injected in very small amounts into the skin of susceptible persons induces a high degree of resistance to infection with virulent tubercle bacilli. There have been a number of field trials with this vaccine which have conclusively shown that, when small numbers of properly prepared living BCG cells are injected in this manner into human beings, the incidence of tuberculosis can be reduced by as much as 80 per cent. Furthermore, this degree of protection persists for many years (see Table 24–2).

In the United States, BCG vaccination of human beings is not widely practiced. The majority of medical opinion has held that BCG vaccine is neither safe nor effective. Furthermore, since vaccination with BCG induces hypersensitivity to tuberculin in the recipient, a valuable diagnostic tool may be lost. Only the last reason has any validity, and even here the importance of this as a contraindication to vaccination is frequently overestimated. As has been previously noted, extensive field trials of BCG vaccine have been carried out. Table 24–2 summarizes some of the data from a large British study of the effectiveness of BCG vaccine in adolescents. This shows that a high level of immunity can be induced which will persist for as long as 10 years after a single vaccination with BCG. As for safety, the vaccination of hundreds of millions of people in various parts of the world with the appearance of few serious reactions attests to the safety of the vaccine.

A more acceptable reason for avoiding the use of BCG vaccine in the United States, at least in certain regions, derives from the fact that in many rural areas the prevalence of infection with *Mycobacterium tuberculosis* is so low (less than 5 per cent of persons) and therefore the risk of exposure to an active case of the disease so remote, that it does not justify the labor and expense of attempting universal vaccination. However, even this attitude may eventually require modification. The low prevalence of infection with *M. tuberculosis* and of tuberculous disease in the populations just referred to means that a high proportion of the people are highly susceptible. One can reason that the introduction of an active case of tuberculosis might have catastrophic consequences. This is confirmed by the increasing number of severe localized epidemics which have occurred in school children and personnel of the United States' armed forces following accidental exposure to an active case (e.g., in a school teacher). Therefore, there may eventually be a need for BCG vaccination even in areas of very low incidence. In addition, any event which would severely disrupt the society and economy of the United States for a prolonged period would increase the risk to these nonimmune people. This was clearly shown by the enormous increase in the incidence of tuberculosis which occurred in the peoples of western Europe during and after the last World War.

Attempts have been made to prevent tuberculosis by the prophylactic use of a chemotherapeutic agent, a procedure called, appropriately, *chemoprophylaxis*. It has been demonstrated that isoniazid administered in appropriate doses daily to populations of human beings at risk of infection significantly reduces the occurrence of active tuberculosis as compared with similar populations not so treated. Isoniazid chemoprophylaxis usually is employed in any child who develops a positive tuberculin test before four years of age, in tuberculin-positive individuals found to be or to have been in close contact with cases of tuberculosis, or in clinically well persons in special settings (e.g., physicians, nurses, hospital attendants) whose tuberculin tests have recently turned positive. The worried medical student or house officer often asks how soon he might be expected to exhibit positive tuberculin reactivity or pulmonary abnormalities in chest x-rays, should intimate contact with a patient with tuberculosis lead to active disease. Although there is considerable individual variation, three weeks and six weeks, respectively, would appear to be reasonable time periods to consider from the practical standpoint of tuberculin skin testing and securing of chest x-rays.

Chemoprophylaxis is often employed for patients known to have a positive tuberculin test and to be either suffering from disease or receiving drugs which alter host resistance and predispose to activation of subclinical or apparently healed tuberculosis. The diseases involved include leukemia, lymphoma, or lymphosarcoma. The drugs include corticosteroids and any of the immunosuppressive agents (e.g., those routinely used in patients receiving renal or cardiac allografts). However, chemoprophylaxis is a completely unsatisfactory method for the prevention of tuberculosis in large numbers of people such as found in entire communities. The requirement that a pill be taken daily over periods of months or years cannot be met by the majority of the people who are in the greatest need of protection. BCG vaccination, which is given only once and which provides protection for years, is the prophylactic method of choice for large numbers of people.

Treatment

The treatment of tuberculosis is a vast and complex subject and cannot be dealt with completely here. The modern therapeutic era began in 1944 with the discovery of streptomycin by Schatz and Waksman. Streptomycin was then found to be effective for the treatment of tuberculosis in lower animals and in man by Feldman and Hinshaw in 1945. Since that time, a number of other antimicrobial agents suitable for treatment of this disease in humans have been developed.

At the present time, the first-line drugs, those used most commonly for initial treatment, consist of isoniazid, rifampin, ethambutol, and streptomycin. Second-line drugs, those used for retreatment or whenever first-line drugs are not suitable, are orally administered ethionamide, cycloserine, pyrazinamide, and para-aminosalicylic acid (PAS). When parenteral use is required, capreomycin, viomycin, and kanamycin are available.

The foundation of therapy of tuberculosis is the use of isoniazid plus a companion drug, usually either ethambutol or streptomycin. Rifampin can also be used but, while it is a highly effective drug even when used alone, a significant number of patients show signs of hepatotoxicity. This appears to be especially noticeable when rifampin is given together with isoniazid. Isoniazid itself when used alone can result in serious liver disease in a small proportion of patients; therefore, since the incidence of liver disease is higher when using rifampin together with isoniazid, this combination of drugs should be avoided.

Streptomycin is an effective drug but should be used with care in persons over 50 years of age because of its adverse effect on the vestibular portion of the eighth nerve.

The reason for the use of two drugs instead of a single highly effective drug such as isoniazid or rifampin is that drug-resistant tubercle bacilli emerge fairly rapidly when only a single drug is employed. The use of a companion drug such as ethambutol or para-aminosalicylic acid markedly reduces the likelihood of the emergence of drug-resistant virulent tubercle bacilli. The administration of as many as three drugs is indicated for serious tuberculous disease such as far-advanced pulmonary disease, miliary tuberculosis, tuberculous meningitis, and tuberculous disease of the genitourinary system.

Treatment of tuberculosis must be prolonged. Even minimal, and certainly moderately advanced, disease without complications will require, for example, isoniazid and ethambutol treatment for at least two years. For advanced or disseminated disease not only may three drugs be given but also drug therapy can be continued for as long as three years.

It is not always necessary to give tuberculous drugs in multiple daily doses. Most of the orally administered antituberculous drugs may be given in a single dose daily rather than in multiple doses. Divided doses, however, should be used with drugs such as cycloserine, ethionamide, and para-aminosalicylic acid in order to reduce the likelihood of toxic reactions and gastrointestinal tract side effects.

In populations of human beings in which it is difficult to supervise administration of drugs, intermittent therapy can be given. For example, after a period of several months of daily treatment, the doses of isoniazid, 15 mg per kilogram orally, and streptomycin, 20 to 25 mg per kilogram intramuscularly, can be given twice weekly. The therapeutic effect is not as great as with daily administration, but significant improvement will be found in most patients so treated. Rifampin should not be given intermittently, however. It has been found that there is a high proportion of allergic reactions in patients who receive rifampin only once or twice a week. Reactions may occur in such a large number of patients and be of such severity that rifampin therapy must be discontinued. The incidence of such reactions is greatly reduced when rifampin is given daily.

The treatment of disease caused by the atypical mycobacteria poses special problems because of the generally greater natural drug resistance of these microorganisms. *Mycobacterium kansasii,* however, is highly susceptible to rifampin and only slightly more resistant than *Mycobacterium tuberculosis* to isoniazid (see Chap. 25). Regimens using three drugs are usually employed.

Mycobacterium intracellulare is quite resistant to all of the antituberculous drugs. Best treatment consists of at least four drugs chosen from isoniazid, rifampin, ethambutol, thionamide, and either streptomycin, capreomycin, or kanamycin (see Chap. 25).

The other atypical mycobacteria tend to be more resistant to the antituberculous drugs and may pose special therapeutic problems.

Advantage is taken of the antimicrobial potency and low toxicity of isoniazid to treat recent tuberculin converters. This therapy is usually referred to as chemoprophylaxis but more properly should be called treatment. The appearance of tuberculin hypersensitivity in previously tuberculin-negative persons indicates recent infection with *Mycobacterium tuberculosis.* It also means that the tubercle bacilli have multiplied and may still be multiplying even though no overt signs of disease may have appeared. Therefore, the drug is being used to treat an active process and this constitutes therapy. This is an effective way of preventing the development of serious disease in people who, because of the appearance of tuberculin hypersensitivity, are known to have been recently infected with *M. tuberculosis*.

Some physicians recommend treatment of all persons with a high degree of tuberculin hypersensitivity regardless of whether the infection was acquired recently or many years before. It has been pointed out previously that there is a direct relationship between the degree of tuberculin sensitivity as indicated by the size of the reaction obtained following injection of the low or the intermediate dose of purified protein derivative and the eventual occurrence of grossly evident tuberculous disease. It would appear logical, therefore, to reduce by the administration of isoniazid the risk of the development of destructive disease when a high degree of tuberculin hypersensitivity is present in persons undergoing treatment with immuno-suppressive drugs, or in those persons whose acquired cellular immunity may be compromised by other disease.

CASE PRESENTATION

A 71-year-old black female was hospitalized with an illness of at least eight days' duration which was characterized by fever, cough, and dypsnea. Despite prior injections of penicillin, her cough had become more productive of thick yellow sputum with intermittent blood streaking. Fever, as well as the shortness of breath, had increased in intensity. The patient had lived most of her life in an urban-metropolitan setting under impoverished circum-stances. A left radical mastectomy had been performed eight years previously for breast cancer.

Admission physical examination revealed an oral temperature of 98.8°F; pulse, 100 per minute; respirations, 26 per minute; and blood pressure, 156/80. Signs of consolidation were demonstrable anteriorly over the right upper and right middle lobes.

Laboratory data obtained at the time of and during the first few days after the patient's admission to the hospital included the following: Gram stain of sputum which showed many neutrophils, scattered gram positive cocci, and a few gram negative cocci and rods; white blood cell count of 6300 per cubic millimeter with 64 per cent mature neutrophils, 24 per cent small lymphoctyes, 10 per cent monocytes, and 2 per cent eosinophils; hematocrit, 42 per cent; and a normal urinalysis except for 10 to 20 leukocytes per high power field. Two blood cultures were reported to show no evidence of bacterial growth at 24 hours. Sputum culture yielded a moderate growth of Pseudomonas species and a few colonies of *Enterobacter aerogenes*.

The admission posteroanterior and lateral chest roentgenograms showed a dense infiltrate within the right upper lobe, within which could be discerned a "highlight" consistent with a cavity. An infiltrate also was present in the superior segment of the right middle lobe.

The medical resident ordered a tuberculin skin test. Because of the "normal" body temperature and leukocyte count and evidence of what appeared to be normal bacterial flora in the sputum, antimicrobial therapy was not initiated. The day after admission, the attending physician ordered intramuscular procaine penicillin, 600,000 units every six hours, after noting that the patient was spiking fever to 101°F and that she was acutely ill with a respiratory rate of 28 to 32 per minute. Forty hours after admission, the tuberculin skin test showed 18 mm induration. Upon receiving this information, the physician ordered acid-fast stains of sputum and sputum cultures for mycobacteria. Each of two acid-fast stains of sputum specimens revealed a moderate number of acid-fast rods which morphologically resembled mycobacteria. Antituberculous therapy with isoniazid and ethambutol was initiated; procaine penicillin was discontinued. Culture of each of the two sputum specimens containing acid-fast bacteria was reported 21 days later to have yielded *Mycobacterium tuberculosis.*

The diagnostic thinking springing from the data base for this patient procured soon after admission to the hospital should have focused primarily on pulmonary tuberculosis. The patient's age, socioeconomic-environmental status, and the upper lobe infiltrative process with what appeared to be a cavity represent important signposts pointing to tuberculosis of the lungs. The differential leukocyte count indicating an abnormal number of circulating monocytes provides an additional clue pointing towards tuberculosis.

The admitting physician was too slow to consider that the patient's problem might have an infectious cause, probably owing to the fact that the patient's body temperature was initially reported as normal and the total leukocyte count was within normal limits. Patients in this age group may exhibit surprisingly little fever or none at all, even in the face of well-established infectious disorders. Another reason for a spuriously low temperature recording, especially in older individuals, in whom deteriorating renal function is not uncommon, is metabolic acidosis. This alteration in metabolic status appears to suppress the capacity of the nervous system to respond to pyrogenic stimuli (see Chap. 8). Still another explanation for an unexpectedly low body temperature, and perhaps the most likely one in the case under discussion, is the inability to measure oral temperature accurately in any individual with dyspnea, irrespective of its cause, simply because rapid breathing makes it difficult to close the lips firmly around an oral thermometer. The patient's temperature should have been recorded using a rectal thermometer.

The presence of a cavity within the dense pulmonary infiltrate, together with the presence of gram negative bacillary rods in the sputum, might well have raised the question of bacterial pneumonia with early abscess formation. Specific microorganisms capable of causing this picture would include *Klebsiella pneumoniae* or, because of the patient's age, *Haemophilus influenzae* (see Chap. 21).

The presence of a cavitary process would have excluded pneumonia due to *Streptococcus pneumoniae* since pneumococcal pneumonia simply does not lead to abscess formation. It should be stressed that the initial data base in no way excludes an acute pneumococcal pneumonia being superimposed on a preexistent active pulmonary tuberculous infection, the latter process accounting for the cavitation. The small numbers of gram negative rods in the sputum would argue against infection due to *Klebsiella pneumoniae* or *Haemophilus influenzae* and far more likely represent an alteration in the microbial flora of the upper respiratory tract associated with prior administration of penicillin. It is not generally appreciated that unsuccessful demonstration of *S. pneumoniae* in the sputum by smear or culture in no way excludes infection due to this microorganism. In patients with classic lobar pneumonia due to *S. pneumoniae,* as evidenced by positive blood cultures, sputum specimens in approximately one half of patients do not contain demonstrable *S. pneumoniae* when cultured according to the routine followed by most bacteriologic laboratories. The explanation for this most likely lies in relatively few *S. pneumoniae* being present in the ordinary sputum specimen and being overgrown on the routine streak plate or in broth cultures to such a degree by other microorganisms as to remain undetected. Intraperitoneal inoculation of mice with freshly collected sputum is an important ancillary method for demonstrating *S. pneumoniae* (see Chaps. 10 and 20).

It is interesting to note that it was the positive tuberculin skin test rather than the clinical setting that triggered the order for acid-fast stains of sputum. Acid-fast stains should have been done at the time of the patient's admission to the hospital, when inspection of the chest roentgenogram revealed an upper lobe cavitary process. The admitting physician's failure to consider tuberculosis as a diagnostic possibility is not uncommon in today's clinical arena owing to the mistaken idea that tuberculosis has become an uncommon disease as the result of the impact of antituberculous drugs and improved standards of living. The failure of a physician to consider tuberculosis as a diagnostic possibility underlines the hazard of admitting to the hospital for reasons other than pulmonary disease patients who are shedding mycobacteria and thereby providing a dangerous source of infection for hospital attendants and even other patients before their infection and communicability is recognized. The attending physician might well have considered other types of pneumonias, viz., aspiration pneumonia, or infection of the lung due to fungi or a viral agent. However, the absence of any history suggesting chronic alcoholism or unconscious episodes would argue against aspiration of foreign material, and the presence of a cavitary process together with the physical findings of consolidation would constitute strong evidence against viral pneumonia. Finally, the relatively acute onset and the demonstration of acid-fast bacilli in the sputum, together with lack of any epidemiologic data to point to fungal infection, permitted exclusion of this etiologic possibility with ease.

References

Books

Beeson, P. B., and McDermott, W. (eds.): Textbook of Medicine. 14th ed. Philadelphia, W. B. Saunders Co., 1975, p. 391.

Canetti, G.: The Tubercle Bacillus in the Pulmonary Lesion of Man. New York, Springer Publishing Co., Inc., 1955.

Davis, B. D., Dulbecco, R., Eisen, H. N., Ginsberg, H. S., and Wood, W. B., Jr.: Microbiology. 2nd ed. Hagerstown, Maryland, Harper and Row, 1973.

Gerbeaux, J.: Primary Tuberculosis in Childhood. Springfield, Illinois, Charles C Thomas, 1970.

Rich, A. R.: The Pathogenesis of Tuberculosis. 2nd ed. Springfeld, Illinois, Charles C Thomas, 1951.

Rosenthal, S. R.: BCG Vaccination Against Tuberculosis. Boston, Little, Brown and Company, 1957.

Smith, D., Conant, N. F., and Willett, H. P.: Zinsser Microbiology. 14th ed. New York, Appleton-Century-Crofts, 1968, pp. 520, 531, 564.

Sommers, H. B., and Russell, J. P.: Manual for the Clinically Significant Mycobacteria. Their Recognition and Identification. Commission on Continuing Education Council on Microbiology. American Society of Clinical Pathologists, 1967.

Review Articles

Youmans, G. P.: Relation between delayed hypersensitivity and immunity in tuberculosis. Am. Rev. Resp. Dis. *111:*109, 1975.

Youmans, G. P., and Youmans, A. S.: Recent studies on acquired immunity in tuberculosis. Curr. Top. Microbiol. Immunol. *48:*129, 1969.

Original Articles

Bates, H. H., and Stead, W. W.: Effect of chemotherapy on infectiousness of tuberculosis. N. Engl. J. Med. *290:*459, 1974.

Feldman, W. H., and Hinshaw, H. C.: Effects of streptomycin on experimental tuberculosis in guinea pigs: a preliminary report. Proc. Mayo Clin. *19:*593, 1944.

Frenkel, J. K., and Caldwell, S. A.: Specific immunity and nonspecific resistance to infection: Listeria, protozoa, and viruses in mice and hamsters. J. Infect. Dis. *131:*201, 1975.

Hinshaw, H. C., and Feldman, W. H.: Streptomycin treatment of clinical tuberculosis: a preliminary report. Proc. Mayo Clin. *20:*313, 1945.

Patterson, R. J., and Youmans, G. P.: Multiplication of Mycobacterium tuberculosis within normal and "immune" mouse macrophages cultivated with and without streptomycin. Infect. Immun. *1:*30, 1970.

Patterson, R. J. and Youmans, G. P.: Demonstration in tissue culture of lymphocyte-mediated immunity to tuberculosis. Infect. Immun. *1:*600, 1970.

Smith, D. T.: Diagnostic and prognostic significance of quantitative tuberculin tests. Ann. Intern. Med. *67:*919, 1967.

Stead, W. W.: Pathogenesis of the sporadic case of tuberculosis. N. Engl. J. Med. *277:*1008, 1967.

Wolinsky, E.: New antituberculosis drugs and concepts of prophylaxis. Med. Clin. North Am. *58:*697, 1974.

Wolinsky, E.: Nontuberculous mycobacterial infections of man. Med. Clin. North Am. *58:*639, 1974.

Chapter 25

DISEASE DUE TO MYCOBACTERIA OTHER THAN MYCOBACTERIUM TUBERCULOSIS

Introduction

It long has been recognized that acid-fast microorganisms different from *Mycobacterium tuberculosis* are sometimes associated with pulmonary disease in human beings. Until recently, little thought had been given to the possibility that some of these might be etiologically related to the pulmonary pathology, in spite of descriptions in the earlier literature of cases which supported this possibility. During about the last 20 years, however, we have become fully aware that a significant proportion of cases diagnosed as tuberculosis may be caused by acid-fast microorganisms so different from *M. tuberculosis* that they represent separate mycobacterial species.

Of equal importance, and of special significance to the epidemiology and immunology of the mycobacterial diseases, is the relatively recent accumulation of evidence which strongly suggests that large numbers of persons in the United States, and probably in other countries, may become naturally infected with one or more of these other mycobacteria at some period in their lives, even though the great majority of those so infected never show evidence of disease.

The reasons for this tardy recognition of the role of other mycobacteria in latent infection and pulmonary disease are several. First, for many years following the initial isolation of *Mycobacterium tuberculosis* by Koch in 1882, the incidence of pulmonary disease due to *M. tuberculosis* was so great that the relatively few cases which may have been caused by other mycobacteria were not apparent. Therefore, the doctrine became firmly established that tuberculosis was caused only by one fairly characteristic microbe, *M. tuberculosis;* later, it was found that *Mycobacterium bovis* also could cause pulmonary disease in man. Secondly, this state of obscurity of the other pathogenic mycobacteria was maintained, in part, by the failure of workers in diagnostic laboratories to isolate and cultivate routinely the acid-fast bacteria present in the sputum or infected tissue of persons suffering from pulmonary disease; smears and Ziehl-Neelson stain were considered adequate bacteriologic control procedures. Thirdly, the recognition of the pathogenic propensities of other mycobacteria has been hindered by the fact that most of them are not pathogenic for guinea pigs as are *M. tuberculosis* and *M. bovis.* Finally, pigmented and nonpigmented acid-fast organisms are widely distributed in nature (soil, water, etc.) and may be found in association with tubercle bacilli in sputum or gastric washings. It is not surprising that when similarly appearing microorganisms have been encountered alone their etiologic significance has been regarded with skepticism.

In this chapter the events and the findings which have contributed to the present understanding of the role of other mycobacteria in the production of pulmonary disease in human beings are given. Similarly, the evidence which supports the concept that latent subclinical infection with certain atypical mycobacteria is widespread in our population is detailed. Finally, the significance of these findings to the epidemiology, immunology, diagnosis, and treatment of mycobacterial disease is discussed. In addition, some of the nonpulmonary diseases caused by mycobacteria other than *Mycobacterium tuberculosis* or *Mycobacterium bovis* are mentioned.

It has been traditional to refer to mycobacteria which differ appreciably from *Mycobacterium tuberculosis* but which are found in association with pulmonary disease in man as "atypical"; some clinicians called them "anonymous" or "unclassified" mycobacteria. A few of these atypical mycobacteria have now been given species names. These are *Mycobacterium kansasii* (yellow bacillus), *Mycobacterium intracellulare* (Battey bacillus), *Mycobacterium marinum (Mycobacterium balnei), Mycobacterium scrofulaceum, Mycobacterium ulcerans,* and *Mycobacterium fortuitum.*

Pulmonary Disease Caused by Mycobacterium kansasii and Mycobacterium intracellulare

The role of mycobacteria other than *Mycobacterium tuberculosis* and *Mycobacterium bovis* in the production of pulmonary and other disease in man probably could not have become apparent until the two following conditions existed. First, it would be necessary for the incidence of infection and disease caused by *Mycobacterium tuberculosis* to be very low as compared with that which occurred during the earlier years of this century. Second, it also would be necessary for the isolation, cultivation, and characterization of the microorganisms found in pathologic material from patients with chronic pulmonary disease to be widely, even if not routinely, practiced. These two situations fortuitously prevailed in the United States in the early 1950s, both as a result of a half century of intensive effort to control tuberculosis by public health measures and because of the impact of chemotherapy. Chemotherapy played a dual role. Not only did it contribute significantly to the decrease in the incidence and prevalence of tuberculous disease but, once it was realized that *M. tuberculosis* could readily develop a high degree of resistance to the antimicrobial drugs employed at that time, there was a marked increase in the routine use of procedures for the isolation, cultivation, and characterization of the acid-fast bacteria present in the pathologic material obtained from patients. Initially, these procedures were carried out primarily to permit the determination of the sensitivity of the microorganisms to chemotherapeutic agents, but they functioned equally well in revealing the presence of atypical mycobacteria.

The publications of Pollak and Buhler in 1953 and 1955 were among the first to report the isolation of an atypical mycobacterium from patients with pulmonary tuberculosis. This microorganism grew on the usual isolation media, producing yellow to orange-yellow colonies (yellow bacillus). The mycobacterium did not produce progressive disease in guinea pigs inoculated subcutaneously but did produce generalized infection in some mice following intraperitoneal inoculation.

Timpe and Runyon in 1954 described atypical mycobacteria which had been isolated from 120 patients; 93 of the strains were isolated by the authors from original specimens, the remainder were isolated by others and sent to the authors for examination. None of the atypical mycobacteria were pathogenic for guinea pigs following subcutaneous inoculation, although the pigmented strains produced pulmonary disease in mice following intravenous inoculation. Many of these microorganisms were etiologically related to pulmonary disease in the humans from whom they were isolated, not only because no other mycobacterium could be found in sputum but also because they were the only ones obtained from pleural fluid and diseased lung tissue. From the cultural characteristics and the development of pigmentation when exposed to light, it was possible for Runyon to divide these atypical mycobacteria into four large goups and to make certain correlations between the members of two of the groups and their pathogenicity for man. (See Table 25–1 for the nomenclature.)

Pathogenesis of Disease Caused by Mycobacterium kansasii and Mycobacterium intracellulare

The capacity to produce pulmonary disease in man has been fully demonstrated for microorganisms found in Groups I and III. However, there is evidence which indicates that microorganisms found in Groups II and IV also may be involved in pulmonary disease.

Group I microorganisms constitute a reasonably homogeneous group and appear the same regardless of where they are found. This microorganism is the "yellow bacillus" of Pollak and Buhler and has now been designated *Mycobacterium kansasii.*

The outstanding characteristic of this microbe is its capacity to develop a bright lemon yellow or orange pigment when exposed to light. If the microorganism is cultivated only in the dark, this pigmentation will not appear, and the cultures may then easily be mistaken for *Mycobacterium tuberculosis.*

TABLE 25-1. Nomenclature of Mycobacteria

Legitimate Name	Relative Pathogenicity for Man	Equivalent of Runyon Group	Acceptable Common Name	Names Without Legitimate Standing and Comments
M. africanum	+++			Intermediate between *M. bovis* and *M. tuberculosis*
M. asiaticum	++	Group I photochromogen		Similar to *M. simiae* but differs antigenically
M. avium	+++	Group III nonphotochromogen	Avian tubercle bacillus	Closely related to *M. intracellulare*
M. bovis	++++	Bovine tuberculosis	Bovine tubercle bacillus	
M. chelonei	+	Group IV rapid grower		*M. abscessus, M. borstelense* – may cause occasional skin disease
M. fortuitum	+	Group IV rapid grower		*M. ranae; M. minetti* skin infection –may cause disease in immune suppressed host
M. gastri	0	Group III nonphotochromogen		Not known to be pathogenic for man
M. gordonae	0	Group II scotochromogen	"Tap-water" scotochromogens	*M. aquae*—rarely, if ever, pathogenic for man
M. intracellulare	++	Group III nonphotochromogen		*M. batteyi, M. battey*
M. kansasii	+++	Group I photochromogen		Rare, non-pigmented, scotochromogenic, and niacin positive strains
M. marinum	+++	Group I photochromogen		*M. balnei, M. platypeocilus*
M. scrofulaceum	++	Group II scotochromogen		*M. marianum*
M. simiae	++	Group I photochromogen		Facultatively pathogenic; photo-chromogenicity may be unstable
M. szulgai	+++	Photochromogenic at 25°C Scotochromogenic at 37°C		Associated with chronic, pulmonary, and extrapulmonary disease. Distinctive lipid composition
M. terrae	Rare	Group III nonphotochromogen	Radish bacillus	May be closely related to *M. triviale*
M. triviale	0	Group III nonphotochromogen	"V" bacillus	Has been called "atypical-atypical" mycobacterium
M. tuberculosis	++++	Human tuberculosis	Human tubercle bacillus	
M. ulcerans	++++	*M. buruli*		Associated with skin infections in tropics
M. xenopi	++	Group III nonphotochromogen		*M. littorale, M. xenopei* slow growth –best at 42°C

It is nonpathogenic for guinea pigs, regardless of the route of administration. Nevertheless, progressive disease can be produced in hamsters and sometimes in mice.

Following the initial demonstration of the etiologic relationship of *Mycobacterium kansasii* to pulmonary disease in man, the incidence of pulmonary disease due to this organism in humans has been found to be high. Numerous reports have appeared showing the wide distribution of this disease in the United States and other parts of the world. In some areas, the incidence of infection with this microorganism in patients suspected of having tuberculosis may be quite high; in others, it is apparently quite low. For example, in 1958, Lester and his colleagues reported that 55 (18.3 per cent) of 929 consecutive culture-positive cases of tuberculosis studied in the Suburban Cook County Tuberculosis Hospital Sanitorium, Hinsdale, Illinois, were due to photochromogenic strains, probably *M. kansasii.* On the other hand, the overall occurrence of pulmonary disease due to other mycobacteria in the patient population in the Florida State Tuberculosis Hospitals was only 2 per cent, of which only 7 per cent constituted infections caused by *M. kansasii.*

Of particular interest are the observations of Lester et al, who made an epidemiologic analysis of 49 of 55 cases of infection with this microorganism. These authors found that the incidence of infection with *Mycobacterium kansasii* in the Chicago suburbs of Cicero, Berwyn, and Oak Park, having a total population of 184,129, was 10.7 per cent, whereas the incidence of infection in the remainder of Cook County, with a population of 940,000, was only 1.4 per cent. They also noted that whereas the incidence of disease caused by *Mycobacterium tuberculosis* was 67.5 per cent in males and 32.5 per cent in females, the incidence of *M. kansasii* infection was 85 per cent in males and 15 per cent in females. This finding illustrates what has been the general experience; *M. kansasii* infections occur predominantly in older white males. In this study, a careful survey was also made of the families and the contacts of these patients with *M. kansasii* infection, and no secondary cases were found. This is similar to the findings of other investigators.

The absence of household or other contact cases indicates not only that the disease is not highly communicable but also that the epidemiologic pattern is quite different from that of the disease caused by *Mycobacterium tuberculosis.* (This matter is discussed further in the next section.)

There is nothing at present to indicate that there is a particular predisposing disease or environmental condition, nor is there a significant relationship to any occupation.

Pulmonary disease, as well as its complications, produced by *Mycobacterium kansasii* is indistinguishable from that caused by *Mycobacterium tuberculosis,* but it follows a somewhat milder and more chronic course. Therapy is more difficult because of the higher resistance of *M. kansasii* to the bacteriostatic activity of the drugs currently available for the treatment of mycobacterial disease.

Group III atypical mycobacteria, on the other hand, do not constitute a homogeneous group. This group comprises a variety of mycobacteria placed together because they do not develop pigmentation when exposed to light. Many of them are closely related to *Mycobacterium avium* except that they are not pathogenic for fowl. Experimentally, these microorganisms do not produce infection in guinea pigs, although some have been reported to be pathogenic for mice.

Numerous cases of infection with Group III microorganisms have been found, although the overall incidence of disease seems to be lower than that caused by *Mycobacterium kansasii.* Many cases have been recognized at the Battey State Hospital, Rome, Georgia, by Crow and his associates, and the microorganism isolated from these cases, therefore, is frequently referred to as the "Battey" bacillus. Of major epidemiologic interest is the finding that the majority of cases occur in the southeastern United States, although isolations have been made in eastern, midwestern, and western states, as well as in other countries.

Clinically, pulmonary disease due to *Mycobacterium intracellulare* is indistinguishable from that produced by *Mycobacterium tuberculosis* or *Mycobacterium kansasii,* and, as in the case of the latter, infection occurs primarily in older white males. In addition, as in *M. kansasii* infection, there is little evidence to indicate that contact infection occurs. In spite of close and intimate contact, members of families of patients do not contract the disease.

From the foregoing it is apparent that a significant amount of pulmonary disease in human beings can be caused by mycobacteria possessing characteristics which clearly set them apart from *Mycobacterium tuberculosis* or *Mycobacterium bovis.* The major differential characteristics are (1) the capacity to grow at least slowly at lower temperatures (room temperature); (2) significantly increased resistance to the antimicrobial actions of streptomycin, PAS, and isoniazid; (3) a lowered degree of pathogenicity for all experimental animals but, of particular importance, the absence of capacity to produce progressive disease in guinea pigs, rabbits, and fowl; (4) frequently, a high catalase activity in spite of increased resistance to isoniazid; and (5) some, those in Groups I and II, are highly pigmented, either yellow or orange, and *Mycobacterium kansasii* is photochromogenic (see Tables 25–1 and 25–2).

These mycobacteria may be microorganisms that have existed for many years and have only recently been recognized, or they may represent strains that have recently appeared, possibly as mutants of *Mycobacterium tuberculosis,* which have been selected and become prominent in certain patients because of their higher drug resistance. This last hypothesis has been proposed by some investigators, but it has been discounted by others for the following reasons: (1) many of these organisms were recognized long before the use of streptomycin, the first antimycobacterial drug, (2) in no case have closely similar drug-resistant mutants been detected in vitro following long or repeated exposure of *M. tuberculosis* to chemotherapeutic agents, (3) when the total number of tuberculous patients who have been treated with chemotherapeutic agents is considered, the number of isolations from them of mycobacteria other than *M. tuberculosis* has been very small, and (4) it is clear, from data which are presented in the next section, that there is a very wide distribution of these atypical organisms in nature, and this in itself makes it unlikely that they are mutants which have recently appeared.

Accepting the more reasonable view that these other mycobacteria do not represent newly derived species, the question concerning the source of those

TABLE 25–2. Identification Characteristics of Mycobacteria*

Organism	Best Isolation Temperature and Rate of Growth in Dark	Colony Color Growth in Light	Colony Color Growth in Dark	Niacin Test	Nitrate Reduction	Catalase Semi-quantitative[1]	Catalase pH 7.0 68°C	Tween 80 Hydrolysis 5 or 10 Days	Arylsulfatase 3 Days	Tellurite Reduction 3 Days	Urease	Resistance to T_2H 1 µg/ml	Growth on 5% NaCl
M. tuberculosis	37°C 12–25	Buff	Buff	+	3–5+	<40[2]	–	∓	–	–	+	+	–
M. africanum	37°C 12–28	Buff	Buff	+	V	<20	–	–	–	–	+	+	–
M. bovis	37°C 24–40	Buff	Buff	–	–	<20	–	–	–	–	+	+	–
M. ulcerans	32°C 21–48	Buff	Buff	–	–	>50	+	–	–		–	+	
M. kansasii	37°C 10–20	Yellow	Buff	∓	3–5+	>50	+	+[3]	–	–	+	+	–
M. marinum	31–32°C 5–14	Yellow	Buff	∓	–	<40	∓	+	–	∓		+	–
M. simiae	37°C 7–14	Yellow[4]	Buff	+	–	>50	+	–	±	–		+	–
M. szulgai	37°C 12–25	Yellow to orange	Yellow–37°C Buff–25°C	–	+	>50	+	∓	±	–		+	
M. scrofulaceum	37°C 10+	Yellow	Yellow	–	–	>50	+	–	–	–	+	+	–
M. gordonae	37°C 10+	Yellow to orange	Yellow	–	–	>50	+	+	±	–	–	+	–
M. xenopi	42°C 14–28	Yellow	Yellow	–	–	<40	+	–	±	–	–	+	–
M. intracellulare-avian complex	37°C 10–21	Buff to pale yellow	Buff to pale yellow	–	–	<40	+	–	–	±	–	+	–
M. gastri	37°C 10–21	Buff	Buff	–	–	<40	–	+	–	–	+	+	–
M. terrae complex	37°C 10–21	Buff	Buff	–	+	>50	+	+	–	–	–	+	–
M. triviale	37°C 10–21	Buff	Buff	–	+	>50	+	+	∓	–	–	+	+
M. fortuitum	37°C 3–5	Buff	Buff	–	+	>50	+	±	+	±	+	+	+
M. chelonei	37°C 3–5	Buff	Buff	V	–	>50	+	–	+	∓	+	+	–
subspecies abscessus	37°C 3–5	Buff	Buff	V	–	>50	+	–	+	∓	+	+	+
M. smegmatis	37°C 3–5	Buff to yellow	Buff to yellow	–	+	>50	±	+	–	+	+	+	+

*Adapted from Kubica, G. P.: Identification of mycobacteria. Am. Rev. Resp. Dis. 107, 1973, and Diagnostic Standards 1974 edition. New York, American Thoracic Society.
Key to results: + = 84 per cent of strains +; ± = 50–84 per cent; ∓ = 16–49 per cent; – = 16 per cent of strains +; V = variable; blank spaces = little or no data.
[1] Numbers indicate millimeters of bubbles.
[2] INH resistant strains may be negative.
[3] Positive (most) in 24–48 hours.
[4] Photochromogenicity unstable with repeated subcultures.

which do produce clinical disease in man remains to be answered. We shall be concerned in this respect primarily with *Mycobacterium kansasii* and *Mycobacterium intracellulare* and related organisms. Many of the myco-bacteria in Groups II and IV are microorganisms which have been long known to be widely distributed in nature as acid-fast saprophytes. They are frequently encountered in soil, water, and other places. The significance of these bacteria in the production of disease is slight.

Some of the features of pulmonary disease caused by *Mycobacterium kansasii* and *Mycobacterium intracellulare* are interesting and unusual. We have already noted that the geographic distribution of disease due to these microorganisms is not uniform, that there is little or no evidence for transmission from open cases to contacts, and that the disease is seen most frequently in white males over 40 years of age. How can these puzzling features be explained, especially the lack of contagiousness, since a high degree of contagiousness is one of the outstanding features of the disease caused by *Mycobacterium tuberculosis*? A clue may lie in the low degree of pathogenicity of these microorganisms for experimental animals, even though viable cells may persist in the tissues of these animals for extended periods following injection. If pathogenicity is also very low for human beings, large numbers of human beings might become infected with atypical mycobacteria of Group I or Group III, or both, at some period in their lives, without developing clinically recognizable disease. Subsequently, an occasional infected person might, however, develop disease under conditions which would so lower local or general resistance that the atypical mycobacteria already in the body would begin to proliferate. Once a focal area of necrosis appears, the disease might become slowly progressive.

The production of disease by the mycobacteria found in Runyon's Groups I, II, III, and IV emphasizes the importance of host susceptibility. It is probably safe to postulate, as was done with histoplasmosis, that progressive disease due to these other mycobacteria probably will occur only in the abnormal host. The abnormality may be caused by other local or systemic disease or by one or more of the factors which are known to reduce cellular immunity to infection (see Chaps. 2 and 3). In general, the mycobacteria included within the Runyon groups should be regarded as opportunists rather than as primary pathogens capable of producing progressive disease in the normal host. *Mycobacterium tuberculosis* and *Mycobacterium bovis* would fall into the latter category. Evidence is presented in the following section which indicates that a broad base of latent infection with some of these microorganisms may exist in certain human populations.

Latent Infection with Mycobacteria

Following exposure of human beings to *Mycobacterium tuberculosis*, disease may develop or the microorganisms may persist in the tissues for long periods of time without producing evidence of illness. We have already seen that one of the major consequences is the development of a high degree of delayed hypersensitivity to certain protein products of the tubercle bacillus.

In 1941, Furcolow and associates, using quantitative skin testing procedures, reported that all patients with tuberculosis and most persons in contact with patients with tuberculosis showed positive skin tests when given 5 TU (tuberculin units) of purified protein derivative (PPD). On the other hand, those persons who had no known contact with the tubercle bacillus were relatively insensitive to tuberculin; only through the use of large doses of PPD were reactions produced. These authors suggested that the reactions obtained only with the large doses might well be nonspecific.

In 1950, investigators from the United States Public Health Service reported the results of a six-year study conducted among thousands of young white women attending nursing training school in 10 metropolitan areas in the United States. The students were first tested with 5 TU of PPD-S (World Health Organization standard PPD); those students who did not react to the 5 TU dose were then given a larger dose, 250 TU. The frequencies of reactors to the 5 TU test dose ranged from 6 per cent to 27 per cent in the different states and also showed a close correlation with the tuberculosis mortality rates in these areas. On the other hand, the frequencies of reactors to the 250-TU dose ranged from 14 to 70 per cent, with the highest rate being concentrated in the southeastern part of the United States. Furthermore, the frequency of reactors to the larger dose was not related to the frequency of reactors to the small dose, nor to the tuberculosis mortality rate in the area. In all the student nurses tested, approximately three fourths of those who reacted responded only to the larger dose. In addition, the percentage of reactors to the small dose was higher among nurses who came from cities than among those who came from rural areas; this would be expected because both tuberculosis morbidity and mortality are higher in urban than in rural populations. In contrast, those who reacted only to the larger dose were more frequently from rural areas than from cities; this was particularly noticeable in the southeastern part of the United States. For example, 9 per cent of the girls from farms in Louisiana reacted to the small dose, but 72 per cent reacted only to the larger dose. Furthermore, tuberculous disease and history of contact with known tuberculosis among these nurses was closely correlated with positive reactions to the small dose of PPD-S but not with reactions to the large dose of PPD-S.

These findings were clearly in conflict with the traditional notion that a reaction to any dose of tuberculin is specific for tuberculous infection. The hypothesis which would most reasonably explain these findings was one which proposed that the majority of the reactions obtained only with the large dose of PPD were nonspecific; i.e., nonspecific in the sense that a lower degree of hypersensitivity had been engendered in these individuals by infection with some mycobacterium other than *Mycobacterium tuberculosis*, but one which was antigenically related. Some support for this hypothesis came from the knowledge that in lower animals low grades of tuberculin hypersensitivity could be induced by heterologous mycobacteria.

Subsequent studies revealed that similar patterns of reaction to small and large doses of PPD-S prevailed in other parts of the world. Studies in India, the Philippines, Egypt, England, and other areas showed that a much higher proportion of the population reacted to the large doses without any correlation being found with the incidence of active tuberculous disease. On the other hand, a much smaller proportion reacted to the small dose of PPD, and a direct correlation did exist between the number of these reactors and the incidence of tuberculous disease in the population being studied.

The results of these studies provided strong presumptive evidence that appreciable numbers of people in different parts of the world were infected with mycobacteria different from but antigenically related to *Mycobacterium tuberculosis*. However, direct evidence for this was lacking, since another mycobacterium which might be responsible for such a wide degree of infection in human beings had not been identified.

During the 1950s, as has been outlined in the preceding section, investigators gradually became aware that certain atypical mycobacteria were capable of causing pulmonary disease in man. The significance of this development was not lost upon the workers from the United State Public Health Service, and they soon initiated studies in which the sensitivity of experimental animals infected with "atypical" mycobacteria, as well as of various human population groups, was tested with "tuberculins" prepared from cultures of a number of these atypical mycobacteria. A variety of "tuberculins" were used, but the most important results were obtained with PPD (PPD-B) prepared from cultures of the *Mycobacterium intracellulare* (Battey bacillus).

Experimental studies in guinea pigs injected with the living Battey bacillus and with living cultures of the bovine strain BCG showed that infection with these two organisms could be clearly distinguished by "tuberculin" testing; i.e., the reactions following injection of 25 TU intracutaneously into the guinea pigs were consistently larger and more intense with the homologous preparation.

Similar results were obtained when tests were performed on patients in the Battey State Hospital. Comparative tests with 5 TU of PPD-S and PPD-B differentiated in the same way patients with pulmonary disease caused by the Battey bacillus from those patients with disease caused by *Mycobacterium tuberculosis*. Most of the patients infected with the Battey bacillus gave larger reactions to PPD-B than to PPD-S, and most of the patients with human-type tuberculosis gave larger reactions to PPD-S than to PPD-B.

Healthy population groups were also tested, among them large numbers of naval recruits. Only 6 per cent of these reacted to PPD-S, whereas 25.3 per cent of them gave positive reactions with PPD-B. Furthermore, a much higher proportion of positive reactors to PPD-B was found in those naval recruits coming from the southeastern part of the United States than in those from other areas. It should be recalled in this connection that this finding paralleled the greater frequency of pulmonary disease caused by the Battey bacillus in the southeastern part of the United States. In these studies, the frequency and size of reactions obtained with PPD-B were also compared with those obtained with tuberculin prepared from *Mycobacterium avium*. They were similar, thus furnishing evidence for a close relationship between these two microorganisms. These results provided direct support for the earlier hypothesis which stated that a large proportion of those people who showed a low degree of hypersensitivity to PPD-S actually may have been infected with a related but different mycobacterium and, furthermore, a mycobacterium with a capacity to produce clinical disease in human beings that is much lower than that of *Mycobacterium tuberculosis*.

Later studies have confirmed these findings and, in addition, have shown that human adults may be highly sensitive not only to PPD prepared from a variety of mycobacteria but also to the PPD-S prepared from such well-recognized species as *Mycobacterium phlei, Mycobacterium smegmatis,* and *Mycobacterium fortuitum* (see Table 25–3).

TABLE 25–3. Frequency and Mean Size of Reactions Among Navy Recruits to 0.0001 mg of PPD Antigens Prepared from Various Strains of Mycobacteria*

PPD antigen	Prepared from	Number Tested	Reactions of 2 mm or more	
			Percentage	Mean size (millimeter)
PPD-S	M. tuberculosis	212,462	8.6	10.3
PPD-F	M. fortuitum	3,415	7.7	4.8
PPD-240	Unclassified; group 3	3,729	12.0	5.8
PPD-Y	M. kansasii	13,913	13.1	6.2
PPD-63	Unclassified; group 3	9,473	17.5	7.0
PPD-sm	M. smegmatis	14,239	18.3	5.7
PPD-ph	M. phlei	15,229	23.1	6.4
PPD-216	Unclassified; group 2	10,060	28.4	9.0
PPD-A	M. avium	10,769	30.5	6.7
PPD-B	Unclassified; (Battery type)	212,462	35.1	7.7
PPD-269	Unclssified; group 3	8,402	39.0	7.2
PPD-G	Unclassified; group 2	29,540	48.7	10.3

*From Edwards, L. B.: Current status of the tuberculin test. Ann. N. Y. Acad. Sci. *106:* 32, 1963.

The results given in Table 25–3 reveal that an unusually large number (48.7 per cent) of naval recruits were highly sensitive to PPD-G (PPD prepared from a scotochromogen strain isolated from a lymph node of a child with cervical lymphadenitis). Furthermore, the frequency of reactions of 6.0 mm or more to PPD-G among the naval recruits ranged from 22 per cent for lifetime residents of the northwestern states of Oregon and Washington to 83 per cent for recruits who had lived all their lives in Florida. This provides additional evidence of the wide variation in the incidence of latent infection with mycobacteria in man in the United States and of the concentration of such infection in certain geographic areas.

Tuberculin testing studies have also been conducted in human beings using PPD prepared from *Mycobacterium kansasii,* but the clear-cut differential reactions noted with the other skin testing antigens were not obtained.

Apparently, the antigenic relationship of *Mycobacterium kansasii* to *Mycobacterium tuberculosis* is much closer than is that of the other mycobacteria concerned in such studies.

It must not be concluded from these studies, however, that a positive reaction obtained with a 5-TU dose of one of the "tuberculins" shown in Table 25–3 always indicates latent infection with the species of mycobacterium from which the PPD was prepared. Cross-reactions do occur, and there is evidence which suggests that in both animals and in man infection with, e.g., a scotochromogen may produce a degree of sensitization such that a 5-TU dose of tuberculin prepared from other mycobacteria will cause a cutaneous reaction. The size of reactions, however, will be smaller to the heterologous PPD.

Thus, certain features of the epidemiology of pulmonary diseases in man caused by *Mycobacterium kansasii* and *Mycobacterium intracellulare* may become clearer. There is apparently a broad base of latent subclinical infection in the human population with one or more of these microorganisms. It would be reasonable to propose that disease might result when immunity wanes in certain persons later in life as a result of either age or some as yet unknown predisposing factor or factors; hence, the observed pattern of a greater incidence of disease in older people and the lack of relationship between cases. No explanation is currently available, however, for the predominance of pulmonary disease due to these microorganisms in white males. This may represent a racial predisposition, an occupational hazard not shared by colored races, or merely a higher incidence of initial infection.

The appreciably higher incidence of latent infection due to the Group II scotochromogens is most probably a reflection of their greater ubiquitousness in nature. The very low incidence of actual disease due to Group II microorganisms is probably, in turn, a reflection of their much lower pathogenicity for man. The low incidence of latent infection due to *Mycobacterium kansasii* but the relatively high incidence of pulmonary disease may indicate a degree of pathogenicity of *Mycobacterium kansasii* that is higher for man than is that of *Mycobacterium intracellulare* or Group II mycobacteria.

The source of infection for man with these atypical mycobacteria has not been firmly established. Contact with Group II scotochromogenic atypical mycobacteria undoubtedly is frequent because of their wide distribution in nature, i.e., in water, soil, etc. These microorganisms have also been isolated from secretions of the upper respiratory tract of man; therefore, they may, under certain conditions, be normal microbial inhabitants of this area. It should be emphasized in this connection, however, that the high degree of tuberculin sensitivity to PPD prepared from these microorganisms indicates actual infection. Such infection might occur following the ingestion of the microorganism in water or food, following inhalation of the microorganism in dust or in droplets, or as a consequence of invasion from a habitat in the upper respiratory tract by way of the regional lymphatics. No clarifying information is available on this point.

There is a close relationship between Group III nonphotochromogenic atypical mycobacteria and *Mycobacterium avium*. This suggests that man may become infected with these microorganisms from sources in which one would expect to find *M. avium*. Infected fowl are known to distribute these bacteria widely in their environment, and it is known also that these microorganisms may persist for long periods in the soil, where they may even multiply. Although pulmonary infection in man caused by *M. avium* is rare, swine are frequently infected. Low-grade infection can occur in cattle and possibly in sheep. The greater incidence of tuberculin sensitivity to PPD-B in rural areas adds support to the possibility that humans may become infected directly from domestic animals or indirectly from soil contaminated by infected domestic animals, although the lack of pathogenicity of the Group III nonphotochromogenic atypical mycobacteria for experimental animals does not lend support to this hypothesis. Many of the atypical mycobacteria may reside in soil and be carried from there to water supplies and hence to man or animals by either inhalation or ingestion. Microorganisms similar to *Mycobacterium intracellulare* also have been isolated from the upper respiratory tract of healthy humans. Conceivably this microorganism may colonize the oropharynx of human beings on occasion and become part of the indigenous microbiota. A ready source of pulmonary infection would thus be provided.

Mycobacterium kansasii, on the other hand, has not been found in association with any disease of lower animals, nor have there been reports of it being found in the upper respiratory tract of man.

Mycobacterial Infection and Immunity to Tuberculosis

The existence of a large number of people in the United States who have become naturally infected with a variety of mycobacteria raises a question of great practical importance. Have the people who have become so infected, in addition to having developed a high degree of tuberculin allergy, also developed an increased resistance (acquired cellular immunity) to infection with *Mycobacterium tuberculosis*?

In view of the close antigenic relationships which exist between some of the other microorganisms and *Mycobacterium tuberculosis*, cross-immunization might also occur. This is especially pertinent since BCG vaccine, an attenuated strain of *Mycobacterium bovis*, will induce a high degree of immunity to *M. tuberculosis* in man and animals (see Chap. 24).

If the answer to this question should be in the affirmative, the implications, especially in regard to the epidemiology and control of tuberculosis, would be far reaching.

Information pertinent to the answer of the above question is difficult to obtain in human beings. However, this problem has been approached from the experimental standpoint by immunizing laboratory animals with other mycobacteria and then measuring the degree of immunity by challenging the animals with virulent cultures of *Mycobacterium tuberculosis*.

Such studies have demonstrated that mycobacteria of certain Groups (I, II, and III) will stimulate the production in experimental animals of an appreciable degree of acquired immunity to subsequent infection with virulent human tubercle bacilli. These data do not, however, indicate whether these microorganisms would be equally immunogenic for human beings, but there is every reason to think that they would.

Direct evidence for the presence of a large nonspecifically immunized human population in the United States because of inapparent infection with mycobacteria is at present completely lacking. Hopefully, data will be accumulated in the future which will show whether the incidence of tuberculosis is appreciably less in people who are naturally infected with one or more of these other mycobacteria than in persons not so infected.

The very real possibility, however, that large numbers of people exist in the United States who are naturally actively immunized due to infection with atypical mycobacteria raises the interesting question of what influence this situation may have had on the steady decline in the incidence in tuberculosis which has been evident in this country ever since reasonably reliable morbidity rates have been available. All of the factors responsible for this persistent decline have never been clearly understood, but the presence of a large, and possibly gradually increasing, nonspecifically partially immunized population because of natural infection with a variety of mycobacteria might provide part of the explanation.

CASE PRESENTATION

A 24-year-old single white female was hospitalized with a 10-day history of increasing fever, one or two severe shaking chills daily, and progressive weakness. A chronic, nonproductive cough, which the patient attributed to moderately heavy cigarette smoking, probably had become more prominent during the two or three weeks preceding hospitalization. A diagnosis of primary thrombocythemia had been established approximately one year previously, based on the presence of splenomegaly and a markedly elevated platelet count. Although the patient had been treated with Myleran for this disease for some time, no immunosuppressive therapy had been administered during the four months preceding onset of the present illness. A chest roentgenogram at the time the diagnosis of primary thrombocythemia was made showed no abnormalities.

Initial physical findings included a temperature of 102°F orally, a pulse of 110 per minute, respirations 24 per minute, and a blood pressure of 110/70 mm Hg. The patient appeared acutely ill, dyspneic, and extremely apprehensive. Conversation was difficult because of intermittent paroxysms of coughing, which produced no sputum. Several nontender lymph nodes, up to 1 cm in diameter, were readily palpable in each axilla. The spleen was enlarged, with a firm nontender edge descending at least 6 cm below the left costal margin on deep inspiration. A grade 2/6 systolic murmur was audible over the apical regions of the heart as well as along the left sternal border. The lungs were free of any physical signs of pulmonary disease.

Initial laboratory data included a total leukocyte count of 20,800 per cubic millimeter, a differential count of 42 per cent neutrophils, 25 per cent band forms, and 19 per cent lymphocytes, and a hematocrit of 42 volumes per cent; the platelet count was 2,120,000 per cubic millimeter. Chest roentgenogram revealed a moderately dense pulmonary infiltrate extending out from the right hilum into the right lower lobe. One of two initial blood cultures obtained at the time of admission to the hospital and before any antimicrobial agents were administered yielded a slow-growing, gram negative bacillary rod. It ultimately was identified as a Pseudomonas species.

The attending physician elected to initiate antimicrobial therapy with penicillin G administered intravenously, 2.5 million units every six hours. Because of a febrile course, with spiking fever ranging as high as 105.6°F, evidence of an increase in the right lower lobe infiltrate on a subsequent chest roentgenogram, and the report of a gram negative bacillary rod in one of two blood cultures, penicillin therapy was discontinued and cephalothin therapy was initiated on the third hospital day. With identification of the gram negative rod as a Pseudomonas species on the seventh hospital day, cephalothin was discontinued and gentamicin therapy substituted. During this period, there was a progressive increase in the right lower lobe infiltrate. Other diagnostic studies included a negative intermediate-strength PPD tuberculin skin test, examination of cerebrospinal fluid, and an intravenous pyelogram; both were within normal limits. The spinal fluid remained sterile on culture. Myleran therapy was instituted in order to reduce the platelet count and lessen the chance of thrombosis. Approximately three weeks after admission to the hospital, bronchial brushing was done. A right supraclavicular lymph node was removed the following day and was reported to show histopathologic changes of chronic lymphadenitis. A lung biopsy of the right lower lobe was performed the next day. The specimen revealed many focal granulomas consisting largely of histiocytes and epithelioid cells with some areas of necrosis and caseation. Innumerable acid-fast bacilli were present.

Two lines of differential diagnostic thinking should have been stimulated by the patient's initial information. First and foremost was the possibility that all of the manifestations of her current illness reflected a progression of her underlying hematoproliferative disease, primary thrombocythemia. The second line of thinking concerned the possibility that a second disease was responsible for the fever and pulmonary infiltrate and superimposed on the patient's hematologic disorder.

Increasing cough, together with roentgenographic evidence of an infiltrative process in the right lower lung field, clearly pointed to the lower respiratory tract as one organ system which was at least in part responsible for the recent onset of fever. The presence of splenomegaly, known to have existed previously, was thought only to confirm the original diagnosis of thrombocythemia. The prominent axillary adenopathy was a new development and raised the question of whether the process manifesting itself in the lungs really was a systemic one involving multiple organ systems.

The notorious propensity of the hematoproliferative diseases to be associated with host immunologic disorders of one type or another would make a physician alert to the strong possibility of opportunistic infection in a compromised host. While the patient's underlying proliferative disorder is a rare one and not yet identified with any definitive immunologic deficiency in so far as is known, the fact that it does indeed involve uncontrolled proliferative changes in one hematologic stem cell line makes this possibility a real one.

The course of events in this patient illustrates well how difficult it is to attempt to establish a definitive diagnosis of a nondescript pulmonary infiltrative process without tissue biopsy. The initial clinical and laboratory data and the responses by physicians caring for this patient also are worth noting. The pulmonary infiltrate precipitated the use of penicillin, on the premise that a bacterial infection was present. Yet there was no sputum and no evidence of consolidation of the lungs or "air space" involvement on physical examination, and both the clinical picture and roentgenographic data pointed to an interstitial-type pulmonary process which would be uncommonly associated with usual types of penicillin-susceptible bacteria. A single blood culture was then reported positive for a gram negative rod, and the physician immediately switched to an antimicrobial agent with a broader based action than that of penicillin, viz., cephalothin. The blood culture isolate was reported to be a Pseudomonas species, and this caused the attending physician to prescribe a "pseudomonas antibiotic," viz., gentamicin.

The presence of a heart murmur, together with spiking fever and chills, and the report of a blood culture isolate identified as a Pseudomonas species did raise the question of bacterial endocarditis. However, it should be emphasized that in this disease, especially when caused by gram negative microorganisms, all blood cultures would be expected to be positive and to exhibit evidence of bacterial growth in a day or so rather than in a week. Furthermore, one would expect a more pathogenic representative of Pseudomonas to be present, e.g., *Pseudomonas aeruginosa.* The slow-growing Pseudomonas species reported in this patient most likely represented a "pseudomonad," which is often found on the skin and causes contamination of blood cultures. Pseudomonas is the most common gram negative microorganism causing bacterial endocarditis. However, the clinical setting for this condition usually involves an opiate addict, usually a heroin "main liner," and drug abuse was never raised as an issue in the patient under consideration. Furthermore, a progressive pulmonary infiltrate and prominent adenopathy would be uncommon presentations for endocardial infection, irrespective of its specific cause.

One other facet to be considered is the negative tuberculin skin test. There is increasing evidence that even in patients with active tuberculosis that is confined to a small part of the lungs, the PPD skin test may be negative. Disseminated tuberculosis, conceivably a diagnostic consideration in the case under discussion, only increases the likelihood of anergy and a false negative PPD skin test result (see Chap. 24).

The diagnostic maneuvers employed by the attending physicians in arriving at the correct diagnosis in this case are exactly those destined to yield the greatest amount of information with the least risk, i.e., bronchial brushings, removal of a lymph node, and finally lung biopsy by either closed or open means.

As a follow-up, culture of secretions obtained by bronchial brushing and the bone marrow and lymph node cultures were recorded as showing no growth at two weeks but were positive at four weeks. The culture of the lung biopsy grew out at three weeks. Despite the long period required for growth to appear on primary culture, subcultures of the microorganism from all four sources grew luxuriantly in less than a week. The microorganism was identified as *M. kansasii,* an atypical mycobacterium which commonly infects residents of the midwest, especially the Chicago region. Because a high proportion of atypical mycobacteria are isoniazid-resistant and there was no clinical response after employing isoniazid therapy for 10 days, it was decided to administer rifampin. The patient slowly responded to rifampin therapy, her fever was reduced, the lung infiltrate cleared, and the axillary lymph nodes receded in size.

References

Books

Chapman, J. S. (ed.): The Anonymous Mycobacteria in Human Disease. Springfield, Illinois, Charles C Thomas, 1960.
Sommers, H. M., and Russell, J. P.: Manual for the Clinically Significant Mycobacteria: Their Recognition and Identification. Chicago, Illinois, American Society of Clinical Pathologists, 1967.

Review Articles

Grigg, E. R. N.: The arcana of tuberculosis. Am. Rev. Tuberc. Pulmonary Diseases *78:*151–72 (Parts I and II), 426–454 (Part III), 583–604 (Part IV).
Runyon, E. H.: Pathogenic mycobacteria. Adv. Tuberc. Res. *14:*235, 1965.
Youmans, G. P.: The pathogenic "atypical" mycobacteria. Annu. Rev. Microbiol. *17:*473, 1963.

Original Articles

Buhler, V. B., and Pollack, A.: Human infection with atypical acid-fast organisms. Am. J. Clin. Pathol. *23:*363, 1953.
Collins, C. H.: Revised classification of anonymous mycobacteria. J. Clin. Pathol. *19:*433, 1966.
Edwards, L. B.: Current status of the tuberculin test. Ann. N. Y. Acad. Sci. *106:*32, 1963.
Furcolow, M. L., Hewell, B., Nelson, W. E., and Palmer, C. E.: Quantitative Studies of the Tuberculin Reaction. I. Titration of Tuberculin Sensitivity and its Relation to Tuberculous Infection. U. S. Public Health Reports *561:*1082, 1941.
Lester, W., Botkin, J., and Colton, R.: An analysis of forty-nine cases of pulmonary disease caused by photochromogenic mycobacteria. Trans. 17th Conf. Chemoth. Tuberc., Memphis. Washington, Veterans Administration, 1958, 289–294.
Pollack, A., and Buhler, V. B.: The cultural characteristics and animal pathogenicity of an atypical acid-fast organism which causes human disease. Am. Rev. Tuberc. *71:*74, 1955.
Palmer, C. E., and Edwards, L. B.: Geographic variations in the prevalence of sensitivity to tuberculin (PPD-S) and to the Battey antigen (PPD-B) throughout the United States. Bull. Int. Union Tuberc. *32:*373, 1962.
Timpe, A., and Runyon, E. H.: The relationship of "atypical" acid-fast bacteria to human disease. J. Lab. Clin. Med. *44:*202, 1954.

Chapter 26

HISTOPLASMOSIS, COCCIDIOIDOMYCOSIS, BLASTOMYCOSIS

Introduction

Thousands of species of fungi are found in nature, a few of which are capable of producing disease in man or lower animals. The fungal diseases of man are usually divided into two groups, the superficial mycoses and the deep mycoses. The superficial mycoses are limited for the most part to the skin, mucous membranes, nails, and hair. The microorganisms which cause the superficial mycoses seldom invade deeper tissues, although subcutaneous lesions are sometimes found. The superficial mycoses are not dealt with further here since they are discussed in textbooks of dermatology.

The deep mycoses include those fungal diseases in which there is involvement by the parasite of deeper tissues and internal organs. Several of these are of importance in the production of disease in man. In this chapter, three of the major deep mycoses, histoplasmosis, coccidioidomycosis, and blastomycosis, are considered.

Histoplasmosis

Introduction

Histoplasmosis is a disease which may appear in a number of forms in man and is caused by a fungus named *Histoplasma capsulatum,* a facultative intracellular parasite. This parasite was first described by Darling in 1904. Darling called it *Histoplasma capsulatum* because the parasite was seen within histiocytes as round, protozoan-like cells which appeared to have capsules (Fig. 26–1). It is now known that *H. capsulatum* is not a protozoan but is instead a dimorphic fungus which appears in the form of a yeast when producing infection in man, and it does not possess a capsule. When grown in vitro at 25°C on an appropriate solid medium, the fungus appears in a mycelial form and produces two types of characteristic spores, chlamydospores which are tuberculate in appearance and microconidia (Fig. 26–2).

The fungus grows in soil in the mycelial form and produces spores which are carried by air currents; man is infected by inhaling these spores. Because of their smaller size (2 to 3 microns in diameter), the microconidia are probably more important as a source of infection than are the tuberculate chlamydospores (10 to 15 microns in diameter).

Types of Disease

Table 26–1 provides a useful clinical classification of histoplasmosis. This table demonstrates a number of important points. First, it emphasizes that pulmonary histoplasmosis is usually a benign disease regardless of whether the primary infection is due to exposure to a few spores or exposure to large

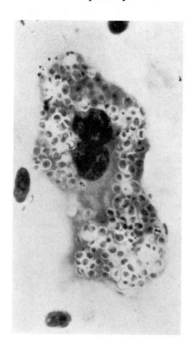

Figure 26–1. Illustration from Darling's original description of histoplasmosis shows an endothelial cell from the liver (macrophage) distended with yeast cells of *Histoplasma capsulatum.* (From J. Exp. Med. *11:*515, 1909.)

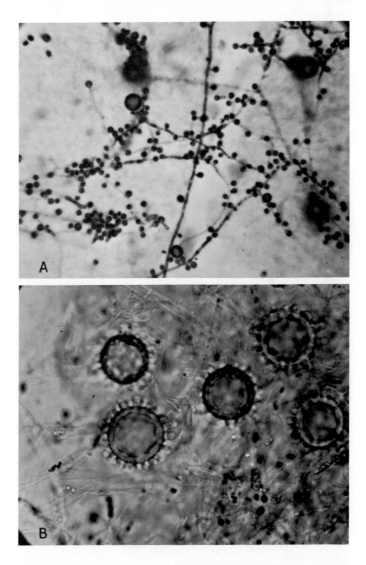

Figure 26–2. *Histoplasma capsulatum* from Sabouraud's glucose agar. *A,* Small, smooth, round to pyriform conidia. (× 600.) *B,* Large, thick-walled, round, tuberculate macroconidia. (× 1150.) (From Conant, N. F., Smith, D. T., Baker, R. G., and Calloway, J. L.: Manual of Clinical Mycology. Philadelphia, W. B. Saunders Co., 1974.)

numbers of spores. It also differentiates between the response to infection of the so-called normal and the abnormal host. In a normal host, both primary infection and reinfection are usually self-limited. This classification emphasizes, and this is particularly important, that progressive histoplasmosis probably occurs only in the abnormal host. By "abnormal" we mean that there most likely is some other disease or abnormality, or a defect of immunologic response, in particular cellular immunity. This certainly would be the case in infants and young children in whom it is recognized that the capacity to react immunologically is not well developed. This is also clearly the case in tuberculosis, another disease in which cellular immunity is critical for recovery (see Chap. 24). Disseminated histoplasmosis in the adult frequently is associated with demonstrable defects of the immune mechanism, and it is a reasonable hypothesis that when adults with this condition do not readily demonstrate these defects, it is merely because the techniques are not available for bringing the defects to light. No immunologic or cellular defect can be detected in patients with chronic pulmonary histoplasmosis, and immune mechanisms are apparently competent as indicated by the fact that dissemination from established chronic pulmonary histoplasmosis seldom if ever occurs. It is important in this connection to know that chronic pulmonary histoplasmosis is seen predominantly in white middle-aged or older males, and that most of these individuals have underlying chronic obstructive pulmonary disease. Thus, even though the defect may not be in the immunologic system, the underlying pathologic condition would reduce resistance in the pulmonary tree. The parallel to pulmonary disease caused by *Mycobacterium kansasii* and *Mycobacterium intracellulare* should be apparent (see Chaps. 24 and 25).

TABLE 26-1. A Classification of Histoplasmosis*

Usual benign infection of the normal host
  Primary infection
    Light exposure (asymptomatic)
    Heavy exposure (acute histoplasmosis, primary type)
  Reinfection
    Light exposure (asymptomatic)
    Heavy exposure (acute histoplasmosis, reinfection type)

Potentially progressive disease of the abnormal host
  Childhood infection
  Disseminated histoplasmosis in the adult
    Clinically disseminated (nonreactive)
    Clinically localized (partially reactive)
  Pulmonary histoplasmosis

Complications of healed primary infection
  Histoplasmomas
  Mediastinal fibrosis
  Broncholithiasis

---

*From Goodwin, R. J., Jr., and DesPrez, R. M.: Pathogenesis and clinical spectrum of histoplasmosis. South. Med. J. *66:*13, 1973.

Pathogenesis

After inhalation, the spores are probably phagocytized by alveolar macrophages within which they germinate and form yeast cells which then multiply by budding. In the previously uninfected healthy person, a primary-type disease develops which in almost every respect is similar to that found in primary tuberculosis. There is local multiplication of the parasite, with early involvement of the regional lymphatics and very early dissemination by way of the lymphatics and blood into other organs and tissues. Most of the yeast cells which are spread hematogenously are phagocytosed by reticuloendothelial cells, particularly in the liver, spleen, and bone marrow.

Growth also occurs at these secondary sites of infection. As in tuberculosis, the fate of the disease in this type of person depends upon the time it takes for the development of cellular immunity to infection and of delayed hypersensitivity to proteins of *Histoplasma capsulatum. H. capsulatum* multiplies more rapidly than *Mycobacterium tuberculosis;* therefore, there is a greater and earlier stimulation of immune mechanisms. The time until immunity and hypersensitivity develop probably varies between 7 and 21 days. As in tuberculosis, necrosis occurs, following the appearance of hypersensitivity, at the initial sites of infection in the lung, in the regional lymph nodes, and most likely at secondary foci of infection. As a consequence of the cellular immunity, further multiplication of the yeast cells is inhibited, and healing takes place by fibrous encapsulation. Eventually, these sites of infection will calcify and yield residual small areas of calcification. The calcified original parenchymal focus in the lung and in the hilar lymph nodes constitutes a Ghon complex which is similar to that seen following primary tuberculosis. In histoplasmosis, in contrast to tuberculosis, usually there are more numerous parenchymal calcified areas, and there is more enlargement and calcification of the hilar lymph nodes.

The sequence of events following reinfection in the normal host may be similar to or different from tuberculosis. When reinfection is light, there are no symptoms of disease because the immune mechanisms are sufficient to cope with the infection. This parallels that which occurs in light reinfection tuberculosis. In persons suffering heavy reinfection, the clinical picture may be quite different. Symptoms will appear soon after exposure, usually in three to four days. The temperature may be high, as much as 105°F, and the disease can be mistaken for influenza. Instead of the multiple areas of patchy pneumonitis which characterize primary histoplasmosis in the nonsensitized individual, the chest x-ray will usually show fine nodulation characteristic of a miliary type granulomatosis. Hilar adenopathy is not found, and pleural reactions are not noted. The changes on the chest x-ray may lag several days to a week behind the clinical symptoms. Accordingly, the initial radiologic examination following onset of symptoms may be negative, and abnormal changes may not appear until the patient has become asymptomatic. It is most likely, since recovery is rapid, that both symptoms and pulmonary findings represent a delayed-type allergic reaction in a previously sensitized host to a massive exposure to *Histoplasma capsulatum* spores. While the usual pattern is spontaneous recovery, progressive histoplasmosis may develop in a certain number of such patients. No such picture as this is seen in reinfection tuberculosis, probably because the likelihood of exposure to enormous numbers of tubercle bacilli is infinitesimal. By contrast, a person can accidently encounter an area of soil which contains enormous numbers of *H. capsulatum* spores.

The pathogenesis of histoplasmosis in the abnormal host also shows many parallels to tuberculosis. These parallels occur because the person who does not cope well with either a primary- or reinfection-type tuberculosis probably fails to do so because of compromised defense mechanisms. In the abnormal host, the outcome of histoplasmosis infection depends in part on the size of the infecting dose. Disseminated histoplasmosis in the child is equivalent to disseminated tuberculosis (miliary tuberculosis).

Disseminated histoplasmosis in the adult is not common but does occur in persons whose immune mechanisms are depressed by immunosuppressive drugs or by diseases which affect cellular immune mechanisms. It is of importance to recognize that disseminated histoplasmosis in the adult may frequently be associated with the incapacity of the patient to show reactions of delayed hypersensitivity either to histoplasmin or to other agents that will elicit delayed reactions in most adults. However, disseminated histoplasmosis is not always generalized, since only local lesions may occur. In patients with local lesions, cellular immune mechanisms seem to function. The cellular immune mechanisms, operating at the focus of infection, prevent generalized histoplasmosis but are unable, for reasons not known, to cope completely with the local disease. The similarity to localized tuberculous disease is striking.

In chronic pulmonary histoplasmosis, the infection is localized in the lung and probably superimposed upon some pulmonary defect. The disease persists because of the underlying pulmonary defect but does not disseminate because of adequate cellular immunity.

It has already been pointed out that histoplasmosis strikingly resembles tuberculosis, although the parasites are very different; both induce a high degree of delayed hypersensitivity to protein constituents of the parasitic cells, and in both the host depends upon the rapid acquisition of cellular immunity to infection to resolve the disease process. This favorable resolution occurs more readily and more frequently in histoplasmosis than in tuberculosis; this is probably due to some difference in the nature of the parasite. Reinfection histoplasmosis parallels in most respects reinfection tuberculosis, since in both diseases cellular immunity to infection predominates and progressive disease usually does not occur.

Diagnosis

Insofar as clinical signs and symptoms are concerned, there is nothing that distinguishes pulmonary histoplasmosis from pulmonary tuberculosis, coccidioidomycosis, or a number of other fungal diseases. Therefore, the diagnosis of histoplasmosis cannot be made without the detection of the causative agent in tissues or exudates. Preferably, this should be done by isolation upon a suitable medium and identification of the parasite by the characteristic growth and by the presence of the asexual spores. In tissue and biopsy specimens, the typical yeast form should be demonstrated within macrophages. Details of the procedures involved can be found in several textbooks and manuals.

Immunologic tests are useful in the diagnosis of histoplasmosis. One test, equivalent to the tuberculin test used for the detection of tuberculous infection, is called the *histoplasmin skin test*. Histoplasmin is prepared from broth medium upon which *Histoplasma capsulatum* has been grown. This is concentrated and is roughly equivalent to old tuberculin still used sometimes for the tuberculin test. Secondly, serologic tests for the detection of circulating antibody in the serum of persons suspected of having histoplasmosis are particularly useful. Much more so, in fact, than equivalent serologic tests in tuberculosis.

The significance of a positive histoplasmin test is much the same as the significance of a positive tuberculin test but its usefulness is much more limited. A positive histoplasmin test in an adult may indicate present infection or disease, or past infection or disease. Negative histoplasmin tests occur more frequently in adults who have active histoplasmosis than do negative tuberculin tests in those who have tuberculosis; therefore, a negative histoplasmin test does not necessarily mean absence of active disease. As in a positive test for tuberculosis, a positive histoplasmin test in very young children has greater significance since it more frequently means the presence of active disease. A major defect of the histoplasmin test is that cross-reactions are common in persons suffering other fungal infections such as blastomycosis and coccidioidomycosis. In contrast to the tuberculin test, therefore, the histoplasmin test is quite nonspecific. One of the most serious drawbacks that accompanies the use of the histoplasmin skin test for the diagnosis of histoplasmosis is that the test material itself, after injection into the skin, may stimulate the immune system and increase antibody levels in the serum. A skin test with histoplasmin, therefore, seriously affects the interpretation of the results of serologic tests. Realizing this, physicians should obtain a sample of blood for serologic tests before doing the histoplasmin test. In this way, the antibody titer of the serum sample is not affected. Serologic tests are most useful, when employed over a period of time, in following the antibody response of the patient. This surveillance requires serial samples of serum, and a histoplasmin skin test applied anytime prior to the taking of any blood sample might make it impossible to determine whether the patient had a rising titer. The detection of a rising circulating antibody titer is of great importance, since it strongly indicates the presence of an active disease process.

For the above reasons, it is recommended that the histoplasmin test not be used for the diagnosis of histoplasmosis. Instead, more reliance should be placed upon serologic tests. A number of serologic tests are available, but the most common is a complement-fixation reaction, using either yeast phase or mycelial phase antigen, or both. Antibody to yeast phase antigen is more likely to be present in acute cases, whereas antibody detected by the complement-fixation test using mycelial phase antigen is somewhat more likely to be present in patients with chronic histoplasmosis. It must be remembered that a negative complement-fixation test does not rule out disease, but, as already mentioned, demonstration of a rising titer is of great diagnostic significance. Care must be taken in interpretation of results because cross-reactions may be obtained in cases of other fungal infection. In the absence of a rising titer, a high titer of 1:16 or more is considered to be highly suggestive of active disease.

It is important to emphasize a difference between histoplasmosis and tuberculosis. In tuberculosis, serologic tests are of no value for the diagnosis of disease since there is no correlation between serum antibody content and disease activity. Furthermore, a fairly large number of patients with tuberculosis do not show a significant antibody response. The skin test, because of the specificity, is of considerable usefulness in tuberculosis and, since serologic tests are of no use in the diagnosis, we need not be concerned about the effect of skin testing on the antibody response. Therefore, the situation in tuberculosis is the reverse of that in histoplasmosis.

Other serologic tests have been used in histoplasmosis. These consist of the histoplasmin latex agglutination test, agar gel double diffusion, hemagglutination, and fluorescent antibody. These four tests are not used routinely. In fact, the last three can only be performed in a few highly specialized laboratories.

Epidemiology

The greatest usefulness of the histoplasmin skin test is in determining the incidence of histoplasmin infection in large populations of human beings. It is in this manner that the geographic distribution of *Histoplasma capsulatum* infection has been determined (Fig. 26–3). In these areas, the fungus grows in the mycelial form in soil producing the spores, which are then carried by air currents and inhaled by man and lower animals. In the majority of people infected in this manner, the infection either is so mild it is passed off or it goes unnoticed. As previously noted, heavy exposure to *H. capsulatum* spores can result in clinically evident and sometimes progressive disease. Epidemics of acute histoplasmosis may occur. These usually are found in the periphery of the endemic area and among groups of people who encounter an unusually large concentration of *H. capsulatum* spores. For unknown reasons, this fungus grows, multiplies, and produces spores particularly well in soil that has been heavily contaminated with fowl excreta. Epidemics have been reported following exposure of susceptible people to heavy concentrations of spores in chicken houses, areas under starling roosts, pigeon roosts, hollow trees, and water towers, or any area where large numbers of fowl congregate. The fowl are not infected, probably because of their higher body temperature. Bats can become infected, and areas of deposition of bat feces, such as caves, attics, and hollow trees, may be extremely infectious because of the high concentration of spores (see Chap. 42).

Prevention

The disease could be prevented if infected soil were able to be decontaminated. Unfortunately, there are no good methods for the decontamination of the enormous areas of soil involved in the endemic regions. Vaccination to raise the level of resistance to infection of the population at risk might be useful. To date, however, no effective vaccine has been developed. Since histoplasmosis in the normal person does not carry much risk, prevention probably should be limited to attempts to raise the resistance of the immunologically compromised person or of those individuals with known pulmonary or other defects that might lower resistance. All persons should avoid those places having high concentrations of fowl or bat excreta.

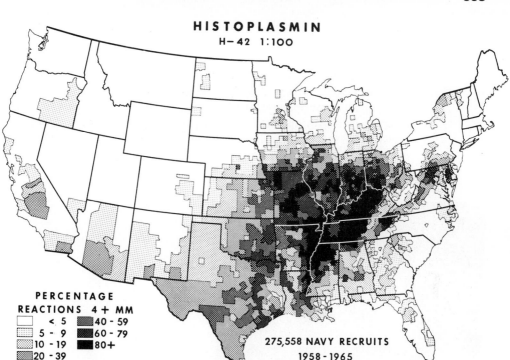

Figure 26-3. Map shows incidence of skin reactivity to histoplasmin among naval recruits. In southern Kentucky, middle Tennessee, and other areas, the incidence of skin reactivity is as high as 90 to 95 per cent. (From Edwards, L. B., Acquaviva, F. A., Livesay, V. T., et al.: An atlas of sensitivity of tuberculin, PPD-B, and histoplasmosis in the United States. Amer. Rev. Resp. Dis. *99:*1, 1969.)

Treatment

Amphotericin B is the only drug at the moment which will favorably affect the course of histoplasmosis. This drug is very toxic and should be used only in those cases in which there is some question of a favorable outcome, whether the disease is of the primary or reinfection type, since both are ordinarily self-limited infections. Occasionally, however, short courses of treatment with amphotericin B can be given in the rare unusually prolonged or relapsing infection.

Full dosages of amphotericin B should be given to all patients with disseminated histoplasmosis. It has been estimated that approximately 50 per cent of such severe infections can be controlled with this treatment.

Coccidioidomycosis

Introduction

Coccidioidomycosis (coccidiomycosis, valley fever, San Joaquin fever) is caused by the dimorphic fungus *Coccidioides immitis*. As with *Histoplasma capsulatum,* this fungus grows in the soil and produces spores (arthrospores) which are carried by air currents and inhaled by human beings and lower animals. In the infected host, the arthrospores develop into spherules (sporangia) which are from 20 to 100 microns in diameter. The cytoplasm and the nucleus within the spherules divide to produce thousands of endospores (sporangiospores), each about 2 to 3 microns in diameter. The spherules eventually rupture, and endospores are liberated. Each endospore, unless destroyed, again will develop into a spherule which in turn will produce more endospores. When growing at lower temperatures in soil, or on culture the fungus appears in a mycelial form (Figs. 26–4 and 26–5).

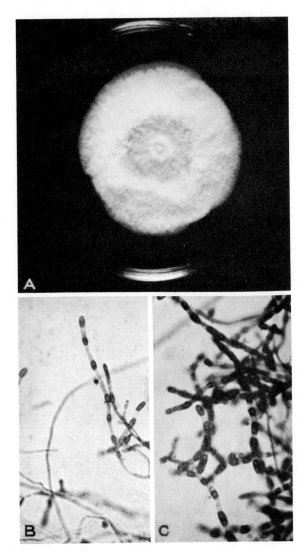

Figure 26–4. *Coccidioides immitis. A,* Culture on Sabouraud's glucose agar, 19 days, at room temperature. *B,* Arthrospore formation in young culture. (X 580.) *C,* Arthrospore formation in old culture. (X 700.) (From Conant, N. F., Smith, D. T., Baker, R. G., and Calloway, J. L.: Manual of Clinical Mycology. Philadelphia, W. B. Saunders Co., 1974.)

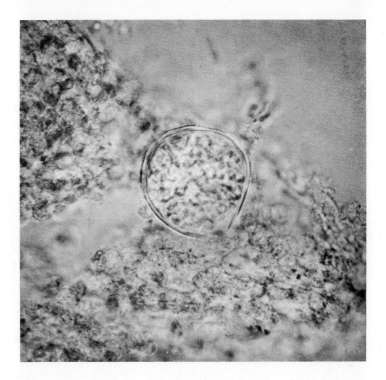

Figure 26–5. *Coccidioides immitis.* Round, thick-walled endospore-filled spherule in sputum. (× 700.) (From Conant, N. F.: Laboratory diagnosis of pulmonary mycoses. Am. Rev. Tuberc. *61:*690, 1950.)

In contrast to histoplasmosis, coccidioidomycosis is limited to the New World and to well-defined areas in the southwestern United States, Mexico, and South America.

Types of Disease

There is no clinical classification of coccidioidomycosis equivalent to that given in the preceding section for histoplasmosis. Little question exists, however, that the same factors operate in the development of active disease in coccidioidomycosis as in histoplasmosis, and a clinical classification similar to that given for histoplasmosis no doubt could be constructed. Of all the people who become infected, only a small number will show signs of clinical disease, and whether they do or not is related to the number of arthrospores inhaled and to the immune status of the host.

The primary lesion is usually pulmonary and, following an incubation period of 7 to 28 days, averaging 10 to 16 days, clinical symptoms of fever, malaise, slight dry cough, and chest pain occur. Night sweats and anorexia may be present. The disease is usually self-limited, particularly in adults, but approximately 5 per cent of such patients may develop residual cavitary disease, and sometimes nodules or pulmonary abscesses. The pulmonary cavities are usually thin walled and heal spontaneously. Chronic progressive pulmonary disease, resembling histoplasmosis or tuberculosis, may occur (Figs. 26–6 to 26-8).

Allergic manifestations are found more frequently in coccidioidomycosis than in histoplasmosis or tuberculosis. Erythema nodosum or erythema multiforme may occur a few days or a few weeks after infection. The appearance of these manifestations coincides with the development of delayed hypersensitivity to proteins of the infecting fungus. Delayed hypersensitivity in this disease is an outstanding feature, as it is in tuberculosis and histoplasmosis. Disseminated progressive disease occurs only in a very small number of persons infected or in persons showing some evidence of primary pulmonary disease. Almost any tissue or organ can be involved, and detailed descriptions of these secondary manifestations can be found in standard textbooks of medicine. Although direct evidence is lacking, it is extremely probable that, as in histoplasmosis and tuberculosis, disseminated disease or progressive chronic pulmonary disease occurs only in the person who is immunologically compromised, or in persons with an underlying disease that lowers resistance.

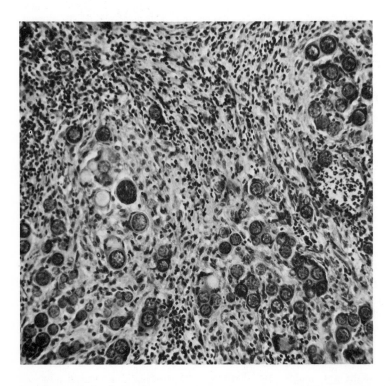

Figure 26–6. Coccidioidal granuloma. Lymph node with much scarring. The spherules are largely in a stage that does not show the endospores. Hematoxylin and eosin stain. (X 200.) (From Conant, N. F., Smith, D. T., Baker, R. G., and Calloway, J. L.: Manual of Clinical Mycology. Philadelphia, W. B. Saunders Co., 1974.)

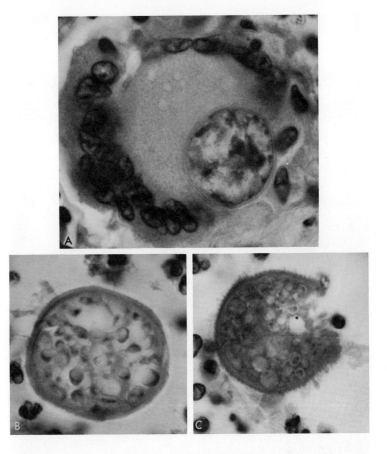

Figure 26–7. Coccidioidal granuloma. *A,* Giant cell containing a rounded, thick-walled form easily confused with similar forms in blastomycosis and paracoccidioidomycosis. Lymph node. Case of fatal coccidioidal granuloma. Hematoxylin and eosin stain. (X 1200.) *B,* Endosporulating spherule in an abscess of a lymph node. Hematoxylin and eosin stain. (X 1200.) *C,* Endosporulating spherule ruptured on one side. Note the peripheral spines. From same lymph node. Hematoxylin and eosin stain. (X 1200.) (From Conant, N. F., Smith, D. T., Baker, R. G., and Calloway, J. L.: Manual of Clinical Mycology. Philadelphia, W. B. Saunders Co., 1974.)

Pathogenesis

Although there is no evidence indicating what occurs in human beings immediately following infection, data from studies using experimental animals suggest that the events are very similar to those which follow infection with virulent tubercle bacilli or with *Histoplasma capsulatum.* The arthrospores reach the alveoli, where they are probably phagocytized. Being facultative intracellular parasites, the arthrospores grow, metabolize, and develop into spherules within 48 to 72 hours. The endospores are disseminated during the preallergic and preimmune stage by way of the lymphatics and blood to many regions of the body. Dissemination is indicated by the marked hilar adenopathy which develops and by the fact

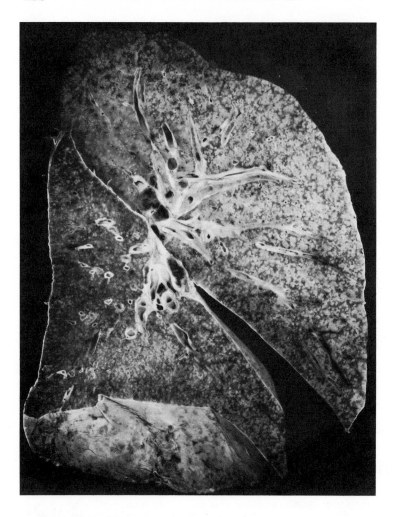

Figure 26–8. Miliary coccidioidomycosis of the lung. (From Forbus, W. D., and Bestebreurtje, A. M.: Coccidioidomycosis. A study of 95 cases of disseminated type with special reference to the pathogenesis of the disease. Milit. Surg. *99:*653, 1946.)

that fungi have been isolated from lymph nodes. The pulmonary disease is pneumonic in character, and necrosis and cavitation may occur after the development of delayed hypersensitivity. With the early appearance of cellular immunity to infection, the disease process will be controlled and resolved in the majority of persons. It should be reemphasized here that progressive disseminated coccidioidomycosis or progressive pulmonary disease most likely occurs only in those hosts whose capacities to resist infection or to develop immunity have been compromised in one way or another. In this regard it is of interest to note that progressive disseminated disease is in part genetically determined. It occurs about 50 times more often in Philippine men, and 10 times more often in black men, than it does in white men. Dissemination among Mexican and American Indians appears to be only slightly more common than among whites. This relatively increased susceptibility to progressive disease parallels the susceptibility of these groups of people to tuberculosis. It seems likely, on the basis of recent experimental evidence, that the increased susceptibility of some races to diseases such as coccidioidomycosis and tuberculosis is due to a genetically determined impairment of the capacity to develop cellular immunity to infection.

Diagnosis

The clinical manifestations and the radiologic findings in coccidioidomycosis may closely resemble those of influenza, bacterial or other mycotic pneumonia, acute or chronic tuberculosis and histoplasmosis, sarcoidosis, lymphomas, and other neoplasms. Therefore, a diagnosis can be made only by identification of the presence of the parasite in the affected tissue. While direct examination, e.g., of sputum, may reveal the presence of the characteristic spherules, this is not definitive because artifacts may be present which resemble spherules. Isolation of the fungus by cultivation on appropriate culture mediums and detection of the characteristic growth, together with a determination of the pathogenicity of the fungus for laboratory animals, may be necessary.

Isolation and cultivation of *Coccidioides immitis* take a great deal of time, however, and the spore-forming mycelial cultures are very dangerous to handle, since the spores are highly infectious for laboratory personnel. Therefore, the usual procedure is to rely on skin tests for delayed hypersensitivity to coccidioidin and upon serologic tests for diagnosis.

A skin-testing material, *coccidioidin,* is available and is especially useful for epidemiologic studies. It also can be used in patients suspected of having coccidioidomycosis and is somewhat more specific than the histoplasmin test. Basically, the interpretation of the significance of the positive skin test has all of the limitations already mentioned for the tuberculin and histoplasmin tests.

Skin tests using coccidioidin are somewhat more useful than those using histoplasmin, mainly because injecting coccidioidin into the skin does not stimulate the formation of antibodies which will react in serologic tests.

A number of tests for the presence of circulating antibody in the serum of patients have been devised. The complement-fixation test is the one most commonly employed and is of particular value in following the stages of progressive disease, since it also has considerable prognostic significance. Almost invariably, patients with progressive and severe coccidioidomycosis show a high complement-fixation titer. In general, a rising complement-fixing titer of more than 1:16 or 1:32 coincides with the spread of the disease, particularly extrapulmonary spread. Conversely, a decreasing titer is a favorable sign.

Epidemiology

Coccidioides immitis is found growing in the soil only in certain rather limited areas in the Western Hemisphere (Fig. 26–9). The endemic areas include central San Joaquin Valley, certain southern counties of California,

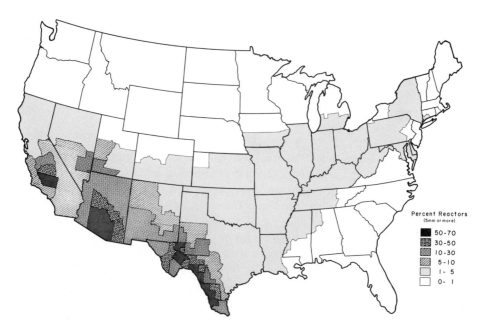

Figure 26–9. Geographic distribution of frequency of coccidioidin reactors among 48,676 young adults. *Coccidioides immitis* is known to exist in areas of high incidence. A low incidence of positive reactions occurs in areas where histoplasmosis is endemic. (From Edwards, P. Q., and Palmer, C. E.: Prevalence of sensitivity to coccidioidin, with special reference to specific and nonspecific reactions to coccidioidin and to histoplasmin. Dis. Chest. *31:*35, 1957.)

southern Arizona, New Mexico, southwestern Texas, Mexico, parts of Guatemala, Honduras, Venezuela, Paraguay, Columbia, and Argentina. These endemic areas encompass what is referred to as the geologic Lower Sonoran Life Zone (Fig. 26–10). This includes semiarid areas that are low in altitude and have hot summers, moderately wet winters, and infrequent freezes. In these areas, the fungus persists in soil as spores over the winter and, following the winter rains, again develops and produces more spores. For these reasons, the incidence of disease is higher in the summer months, particularly in summers that follow wet winters. As in histoplasmosis, certain areas seem to be highly infected because small epidemics have occurred as a result of disturbance of the soil through agricultural operations, housing excavations, archaeologic diggings, or merely through the playing activities of children.

Other animal species, e.g., wild rodents, dogs, cats, sheep, cattle, and even horses, are infected by inhalation of the arthrospores. To the best of our knowledge, however, man-to-man, animal-to-man, or animal-to-animal transmission occurs rarely. Apparently, the fragility of the endospore is too great to permit the survival necessary for easy transmission from person to person, or from animal to person.

Even though the disease occurs predominantly in endemic areas, it may be found anywhere in the world. Persons may be exposed to the disease while in an endemic area and then arrive in a nonendemic area before symptoms develop. Arthrospores may be transmitted long distances on clothes or other inanimate objects that have been contaminated in the endemic areas and then

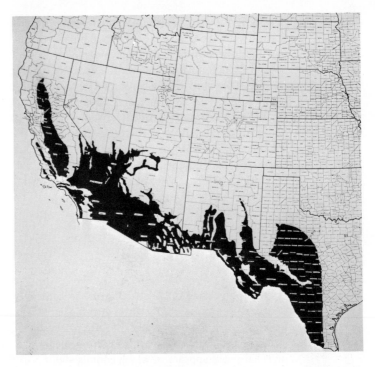

Figure 26–10. Lower Sonoran Life Zone. (From Maddy, K. T.: Disseminated coccidioidomycosis of the dog. J.A.V.M.A. *132:*483, 1958.)

transported to nonendemic areas. Such cases have occurred in Great Britain and Italy.

It has been shown, by using skin tests to detect present or previous infection, that about 15 to 50 per cent of susceptible persons arriving for the first time in an endemic area will be infected within the first 12 months. The incidence rises to 80 per cent or better within five years. As in histoplasmosis, the majority of infections with *Coccidioides immitis* are detected only by the appearance of a positive skin test. At least 60 per cent of persons infected show no clinical signs or symptoms.

Prevention

Factors involved in prevention of coccidioidomycosis are identical with those in histoplasmosis. Avoidance of infection in epidemic areas is impossible, disinfection of soil is equally difficult, and no really adequate vaccine to raise the level of resistance has been developed.

Treatment

Treatment of coccidioidomycosis parallels treatment of histoplasmosis. In those white patients who develop symptoms, no treatment is required for mild or moderate primary coccidioidomycosis. Treatment with amphotericin B is probably indicated in several situations, e.g., severe primary infections or patients in whom there is a high probability of dissemination either because of racial predisposition or on the basis of serologic and other laboratory findings. Disseminated disease should be treated with amphotericin B. Women in the third trimester of pregnancy suffering from coccidioidomycosis should receive amphotericin B, since resistance apparently is lower at that time. Patients who are taking corticosteroids for another condition or are receiving treatment which has an immunosuppressive effect should receive amphotericin B. Amphotericin B is the only drug currently available which is effective for the treatment of coccidioidomycosis.

Blastomycosis

Introduction

Blastomycosis (Gilchrist's disease) is caused by the dimorphic fungus, *Blastomyces dermatitidis*. When growing in tissue at 37°C, it appears as a budding yeast, approximately 8 to 15 microns in diameter, which has a thick refractile cell wall. On artificial culture media and at room temperature, a mycelial phase appears in which conidia about 3 to 4 microns in diameter are produced (Figs. 26–11 to 26–13).

Blastomycosis occurs primarily in the southeastern and central portions of the United States and is frequently referred to as North American blastomycosis. A clinically somewhat similar disease called South American blastomycosis is found in Central and South America. The cause of South American blastomycosis is a similar-appearing fungus, *Paracoccidioides brasiliensis*. It was originally given this name because it appeared to resemble *Coccidioides immitis*. However, it is now recognized that it is more closely related to *Blastomyces dermatitidis*.

Types of Disease

In blastomycosis, the cutaneous manifestations constitute the outstanding clinical feature. These appear initially as small papular or pustular lesions usually occurring on the exposed parts of the body, such as the hands and face, but may be seen elsewhere. The lesions enlarge peripherally and may become raised and verrucous in character. They develop slowly and usually are not painful and do not itch (Figs. 26–14 to 26–16).

Pulmonary disease is frequent but is usually mild and nonprogressive. Progressive pulmonary disease, when it occurs, is clinically indistinguishable from pulmonary tuberculosis, histoplasmosis, or coccidioidomycosis. In patients showing cutaneous lesions, pulmonary disease may or may not be readily demonstrable (Fig. 26–17).

In contrast to other fungi causing systemic infections, *Blastomyces dermatitidis* may affect the male genital tract, including the prostate, epididymis, and testis.

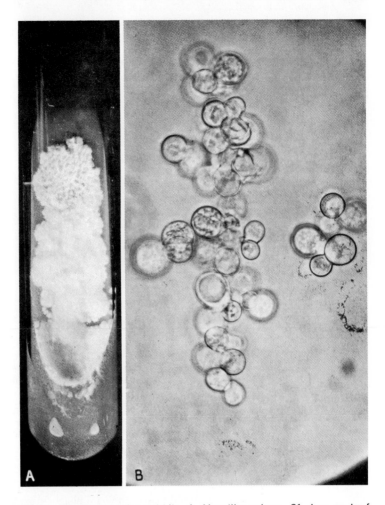

Figure 26–11. *Blastomyces dermatitidis. A,* Yeastlike culture, 21 days on beef infusion glucose agar at 37°C. *B,* Budding yeast cells from beef infusion glucose agar at 37°C. (× 700.) (From Conant, N. F., Smith, D. T., Baker, R. G., and Calloway, J. L.: Manual of Clinical Mycology. Philadelphia, W. B. Saunders Co., 1974.)

Infections of the bone also occur, and these lesions frequently can be demonstrated radiographically. The spine is most commonly affected, but the long bones of the lower extremities and the bones of the pelvis and ribs may also become diseased.

A variety of other organs and tissues may be affected, leading to meningitis, cerebral abscesses, involvement of the adrenal glands, pericarditis, and endocarditis.

Pathogenesis

The prominence of the cutaneous lesions and the fact that the first evidence of blastomycosis may be the appearance of cutaneous disease led to the early belief that these were primary lesions and other forms of the disease

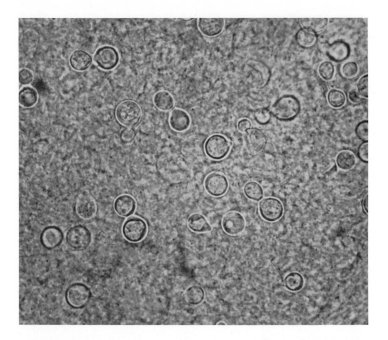

Figure 26–12. *Blastomyces dermatitidis.* Round, thick-walled, budding yeast-like cells in pus from subcutaneous abscess. (X 700.) (From Conant, N. F., Smith, D. T., Baker, R. G., and Calloway, J. L.: Manual of Clinical Mycology. Philadelphia, W. B. Saunders Co., 1974.)

in other tissues were secondary to the cutaneous lesions. It is now recognized that the pathogenesis of blastomycosis probably parallels the pathogenesis of tuberculosis, histoplasmosis, and coccidioidomycosis; therefore, the most likely initial site of infection is the lung. Presumably, spores are inhaled and deposited in the alveoli, where they are phagocytosed. Local disease will then develop which may be too mild to be clinically evident. During this primary infection, there is widespread dissemination by way of the lymphatics and blood; eventually, secondary manifestations either may or may not develop. The cutaneous lesions, therefore, represent metastatic infections from primary pulmonary disease, and further dissemination from the metastatic lesions may occur.

Much evidence suggests that the above picture of the pathogenesis of blastomycosis is correct. First, if careful search is made for evidence of pulmonary infection in patients with cutaneous lesions, infection frequently can be found. Second, if the primary lesion of blastomycosis is due to inoculation of the skin, the cutaneous lesions would be expected to occur most frequently on the hands and feet as do those of other inoculation diseases such as plague, tularemia, or sporotrichosis. Actually, a majority of blastomycotic dermal lesions are found on the face and trunk. In addition, in several cases in which laboratory technicians or physicians have been accidentally infected by direct inoculation of the skin, primary cutaneous blastomycosis developed but the lesions did not resemble "typical" cutaneous lesions seen in patients naturally infected. Instead, the disease resembled primary inoculation tuberculosis and consisted of an ulcerated local lesion,

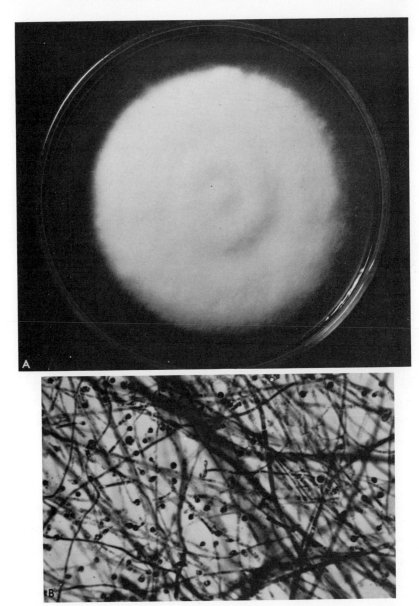

Figure 26–13. *Blastomyces dermatitidis.* *A,* Filamentous colony on Sabouraud's glucose agar, 23 days at room temperature. *B,* Round and pyriform conidia found in filamentous stage from Sabouraud's glucose agar at room temperature. (X 700.) (From Conant, N. F., Smith, D. T., Baker, R. G., and Calloway, J. L.: Manual of Clinical Mycology. Philadelphia, W. B. Saunders Co., 1974.)

lymphangitis, and regional lymphadenopathy. In these cases, the disease tends to be mild and self-limited.

The typical, slowly progressing lesions of cutaneous blastomycosis are quite different from those of the other systemic mycoses; this can be accounted for by postulating that these lesions occur in persons who have had previous experience (infection) with *Blastomyces dermatitidis* and have

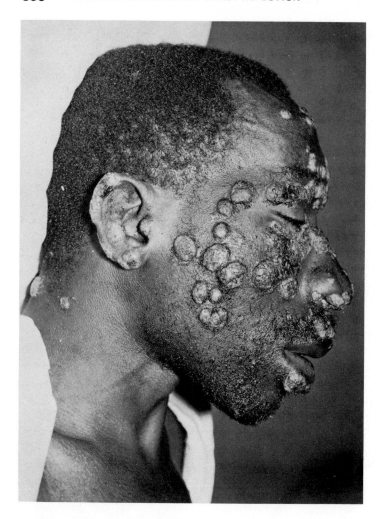

Figure 26–14. Blastomycosis of the skin. Primary lesions of the face showing multiple, discrete, elevated, granulomatous lesions. (From Conant, N. F., Smith, D. T., Baker, R. G., and Calloway, J. L.: Manual of Clinical Mycology. Philadelphia, W. B. Saunders Co., 1974.)

developed both delayed hypersensitivity and cellular immunity to infection. The inflammatory response is a consequence of reactions of delayed hypersensitivity, and the localization, without extensive involvement of the lymphatics, can best be explained by the operation of the forces of cellular immunity to infection. Thus, delayed hypersensitivity and cellular immunity to infection account, respectively, for the localized inflammatory reaction and for the slow progression of the lesion. The parallel here to secondary tuberculosis is almost complete; the major difference is that in tuberculosis the process most commonly involves the lung, while in blastomycosis the process most often involves the skin.

The above discussion does not mean that inoculation blastomycosis cannot occur from either an endogenous or an exogenous source. However, in

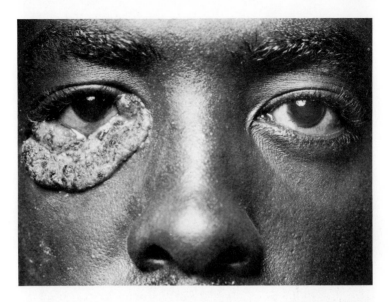

Figure 26–15. Blastomycosis. Primary lesion of the right lower eyelid following injury with a sliver of steel. (From Conant, N. F., Smith, D. T., Baker, R. G., and Calloway, J. L.: Manual of Clinical Mycology. Philadelphia, W. B. Saunders Co., 1974.)

order to obtain typical cutaneous lesions, the parasite would have to be introduced into the skin of a person who had had enough previous experience with the microorganism to have already developed both delayed hypersensitivity and cellular immunity to infection.

Although supportive evidence is not available, there is justification in assuming that progressive pulmonary or disseminated disease does not occur except in the presence of underlying host deficiencies or compromised cellular immunity.

Diagnosis

A diagnosis of blastomycosis can be made only by demonstration of the causative agent in tissue specimens or material such as sputum. This can best be done by cultivation upon artificial culture mediums and identification of the fungus by its characteristic morphologic appearance. *Blastomyces dermatitidis* grows readily on a variety of culture media and can be handled easily and safely in the laboratory.

Neither serologic tests nor skin tests for delayed hypersensitivity are of much help in diagnosis of this disease. Many patients with active disease do not show circulating antibody in significant amounts, and, although a blastomycin skin-testing material has been used, many nonspecific reactions occur.

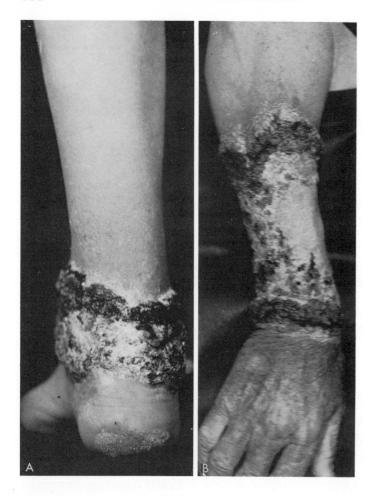

Figure 26–16. Blastomycosis of the arm and leg. *A,* The leg shows an open granulating ulcer. *B,* The arm illustrates a verrucous edge to the lesion with healing in the center. (From Martin, D. S., and Smith, D. T.: Blastomycosis. I. A review of the literature. II. A report of 13 new cases. Am. Rev. Tuberc. *39:*275, 488, 1939.)

Epidemiology

The source of infection with *Blastomyces dermatitidis* is not definitely known. It is assumed, because of the limited geographic distribution (Fig. 26–18), the nature of the parasite, and the parallels between this disease and histoplasmosis and coccidioidomycosis, that the microorganism lives and grows in soil, producing the spores which are carried by air currents and inhaled by man and other animals. *B. dermatitidis* has been isolated occasionally but not consistently from soil samples in endemic areas. It is, therefore, difficult to assess the significance of the few instances in which it has been found in soil. The possibility of transmission from infected lower animals cannot be excluded, since dogs have been shown to acquire the disease. Man-to-man transmission apparently does not occur; therefore, it is unlikely that infected lower animals would transmit the disease to man.

All races appear to be equally susceptible, but the disease occurs about nine times more frequently in males than in females.

Prevention

Without a knowledge of the source of the infection, no direct method for control can be undertaken. In addition, if the causative microorganism is truly a soil inhabitant, attempts at indirect control, as in coccidioidomycosis and histoplasmosis, would be futile. No vaccine suitable for use in human beings has been developed.

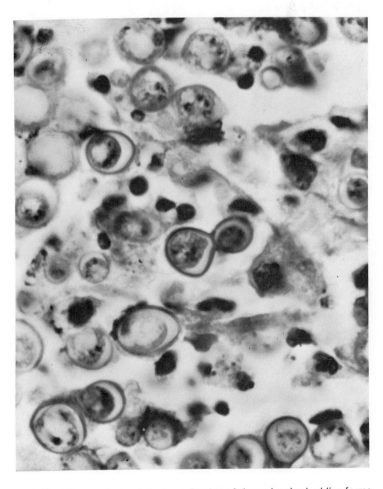

Figure 26–17. Blastomycosis of the lung. Section of tissue showing budding forms. Periodic acid–Schiff stain. (X 1500.) (From Conant, N. F., Smith, D. T., Baker, R. G., and Calloway, J. L.: Manual of Clinical Mycology. Philadelphia, W. B. Saunders Co., 1974.)

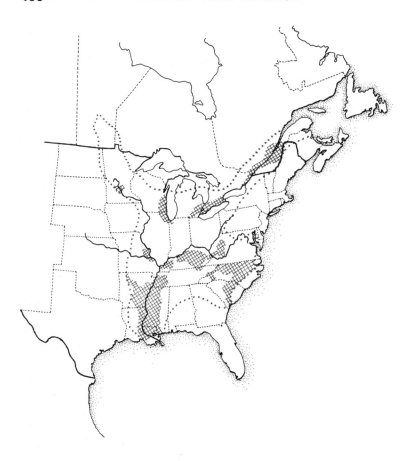

Figure 26–18. Blastomycosis. Incidence and prevalence of blastomycosis in North America. The dotted line indicates the known endemic region. The hatched areas are those with the highest incidence. (From Rippon, J. W.: Medical Mycology. Philadelphia, W. B. Saunders Co., 1974.)

Treatment

The principles that govern the treatment of the other systemic mycoses also govern the treatment of blastomycosis. The general supportive measures are the same, and surgical intervention can be of value in selected cases.

Drug therapy has its place, and, in addition to amphotericin B, 2-hydroxystilbamidine has been found to be effective. Both drugs may be quite toxic, however.

Summary

In this chapter, we have considered the three systemic fungal diseases — histoplasmosis, coccidioidomycosis and blastomycosis — which occur with some frequency in the United States. There are other systemic diseases caused by fungi. These include actinomycosis, nocardiosis, paracoccidioidomycosis, African histoplasmosis, cryptococcosis, candidiasis, geotrichosis, aspergillosis, phycomycosis, and sporotrichosis.

Consideration of the features and the pathogenesis of histoplasmosis, coccidioidomycosis, and blastomycosis, however, allows certain generalizations which may be applicable to all systemic mycotic diseases. First, whether the portal of entry of the parasite is by way of the lung, skin, or gastrointestinal tract, the sequence of events is the same. Since these parasites are all facultative intracellular microorganisms, they are initially phagocytosed. They grow within the phagocytic cells and are then disseminated readily to other parts of the body by way of the lymphatics and blood. This initial primary infection is usually rather mild and in many cases may not even give rise to symptoms. The host responds to this primary infection by rapidly developing delayed hypersensitivity to proteins of the parasite and a cellular type of immunity to infection. The forces responsible for cellular immunity to infection usually prevail, and the multiplication of the parasites at the site of initial invasion and at those areas to which they have metastasized will be controlled; eventually, the parasites may be killed. In a certain number of patients, chronic progressive disease may develop, even in the face of cellular immunity to infection, and this disease may be localized or disseminated in character. When progressive disease develops, delayed hypersensitivity usually plays a large role in the genesis of the inflammatory and necrotic lesions which occur. A possible exception may be cryptococcosis, a disease in which the relative roles of anticapsular antibody and cellular immunity in controlling infection are poorly understood.

Progressive systemic mycotic disease, whether local or disseminated, probably occurs only in the person who has some other disease or abnormality which lowers host resistance or in the person whose capacity to develop cellular immunity to infection is low or has been reduced by any one of a number of factors. Stated another way, progressive fungal disease probably will occur only in the abnormal host.

Evidence is not at hand to permit documentation of all of the above generalizations for all systemic fungal diseases, but the similarities between the parasites, the epidemiology, the pathogenesis, the development of active disease, and the disease manifestations strongly suggest that the generalizations are valid.

It is also worth emphasizing that the pathogenesis of the three diseases reviewed in this chapter closely parallels the pathogenesis of tuberculosis. Therefore, if the pathogenesis of tuberculosis is thoroughly understood, the pathogenesis of all of the systemic mycoses becomes clear. We might, therefore, speak of the "tuberculosis-like infectious diseases." These would include all of the systemic mycotic diseases as well as certain other bacterial diseases some of which are covered in later chapters.

Finally, a number of the other fungal diseases are discussed in Chapter 43. The microorganisms involved in these conditions are particularly prone to take advantage of compromised immune responses of the host.

CASE PRESENTATION 1

A 20-year-old white female who had lived and worked all her life in northern Indiana was admitted to the hospital for investigation of a pulmonary density. Six months prior to admission she injured her back by falling down a staircase. Chest roentgenograms at that time revealed thoracic vertebral fractures. As an incidental finding, a hilar lung density was noted. The density was thought to be pneumonia, and antimicrobial therapy was given. During the intervening six months, the patient had no complaints and was ambulatory. There were no cough, hemoptysis, or fatigue. In follow-up chest roentgenograms, the density had not changed in size but proved to be persistent. She was hospitalized for further studies to determine the cause of the lung density.

Physical examination revealed no abnormalities. Additional chest roentgenograms demonstrated focal atelectasis of the right lower lobe and a mass in the right hilum. Bronchoscopy was performed, but no abnormalities were detected. A right scalene lymph node was removed, and microscopic examination revealed nonspecific changes; no cultures were made.

Because of the possibility of a lymphoma or Hodgkin's disease, a thoracotomy was performed. The mass in the right hilum was exposed and found to be composed of caseous necrotic material. A tissue specimen was sent to the laboratory for culture and histopathologic examination. A lymph node contiguous with the hilar mass also was removed. The mass demonstrated nonspecific granulomatous inflammation. There also were focal areas of necrosis in the excised lymph node. Direct and histochemical stains of the caseous material and sections of the lymph node for mycobacteria and fungi failed to reveal any recognizable microorganisms. Upon culture of the hilar mass, a microorganism was isolated which was identified as *Histoplasma capsulatum*.

For an analysis of this case, see the discussion which follows Case Presentation 3.

CASE PRESENTATION 2

The patient, a 38-year-old white female, was admitted to the hospital for investigation of a left lower pulmonary mass. She had lived in Chicago all her life except for the period from 1966 to 1969, when she had worked in Phoenix, Arizona. Three months prior to admission to the hospital, the patient had had a job interview, and a routine chest roentgenogram performed at that time revealed a mass in the left lower lobe of the lung.

At the time of admission there was no history of shortness of breath or fever. The patient has been very active physically and in general had no complaints, except for a slight chronic cough which she associated with smoking one package of cigarettes a day. Physical examination revealed a well-nourished female with no obvious abnormalities. Chest roentgenograms demonstrated a well-delineated, round density measuring approximately 3 cm in diameter in the lower lobe of the left lung (Fig. 26–19); there appeared to be a small cavity in the center of the pulmonary density. Bronchoscopic examination and tomography were performed but provided no clues to the nature of the lesion.

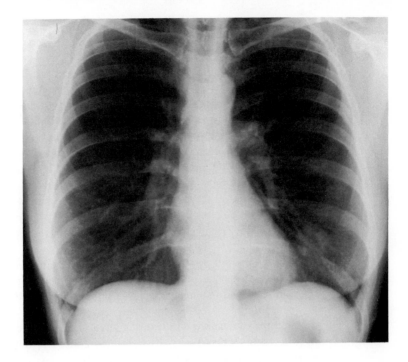

Figure 26–19.

Surgery was recommended, and on the second hospital day a wedge resection of the lesion in the left lower lobe was done. The patient's postoperative course was uneventful, and she was discharged feeling well 10 days later.

Examination of the resected tissue revealed a nodule approximately 3 cm in diameter in the central portion of the specimen. This nodule was sharply circumscribed from the surrounding lung and had a mottled tan and gray cut surface. Upon sectioning this nodule, it was found to contain a cavity which, when examined microscopically, revealed spherules and hyphae consistent with *Coccidioides immitis. C. immitis* subsequently was cultivated from this specimen. Cultures and stained smears for mycobacteria were negative.

For an analysis of this case, see the discussion which follows Case Presentation 3.

CASE PRESENTATION 3

A 58-year-old white male was admitted to the hospital because of high blood pressure, weight loss, and a chronic cough. Hypertension had been detected six months previously, and the patient had been taking diuretics since then. He had noted a 12-pound weight loss over the preceding two months in spite of normal appetite and food intake. The patient had no other complaints except for a chronic cough productive of some sputum. He smoked two to three packages of cigarettes a day.

Findings on physical examination were within normal limits except for an undescended right testicle and a blood pressure reading of 160/110 mm Hg.

A chest roentgenogram showed the heart and great vessels to be of normal size and shape. A homogeneous mass which had hazy borders and was not segmented was seen in the right hilum. No lymphadenopathy was noted.

Because of the possibility of carcinoma, surgery was recommended and a thoracotomy, followed by resection of the right middle and lower lobes of the lung, was performed. Histologic examination of the resected lobes revealed extensive chronic granulomatous inflammation with many giant cells which contained budding yeasts (Fig. 26–17). In addition to the granulomatous inflammation, there were many microabscesses and areas of necrosis. The appearance of the budding yeast was compatible with that of *Blastomyces dermatitidis.* Subsequently, *B. dermatitidis* was isolated by culture from the specimen.

These cases illustrate well the subtle presentations and diagnostic problems appearing in fungal diseases, especially when they occur, as in Case Presentation 2, in nonendemic areas. There is no way to distinguish clinically between pulmonary lesions caused by any of a number of fungi. The most common microorganism which might serve as an etiologic agent is, of course, *Mycobacterium tuberculosis.* In Case Presentation 2, the history of several years residency in Phoenix, Arizona, might have provided a clue and retrospectively explained the occurrence of coccidioidomycosis in a Chicago resident. Serologic tests might also have been useful. In the final analysis, the resolution of the nature of the lesions may have required excision of the pulmonary lesions in question and appropriate histopathologic and bacteriologic examination which, hopefully, would result in the cultivation and isolation of the offending microorganism.

In all of these cases, a primary concern to the physician was the possibility that the pulmonary densities might represent malignancies, either primary or metastatic. In all three cases, this possibility was entertained almost to the exclusion of the possibility of an infectious agent being responsible, since almost no studies were carried out in each patient to establish an infectious agent.

In Case Presentation 1, the roentgenographic abnormality was initially considered to be due to pneumonia, and antimicrobial therapy was prescribed even though none of the symptoms and physical findings usually expected in acute forms of pneumonia were present. One should note the lack of any studies, viz., intrabronchial brushing or translaryngeal aspiration as a means of selectively obtaining pulmonary secretions for morphologic studies and cultures, which conceivably might have yielded the causative agent. PPD skin testing was not performed prior to surgery despite the fact that tuberculosis is a cause of pulmonary disease even in young patients. In view of the patient's age, primary consideration was given to the possibility of lymphoma or Hodgkin's disease.

In Case Presentation 2, a primary carcinoma of the lung was not a very likely possibility, even in the face of a history of cigarette smoking, because of the relatively young age of the patient. Additional studies should have been undertaken in efforts to rule in or out an infectious process. In this instance, the history of residence in a geographic area where coccidioidomycosis is endemic should have suggested skin testing or serologic tests specially directed at the causative fungal agent.

In Case Presentation 3, bronchogenic carcinoma of the lung was a real concern. The patient was a heavy cigarette smoker and was in an age group that experiences high incidence of this malignancy. Once again, diagnostic procedures that might have provided meaningful clues to the diagnosis before major lung surgery was performed were not done. Intrabronchial brushing is a reasonably reliable method for obtaining lower respiratory tract cells for morphologic studies and secretions for smears and cultures. The same applies to translaryngeal aspiration.

Infections due to fungal agents such as *Histoplasma capsulatum, Coccidioides immitis,* and *Blastomyces dermatitidis* are not commonly seen in large urban hospitals in the northern United States. However, these three cases illustrate the fact that such infections do occur and show that the possibility of a fungal cause should be entertained when considering the differential diagnosis of obscure pulmonary disease.

References

Books

Ajello, L.: Coccidioidomycosis. Tucson, University of Arizona Press, 1967.

Beeson, P. B., and McDermott, W. (eds.): Textbook of Medicine. 14th ed. Philadelphia, W. B. Saunders Co., 1975.

Conant, N. F., Smith, D. T., Baker, R. G., and Calloway, J. L.: Manual of Clinical Mycology. Philadelphia, W. B. Saunders Co., 1971.

Hoeprich, P. D. (ed.): Infectious Diseases. Hagerstown, Maryland, Harper and Row, 1972.

Hunter, G. W., III, Swartzwelder, J. C., and Clyde, D. F.: Tropical Medicine. 5th ed. Philadelphia, W. B. Saunders Co., 1975.

Rippon, J. W.: Medical Mycology. Philadelphia, W. B. Saunders Co., 1974.

Original Articles

Buechner, H. A., Seabury, J. H., Campbell, C. C., Georg, L. K., Kaufman, L., and Kaplan, W.: The current status of serologic, immunologic and skin tests in the diagnosis of pulmonary mycoses. Chest *63:*259, 1973.

Goodwin, R. A., Jr., and DesPrez, R. M.: Pathogenesis and clinical spectrum of histoplasmosis. South. Med. J. *66:*13, 1973.

Kaufman, L., Terry, R. T., Schubert, J. H., and McLaughlin, D.: Effect of a single histoplasmin skin test on the serological diagnosis of histoplasmosis. J. Bacteriol. *94:*798, 1967.

Schwarz, J., and Baum, G. L.: Blastomycosis. Am. J. Clin. Pathol. *21:*999, 1951.

Witorsch, P., and Utz, J. P.: North American blastomycosis: A study of 40 patients. Medicine *47:*169, 1968.

V

GENITOURINARY TRACT INFECTION

Chapter 27

URINARY TRACT INFECTIONS: GENERAL CONSIDERATIONS

Introduction and Terminology

Infection of urinary tract tissues may result in a wide variety of clinical presentations. At one end of the spectrum, infection commonly is completely asymptomatic and recognized only by shedding of bacteria in the urine, i.e., significant bacteriuria, as discussed in Chapter 28. Asymptomatic bacteriuria probably reflects restriction of multiplication of bacteria to the mucosal surface of the bladder or bladder urine. In a sense, this form of infection represents "colonization" of the lower urinary tract analogous to the colonization responsible for the normal microbial flora of other organ systems, e.g., the upper respiratory tract, skin, and lower portions of the gastrointestinal tract.

At the other end of the spectrum, bacteria may penetrate the deeper layers of the bladder and cause low grade fever, frequent and urgent urination, and painful micturation, i.e., dysuria. These are the expected clinical manifestations of cystitis. In a very small proportion of patients, the bacteria in the bladder may gain access to the upper urinary tract, invade the mucosa of the renal pelvis, extend into the interstitial tissue of one or both kidneys, and cause acute pyelonephritis. Patients with acute pyelonephritis are usually very ill, with shaking chills, temperature spikes to 104 or 105°F, paralytic ileus of a degree simulating an acute surgical abdomen, and excruciating pain in one or both flanks. The urine contains innumerable bacteria and leukocytes, i.e., pyuria.

Acute pyelonephritis often follows interference with normal urine flow secondary to mechanical obstruction caused by a renal stone, tumor, or an

409

enlarged prostate gland. Altered urine flow also may result from neurophysiologic dysfunction with impaired ureteral contractions and imperfect bladder emptying, e.g., diabetic neuropathy. If flow of urine through a ureter becomes totally obstructed, a grave emergency can arise, since the obstruction must be relieved within at least 36 hours if function of the affected kidney is to be preserved.

One of the most tragic situations encountered in the treatment of urinary tract infections occurs when the urine of a patient with typical pyelonephritis begins to clear of leukocytes and bacteria soon after antimicrobial therapy is initiated. Because of dramatic clearing of the urine, the patient may be considered to be making a satisfactory response to therapy despite increasing fever, a marked exacerbation of back or flank pain, and more evident spasm of the paraspinal lumbosacral musculature. The unsuspecting physician who assumes that clearing of the urine in this setting is a good omen will not recognize the presence and urgency of total ureteral obstruction. Rapidly developing hydronephrosis and mounting intrarenal pressure can lead to destruction of the affected kidney. Emergency urologic consultation must be requested irrespective of the hour of day or night. Emergency retrograde pyelography is essential as a first step in pinpointing and correcting the site of obstruction. To do otherwise not only results in failure to control the acute pyelonephritis behind the obstruction but also may well result in total loss of functioning renal tissue, and nephrectomy may be required.

The histopathologic changes of acute pyelonephritis are relatively well defined. There is an accumulation of inflammatory cells consisting predominantly of segmented neutrophils that encroach upon and invade the renal tubules, giving rise to "white blood cell casts," and infiltrate the interstitial tissue of the renal medulla with extension into the cortex. The glomeruli usually are not involved and often stand out conspicuously against a background of interstitial fibrosis, tubular dilatation, and degeneration. In most instances, bacteria are demonstrable in the urine or cultures of affected renal tissue.

In chronic pyelonephritis, the identifying histopathologic changes are far less distinct and difficult to define. There is a striking paucity of inflammatory cells. Sparse collections of mononuclear cells are evident around relatively few tubules. Obstructed and dilated tubules are often filled with hyaline material resembling colloid. This can be a prominent finding and is responsible for the term "thyroidization," a condition which was once believed to be pathognomonic for chronic pyelonephritis. Obstruction and loss of collecting ducts and inevitable fibrosis in time result in an irregularly pitted and lobulated kidney of ever decreasing size, the so-called vest pocket kidney, which for decades was considered to be prototypic of endstage chronic renal infection. One of the enigmas of chronic pyelonephritis is the frequent lack of any evidence of infection. The urine may contain neither formed elements nor bacteria and may be considered abnormal only because of persistent trace or 1+ proteinuria. Furthermore, bacteria almost invariably cannot be demonstrated in grossly abnormal areas of affected kidneys. Indeed, the absence of direct evidence supporting a role for bacteria in active chronic pyelonephritis has led several laboratories to search for noninfectious mechanisms that would account for relentless progression of the disease.

Results of these studies are of considerable interest and are briefly summarized in a later section of this chapter.

From a large number of studies involving experimental animals and patients, it is clear that all of the foregoing histopathologic changes, once accepted as characteristic of chronic pyelonephritis, may occur in other diseases of the kidney that do not have an infectious origin. Ischemia secondary to progressive nephrosclerosis, persistent obstruction of the urine outflow tract due to an intrarenal or extrarenal lesion, analgesic nephropathy, and chronic allorenal transplant rejection — all may result in peritubular mononuclear cell infiltration, dilatation of tubules including thyroidization, fibrosis, and microscopic or grossly evident scarring unaccompanied at any time by evidence of bacterial infection. The fact that a multiplicity of pathogenic mechanisms can cause renal injury indistinguishable from that of chronic pyelonephritis explains why the incidence of chronic renal infection, based on autopsy·surveys, has been exaggerated over the years. This new perspective also means that chronic pyelonephritis is probably less important than formerly believed as a determinant of elevated blood pressure and such complications of pregnancy as prematurity and increased morbidity and mortality of newborns.

Efforts to uncover identifying characteristics of chronic pyelonephritis other than histopathologic changes have been made by several research groups with some degree of success. For example, a syndrome of hyperkalemic, hypochloremic acidosis accompanied by a normal blood urea nitrogen level may reflect biochemical changes unique for chronic pyelonephritis. Other studies using indirect immunofluorescence methods to demonstrate the presence of a common bacterial antigen, allegedly shared by all members of the family Enterobacteriaceae, in renal biopsy or autopsy specimens may hold some promise.

Incidence and Prevalence

Several epidemiologic studies using significant bacteriuria, i.e., more than 10^5 bacteria per milliliter of freshly voided or collected urine, as a criterion of urinary tract infection have shown that infection of this organ system often begins early in life and affects a significant number of individuals (see Chap. 28). For example, the incidence of bacteriuria among newborn, pre-school, and school children is approximately 1 to 2 per cent. Noteworthy is the female to male ratio of 30:1, indicative of the predilection of females to urinary tract infection. Available data suggest that approximately 5 per cent of young girls will experience at least one episode of bacteriuria at some point between entering first grade and graduating from high school.

Prevalence of bacteriuria increases progressively among adult females and especially married women, presumably reflecting sexual activity and pregnancy as two important factors predisposing to urinary tract infection. Incidence of infection may reach 10 per cent in elderly women owing in large part to anatomic and physiologic changes in the urinary tract secondary to aging or gynecologic problems. There is also a marked rise in the incidence of urinary tract infection in men 50 or more years in age as a result of the increasing incidence of prostatic obstruction and associated urologic instrumentation and surgery. The incidence of infection is even higher among hospitalized women and men who are suffering from a serious illness.

Several studies have indicated that at least 50 per cent of adult women with significant bacteriuria can be shown to have infection of one or both kidneys and, thus, to be candidates for progressive pyelonephritis and associated complications, i.e., hypertension and secondary cardiovascular complications.

As this section has pointed out, infection of the urinary tract affects a sizable proportion of the population. The challenge it poses is exciting because there is evidence that early detection and eradication of bacteriuria and prevention of recurrence will reduce the incidence of later occurring life-threatening consequences of persistent or repetitive urinary tract infection.

Microbe-Host Relationships

Reservoir of Infection

The overwhelming majority of urinary tract infections are caused by microorganisms constituting the normal intestinal microbial flora. Nearly 90 per cent of all infections occurring in the absence of urinary tract obstruction in nonhospitalized patients are caused by *Escherichia coli.* Other gram negative enteric bacteria as well as gram positive enterococci, e.g., *Streptococcus faecalis,* also have the capacity to invade the urinary tract. There is not much evidence that the numerically superior anaerobic bacteria in the intestinal microbial flora play a significant etiologic role in urinary tract infections. However, it should be added that since attention has been focused so intensely on the aerobic enteric microorganisms, there are relatively few data concerning this point. In addition, virtually nothing is known concerning the potential role of viruses and bacteria acting in concert to cause urinary tract disease in man. Such information as is available from studies of experimental animals indicates that this subject is deserving of more study.

When identification of specific infecting strains of bacteria is possible, e.g., by using a specific antigenic marker such as the O and K antigens of *Escherichia coli,* there is a remarkable degree of concordance of the urinary tract strain isolates with those found simultaneously in the patient's intestinal tract. Such antigenic constituents that permit serotyping of bacteria have proved useful in delineating the epidemiology and pathogenesis of urinary tract infection among ambulatory as well as hospitalized patients.

A wider spectrum of etiologic microorganisms, most commonly including members of the Pseudomonas and Serratia genera, is found among hospitalized patients. This situation in large part is considered to be a reflection of altered host defenses caused by not only the underlying diseases in the hospitalized patients but, more importantly, the impact of specific factors well known to increase susceptibility to urinary tract infections, i.e., indwelling catheter and genitourinary tract surgery.

Epidemiologic studies indicate that surprisingly rapid shifts occur in the intestinal microbial flora following hospitalization. Within one or two days, specific strains of *Escherichia coli* demonstrable in the intestinal flora at the time of admission to the hospital begin to be replaced by increasing numbers of "hospital strains." Presumably the same type of exchange of bacteria occurs for other bacterial species that cannot be followed as precisely because of lack of available serotypes for epidemiologic tracking. Such hospital strains of enteric microorganisms are the products of intensive selection pressures ever present within the environment of the hospital and, consequently, these strains are often more resistant to one or as many as several different antimicrobial agents. The latter point suggests the possibility that episomal transfer of drug resistance occurs among the hospital strains. It also seems likely that such selected strains may well be endowed with virulence factors not represented by the more common enteric strains of bacteria that account for the bulk of urinary tract infections among nonhospitalized patients.

Routes of Infection

Ascending Infection

Prevailing opinion holds that the sequence of events leading to acquisition of urinary tract infection in the majority of individuals is as follows: Enteric bacteria are believed to colonize the perineum, periurethral meatus, and anterior urethra, as well as the vagina and introitus in the female, as a result of imperfect toilet habits, sexual activity, or fecal incontinence. Occurrence of urinary tract infection among newborns and young children who are not toilet trained, as well as elderly individuals with poor sphincter control, is thought to reflect fecal contamination of the perineal and genital areas. Studies in a relatively small number of females revealed that colonization of the vestibule and lower vaginal passages by specific serotypes of *Escherichia coli* occurred prior to development of urinary tract infection by identical serotypes. Such observations suggest that enteric microorganisms may accumulate in significant numbers on the external anatomic surfaces separating the orifices of the intestinal and urinary tracts, respectively. The proximity of these two orifices in the female, together with the extremely short urethral conduit in women, is believed to explain the strikingly greater susceptibility of women to urinary tract infection throughout their entire life span.

How solid is the evidence supporting the sequence of events described above? To be sure, some of the most persuasive evidence comes from thorough studies of sequences and patterns of bacterial colonization in women. However, it is important to note that relatively few female subjects were found in the "infected" and noninfected or "control" group. No comparable studies have been carried out in men. If urinary tract infection merely represents implantation of intestinal bacteria on perineal surfaces and introital tissues in close approximation to the urethral orifice, why does *Escherichia coli* emerge as the most frequent and important pathogen? Numerically speaking, *E. coli* is a "minority" representative of the intestinal microbial flora, being strikingly outnumbered by many other bacterial genera and species (see Chap. 7). Why are there not more urinary tract infections caused by anaerobic bacteria or other bacterial species more numerous in feces than *E. coli*? Is it merely the short length of the urethra that accounts for the increased incidence and prevalence of urinary tract infection among women? Could the fact that urine excreted by clinically well females has a pH and osmolarity that are more favorable for bacterial survival and multiplication compared to those of men be an important host factor? Should not more attention be focused on specific microbial constituents, e.g., capsular K antigens, which may be critical for binding of certain strains of *E. coli* to host cells as a prerequisite for initiating infection? Increasing knowledge of specific microbial and host determinants of colonization and disease undoubtedly will provide greater understanding of pathogenetic mechanisms of urinary tract infection in coming years.

Very little is known about the specific events whereby bacteria migrate upstream through the urethra into the bladder and are able to establish infection of the bladder mucosa. Bladder mucosal cells have a remarkable capacity to ingest foreign particles of various kinds, including bacteria. In this sense they are phagocytic cells. Delayed-type hypersensitivity reactions may occur following injections of specific antigen into the bladder mucosa of an appropriately sensitized host under cystoscopic control. The bladder also is known to synthesize immunoglobulins which presumably are shed by specific secretory pathways into the urine. Thus, in many respects the bladder is an "immunologic organ" with the capacity to generate in situ both humoral and cell-mediated immune responses. For these reasons alone, one might anticipate that those bacteria which successfully implant upon and infect bladder mucosal cells must have specific virulence factors that give them a pathogenic advantage (see below).

Once the bladder mucosa is infected, microorganisms begin to multiply in the bladder urine. Urine can support limited bacterial growth at a pH above approximately 5.5. At such a pH, the stage is set for extension of the infection to the upper urinary tract, viz., the ureters and kidneys.

Large numbers of gram negative bacteria in bladder urine or an equivalent amount of endotoxin have been reported to decrease the competence of the vesicoureteral valves. Malfunction of these valves allows reflux of bacteria-laden bladder urine into the ureters. Once within the ureters, bacteria and endotoxin can compromise normal ureteral peristaltic action. Disrupted peristaltic action may facilitate retrograde movement of microorganisms against the urine flow gradient.

Experimental studies using an artificial urinary tract model system in animals have shown that those microorganisms possessing flagella and exhibiting the property of bacterial motility can move against a moving fluid stream. The assumption is that bacteria gain access to the upper reaches of the urinary tract by active flagellar action. It also is likely that the overwhelming majority of gram negative microorganisms causing upper urinary tract infection, i.e., pyelonephritis, possess flagella and are actively motile bacteria. Mention already has been made of the importance of Group D streptococci, viz., *Streptococcus faecalis*, in urinary tract infections.

However, *S. faecalis* possesses no flagella; it is a nonmotile bacterial species. Yet it is clearly capable of causing pyelonephritis.

Bacteria reaching the renal pelvis presumably infect the pelvic mucosal cells and then invade medullary interstitial tissue via adjacent papillae and the collecting duct system. Recent studies in rats with experimentally induced pyelonephritis, however, indicate that bacteria move from the renal pelvis directly into pyelovenous communications and by this means enter the bloodstream. Once in the bloodstream, the microorganisms recirculate and reenter the kidney to establish infection. Should these findings be confirmed, the classic picture of ascending "retrograde" pyelonephritis may have to be revised, with greater emphasis placed on the hematogenous route as a mechanism for seeding of the kidney by bacteria.

Hematogenous Infection

No one will deny the importance of the hematogenous route in the development of renal infections due to staphylococci, Group A streptococci, and other microorganisms that rarely are implicated in lower urinary tract infection. Seeding of the kidney by such bacteria represents the primary mechanism for development of intrarenal or perirenal abscesses. The mesangium of the glomerulus is endowed with remarkable phagocytic capacity. It readily traps carbon particles and bacteria as well as antigen-antibody immune complexes. Despite the relative frequency of bacteremia and what must be repetitive episodes of bacterial trapping by the glomerular mesangium, bacterial infection of the glomeruli virtually never occurs, and infection of interstitial tissue, i.e., pyelonephritis, due to hematogenous seeding of the kidney is relatively infrequent when considered in the light of how often bacteremia occurs. Clearly, certain species of microorganisms have a far greater capacity to initiate urinary tract infection, irrespective of how they gain access to this organ system. It seems likely that bacteria such as *Escherichia coli* elaborate specific virulence factors which explain their propensity to cause infection.

Bacterial Virulence Factors

Many of the strains of *Escherichia coli* and other microorganisms frequently implicated in urinary tract infection possess pili analogous to those already mentioned for other gram positive and gram negative bacteria. The surface of these pili have important antigenic determinants reactive with specific antibodies. Such antibodies can protect experimental animals against urinary tract infection by the bacteria in question. It is likely that such pili have a role similar to that of the M protein fimbriae on Group A streptococci (see Chap. 13); i.e., they provide a means whereby the bacteria can bind to specific receptor sites on host cells within the urinary tract. If such should prove to be the case, the inordinate frequency of *E. coli* as a cause of urinary tract infections would then have a rational explanation. In this setting, a very important role for secretory IgA could be envisioned, viz., as a factor influencing the extent of *E. coli*–host cell binding.

Strains of *Eschericha coli* elaborate envelope or capsular acidic polysaccharide antigens called K antigens. Specific K antigens are associated with *E. coli* strains implicated in urinary tract infection in general and pyelonephritis in particular. For example, among 30 women experiencing 33 episodes of urinary tract infection caused by *E. coli* serotype O6, 10 of the 33 infections were caused by *E. coli* possessing K-2a and K-2c capsular antigens. No less than 8 of these 10 infections consisted of acute pyelonephritis. The rarity of *E. coli* O6 strains with K-2a and K-2c antigens among the intestinal microbial flora was revealed by studies of fecal specimens provided by these 30 women as well as other subjects. Of 250 fecal samples collected; only 18 strains of *E. coli* O6 could be identified. Of these 18 strains, only one could be shown to have K-2a and K-2c capsular antigens. In several experimental studies of urinary tract infection in mice, it is quite clear that *E. coli* strains elaborating specific K antigens have a striking propensity to cause pyelonephritis in contrast to other strains elaborating either no K antigens or K antigens of other serotypes. These observations collectively suggest that specific K antigens endow strains of *E. coli* with enhanced pathogenetic potential; i.e., either they are themselves virulence factors or they serve as reliable markers for the presence of other determinants intimately associated with virulence of the specific bacterial strains.

Studies from several laboratories indicate that it is not merely the presence of K antigen but the quantity of K antigen synthesized by a given strain of *Escherichia coli* that determines the degree of virulence of that strain. This situation is analogous to that of *Streptococcus pneumoniae* (see Chap. 20). By the use of crossed immunoelectrophoresis assays, quantitation of K antigens has reached a point of high precision. For example, strains of *E. coli* producing pyelonephritis in man have been shown to elaborate from three to five times more K-2a and K-2c antigens than those strains causing only bladder infections, viz., cystitis.

Production of K antigens would appear to account for the relative resistance of such microbial strains to the bactericidal activity of normal serum mediated by immunoglobulins in concert with complement. For reasons unknown, microorganisms producing large amounts of specific K antigens also are less susceptible to killing following ingestion by phagocytic cells. A significant proportion of experimental animals and also patients infected with *E. coli* strains producing certain K antigens appears unable to elaborate specific antibodies against them. The question arises as to whether the K antigens may induce immunologic unresponsiveness or "paralysis" identical to that described decades ago for pneumococcus polysaccharide. Should antibody synthesis and shedding within the urinary tract tissues be important in prevention of colonization by K antigen–elaborating microorganisms, induction of immunologic paralysis by the K antigens could be critical in the acquisition of infection and disease.

Host Factors

Major Defense Mechanisms

Since the turn of the century it has been known that gram negative microorganisms undergo dissolution when coated with specific antibody and exposed to serum complement. This antibody-complement–dependent bacteriolytic effect, observed with most normal sera, is the result of activation of the complement cascade with C8 and C9 producing breaks in the integrity of the bacterial cell wall and membrane, leading to loss of internal contents, swift shifts in oncotic pressure, and bacterial lysis (see Chap. 3). From experimental studies in animals, deposits of bacterial antigen are known to persist in the kidney for long periods of time. Among the infiltrating cells constituting the inflammatory response to infection are fair numbers of plasma cells producing antibody specifically reactive with the bacterial antigen. IgG and IgA are both known to be synthesized by the bladder and kidney tissues and to be shed into the urine. Bacteria infecting the kidney are often coated by IgG as they pass down the ureter and enter the bladder urine. In fact, demonstration of such IgG–coated bacteria in freshly voided urine specimens has been suggested as a means for distinguishing upper urinary tract from lower urinary tract infections. Key questions as yet unanswered include sites and extent of synthesis and shedding of IgM, which is many fold more active in producing bacterial lysis through its greater capacity to bind and activate complement. Can antibody directed against the K antigens be demonstrated? What is the precise role of secretory IgA in host defense against bacterial invasion of urinary tract tissues? Conspicuously lacking in most studies of urinary tract infection is attention to the role of cell-mediated immune host responses. Attention has already been called to the fact that delayed hypersensitivity can be demonstrated in bladder mucosal cells in the same manner one ordinarily performs a skin test. It would seem unlikely that cell-mediated immune responses would not play a role in host defense. It is hoped that studies along such lines will be forthcoming in the near future.

Unique Susceptibility of Renal Medullary Tissues

It is a remarkable fact that *Escherichia coli* and other gram negative enteric microorganisms have an extraordinary propensity for infecting renal peritubular and interstitial tissues whereas they have relatively little capacity to establish serious infections of most other organ systems except under very special clinical conditions. In recent years, a number of factors have been identified which provide tentative explanations for the ease with which such microorganisms can cause disease of the renal medulla. There is a very high solute concentration in the medulla, with values of sodium reaching 425 mM per liter and urea 850 mM per liter. Tubular fluid osmolality ranges from less than 50 to more than 1300 milliosmoles per liter, approximately one sixth to four times the osmolality of plasma. Leukocytes show decreased migration and phagocytic activity in fluids of equivalent hypo- or hypertonicity. The high solute concentrations as well as the hypertonicity of the medullary environment lead to partial inactivation of complement. Furthermore, the production of ammonia is specifically involved in the inactivation of C4, a critical complement component in the classic cascade pathway. These factors may explain why the otherwise potent antibody-complement bacteriolytic system appears relatively ineffective in the milieu of the renal medulla.

Survival of gram negative microorganisms devoid of their rigid cell walls in the form of protoplasts or spheroplasts has been demonstrated to occur in bladder urine with an osmolality of 100 milliosmoles or greater per liter. Presumably such "soft forms" of bacteria would readily survive in the even more hypertonic milieu of the renal medulla. It has been postulated that bacteria injured by antimicrobial agents or the host antibody-complement bacteriolytic system might survive as soft forms, i.e., cell wall–injured or cell wall–deficient bacteria, and account for persistence and remittency of infection. Most studies attempting to demonstrate a capacity of bacterial protoplasts to invade and infect host tissues in animals have been unsuccessful. Furthermore, most protoplasts, even though devoid of most of their cell wall material, still possess critical antigenic constituents, including K antigenic constituents, capable of binding specific antibody. Thus, the host should be able to react with and dispose of bacteria irrespective of whether they are in their classic or soft form stage.

Alternate Mechanisms of Renal Injury

Progression of pyelonephritis in the absence of bacteria in the urine or in biopsy specimens has led to the notion that mechanisms other than infection may be implicated in the production of renal damage. Experimental studies in mice and rats have revealed that microorganisms elaborating large amounts of urease, viz., strains of *Proteus mirabilis* and occasional strains of Klebsiella species, may leave in their wake large deposits of this enzyme following their elimination from host tissues. The deposited enzyme would continue to create a high concentration of ammonia and a very high pH, approaching 8.0 to 8.5 or even greater, in extracellular fluids. Indeed, occurrence of urine with a pH of 6.5 to 7.0 and containing bacteria usually means infection due to *P. mirabilis* or some other urea-splitting microorganism. Such an alkaline extracellular environment is well known to lead to cellular injury. Continued action of bacterial ureases might in this way lead to continued renal injury in the absence of any viable bacteria.

Mention has already been made of deposits of bacterial antigen within the kidney of animals with experimentally induced pyelonephritis. Using indirect immunofluorescence methods, some but not all groups of investigators have also demonstrated variable amounts of antigen, e.g., the so-called common antigen elaborated by most of the members of the family Enterobacteriaceae, in human kidney biopsies or autopsy sections. Among the inflammatory cells in infected renal tissue are immunologically competent cells actively elaborating antibodies specifically reactive with the bacterial antigenic constituents in question. In this manner, the stage could be set for renal cell injury caused by in situ antigen-antibody interactions with or without complement binding and activation contributing to the injurious process.

Certain strains of *Escherichia coli* have been found to elaborate antigenic constituents shared by renal medullary cells of certain experimental animal species. Immune responses of the host to such bacterial antigens might well be expected to result in "autoimmune" renal damage. As yet, specific antibodies directed against kidney cells have not been found in the sera or renal tissue of animals with experimental pyelonephritis.

Very recently, pyelonephritis of rats induced by *Streptococcus faecalis* has been reportedly transferred to normal syngeneic Fisher rats by means of parabiosis. In this work the prospective donors were infected with *S. faecalis* by a method previously established as regularly inducing acute and chronic pyelonephritis in a high proportion of rats. The animals were subsequently treated with an antimicrobial regimen known to eradicate *S. faecalis* from renal tissues. The infected and treated rats were then placed in parabiotic union with normal Fisher recipients. Kidneys of the recipient parabionts were examined histologically at varying times during the 16-week period of parabiosis. Between 40 and 50 per cent of the recipient Fisher rats developed histopathologic changes of pyelonephritis, including interstitial infiltration of mononuclear inflammatory cells, tubular and papillary distortion and degeneration, and fibrosis leading to significant scarring. Since antibodies reactive with normal rat kidney could be demonstrated in the sera of neither the donor rats nor the recipient parabionts, it was assumed that a cell-mediated immune mechanism was responsible for the pyelonephritis that was transferred.

Septic Shock Syndrome and Therapeutic Approaches

One of the most pressing situations in clinical medicine is the patient with the syndrome of septic shock. The cardinal features of this syndrome are relatively easy to recognize and include the following: high fever, altered mentation, pallor, moist skin, fast pulse, and collapsing blood pressure, as well as other physiologic hallmarks of a failing circulation. A small percentage of patients with this syndrome appear mentally alert and exhibit flushed facies and warm dry skin, despite hypotension and other manifestations of circulatory failure. These patients are in special jeopardy because their critical status often is not recognized promptly. Although septic shock may be observed in virtually any type of infection, it is most commonly associated with the presence of gram negative bacteria in the bloodstream. Because bacteremia due to gram negative bacillary microorganisms is such a frequent accompaniment of acute pyelonephritis or a consequence of instrumentation or surgery of the genitourinary tract, it seems appropriate to discuss this syndrome briefly.

Several general statements concerning this syndrome can be made. First, while it is true that septic shock occurs most commonly with endotoxin-producing gram negative microorganisms and the clinical-physiologic features of the syndrome can be induced in animals by injection of endotoxin, one cannot conclude that septic shock is caused solely by endotoxin. The clinical syndrome may be observed in association with bacteremia due to gram positive bacteria that do not elaborate endotoxin. It may also be observed with fulminating disease due to *Streptococcus pneumoniae,* which does not have any known toxin. It also is seen with severe or fulminating infections caused by many different classes of microorganisms, including fungi and viruses. On these grounds one must adopt the view that in addition to endotoxin, other factors can elicit the septic shock syndrome. In all likelihood, the syndrome results from one or more mechanisms operating singly or in concert via a multiplicity of biochemical and physiologic pathways.

Second, despite an enormous amount of investigation, the basic mechanism responsible for septic shock is still unknown. Many important features of the syndrome have been identified, including activation of the clotting cascade, impaired cardiac myofiber contractility, and pooling of blood in the liver. However, none of these physiologic aberrations, either individually or collectively, provides a totally satisfactory explanation for septic shock.

Third, since the basis of septic shock remains undetermined it is not surprising that a great number of therapeutic regimens have been devised which are employed widely in the clinical arena despite lack of evidence of established efficacy. One of the most controversial therapeutic approaches involves corticosteroids. The historic background and rationale leading to the use of one or more of these adrenal hormones or their synthetic derivatives is briefly outlined in Chapter 33, in connection with fulminant meningococcemia, itself a classic manifestation of the septic shock syndrome. Carefully designed double-blind studies pinpointing the clinical efficacy of corticosteroids in the management of life-threatening infections including septic shock were not conducted until long after these hormones had been enthusiastically accepted for therapeutic use.

The results of a multi-hospital study of hydrocortisone (cortisol) as an adjunct to therapy of life-threatening bacterial infections are summarized in Table 27–1. All patients were managed by accepted protocols and received equivalently effective antimicrobial drug therapy. On an alternating basis and

TABLE 27–1. Cortisol and Life-Threatening Bacterial Infections*

Treatment Group	Age of Patients	Mortality Rate	
		Overall	*After first 24 hours**
Cortisol	> 16 years	54/96 (56%)†	32/80 (40%)
	≤ 16 years	5/74 (7%)	
Placebo	> 16 years	32/98 (43%)	33/89 (37%)
	≤ 16 years	4/61 (7%)	

*Adapted from published data of the Cooperative Study Group, Trans. Assoc. Am. Physicians *75:*198, 1962; and J.A.M.A. *183:*462, 1963.

**Data for 25 adult patients dying during first 24 hours following hospitalization has been excluded.

†Numerator = number of patients dying; denominator = number of patients in treatment group.

by code, patients received intravenous hydrocortisone for three days in those doses considered effective for management of septic shock and in wide use at the time the study was conducted. The steroid was started at the time antimicrobial therapy was initiated. Patients in the placebo group received a preparation indistinguishable from hydrocortisone for a similar period of time. As indicated in Table 27–1, no advantage of hydrocortisone supplementation could be discerned as judged by the proportion of patients dying after only 24 hours of therapy or by the overall mortality rate. Hydrocortisone also did not offer any beneficial effect with respect to other parameters of infection that were monitored, e.g., days of fever and days of hospitalization.

A second double-blind study conducted more recently and using betamethasone, a beta form of dexamethasone with biologic activity 25-fold greater than hydrocortisone, is summarized in Table 27–2. Betamethasone or placebo was initiated at the time antimicrobial drug therapy was started. Once again (Table. 27–2) judging by the criteria for successful clinical and bacteriologic responses as defined by the physicians conducting this study, the supplemental steroid appeared to offer no detectable beneficial influence on immediate or eventual outcome. Indeed, if anything the steroid group fared less well.

TABLE 27–2. Betamethasone and Life-Threatening Bacterial Infections*

Results	Treatment Group	
	Betamethasone	Placebo
Number of patients	25	25
Number of therapeutic successes	12	17
Number of therapeutic failures	13	8
Number of patients with vasomotor collapse	4	3

*Adapted from Klastersky, J., and Cappel, R.: Adreno-corticosteroids in the treatment of bacterial sepsis: a double-blind study with pharmacological doses. Antimicrob. Agents Chemother. *10:*175, 1970; and Klastersky, J., et al.: Effectiveness of betamethasone in management of severe infections. N. Engl. J. Med. *284:*1248, 1971.

Fourth, most infectious disease consultants agree that the most effective therapy consists of prompt clearing of the blood of microorganisms and eradication of the underlying infection. To be successful, this approach demands rapid initiation of treatment with effective antimicrobial agents as soon as a provisional diagnosis of bacteremia is made and the early development of septic shock is suspected or recognized as present. Since such decision making will occur at least many hours and more likely several days before initial results of bacteriologic cultures and definitive antimicrobial susceptibility data are in hand, it is customary to employ two or sometimes three different antimicrobial drugs for initial therapy. This is done in order to increase the probability that the causative microorganisms will be moderately or highly susceptible to at least one of the drugs initially selected for use.

The important issue of what specific antimicrobial agents to employ in combination, as dictated by the clinical setting, is discussed in Chapter 46. If at least one drug is used to which in retrospect the etiologic microorganism is shown to be susceptible, there is a statistically significant increased chance that the patient will survive. The initial therapy of septic shock is one of the very few situations in clinical infectious diseases in which combination antimicrobial therapy is warranted until such time as bacteriologic data permit revision of the program and reliance being placed on only one antimicrobial agent.

Fifth, there are already exciting hints that an immunologic approach to the problem of gram negative bacteremia—septic shock may have therapeutic merit for patients known to be at special risk. Two different but related studies, both concerning infection with *Pseudomonas aeruginosa*, will serve as examples.

Pseudomonas aeruginosa isolates can be serotyped using antibody reactive with their antigenically specific somatic cell wall polysaccharide. Hospital epidemiologic studies have revealed that seven distinct serotypes account for approximately 95 per cent of bacteremic episodes of *P. aeruginosa* infection in patients with malignant diseases and impaired immunologic defenses caused at least in part by their medical treatment. Since an important host defense in resistance to infections due to *P. aeruginosa* and other gram negative microorganisms resides in a suitable level of antipolysaccharide opsonizing antibody that augments phagocytosis of these bacteria, patients were actively immunized with a pseudomonas vaccine representing all seven serotypes. The vaccine was administered well before or at least concomitantly with institution of medical therapy (cytolytic drugs, corticosteroids) which would predictably compromise host defenses. A statistically significant reduction in the incidence of *P. aeruginosa* infections and associated mortality was observed among the vaccinated as opposed to the nonvaccinated patient groups.

The second approach concerning treatment of infections with *Pseudomonas aeruginosa* has so far been limited to experimental animals, but the results are so striking that trials in patient can be anticipated in the very near future. A mutant of *Escherichia coli* serotype O111, termed J5, lacks the capacity to link O-somatic polysaccharide side chains to the cell wall lipopolysaccharide core because of a deficiency in UDP-galactose epimerase. The J5 mutant contains the core but no O side chains. Injection of inactivated J5 microorganisms into animals or human volunteers has induced antibody reactive with the lipopolysaccharide core. High titer antibody to the core appears to result because of the absence of competing antigenic O-polysaccharide side chains. The antibodies induced by J5 not only "neutralize" the endotoxic activity of J5 lipopolysaccharide core but also are able to "neutralize" the activity of cores of other gram negative bacteria, including *P. aeruginosa*. Injection of J5 antiserum has proved efficacious in reducing or abrogating mortality among rabbits rendered neutropenic by nitrogen mustard and given a lethal challenge of *P. aeruginosa* microorganisms.

These findings reveal a heretofore unsuspected degree of antigenic similarity among the lipopolysaccharide cores of gram negative bacteria of widely diverse origins. The experimental work in rabbits suggests that prospective active immunization with J5 vaccine may be useful in protecting selected patients against development of gram negative bacteremia. Conceivably, administration of J5 antiserum to patients already exhibiting evidence of gram negative bacteremia might diminish the morbidity and mortality associated with the septic shock syndrome.

References

Book

Kunin, C. M.: Detection, Prevention and Management of Urinary Tract Infections. Philadelphia, Lea and Febiger, 1972.

Review Articles

Beeson, P. B.: Urinary tract infection and pyelonephritis. *In* Black, D. A. K. (ed.): Renal Disease. 2nd ed. Oxford, Blackwell Scientific Publications Ltd., 1967.

Hepinstall, R. H.: The limitations of the pathological diagnosis of chronic pyelonephritis. *In* Black, D. A. K. (ed.): Renal Disease. 2nd ed. Oxford, Blackwell Scientific Publications Ltd., 1967.

Original Articles

Andriole, V. T.: Acceleration of the inflammatory response of the renal medulla by water diuresis. J. Clin. Invest. *45:*847, 1966.

Andriole, V. T.: Water, acidosis, and experimental pyelonephritis. J. Clin. Invest. *49:*21, 1970.

Angell, M. E., Relman, A. S., and Robbins, S. L.: "Active" chronic pyelonephritis without evidence of bacterial infection. N. Engl. J. Med. *278:*1303, 1968.

Aoki, S., Imamura, S., Aoki, M., and McCabe, W. R.: "Abacterial" and bacterial pyelonephritis. Immunofluorescent localization of bacterial antigen. N. Engl. J. Med. *281:*1375, 1969.

Asscher, A. W., Sussman, M., Waters, W. E., Davis, R. H., and Chick, S.: Urine as a medium for bacterial growth. Lancet *2:*1037, 1966.

Asscher, A. W.: Urinary-tract infection. Lancet *2:*1365, 1974.

Beeson, P. B., and Rowley, D.: The anticomplementary effect of kidney tissue. Its association with ammonia production. J. Exp. Med. *110:*685, 1959.

Bennett, I. L., Jr. Finland, M., Hamburger, M., Kass, E. H., Lepper, M., and Waisbren, B. A.: A double-blind study of the effectiveness of cortisol in the management of severe infections. Trans. Assoc. Am. Physicians *75:*198, 1962.

Bennett, I. L., Jr., Finland, M., Hamburger, M., Kass, E. H., Lepper, M., and Waisbren, B. A.: The effectiveness of hydrocortisone in the management of severe infections. A double-blind study. J.A.M.A. *183:*462, 1963.

Braude, A. I.: Current concepts of pyelonephritis. Medicine *52:*257, 1973.

Bryant, R. E., Sutcliffe, M. C., and McGee, Z. A.: Human polymorphonuclear leukocyte function in urine. Yale J. Biol. Med. *46:*113, 1973.

Carroll, H. J., and Farber, S. J.: Hyperkalemia and hyperchloremic acidosis in chronic pyelonephritis. Metabolism *13:*808, 1964.

Chernew, I., and Braude, A. I.: Depression of phagocytosis by solutes in concentrations found in the kidney and urine. J. Clin. Invest. *41:*1945, 1962.

Fierer, J., Talner, L., and Braude, A. I.: Bacteremia in the pathogenesis of retrograde *E. coli* pyelonephritis in the rat. Am. J. Pathol. *64:*443, 1971.

Freedman, L. R.: Experimental pyelonephritis. XII. Changes mimicking chronic pyelonephritis as a consequence of renal vascular occlusion in the rat. Yale J. Biol. Med. *39:*113, 1966.

Ginder, D. R.: Urinary tract infection and pyelonephritis due to Escherichia coli in dogs infected with canine adenovirus. J. Infect. Dis. *129:*715, 1974.

Glassock, R. J., Kalmanson, G. M., and Guze, L. B.: Pyelonephritis. XVIII. Effect of treatment on the pathology of enterococcal pyelonephritis in the rat. Am. J. Pathol. *76:*49, 1974.

Glynn, A. A., and Nicholson, A. M.: Urinary-tract infection: localization and virulence of Escherichia coli. Lancet *1:*270, 1975.

Gutmen, L. T., Turck, M., Petersdorf, R. G., and Wedgwood, R. J.: Significance of bacterial variants in urine of patients with chronic bacteriuria. J. Clin. Invest. *44:*1945, 1965.

Hand, W. L., Smith, J. W., Miller, T. E., Barnett, J. A., and Sanford, J. P.: Immunoglobulin synthesis in lower urinary tract infection. J. Lab. Clin. Med. *75:*19, 1970.

Hanson, L. A.: Host-parasite relationships in urinary tract infections. J. Infect. Dis. *127:*726, 1973.

Jones, S. R., Smith, J. W., and Sanford, J. P.: Localization of urinary-tract infections by detection of antibody-coated bacteria in urine sediment. N. Engl. J. Med. *290:*591, 1974.

Kaijser, B.: Immunology of Escherichia coli: K antigen and its relation to urinary-tract infection. J. Infect. Dis. *127:*670, 1973.

Kalmanson, G. M., and Guze, L. B.: Role of protoplasts in pathogenesis of pyelonephritis. J.A.M.A. *190:*1107, 1964.

Kalmanson, G. M., Glassock, R. J., Montgomerie, J. Z., and Guze, L. B.: Pyelonephritis transferred by parabiosis. Proc. Soc. Exp. Biol. Med. *146:*1097, 1974.

Klastersky, J., and Cappel, R.: Adreno-corticosteroids in the treatment of bacterial sepsis: a double-blind study with pharmacological doses. Antimicrob. Agents Chemother. *10:*175, 1971.

Klastersky, J., Cappel, R., and Debusscher, L.: Effectiveness of betamethasone in management of severe infections. N. Engl. J. Med. *284:*1248, 1971.

Lehmann, J. D., Smith, J. W., Miller, T. E., Barnett, J. A., and Sanford, J. P.: Local immune response in experimental pyelonephritis. J. Clin. Invest. *47:*2541, 1968.

Levison, S. P., and Kaye, D.: Influence of water diuresis on antimicrobial treatment of enterococcal pyelonephritis. J. Clin. Invest. *51:*2408, 1972.

McCabe, W. R., Carling, P. C., Bruins, S., and Greely, A.: The relation of K-antigen to virulence of Escherichia coli. J. Infect. Dis. *131:*6, 1975.

Numazaki, Y., Kumasaka, T., Yano, N., Yamanaka, M., Miyazawa, T., Takai, S., and Ishida, N.: Further study on acute hemorrhagic cystitis due to adenovirus type 11. N. Engl. J. Med. *289:*344, 1973.

Parker, J., and Kunin, C.: Pyelonephritis in young women. A 10- to 20-year follow-up. J.A.M.A. *224:*585, 1973.

Schwartz, M. M., and Cotran, R. S.: Common enterobacterial antigen in human chronic pyelonephritis and interstitial nephritis. An immunofluorescent study. N. Engl. J. Med. *289:*830, 1973.

Thomsen, O. F., and Hjort, T.: Immunofluorescent demonstration of bacterial antigen in experimental pyelonephritis with antiserum against common enterobacterial antigen. Acta Pathol. Microbiol. Scand. *81:*474, 1973.

Virus infection of the kidney and urinary tract. (Editorial); Lancet *1:*19, 1974.

Young, L. S., Meyer, R. D., and Armstrong, D.: Pseudomonas aeruginosa vaccine in cancer patients. Ann. Intern. Med. *79:*518, 1973.

Ziegler, E. J., Douglas, H., and Braude, A. I.: Prevention of lethal Pseudomonas bacteremia with epimerase-deficient E. coli antiserum. Clin. Res. *23:*445A, 1975.

CYSTITIS AND PYELONEPHRITIS

Introduction

Infection of the urinary tract is a common problem affecting men and women of all ages. Numerically, women are affected more frequently, especially during adolescence and childbearing years. Although urinary tract infection has been the subject of several studies over the past two decades, many important questions concerning this condition, including what relationship exists between asymptomatic bacteriuria and chronic pyelonephritis, and what role infection of the urinary tract plays in the development of hypertension and chronic renal failure, remain unanswered.

Infection of the urinary tract is produced primarily by enteric gram negative bacilli. Of these, *Escherichia coli* is the most frequently isolated causative agent. There are many antimicrobial agents which are effective in the treatment of bacillary infections of the urinary tract. After completion of therapy, most patients are asymptomatic, and cultures of their urine are sterile. Unfortunately, relapse of the original infection or acquisition of a new infection is all too common.

The patient who has repeated episodes of symptomatic urinary tract infection over a short period of time poses a most difficult problem in regard to medical management. Much of the problem is due to the fact that both the patient and physician tend to view each episode as an isolated event. It is hoped that with a better understanding of the pathogenesis and natural history of urinary tract infection, greater success can be attained and some of the frustration reduced in treatment of this problem. It is the purpose of this chapter to discuss current concepts of the pathogenesis, diagnosis, and management of urinary tract infection.

Pathogenesis of Urinary Tract Infection

In most patients who develop a urinary tract infection, no host abnormality, neither anatomic nor biochemical, is found. This section discusses the pathogenesis of urinary tract infection in such individuals. The subsequent section deals with some of the anatomic and biochemical abnormalities which predispose certain patients to an increased incidence of urinary tract infection.

Infection of the urinary tract occurs most commonly as an ascending infection. Bacteria first gain entrance through the urethra and then progress upward to invade the bladder and kidneys. Urinary tract infection is much more common in women than men. This predominance in women is probably due to the anatomic differences between the two sexes. In women, the urethra is shorter and wider than in the male. In some women, the meatus of the urethra may have widespread lips, further exposing the periurethral area to potential colonization by bacteria originating in the vagina and rectum. Women frequently experience renewed episodes of symptomatic urinary tract infection following sexual intercourse, suggesting that trauma to the female urethra may also play a role in the pathogenesis of this illness. Males may be protected in part from ascending infection by the presence of a low molecular weight substance in prostatic fluid which is bactericidal to many gram negative and gram positive microorganisms. This substance has not as yet been identified but does not appear to be lysozyme or spermine.

The bacteria that produce urinary tract infection are part of the host's endogenous flora. The reservoir of these bacteria is the fecal flora. Several detailed studies have shown that a microorganism isolated from the urine can also almost invariably be found in the stool. When *Escherichia coli*, the most frequent causative agent of infection, is isolated from the urine, it is usually found that the same serotype of *E. coli* is also the preponderant strain of *E. coli* in the fecal flora.

Since all individuals harbor *E. coli* and other potentially pathogenic enteric microorganisms in the stool, the question arises as to how these microorganisms gain entrance into the bladder. Some explanations have already been mentioned, i.e., the shorter female urethra and sexual intercourse. However, there are other, and perhaps more important, factors in the pathogenesis of urinary tract infection in women. In many women who develop infection, colonization of the periurethral area and vaginal introitus by enteric microorganisms occurs prior to the onset of infection. In 1973, Stamey followed 16 patients in a prospective manner through 37 episodes of bacteriuria. In 25 of these 37 episodes of infection, the microorganisms responsible for the infection were cultured from the vaginal introitus prior to their isolation in significant numbers from the urine. In the remaining 12 episodes of bacteriuria, the vaginal introitus had not been cultured 5 to 180 days prior to the onset of the infection. In some patients, the time between the demonstration of an abnormal vaginal introital flora and the onset of bacteriuria was only a few days. As a control group, 30 women who had no history of urinary tract infection also were studied. Of these, 27 women had no gram negative bacilli isolated from their vaginal introitus; in the three who did, the gram negative microorganisms were present in very low numbers. The results of Stamey's investigation were similar to those found in 1969 by Gruneberg, who was able to isolate the microorganism responsible for bacteriuria from the periurethral flora in 93 per cent and from the vaginal introitus in 90 per cent of the cases studied. From these observations it would appear that bacteria present in the fecal flora of women must first colonize the vaginal introitus and periurethral area prior to the development of ascending urinary tract infection. Women who are free of such colonization rarely develop infection. Changes, i.e., loss and acquisition, in the periurethral and vaginal introital flora occur spontaneously. The local conditions which favor or inhibit the bacterial colonization of the periurethral area and vaginal introitus are not known at this time.

In addition to the mechanisms mentioned thus far, bacteria, as well as fungi and mycobacteria, may invade the kidneys, bladder, or prostate gland by hematogenous spread from a distant focus of infection. In fact, fungal and mycobacterial infections of the urinary tract usually occur by this mechanism; however, bacteria rarely invade the kidney, bladder, or prostate by hematogenous spread. When they do, invasion is usually secondary to extensive systemic infection in which many other organ sites are involved. A classic example of renal infection via bacteremic spread is that which occurs during staphylococcal bacteremia.

Factors Predisposing to Infection

There is no doubt that certain anatomic abnormalities, systemic diseases, and manipulative procedures carry an increased risk of urinary tract infection. A common abnormality is obstruction of urine flow. Once infection is established in the presence of an obstructing lesion, eradication is extremely difficult.

In infants and children, urinary tract infection is frequently associated with anatomic abnormalities. The incidence of abnormalities is the same for both males and females, and appropriate diagnostic studies should be performed if infection occurs in this age group (discussed later in this chapter). The anatomic abnormalities most often encountered include stenosis of the external urethral meatus (usually in males), the presence of urethral valves, periureteral diverticula, and abnormalities of the collecting system.

In adults, congenital defects are less frequently found, and obstructive lesions, when present, are usually acquired. As a general rule, males should be investigated for an anatomic abnormality after their first episode of urinary tract infection. Investigation in the female is usually undertaken after the second or third infection. Some of the more common factors associated with an increase in urinary tract infection are discussed below.

Pregnancy

Pregnancy appears to be associated with an increased incidence of bacteriuria. Five to 7 per cent of pregnant women are found to have asymptomatic bacteriuria when routine screening is performed in the prenatal clinic. If untreated, 20 to 40 per cent of these women will develop acute symptomatic urinary tract infection at some time prior to delivery. It is possible that the increased incidence of asymptomatic bacteriuria is related in part to ureteral dilatation which occurs during pregnancy. Ureteral dilatation may be secondary to hormonal factors or to mechanical pressure of a gravid uterus.

Tumor

Benign and malignant tumors may produce partial or complete obstruction of urine flow. Obstruction may follow compression of the urinary tract by an expanding tumor mass or by direct invasion of the bladder, ureter, or kidneys. In males more than 60 years of age, benign prostatic hypertrophy and carcinoma of the prostate often produce obstruction at the level of the bladder neck. Benign prostatic hypertrophy is the most common lesion predisposing to urinary tract infection in the male.

Calculi

Renal calculi may also be responsible for obstruction of urine flow. Most renal calculi are formed by excessive production and excretion of calcium. Calcium stones are most frequently seen in patients with hyperparathyroidism, hyperthyroidism, metastatic carcinoma, vitamin D intoxication, and renal tubular acidosis, and in those who have experienced prolonged bed rest. Stones may also be formed by other crystalloids, e.g., oxalate. Metabolic products such as uric acid, cystine, and xanthine may be responsible for stone formation in patients with gout, cystinuria, and xanthinuria. Chronic infection of the urinary tract with Proteus microorganisms may lead to the formation of calcium stones in otherwise normal individuals. All Proteus species manufacture a potent urease which is capable of producing ammonia from urea. The resulting alkalization of the urine decreases the solubility of calcium and increases the possibility of precipitation and stone formation.

Neurologic Disorders

Neurologic dysfunction predisposes to urinary tract infection because of the inability to initiate or control bladder emptying. This inability is most frequently seen in patients with spinal cord transection, spinal cord tumors, spina bifida, and diabetic neuropathy. Indwelling bladder catheters are often used in the treatment of these conditions and contribute to the increased incidence of urinary tract infection in these patients.

Diabetes Mellitus

In the past, diabetes has been associated with an increased incidence of urinary tract infection. More recent studies have shown that in well-controlled, nonhospitalized diabetic patients the incidence of bacteriuria is no greater than in age- and sex-matched controls. Diabetic patients who do require hospitalization have an increased incidence of urinary tract infection, but this may be due to many factors, including repeated catheterization to obtain urine specimens. Diabetics who develop pyelonephritis occasionally have more extensive and severe urinary tract infection than is usually seen in the general patient population. Rarely, pyelonephritis in diabetic patients progresses to acute papillary necrosis or perinephric abscess (discussed later in this chapter).

Mechanical Factors

The most common factor predisposing to the development of a urinary tract infection in the hospital is catheterization or instrumentation of the bladder. Surveillance studies over the past four years have revealed that 80 per cent of hospital-acquired urinary tract infections occurred in patients who had been catheterized or instrumented at some time during their hospital stay. In one large study by Kunin and McCormack, 21 per cent of the patients who had an indwelling Foley catheter in place for seven days developed significant bacteriuria. If the catheter was left in place for 14 days, the number of patients who became infected increased to 56 per cent.

Miscellaneous Factors

When obtaining a history from a patient with a urinary tract infection, inquiry should be made about personal hygiene habits, especially the method of toilet wiping and the use of irritant soaps, bubble baths, vaginal douches, or spermicidal agents. Contact inflammation produced by any of these agents may predispose the introital and periurethral areas to colonization and subsequent infection by enteric bacilli.

Diagnosis of Urinary Tract Infection

Urinary tract infection may be defined as the multiplication of bacteria at any site in the urinary tract proximal to the urethra. Since most patients are completely asymptomatic, the diagnosis rests on the demonstration of bacteria in the urine.

The most common method of obtaining urine for culture is the clean-catch midstream technique. After properly washing the labia and periurethral area in women or the glans penis in men, the first portion of the urinary stream is discarded and the middle portion "caught" in a sterile culture bottle. This midstream sample is then submitted for urinalysis and quantitative bacterial culture. Kass and others have found that when the urine from patients with urinary tract infection is cultured, the number of bacteria present is equal to or exceeds 100,000 per milliliter. Even when proper technique is carried out, residual microorganisms present in the periurethral area and meatal orifice in females may contaminate the specimen. Contamination of the collected specimen usually produces colony counts of no greater than 10,000 microorganisms per milliliter. A small percentage of patients, probably less than 5 per cent, may be infected and yet have a urine colony count between 10,000 and 100,000 microorganisms. If infection is suspected but the colony count is low, a repeat urine culture is often helpful.

Occasionally, colony counts below the dividing line of 100,000 microorganisms per milliliter may occur when the rate of urine flow is very high. This is seen most frequently in patients undergoing water- or drug-induced diuresis. The presence of antimicrobial agents in the urine or infection by fastidious microorganisms also may lower the colony count. Rarely, in patients with unilateral renal infection, complete obstruction of the ureter on the same side will prevent bacteria and polymorphonuclear leukocytes from entering the bladder. This situation requires immediate emergency treatment if renal function is to be preserved and the site and nature of the obstructing lesion identified. The type and location of the lesion can best be recognized by intravenous pyelography, which will demonstrate the failure of the intravenously injected dye to traverse the ureter from kidney to bladder on the affected side.

It should be pointed out that acceptance of 100,000 microorganisms or more per millilter of urine as a basis for determining the presence of urinary tract infection holds true only for infection produced by enteric, gram negative bacilli. Studies on the significant number of gram positive cocci, anaerobic bacteria, and fungi present in the urine when infection is produced by these microorganisms have not been carried out.

For obvious reasons, the clean-catch, midstream collection technique is most reliable in cooperative, well-coordinated, nondebilitated patients. Elderly and hospitalized patients often require assistance and clear instruction in order to obtain a meaningful urine culture. Because of the importance of procuring an uncontaminated urine specimen, it is the physician's responsibility to instruct the patient and oversee the collection procedure (see Chap. 10).

Urine is a good growth medium for most bacteria. If a urine specimen is collected and allowed to stand at room temperature, bacterial multiplication will occur, creating falsely elevated colony counts (see Chap. 10). Urine obtained for culture should be plated out on appropriate culture media within one hour of collection. If for any reason this cannot be done, urine may be stored in a refrigerator at 4°C for 12 to 24 hours without a significant change in the colony count.

The vast majority of urinary tract infections are produced by a single microbial species. Rarely, two types of bacteria may be responsible for producing infection. Infection with more than one microorganism should be documented by a repeat urine culture that demonstrates the presence of both microorganisms in concentrations greater than 10^5 per milliliter. When a urine culture is reported to be growing three or more types of bacteria, even if all three are present in significant numbers, this invariably represents improper collection or handling of the specimen. If this is the case, the correct course of action is to repeat the urine culture and not direct antimicrobial therapy against all three microorganisms.

In the event that a patient is too ill to cooperate or has a neurologic disorder which prohibits voiding spontaneoulsy, urine may be obtained for culture by direct catheterization of the bladder. Direct catheterization of the bladder should not be performed routinely on all patients, for this procedure is not without risk. The most frequent complication is the introduction of bacteria into the bladder. Occasionally, minor trauma to the urethra produced by catheterization may be followed by bacteremia and septic shock.

Lastly, bladder urine may be obtained for culture by direct suprapubic percutaneous needle aspiration. In this procedure, the patient is asked to drink a glass of water and refrain from voiding for two hours. After the distended bladder has been palpated, a narrow gauge needle attached to a syringe is inserted through the abdominal wall in the midline 2 cm above the pubic symphysis. This procedure virtually eliminates the problem of urethral contamination, and colony counts below 100,000 microorganisms are frequently significant. The reduction in colony count is due in part to the water diuresis. It is our feeling that this method of obtaining urine for culture is rarely indicated in the adult and should be performed only by a physician well versed in this technique.

An incubation period of 16 to 24 hours is necessary to detect and quantitate bacterial growth. A more rapid method of detecting the presence of significant bacteriuria is a careful microscopic examination of the urine. One or two drops of uncentrifuged, freshly voided urine are placed on a glass slide, dried, and Gram stained. If two or more bacteria are consistently seen in each high power microscopic field, there is an 80 per cent chance that the urine culture will demonstrate the growth of 100,000 microorganisms or more per ml. Only 20 per cent of patients with colony counts between 10,000 and 100,000 will have detectable bacteria on direct microscopic examination. The slide should also be scanned for the presence of segmented neutrophils. Although the presence of neutrophils is a less consistent finding than the presence of bacteria, most patients with acute, symptomatic urinary tract infection will have 5 to 10 segmented neutrophils per high power field. Of patients who have asymptomatic bacteriuria, only 30 to 50 per cent will have this number of leukocytes detectable in the uncentrifuged urine.

In summary, the diagnosis of urinary tract infection is confirmed by demonstrating the growth of greater than 100,000 microorganisms per milliliter of urine. Most problems arise in obtaining a properly collected voided urine and transporting the specimen to the laboratory within one hour for culture. Under certain circumstances, less than 100,000 microorganisms may represent true infection. A carefully performed urinalysis, with the finding of two or more bacteria per high power microscopic field in uncentrifuged urine, is quite helpful in establishing a rapid, presumptive diagnosis of infection of the urinary tract (see Chap. 10).

Symptomatic Urinary Tract Infection

Symptoms of urinary tract infection are often acute in onset and distressing enough for most patients to seek medical attention. Case Presentation 1 (at the end of this chapter) is typical of many of the patients seen with this condition.

Symptoms and Signs of Urinary Tract Infection

Most symptoms of urinary tract infection are a result of inflammation of the bladder wall and posterior urethra. Characteristically, the patient experiences dysuria, urgency, or a burning sensation on voiding. Inflammation of the bladder wall also results in edema and a loss of elasticity. The resulting diminished bladder capacity and a painful sensation on moderate distention are responsible for the symptom of frequency. Some patients feel a need to void as frequently as every hour. Nocturia is present if distention of the bladder is painful enough to wake the patient from sleep.

As in other infectious illnesses, fever and rigors may also be present. Spiking temperature and rigors may coincide with bacteremia. For this reason, several blood cultures should be obtained. Patients with urinary tract infection may also experience flank pain, and tenderness may be elicited on palpation of the costovertebral angle during physical examination. It used to be widely accepted by physicians that the presence of fever (101°F or greater) and costovertebral angle tenderness indicated infection involving the kidneys, and a diagnosis of pyelonephritis was made. Patients with symptoms of bladder inflammation who were afebrile and had no costovertebral angle tenderness on physical examination were thought to have cystitis. Although this division on clinical grounds between upper (pyelonephritis) and lower (cystitis) urinary tract infection is usually valid, recent studies have shown that this is not always the case. Patients with lower urinary tract infection, without renal involvement, may also present with fever and costovertebral angle tenderness.

Localization of Site of Infection

As has been mentioned previously, localization of the site of infection to the kidney or bladder on clinical grounds is not always accurate, and patients with asymptomatic bacteriuria may have renal involvement, also. To determine the site of infection more accurately, various techniques and laboratory studies have been devised. These are discussed briefly below.

Ureteral Catheterization

In this procedure, the ureters under direct cystoscopic visualization are selectively catheterized with small polyethylene catheters. Urine is then collected from both kidneys for culture and urinalysis. A decision as to whether the renal infection is unilateral or bilateral can be made by this technique. Just as do all procedures requiring instrumentation, it carries with it definite risk to the patient. The most serious complications of this procedure are introduction of bacteria into the kidney, bacteremia, and septic shock. For these reasons, this procedure is infrequently used.

Bladder Washout

In this procedure a multilumen catheter is introduced into the bladder, and a baseline urine culture obtained. The bladder is then filled for 30 to 45 minutes with a saline solution containing an aminoglycoside antibiotic and a mucolytic agent. This solution is then washed out with saline, and serial urine cultures are obtained at 10-minute intervals. In most cases of infection confined to the bladder, the post-washout cultures are sterile. If bacteria are detected, and especially if their number increases in the serial post-washout cultures, they are most likely emanating from the kidneys. This technique requires time and also suffers from the complications of all catheterization procedures.

Determination of Serum Antibody to Infecting Microorganism

Patients with pyelonephritis may develop rising antibody titers or have high circulating antibody to their infecting microorganism. Cystitis is thought to be a more superficial surface infection and therefore does not lead to antibody formation. Unfortunately, not all patients with pyelonephritis will develop a rising antibody titer, and normal patients may have persistently elevated antibody titers from prior infection. For this reason, measurement of circulating antibody has not gained favor as a useful diagnostic procedure.

Detection of Antibody-Coated Bacteria in Urine

As an outgrowth of looking for serum antibody, various investigators have turned their attention to the detection of antibody-coated bacteria present in the urine sediment. The sediment, after being washed several times, is smeared out on a glass slide. Antihuman globulin conjugated with fluorescein is then added, and the presence of fluorescence is detected by viewing the bacteria with a microscope illuminated by ultraviolet light. The detection of bacteria coated with antibody has correlated well with the presence of renal bacteriuria as determined by the bladder washout and ureteral catheterization techniques. One explanation for the higher incidence of bacteria coated with antibody in the urine as opposed to circulating antibody is that antibody may be produced locally in the kidney and not gain access to the general circulation. Detection of antibody-coated bacteria requires time and careful attention to technique. The major advantage of this procedure is that it is noninvasive, and preliminary reports indicate that it shows promise in differentiating renal from bladder bacteriuria.

Determination of Maximum Concentrating Ability

Patients with pyelonephritis frequently are unable to concentrate their urine to the same extent as normal controls or patients with cystitis after an overnight fast or following infusion of antidiuretic hormone. There is a significant overlap between patients with pyelonephritis and those with cystitis, and separation is even more difficult when only one kidney is involved. In addition, many noninfectious renal diseases also reduce concentrating ability.

Intravenous Pyelography

There are no characteristic changes in the intravenous pyelogram in acute pyelonephritis. The intravenous pyelogram is useful only in detecting anatomic defects, obstructing lesions, and changes which may occur in chronic pyelonephritis, such as a loss of renal parenchyma or dilated calices. However, even these latter changes are not pathognomonic for pyelonephritis and may be seen in several pathologic conditions affecting the kidney.

Bacteria Isolated from Patients with Urinary Tract Infection

Escherichia coli, followed by *Klebsiella pneumoniae* and *Proteus mirabilis,* is the microorganism most frequently isolated from patients who acquire their infection in the community (nonhospital associated infection). Since other microorganisms may at times be responsible for producing community-acquired urinary tract infection, it is important that the physician obtain a urine culture for bacterial identification and susceptibility testing. Patients who develop their urinary tract infection while in the hospital frequently have serious underlying disease, may be receiving or have previously been treated with antimicrobial agents, or have indwelling bladder catheters. All of these factors make prediction of the nature of the causative microorganism and selection of appropriate antimicrobial therapy difficult. Therefore, a culture is mandatory. Table 28–1 lists bacteria which were isolated from patients with urinary tract infection in the Northwestern Memorial Hospital in 1974. A group of patients with spinal cord injuries, all of whom had indwelling bladder catheters and had received antimicrobial agents on multiple occasions, is included for the purpose of illustrating how these factors can markedly affect the nature of the bacteria responsible for producing infection.

TABLE 28–1. Bacterial Isolates from Hospital-Acquired and Community-Acquired Urinary Tract Infections*

Community-Acquired (438 Patients)		Hospital-Acquired** (388 Patients)		Spinal Cord Injury (102 Patients)	
Organisms	Per Cent	Organisms	Per Cent†	Organisms	Per Cent
Escherichia coli	57	Escherichia coli	39	Proteus rettgeri	30
Klebsiella pneumoniae	13	Proteus mirabilis	18	Pseudomonas aeruginosa	23
Proteus mirabilis	8	Pseudomonas aeruginosa	17	Proteus mirabilis	13
Enterococcus	8	Enterococcus	11	Escherichia coli	8
Pseudomonas aeruginosa	7	Klebsiella pneumoniae	10	Proteus vulgaris	6
Proteus rettgeri	5	Serratia marcescens	8	Klebsiella pneumoniae	6
Others	2				14

*December, 1973 to November, 1974, Northwestern Memorial Hospital.
**Exclusive of patients with spinal cord injury.
†More than one bacterium isolated from a few patients.

Diagnostic Work-Up

After the first infection in males and after the second or third infection in females, a complete diagnostic study is indicated. A thorough history should be obtained, and a careful physical examination given to all patients. Emphasis is placed on any personal habits or medical illness which may predispose the patient to urinary tract infection. Renal function tests should be performed on all patients suspected of having pyelonephritis or prolonged asymptomatic bacteriuria. These should include determination of the blood urea nitrogen and serum creatinine, 24 hour creatinine clearance, and careful examination of the urine sediment.

The most useful study for detecting congenital or acquired lesions that produce obstruction to urine flow is the intravenous pyelogram. Bailey found a major lesion in 9 per cent and a minor lesion in 11 per cent of 204 women studied by intravenous pyelography. In children, voiding cystourethrography with cinephotography is also a useful procedure for identifying those patients who have vesicoureteral reflux, periureteral diverticula, and urethral valves. In a study by Kunin, vesicoureteral reflux was demonstrated by this procedure in 19 per cent of 137 bacteriuric school girls. In some children with vesicoureteral reflux, dye can be followed from the bladder to the renal pelvis. All of the radiographic studies mentioned here are performed in the hope of finding a surgically correctable lesion. In the past, vesicoureteral reflux was treated by surgical reimplantation of the ureters. More recent evidence indicates that the reflux may be secondary to the urinary tract infection. When therapy is directed at eradication of the infection, reflux disappears in the majority of patients.

Asymptomatic Bacteriuria

Most patients with asymptomatic bacteriuria can recall on careful questioning having had urinary tract symptoms at some time in the past. Some of these patients, especially young school girls and young adults, will go on to develop acute symptomatic infection. Mention has been made previously of the high percentage of pregnant women with asymptomatic bacteriuria who will develop acute infection prior to delivery if not treated. In males, asymptomatic bacteriuria is almost always secondary to chronic prostatitis or urinary tract obstruction.

Several investigators have studied the incidence of asymptomatic bacteriuria in the general population. In the newborn, the incidence of asymptomatic bacteriuria is 1 per cent, and the majority of infected newborns are males. This is the only instance in which the sex ratio favors the male. In several of Kunin's studies of school children, 1.2 per cent of the girls were found to have asymptomatic bacteriuria, while only 0.03 per cent of the boys screened had a positive urine culture. In adult women of childbearing age, the incidence of asymptomatic bacteriuria ranges from 4 to 10 per cent. As patients become older and more debilitated, the percentage rises.

Great debate and controversy exist as to the relationship between asymptomatic bacteriuria and chronic pyelonephritis. At this time no proof exists that asymptomatic bacteriuria proceeds to chronic pyelonephritis if left untreated. It is known from bladder washout and ureteral catheterization studies that in 30 to 50 per cent of patients with asymptomatic bacteriuria, the bacteria originate from the kidneys. If this group of patients could be identified and followed on a long-term basis, perhaps the relationship between these two conditions could be established.

Chronic Pyelonephritis

Chronic pyelonephritis is a diffuse interstitial inflammatory disease of the kidneys secondary to bacterial infection. It is not clear how this condition originates. Evidence establishing acute pyelonephritis and chronic asymptomatic bacteriuria as the forerunners of chronic pyelonephritis is insufficient at this time.

There appears to be a more clear-cut relationship between bacteriuria and chronic pyelonephritis in patients with obstruction of urine flow and chronic bacteriuria. Whenever an obstructive lesion is found, surgical correction should be considered.

Many noninfectious diseases can produce a histologic picture almost identical to that of chronic pyelonephritis. This may reflect the fact that the kidney has only a limited capacity to react to a diverse number of insults.

Perinephric Abscess

Abscess formation of the perinephric space is an uncommon problem and is frequently overlooked in the differential diagnosis of patients who present with fever and flank or abdominal pain. Physical findings suggesting this diagnosis include flank tenderness and the palpation of a mass in the flank or abdomen. Some patients with perinephric abscess have no urinary symptoms or localizing signs and are admitted to the hospital with fever of unknown origin. In a recent study of 46 cases of perinephric abscess by Thorley and his colleagues, one third of the cases were diagnosed only at autopsy.

Formation of a perinephric abscess is usually secondary to rupture of an intrarenal abscess into the perinephric space. In most cases, the intrarenal abscess arises from an area of acute pyelonephritis which has progressed to suppuration. This occurs most frequently in patients with urinary tract obstruction or diabetes mellitus. When acute pyelonephritis does accompany the formation of a perinephric abscess, urinary tract symptoms are often present. If the abscess does not communicate with the renal collecting ducts, bacteria do not escape into the urine; therefore, urinary symptoms are absent, and the urine culture will be sterile.

Perinephric abscess may also be produced during the course of bacteremia by implantation of bacteria in the perinephric fat pad from a distant focus of infection.

Associated physical findings may include a flank or intra-abdominal mass. When present, the mass is tender to palpation, and the overlying skin is warm to the touch. In more than half the patients, however, no mass is discovered on physical examination. All patients are febrile, and chills are common. Bacteremia is present in almost half of the patients.

The single most useful study to support the diagnosis of perinephric abscess is the intravenous pyelogram, with additional films taken on inspiration and expiration. Normally, the kidneys descend several centimeters on inspiration and also descend when the patient assumes the upright position (post-voiding film). In the presence of a perinephric abscess, the underlying kidney becomes bound down in the inflammatory process and remains fixed in position. In addition, the intravenous pyelogram may reveal an extrinsic soft tissue mass or poor visualization of the involved kidney. Recently, radioisotope scanning with gallium[67] has proved useful in the localization of cryptic abscesses.

If the perinephric abscess originates as an extention of a pyelonephritic process, the microorganisms isolated are the same as those which produce ascending urinary tract infection (see Table 28-1). Perinephric abscess secondary to bacteremic spread is usually produced by *Staphylococcus aureus.*

The most important aspect of treatment is early recognition and surgical drainage. Antibiotic therapy alone is of little value. The methods of treatment are discussed further in the next section (see also Chap. 46).

Treatment

Acute Symptomatic Infection

Before antimicrobial agents became available for the treatment of bacterial infections, most patients recovered spontaneously from acute urinary tract infection. Eradication of infection in these patients was dependent solely on host factors and the absence of any underlying obstructive uropathy. With the availability of antimicrobial agents, however, more rapid and complete control of infection is now possible, and the mortality rate for those patients whose infection has been complicated by bacteremia has been reduced.

Eradication of bacteria from the urinary tract by antimicrobial agents depends on the agent's ability to produce adequate antibacterial activity in the urine. Most antimicrobial agents excreted by the kidneys are concentrated in the urine and are present in concentrations which are 10 to 100 times greater than their peak serum levels. Antimicrobial agents that are not primarily excreted by the kidneys, e.g., chloramphenicol, may not reach therapeutic concentrations in the urine, especially in patients with diminished renal function. It seems to make little difference whether the mode of action of the antimicrobial agent is bacteriostatic or bactericidal as long as the microorganism isolated is sensitive to the agent chosen.

Initial evaluation of the patient is most important, for a prompt decision must be made as to whether the patient can be treated on an outpatient basis or whether hospitalization is necessary. Those patients who appear seriously ill because of the presence of high fever, shaking chills, and costovertebral angle tenderness and are suspected of having associated bacteremia should be admitted to the hospital. Hospitalization may also be necessary so that antimicrobial agents may be given parenterally; absorption of antimicrobial agents may be erratic or impeded by associated nausea, vomiting, or delayed gastric emptying.

For the patient who requires hospitalization, initial therapy should be given not only by the parenteral route but also in high dosage. This is to assure the attainment of therapeutic serum levels, should coexisting bacteremia be present. Those patients who have acquired their urinary tract infection in the community and who have no underlying disease and have not received antimicrobial agents in the recent past are usually infected with *Escherichia coli* (see Table 28–1). Therapy in these patients is generally begun with ampicillin or a cephalosporin until the results of the urine culture and susceptibility testing are known. Treatment is usually continued for 10 to 14 days. Some physicians believe that renal involvement is more difficult to eradicate than bladder infection, and that the duration of therapy should be extended beyond 14 days in patients with acute pyelonephritis. There is, however, no hard evidence to substantiate the premise that extension of therapy is necessary or improves the overall cure rate in these patients. Eighty-five per cent of the patients who are treated with an appropriate antimicrobial agent are free of bacteriuria at the conclusion of 10 days of therapy.

Patients who are not very ill and have dysuria and urinary frequency and are afebrile or have only a mild elevation of their temperature can be managed on an outpatient basis. As mentioned previously, these patients may have upper urinary tract infection, but they almost always respond to appropriate oral antimicrobial therapy. In this situation a sulfonamide is as efficacious as any of the newer, more expensive antimicrobial agents. However, if the patient fails to respond, and the results of the urine culture and susceptibility testing reveal that the isolated microorganism is resistant to sulfonamides, another agent should be given. Most frequently, ampicillin or an oral cephalosporin will prove effective. Care must be taken in interpreting results of tests for susceptibility to sulfa drugs. Most media used in susceptibility testing contain para-aminobenzoic acid, which interferes with the antibacterial activity of sulfonamides. Thus, microorganisms sensitive to sulfa drugs may be reported to be resistant to these drugs if this is not kept in mind.

Selection of initial antimicrobial therapy in the hospitalized patient is much more difficult because of the wide range of bacteria which may produce infection and the frequency with which these microorganisms are resistant to antimicrobial agents (see Table 28–1). For those patients who develop their infection while receiving antimicrobial agents or who are known to have obstructive uropathy, gentamicin is usually given until the results of the urine culture and susceptibility testing are known. If, at that point, the microorganism isolated is sensitive to a less toxic antimicrobial agent, a change in therapy can be safely made (see Chap. 46).

Asymptomatic Bacteriuria

Although controversy exists as to whether all patients with asymptomatic bacteriuria should be treated with antimicrobial agents, there is agreement that certain groups of patients should definitely be treated. These include children, young adults, and pregnant women. If left untreated, most of these patients will eventually develop acute symptomatic infection. Several studies have shown that in approximately 30 to 50 per cent of patients with asymptomatic bacteriuria, the bacteria originate from the kidney. If this group of patients could be identified, a reasonable argument for treatment could be made, even though these individuals are asymptomatic.

Follow-Up of Patients with Urinary Tract Infection

Unlike many infectious illnesses, the disappearance of symptoms and a return to a sense of well-being in a patient with urinary tract infection do not necessarily imply that the patient has been cured. At the point when the patient is free of symptoms, asymptomatic bacteriuria may still exist. For this reason, urinary tract infection should be viewed not as an isolated event but as a possible recurrent or chronic infection that requires periodic follow-up investigation. Patients should have a urinalysis and culture performed two weeks and three and six months after completion of antimicrobial therapy in order to determine if a relapse or reinfection has occurred. In the past, a relapse was defined as the reisolation in the urine of the same microorganism that caused the original infection; in the case of *Escherichia coli,* it is the reisolation of the same serotype. Reinfection was defined as the appearance of a different microorganism or a new serotype of the same species. From the previous discussion on the pathogenesis of urinary tract infection, it is evident that these definitions are not always reliable. Antimicrobial therapy does not eradicate the pathogenic microorganism from the fecal flora and vaginal introitus. It is, therefore, possible that a patient may be reinfected with the same microorganism which produced the original infection without postulating a failure to eradicate the original infection.

Protracted suppressive therapy is indicated for patients who experience several attacks of symptomatic urinary tract infection during a single year or for those patients who develop asymptomatic bacteriuria between their acute attacks. This type of therapy is most frequently accomplished by urinary acidification with mandelamine and ascorbic acid, or by the use of antimicrobial agents such as nitrofurantoin or sulfa drugs. The duration of suppressive therapy is variable, but it is usually continued for three months to one year. Urine cultures should be obtained at periodic intervals while the patient is on one of the above outlined regimens in order to determine if suppressive therapy has been successful.

CASE PRESENTATION 1

A 24-year-old married woman was admitted to the hospital because of fever, shaking chills, low back pain, and frequency and burning on urination. These symptoms began approximately 12 hours prior to admission. In the past she had been in excellent health, and she had no history of urinary infection during childhood or adolescence. The patient was married at age 21 and one month after her marriage was treated by her private physician and given an antimicrobial agent for frequency and burning on urination. Two weeks after delivery of her first child at age 23 the patient again developed urinary frequency, awakening at night to pass her urine (nocturia), and complained of pain on urination (dysuria). She was again seen and treated by her private physician for a urinary tract infection. The results of her urine cultures on these two prior occasions were not known at the time of admission. Personal hygiene habits were unremarkable, and the patient had been taking no medication prior to this admission. Physical examination revealed a well-developed woman who appeared acutely ill. Her blood pressure was 128/78; pulse rate, 102 per minute; respirations, 21 per minute; and her temperature was 103.4°F. The rest of the physical examination was normal except for tenderness of both costovertebral angles on palpation. Laboratory studies revealed a white blood count of 14,500, with a predominance of segmented neutrophils. Hemoglobin and hematocrit were normal. Urinalysis demonstrated 12 to 30 leukocytes per high power field in uncentrifuged urine, and Gram stain revealed 2 to 5 gram negative rods per high power field. A few white blood cell and granular casts were seen in the centrifuged urine sediment. A portion of the clean-catch midstream urine was also sent for culture. Three blood cultures were obtained.

Therapy was begun with ampicillin 1.5 gm every six hours by intravenous infusion. The results of the urine culture obtained at the time of admission were reported on the second hospital day and revealed growth of *Escherichia coli* greater than 100,000 microorganisms per milliliter and sensitivity of *E. coli* to ampicillin at 2.0 µg per ml. One of the three blood cultures was also reported to be positive for *E. coli* with the same antibiotic sensitivities as the

E. coli isolated from the urine. The patient became afebrile and felt much better by the fourth hospital day. At this point ampicillin was given orally, and the intraveous infusion was discontinued. The total duration of ampicillin therapy was 10 days. The patient was asked to return to the hospital in one month for a repeat urine culture and intravenous pyelogram.

The patient's presenting signs and symptoms were highly suggestive of urinary tract infection. Rapid confirmation of the diagnosis was obtained by examination of the unspun urine. Since the patient acquired her infection outside the hospital, the most likely causative microorganism statistically was *Escherichia coli.* Because most strains of *E. coli* are sensitive to ampicillin, this antimicrobial agent was chosen to initiate therapy. The attending physician suspected the possibility of associated bacteremia because of the high fever and shaking chills. When associated bacteremia is suspected, several (two to four) blood cultures should be obtained. Ampicillin was administered intravenously to avoid the vagaries of oral administration in a seriously ill patient and to assure therapeutic blood levels if bacteremia did coexist with infection of the urinary tract. The choice of 10 days for the duration of therapy, although not agreed upon by all authorities, is usually adequate for the eradication of infection.

Because the patient had a history of several episodes of urinary tract infection, an intravenous pyelogram was performed when the patient became asymptomatic to rule out the possibility of an underlying anatomic defect predisposing this patient to infection. It is also good medical practice to obtain a follow-up urine culture one to four weeks after completion of therapy to assure that the infection has been eradicated. The absence of symptoms is not synonymous with a sterile urine culture. Urine cultures should be obtained three, six, and 12 months following completion of therapy, regardless of the absence of symptoms. Only in this manner can a true picture of the problem of urinary tract infection in this patient be obtained.

CASE PRESENTATION 2

A 19-year-old heroin addict was admitted to the hospital because of fever, shaking chills, and left flank pain of one week's duration. He had no prior history of urinary tract infection and no urinary symptoms at the time of admission. He had had hepatitis 18 months previously, for which he had been hospitalized for one month at another hospital. In all other respects he had been in good health.

On physical examination, the patient appeared acutely ill and resisted movement because of back pain. His temperature was 103.2°F; blood pressure, 124/82; pulse, 88 per minute; and respirations, 20 per minute. Abnormal physical findings were confined to the back, where there was a loss of the normal lumbar lordotic curve. A tender mass, 6 x 8 cm, was palpable just below the left costovertebral angle. Laboratory studies revealed a white blood count of 17,500, with 87 per cent segmented neutrophils. Hematocrit was 37 ml per 100 ml, and hemoglobin was 12.5 gm per 100 ml. Routine urinalysis was normal, and urine culture revealed no growth. Chest x-ray, scout film of the abdomen, and x-rays of the thoracic-lumbar vertebrae were interpreted as normal. Two of four blood cultures taken on admission were reported 48 hours later to be growing *Staphylococcus aureus* which was resistant to penicillin but sensitive to all the semisynthetic penicillinase-resistant penicillins.

After these results were known, treatment was begun with nafcillin 1.5 gm intravenously every four hours. At this point, many diagnostic possibilities, including retroperitoneal, intrahepatic, and perinephric abscess and acute staphylococcal endocarditis, were being considered by the house staff. To further delineate the problem, an intravenous pyelogram was performed, with additional films taken on inspiration and expiration. These revealed that the right kidney moved 3 cm downward on inspiration, but the left kidney remained fixed in position. A four-hour gallium[67] scan performed later the same day showed increased uptake in the area of the left kidney, suggesting an abscess. On the basis of these findings, the patient was taken to the operating room, where a large perinephric abscess was incised and drained through a left flank incision. Culture of the exudate drained at the time of surgery grew *Staphylococcus aureus* with an antimicrobial susceptibility pattern identical to that of the *S. aureus* grown from the blood cultures. The patient was treated for a total of four weeks with intravenous nafcillin and made an uneventful recovery.

References

Aoki, S., Imamura, S., Aoki, M., and McCabe, W. R.: "Abacterial" and bacterial pyelonephritis. N. Engl. J. Med. *281:*1375, 1969.

Bailey, R. R.: Urinary tract infection – Some recent concepts. Can. Med. Assoc. J. *107:*316, 1972.

Beard, R. W., and Roberts, A. P.: Asymptomatic bacteriuria during pregnancy. Br. Med. J. *24:*44, 1968.

Braude, A. I.: Current concepts of pyelonephritis. Medicine *52:*257, 1973.

Gruneberg, R. N.: Relationship of infecting urinary organism to the faecal flora in patients with asymptomatic urinary infection. Lancet *2:*766, 1969.

Harding, G. K. M., and Ronald, A. R.: A controlled study of antimicrobial prophylaxis of recurrent urinary infection in women. N. Engl. J. Med. *291:*597, 1974.

Hinman, F.: Urethrovesical dysfunction and infection. Annu. Rev. Med. *24:*83, 1973.

Jones, S. R., Smith, J. W., and Sanford, J. P.: Localization of urinary-tract infections by detection of antibody-coated bacteria in urine sediment. N. Engl. J. Med. *290:*591, 1974.

Kass, E. H., and Finland, M.: Asymptomatic infections of the urinary tract. Trans. Assoc. Am. Physicians *69:*56, 1956.

Kunin, C. M.: Epidemiology and natural history of urinary tract infection in school age children. Pediatr. Clin. North Am. *18:*509, 1971.

Kunin, C. M., and McCormack, R. C.: Prevention of catheter-induced urinary tract infections by sterile closed drainage. N. Engl. J. Med. *274:*1155, 1966.

Martin, C. M., and Bookrajian, E. N.: Bacteriuria prevention after indwelling urinary catheterization. Arch. Intern. Med. *110:*703, 1962.

Mulholland, S. G., and Bruun, J. N.: A study of hospital urinary tract infections. J. Urol. *110:*245, 1973.

Savage, W. E., Hajj, S. N., and Kass, E. H.: Demographic and prognostic characteristics of bacteriuria in pregnancy. Medicine *46:*385, 1967.

Stamey, T. A.: The role of introital enterobacteria in recurrent urinary infections. J. Urol. *109:*467, 1973.

Stamey, T. A., Govan, D. E., and Palmer, J. M.: The localization and treatment of urinary tract infections: The role of bactericidal urine levels as opposed to serum levels. Medicine *44:*1, 1965.

Stamey, T. A., Fair, W. R., Timothy, M. M., Millar, M. A., Mihara, G., and Lowery, Y. C.: Serum versus urinary antimicrobial concentrations in cure of urinary-tract infections. N. Engl. J. Med *291:*1159, 1974.

Thomas, V., Shelokov, A., and Forland, M.: Antibody-coated bacteria in the urine and the site of urinary tract infection. N. Engl. J. Med. *290:*588, 1974.

Thorley, J. D., Jones, S. R., and Sanford, J. P.: Perinephric abscess. Medicine *53:*441, 1974.

Turck, M.: Therapeutic principles in the treatment of urinary tract infections and pyelonephritis. Adv. Intern. Med. *18:*141, 1972.

Chapter 29

DIAGNOSIS AND TREATMENT OF SYPHILIS

Introduction

Syphilis is an infectious disease of human beings caused by the spirochaete, *Treponema pallidum*. Although nonvenereal transmission of the disease may occur, in most cases syphilis is spread by sexual contact in one form or another. During the 10-year period between 1956 and 1966, an increase of primary syphilis of 247 per cent was reported in the 15 to 19-year-old age group and of 274 per cent in the 20 to 24-year-old age group (Fig. 29–1). One of the most serious problems has been the rapid increase of syphilis among homosexuals. Of all patients treated for syphilis in the state of Washington in 1971, nearly two thirds were homosexual men.

Syphilis may be a fatal or seriously disabling disease causing irreversible damage to the cardiovascular, central nervous, or musculoskeletal systems. One of every 13 untreated patients with syphilis will develop cardiovascular disease, one of 25 will become crippled or incapacitated, and one of 44 will develop irreversible damage to the central nervous system. One patient in every 200 with syphilis will become blind.

Syphilis has three stages which are related to the time of infection and may or may not be correlated with the appearance of cutaneous or visceral lesions. *Primary syphilis* is the term applied to the disease during the first two to four weeks following infection and is characterized by the appearance of a firm, usually nontender cutaneous ulcer at the site of inoculation of the spirochaete. The ulcer is called a chancre and first appears from five to eight days following penetration by the treponemes at the time of exposure. The chancre lasts for 10 to 14 days before healing spontaneously without leaving

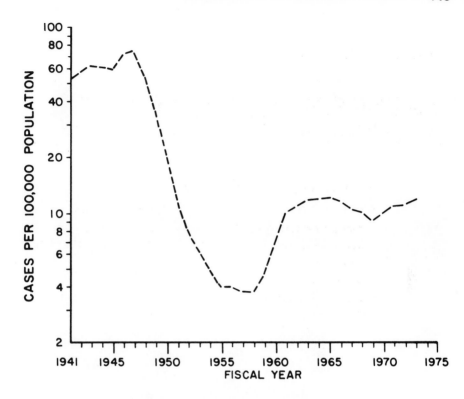

Figure 29-1. Syphilis, primary and secondary. Reported civilian cases in the United States, 1941–1973. (From Center for Disease Control, Morbidity and Mortality Weekly Report, Vol. 22, No. 53, 1973.)

a scar. The *secondary stage of syphilis* develops from two to four weeks later and is characterized by a variety of mucocutaneous eruptions. In some cases, the chancre may still be present with the onset of the skin rash, but usually the chancre has healed. In addition to the skin lesions, secondary syphilis is characterized by diffuse lymphadenopathy, malaise, and fever. The skin eruption may be generalized, and syphilis is one of the few infections that will produce lesions involving the skin of the palms of the hands and the soles of the feet (Fig. 29–2). (For other causes of palmar skin rash, see Chapter 34.) Because of the diffuse skin manifestations of the disease, many patients first seek treatment for syphilis from dermatologists, and until only recently the department of dermatology in many medical schools was called the "Department of Dermatology and Syphilology."

Tertiary *syphilis* is usually not clinically apparent for many years following the spontaneous clearing of the secondary stage. The lesions of tertiary syphilis may involve the cardiovascular (luetic aortitis), the central nervous, and musculoskeletal systems, or gummas (large granulomas characterized by extensive caseation necrosis) may develop at any point in the body. When the lesions of tertiary syphilis appear, it is frequently too late to treat the patient and effect a return to completely normal status. It therefore becomes necessary to find and treat the disease before the onset of the tertiary form if the patient is to be spared permanent, disabling damage or a fatal outcome.

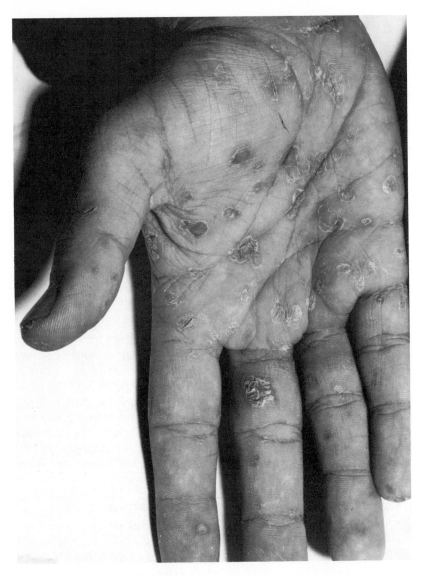

Figure 29–2. Secondary syphilis. For the past six weeks this 22-year-old student has had a scaling papular eruption of the palms and soles, an annular scaling plaque of the scrotum, and a mucous patch on the hard palate. Darkfield examination of the palmar lesions was negative. VDRL serologic test for syphilis was reactive. (From Shelley, W. B.: Consultations in Dermatology II. Philadelphia, W. B. Saunders Co., 1974. Photo by Edward F. Glifort.)

Diagnosis

Darkfield Examination

The diagnosis of syphilis in the primary stage consists of demonstrating motile treponemes from the chancre. Treponemes can usually be found in a chancre from early to the late stages but are very sensitive to penicillin and cannot be found within four hours after the drug is given. Demonstration of treponemes by darkfield examination may be the only way to establish the diagnosis in the initial stage of the disease, as diagnostic serologic changes usually do not begin to appear until 14 to 21 days after contact. Darkfield examinations are simple and easily done. The surface of the chancre is cleaned with a saline-moistened swab to clear away exudate and excessive bacterial contamination. An ether-soaked swab is then applied to the chancre to irritate the surface and cause an outpouring of serum containing treponemes. Using saline, serum is then removed from the surface of the chancre by a small pipette and placed on a microscopic slide, protected by a coverslip, and examined with darkfield illumination. *Treponema pallidum* has an unforgettable, rapid, corkscrew, purposeful motion across the microscopic field (Fig. 29–3). Darkfield preparations for motile treponemes should be examined within 10 to 15 minutes, as the treponemes are susceptible to a decrease in temperature and soon stop moving. The characteristic shape of the microorganism in darkfield illumination is not apparent when it is motionless. Motile treponemes can also be found in both skin lesions and enlarged lymph nodes in patients with secondary syphilis but not in the same numbers as in the primary chancre. Both primary and secondary lesions are contagious.

Serologic Diagnosis

Unfortunately, the cutaneous manifestations of primary and secondary syphilis are inconstant. In many patients, the first warning of the disease is the appearance of the tertiary form. Since the lesions of tertiary syphilis may be irreversible, it becomes increasingly important to recognize the disease and give adequate therapy before tertiary lesions appear. This can be done with a high level of accuracy by using a variety of serologic tests for syphilis (sometimes abbreviated STS).

In the discussion of any serologic test for syphilis, two terms, sensitivity and specificity, should be defined, and the distinction between the two kept clearly in mind. *Sensitivity* is the ability of the test to be reactive in the presence of *all* syphilis. The test will not miss a patient who has syphilis, whether primary, secondary, or tertiary. As long as the test will detect all syphilis, it need not be expected to differentiate between syphilis and similar

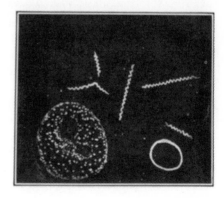

Figure 29–3. *Treponema pallidum.* Diagrammatic sketch of the appearance of this spirochaete under darkfield illumination, drawn to scale in comparison with a red corpuscle and a leukocyte. (From Joklik, W. K., and Smith, D. T. (eds.): Zinsser Microbiology. 15th ed. New York, Appleton-Century-Crofts, Publishing Division of Prentice-Hall, Inc., 1972.)

but nonsyphilitic diseases also reacting with the test. Highly sensitive tests are useful for preliminary screening.

Specificity refers to the ability of a test to reject all cases of nonsyphilis. This test may be applied to reactive cases selected by the sensitivity (screening) test and will discard all cases reactive on some basis other than syphilis. Until such time as a single test will offer both of these characteristics, there is clearly a need for both procedures. The ideal approach for the serologic diagnosis of syphilis is to use a sensitivity test for screening purposes and a specificity test for discrimination between syphilis and nonsyphilis.

Serologic tests for syphilis are divided into two broad categories: (1) tests to detect the presence of an antibody to a cardiolipin antigen, the so-called Wassermann antibody, and (2) tests to detect antibody against treponemal antigens. In general, the tests reactive for Wassermann antibody are useful as screening tests, while those based on detecting treponemal antibody are of help in establishing the specific diagnosis of syphilis.

Wassermann Antibody

In 1906, one year after the treponeme causing syphilis had been identified, Wassermann employed an aqueous extract from the liver of an infant dying of congenital syphilis as an antigen for a complement-fixation test. The liver was shown to contain large numbers of motile treponemes which Wasserman theorized would act as an antigen and combine with antibody in the serum of diseased persons. While the liver antigen worked and did show reactivity with the sera of patients with the disease, it was many years before it was recognized that the reactivity found was not with the treponemes in the liver but with intracellular, nontreponemal components of the liver cells. Similar substances could be isolated from other mammalian and plant sources. This substance is thought to be a component of mitochondrial membranes and has been called cardiolipin. Antibody to this antigen is known as Wassermann antibody or reaginic antibody. It should be emphasized that there is no relation between this antibody and IgE reaginic antibody. For that reason, we will refer to antibody against cardiolipin as Wassermann antibody.

The development of serologic tests for syphilis has followed a long and tortuous path. Inasmuch as a number of different types of tests have been used and the distinctions between these may cause confusion, the following section traces the evolution of these tests to our present practice.

Kahn, in 1922, developed the first precipitating test for syphilis, using an alcoholic extract of beef heart (cardiolipin) in the form of a tube flocculation test. In 1941, Pangborn combined lecithin and cholesterol with cardiolipin and improved both the sensitivity and specificity of the test. This improvement of antigen led to the development of a slide microflocculation test by the Venereal Disease Research Laboratory of the United States Public Health Service (abbreviated as the VDRL test). The VDRL test is simple, inexpensive, and easy to perform on large numbers of sera in a short time. For these reasons, the VDRL has been the mainstay for screening sera for syphilis in many hospitals and municipal, state, and federal public health laboratories since the 1950s.

In addition to the Kahn and VDRL tests, numerous modifications of the Wassermann cardiolipin antigen tests have been developed. The Hinton is a tube flocculation test like the Kahn test, while the Kline and Mazzini tests are slide tests similar to the VDRL. Kolmer adapted the cardiolipin antigen to a complement-fixation test, but it was found to be less sensitive and specific than the VDRL slide test. Quantitation of the amount of the Wassermann antibody can be determined in all tests by making twofold dilutions of the serum until the reaction disappears. Quantitative results of the VDRL test are reported as the reciprocal of the largest dilution of serum which precipitated with antigen. The results of the quantitative test are then reported in terms of "dils," e.g., 4 dils, 8 dils, etc.

Although the cardiolipin antigen tests just described have the advantage of ease, speed, and simplicity in the laboratory, it is necessary to inactivate complement and other inhibitors by heating the serum to be tested to 56°C for 30 minutes. Such a restriction, while not a problem in a well-equipped laboratory, limits application of the test in the field, where controlled test conditions may not be possible. More recently, the cardiolipin-lecithin-cholesterol complex has been stabilized with the addition of ethylenediamine tetraacetic acid and choline chloride to inactivate the inhibiting substances in unheated sera. This modification permits the test to be run under field conditions where minimal laboratory facilities exist to screen large groups of sera. Several commercial variants of this test are available, e.g., the Plasmacrit and RPR (Rapid Plasma Reagin) Card Test. The RPR test is performed by mixing the serum and reagent with an applicator stick on a hard-faced piece of white cardboard. Experience has shown the RPR test to have equal and possibly better sensitivity and specificity than the VDRL test. The reagents for the RPR test are considerably more expensive than the VDRL, a fact which serves to restrict widespread use.

Tests for Wassermann antibody are useful in screening large numbers of individuals for evidence of active syphilis, e.g., those tests performed for marriage license applications, hospital admission tests, or prenatal blood tests for the prevention of congenital syphilis. Positive tests are considered to be diagnostic for syphilis when there is a high or increasing titer or when careful history taking reveals physical lesions consistent with primary or secondary syphilis. Tests for Wassermann antibody are also useful in epidemiologic surveys for the investigation of patient contacts to find otherwise unrecognized active syphilis. In addition, Wassermann antibody tests may be of prognostic aid in following the response to therapy, since the number of VDRL dils will fall over a six- to eight-month period after adequate therapy.

Biologic False Positive Tests

The cardiolipin Wassermann antigen is found in the mitochondrial membranes of many mammalian tissues. Similar antigenic material appears in other microorganisms, including mycoplasma, bacteria, and some yeasts. It should be no surprise that antibodies to the Wassermann antigen should appear in other diseases. Wassermann antibodies may be found in the serum of patients with infectious mononucleosis, hepatitis, and leprosy, and for several months after smallpox vaccinations. Such reactions have been called biologically false positive serologic tests for syphilis.

Antibodies to the Wassermann antigen also occur in several of the so-called collagen diseases — systemic lupus erythematosus, rheumatoid arthritis, and Hashimoto's thyroiditis. The delayed onset of the tertiary stage of syphilis and the similarity of this condition to small vessel disease with evidence of ischemic tissue damage have raised the possibility that the tertiary lesions of syphilis may be a manifestation of autoimmune disease. Further work is needed before this hypothesis can be sustained.

Treponemal Antibody Tests

The second type of serologic test is based on the use of whole treponemes or extracts of treponemes. The treponemes employed for this purpose may be either the virulent *Treponema pallidum,* grown only in rabbit testes, or nonvirulent treponemes that can be cultivated in a special medium, e.g., the Reiter strain of *T. pallidum.*

The first successful treponemal antibody test was developed by Nelson in 1949. Nelson noted that during experiments performed to define growth characteristics of *Treponema pallidum,* serum from patients with active syphilis and added guinea pig complement caused motile treponemes grown in rabbit testes to slow their active, corkscrew-like motion and become immobilized (*Treponema pallidum* immobilization — TPI test). The antibody responsible for immobilization of the treponemes was found to be different from Wassermann antibody in that Wassermann antibody was present in higher concentration during the early phase of the infection, while immobilizing antibody persisted in high titer for many years. The test remained as a standard for many years against which all other serologic tests for syphilis were measured, and until recently was considered to be the ultimate criterion for the presence or absence of antibody to *T. pallidum.* The TPI test is both sensitive and quite specific, but it is difficult to perform and requires closely supervised animal colonies as well as highly trained personnel. Sera tested for TPI are anticomplementary in 25 to 33 per cent of patients, and if penicillin has been given within the preceding month, traces still present in the serum may immobilize the treponemes. The exacting conditions necessary to carry out the TPI test soon limited the number of laboratories offering the service, and at the present time it is performed only once every two months at the Center for Disease Control.

The specificity of the TPI test and the difficulty and expense involved in performing the test spurred efforts to develop a procedure having similar specificity but greater ease of performance and broader applicability. Over the succeeding years, a wide variety of treponemal tests were developed, including the *Treponema pallidum* complement-fixation test (TPCF), the Reiter's protein complement-fixation test (RPCF), the *Treponema pallidum* immune adherence test (TPIA), and a number of others. Of these tests, only the RPCF, or the Kolmer-Reiter protein (KRP) test, performed with any merit. It has now been replaced with the two more sensitive and specific tests described below.

In 1957, Deacon and coworkers at the Venereal Disease Research Laboratory developed a test for antitreponemal antibody based on the principle of the indirect fluorescence procedure. If a virulent *Treponema pallidum* from an infected rabbit testis is placed on a glass microscopic slide and overlaid with serum from a patient with antibody to treponemes, an antigen-antibody reaction will occur, with the antibody binding firmly to the surface of the treponeme. If the treponeme-antibody mixture is then exposed to an antibody against human gamma globulin tagged with fluorescein isothiocyanate and viewed under a strong ultraviolet light, all human antitreponeme antibody binding to the spirochaete will be tagged with fluorescein dye and will outline the treponeme (antigen) (Fig. 29–4). The test was called the fluorescent treponemal antibody test (FTA-1:5, as the serum tested was diluted 1:5). The FTA-1:5 was found to be very sensitive but not very specific, detecting treponemal antibody in approximately 30 per cent of patients with no known history or physical findings of syphilis. Although most such antibody in nonsyphilitics is in low titer, some patients showed positive reactions even when their serum was diluted 1:100. Deacon next suggested that the test be modified by diluting the serum of the test patient 1:200 before running the test. Although a 1:200 dilution of serum was effective in removing false positive reactions, it reduced the sensitivity of the test by a significant factor, missing small quantities of antibody in the serum of patients with active syphilis of many years' duration.

Deacon was not deterred for long and next found that the nonspecific cross-reactions giving false positive tests at 1:5 dilutions were due to antitreponemal antibodies unrelated to *Treponema pallidum*. He and coworkers showed that *Treponema microdentium, Treponema zuelzerae* (a free-growing mud treponeme), the Reiter treponeme, and the virulent *T. pallidum* all shared common nonspecific antigens. By absorption of the patient's serum giving nonspecific reactions with either intact Reiter treponemes or a chemical fraction of the Reiter microorganism containing the common antigen, Deacon found that the nonspecific reactivity could be removed. Absorption with the Reiter extract does not significantly reduce specific antibody to *T. pallidum.* This modification is called the FTA-ABS or fluorescent treponemal antibody absorption test. With absorption of the

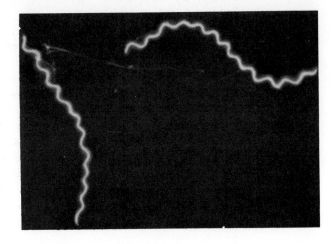

Figure 29–4. Usual spirochaete fluorescence in FTA-ABS test with serum from patients with syphilis. (From Kraus, S. J., Haserick, J. R., and Lantz, M. A.: Atypical FTA-ABS test fluorescence in lupus erythematosus patients. J.A.M.A. *211:*2140, 1970. Copyright 1970, American Medical Association.)

nonspecific treponemal antibodies, sensitivity was regained, as sera now only need to be diluted 1:5 rather than 1:200 (see Table 29–1).

TABLE 29–1. Comparative Tests in Syphilis Serology in Patients
with Biologic False Positive VDRL*

Tests	Serum Categories and Per Cent Reactive	
	Normal (74 Cases)	Biologic False Positive (38 Cases)
VDRL	0	100
KRP (RPCF)	0	0
FTA-200	0	0
FTA–1:5 (saline without absorption)	19.7	31.6
FTA-ABS (1:5 with absorption)	0	0
TPI	0	0

*From Moore, M. B., Jr., and Knox, J. M.: Sensitivity and specificity in syphilis serology: Clinical implications. South. Med. J. *58:*963, 1965.

In contrast to the TPI test, the FTA-ABS can be performed in most clinical laboratories, and results are available within a day. Although the test is not difficult, the number of controls necessary and the experience and time required for reading the individual slides prevent the test from being used as a sensitive screening test as well as a specificity test.

Within the last few years, an automated microhemagglutination assay for antibodies to *Treponema pallidum* (MHA-TP) has been described and evaluated. Results from this test are most encouraging, approaching the specificity achieved by the FTA-ABS and TPI tests. The test is more easily performed than are the standard treponemal tests but depends on an antigen available from a single commercial source in Japan. Limited quantities of the antigen have made widespread application of the procedure impractical at the present time.

Relation of Infection to Conversion of Serologic Tests

Comparison of the reactivity of different serologic tests to sera collected from well-documented cases of clinical syphilis can be helpful in determining the reliability of different serologic tests for syphilis at varying stages of the disease. Table 29–2 lists the results of reactions of different serologic tests of sera from patients with well-documented primary or secondary syphilis. This table shows the FTA-ABS test to be reactive in a significantly higher number of patients with primary syphilis than are any other serologic tests, including the VDRL. Studies subsequent to those listed in Table 29–2 have shown the FTA-ABS test to be reactive in more than 90 per cent of cases of darkfield-positive primary syphilis.

TABLE 29–2. Comparative Tests in Syphilis Serology*

Tests	Serum Categories and Per Cent Reactive	
	Primary Syphilis (76 Cases)	Secondary Syphilis (100 Cases)
VDRL	50.0	100
KRP (RPCF)	48.7	91
FTA-200	52.6	95
FTA–1:5 (saline without absorption)	100.0	100
FTA-ABS (1:5 with absorption)	80.7	100
TPI	36.8	67

*From Moore, J. B., Jr., and Knox, J. M.: Sensitivity and specificity in syphilis serology: Clinical implications. South. Med. J. *58:*963, 1965.

By the time secondary syphilis is well established, all tests give an acceptable result with the exception of the TPI test, which does not reach maximum reactivity until three to four months after the onset of the disease. If specific therapy for syphilis is instituted during the primary stage, and a Wassermann antibody test is positive, the test can be expected to become negative within six to eight months. If therapy is delayed until the onset of the secondary stage of syphilis, 90 to 95 per cent of adequately treated patients can be expected to show a negative reaction within 12 months. If therapy is not started until at least two years after the onset of the disease, treatment will not significantly affect the serologic test, although it can be expected that about half the cases with active syphilis will become Wassermann antibody negative over a 15- to 25-year period.

These findings are in contrast to tests for treponemal antibody of which the TPI and FTA-ABS tests remain positive in a much higher percentage of cases, depending upon what stage the disease was first recognized before therapy was started, and presumably reflect the total time and intensity of antigenic stimulation. Figures 29–5 and 29–6 relate the serologic reactivity of the FTA-ABS, TPI, and VDRL tests relative to the time of onset of the disease and start of therapy.

In assessing the value of different serologic tests for syphilis in long-standing, chronic, and untreated cases, comparison of the serologic findings in a group of patients in the Tuskegee Study for Untreated Syphilis is given in Table 29–3. The relative sensitivity and specificity of the different serologic tests for syphilis are apparent.

Congenital Syphilis

Transmission of the treponeme from the mother to the fetus is still an all too frequent occurrence. The placenta does not offer a barrier to the spirochaete, which can cross and enter the fetal circulation. Once in the fetus, there are few hindrances to growth and multiplication of the spirochaete, so that fetal infections may be severe, frequently resulting in malformations,

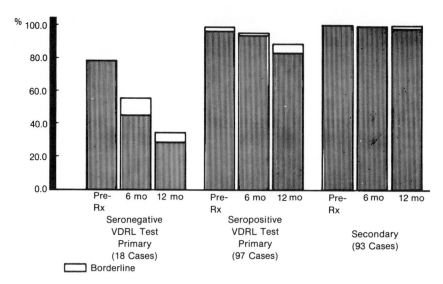

Figure 29–5. Response to FTA-ABS test following adequate treatment of 208 patients observed for 12 months. (From Schroeter, A. L., Lucas, J. B., Price, E. V., and Falcone, V. H.: Treatment for early syphilis and reactivity of serologic tests. J.A.M.A. *221:*471, 1972. Copyright 1972, American Medical Association.)

interstitial keratitis, and rarely in death shortly after birth. Even those infants who survive the primary and secondary stages of the disease are of questionable fortune, as congenital syphilis often produces serious and irreversible damage to the child.

Prevention of fetal infection is the most reasonable approach to control of congenital syphilis. Most states have laws requiring pregnant women to have a serologic test for syphilis, and if positive, treatment is given to the mother while the fetus is in utero. Often, the patients who need this service

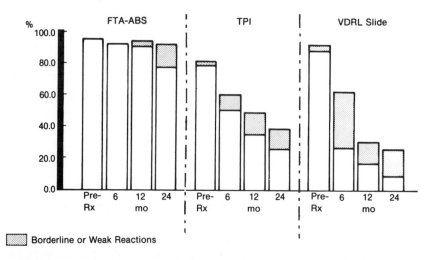

Figure 29–6. Serologic reactivity of 80 patients observed for two years, with use of FTA-ABS, TPI, and VDRL tests. (From Schroeter, A. L., Lucas, J. B., Price, E. V., and Falcone, V. H.: Treatment for early syphilis and reactivity of serologic tests. J.A.M.A. *221:*471, 1972. Copyright 1972, American Medical Association.)

TABLE 29-3. Comparative Serologic Findings in the Tuskegee Study —
1962 Follow-Up (29th Year)*

Tests	Per Cent Reactive	
	Syphilis Patients (46 Cases)	*Nonsyphilitic Controls (36 Cases)*
VDRL	54.4	0
KRP (RPCF)	43.5	0
FTA-200	19.5	0
FTA–1:5 (saline without absorption)	100.0	33.3
FTA-ABS (1:5 with absorption)	100.0	0
TPI	91.2	0

*From Moore, M. B., Jr., and Knox, J. M.: Sensitivity and specificity in syphilis serology: Clinical implications. South. Med. J. *58:*963, 1965.

the most appear to have least access to case finding and treatment, and children continue to be born to mothers having active syphilis. Although fetal blood from the umbilical cord is routinely collected for a serologic test for syphilis in those mothers who do not have the results of a serologic test for syphilis on file during the current pregnancy, the problem remains of how to differentiate treponemal antibody formed by the fetus from antibody that may have been passively transferred from the mother, possibly from an old infection that had been adequently treated.

Recently, the development of a test to differentiate IgG FTA-ABS antibody of the mother from IgM FTA-ABS antibody produced by the fetus permits the differentiation of antibody formed in response to an active infection in the fetus from passively transferred maternal antibodies. IgG antibodies are known to pass the placental barrier, while IgM antibodies cannot. Fetuses will make IgM antibodies against *Treponema pallidum* in response to a stimulus from infection. Therefore, the presence or absence of IgM FTA-ABS antibody in the cord blood of the fetus should be a reliable differentiation between active fetal infection from passively transferred IgG antibody from the mother. Close evaluation of this procedure is currently underway, and preliminary results indicate some restrictions in the interpretation of the test.

Fluorescent Treponemal Antibody–Cerebrospinal Fluid Test

The FTA procedure has now been applied to the detection of antibody against *Treponema pallidum* in cerebrospinal fluid. A test has been developed by the Venereal Disease Research Laboratory which has shown good sensitivity and specificity in the detection of antibody to *T. pallidum* in the cerebrospinal fluid. Cerebrospinal fluid is incubated with lyophilized *T. pallidum* without prior absorption and appears to be the most specific means of detecting central nervous system syphilis.

Fluorescent Treponemal Antibody Absorption Test in Lupus Erythematosus

Recently, it has been recognized that serum from certain patients with systemic lupus erythematosus may give an atypical, beaded appearance of fluorescence on treponemes with the FTA-ABS test. In one study, 11 of 150 patients with lupus erythematosus showed irregular, beaded fluorescent patterns. If the morphologic pattern of the test is not carefully differentiated, it could be confused with a positive test (Fig. 29–7). Perhaps of more importance is the question of the significance of focal localization of human gamma globulin to treponemes in patients with lupus erythematosus. The interpretation of these findings is not yet known.

Treatment

The recommendations for the treatment of syphilis as provided by the United States Public Health Service are listed in Table 29–4.

TABLE 29–4. Recommended Treatment Schedules for Syphilis (1976)*

Early Syphilis

Early syphilis (primary, secondary, latent syphilis of less than one year's duration)

Rx: Benzathine penicillin G—2.4 million units total by intramuscular injection at a single session.

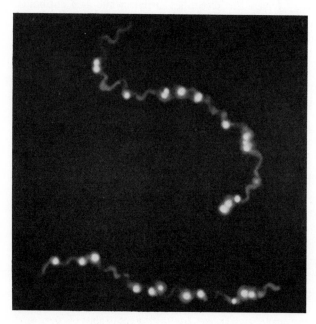

Figure 29–7. Atypical "beaded" spirochaete fluorescence in FTA-ABS test with serum from patients with lupus erythematosus (compare with Figure 29–4). (From Kraus, S. J., Haserick, J. R., and Lantz, M. A.: Atypical FTA-ABS test fluorescence in lupus erythematosus patients. J.A.M.A. *211:*2140, 1970, Copyright 1970, American Medical Association.)

TABLE 29-4. Recommended Treatment Schedules for Syphilis (1976)* *(Continued)*

Benzathine penicillin G is the drug of choice, because it provides effective treatment in a single visit.

or: Aqueous procaine penicillin G–4.8 million units total: 600,000 units by intramuscular injection daily for 8 days.

or: Procaine penicillin G in oil with 2 per cent aluminum monostearate (PAM) – 4.8 million units total by intramuscular injection: 2.4 million units at first visit, and 1.2 million units at each of two subsequent visits 3 days apart.

Although PAM is used in other countries, it is no longer available in the United States.

Patients Who Are Allergic to Penicillin

Rx: Tetracycline hydrochloride** – 500 mg four times a day by mouth for 15 days.

or: Erythromycin (stearate, ethylsuccinate or base) – 500 mg four times a day by mouth for 15 days.

These antibiotics appear to be effective, but have been evaluated less extensively than penicillin.

Syphilis of More Than One Year's Duration

Syphilis of more than one year's duration (latent syphilis of indeterminate or more than one year's duration, cardiovascular, late benign, neurosyphilis)

Rx: Benzathine penicillin G–7.2 million units total: 2.4 million units by intramuscular injection weekly for three successive weeks.

or: Aqueous procaine penicillin G–9.0 million units total: 600,000 units by intramuscular injection daily for 15 days.

Cerebrospinal fluid (CSF) examination is mandatory in patients with suspected, symptomatic neurosyphilis. This examination is also desirable in other patients with syphilis of greater than one year's duration to exclude asymptomatic neurosyphilis.

Patients Who Are Allergic to Penicillin

Rx: Tetracycline hydrochloride – 500 mg four times a day by mouth for 30 days.

or: Erythromycin (stearate, ethylsuccinate or base) – 500 mg four times a day by mouth for 30 days.

There are NO published clinical data which adequately document the efficacy of drugs other than penicillin for syphilis of more than one year's duration. Cerebrospinal fluid examinations are highly recommended before therapy with these regimens.

Syphilis in Pregnancy

Rx: For patients at all stages of pregnancy who are not allergic to penicillin: Penicillin in dosage schedules appropriate for the stage of syphilis as recommended for the treatment of nonpregnant patients.

For patients of all stages of pregnancy who are allergic to penicillin: Erythromycin (stearate, ethylsuccinate or base) in dosage schedules appropriate for the stage of syphilis, as recommended for the treatment of nonpregnant patients. Although these erythromycin schedules appear safe for mother and fetus, their efficacy is not well established. Therefore, the documentation of penicillin allergy is particularly important before treating a pregnant woman with erythromycin.

Erythromycin estolate and tetracycline are not recommended for syphilitic infections in pregnant women because of potential adverse effects on mother and fetus.

Follow Up

Pregnant women who have been treated for syphilis should have monthly quantitative nontreponemal serologic tests for the remainder of the current pregnancy. Women who

TABLE 29–4. Recommended Treatment Schedules for Syphilis (1976)* *(Continued)*

show a fourfold rise in titer should be retreated. After delivery, follow up is as outlined for nonpregnant patients.

Congenital Syphilis

Infants with congenital syphilis should have a CSF examination before treatment.

Infants With Abnormal CSF

Rx: Aqueous crystalline penicillin G, 50,000 units/kg intramuscularly or intravenously daily in two divided doses for a minimum of 10 days.
or: Aqueous procaine penicillin G, 50,000 units/kg intramuscularly daily for a minimum of 10 days.

Infants With Normal CSF

Rx: Benzathine penicillin G, 50,000 units/kg intramuscularly in a single dose.
Although benzathine penicillin has been previously recommended and widely used, published clinical data on its efficacy in congenital neurosyphilis are lacking. If neurosyphilis cannot be excluded, the procaine or aqueous penicillin regimens are recommended. Since cerebrospinal fluid concentrations of penicillin achieved after benzathine penicillin are minimal to nonexistent, these revised recommendations seem more conservative and appropriate until clinical data on the efficacy of benzathine penicillin can be accumulated. Other antibiotics are not recommended for neonatal congenital syphilis.
Penicillin therapy for congenital syphilis after the neonatal period should be with the same dosages used for neonatal congenital syphilis. For larger children, the total dose of penicillin need not exceed the dosage used in adult syphilis of more than one year's duration. After the neonatal period, the dosage of erythromycin and tetracycline for congenital syphilitics who are allergic to penicillin should be individualized but need not exceed dosages used in adult syphilis of more than one year's duration. Tetracycline should not be given to children less than 8 years of age.

Follow Up and Retreatment

All patients with early syphilis and congenital syphilis should be encouraged to return for repeat quantitative nontreponemal tests 3, 6, and 12 months after treatment. Patients with syphilis of more than one year's duration should also have a repeat serologic test months after treatment. Careful follow up serologic testing is particularly important in patients treated with antibiotics other than penicillin. Examination of CSF should be planned as part of the last follow up visit after treatment with alternative antibiotics.

All patients with neurosyphilis must be carefully followed with serologic testing for at least 3 years. In addition, follow up of these patients should include clinical reevaluation at 6-month intervals and repeat CSF examinations, particularly in patients treated with alternative antibiotics.

The possibility of reinfection should always be considered when retreating patients with early syphilis. A CSF examination should be performed before retreatment unless reinfection and a diagnosis of early syphilis can be established.

Retreatment should be considered when:

(1) Clinical signs or symptoms of syphilis persist or recur;
(2) There is a sustained fourfold increase in the titer of a nontreponemal test;
(3) An initially high-titer nontreponemal test fails to decrease fourfold within a year.

Patients should be retreated with the schedules recommended for syphilis of more than one year's duration. In general, only one retreatment course is indicated because patients may maintain stable, low titers of nontreponemal tests or have irreversible anatomical damage.

---

*From the United States Department of Health, Education, and Welfare, Public Health Service, Center for Disease Control, Bureau of State Services, Venereal Disease Branch, Atlanta, Georgia.

**Food and some dairy products interfere with absorption. Oral forms of tetracycline should be given one hour before or two hours after meals.

Historical Notes*

Syphilis — The Beginning

The origin of syphilis is cloaked in myth and hypothetical judgments. Some authorities point to references in the Bible which seem to indicate that syphilis existed in the Middle East, and therefore probably Europe, prior to the birth of Christ. Other scholars cling to the thesis that descriptions of syphilis — as we know the disease — can be found in history only since the voyages of Columbus. The controversy adds considerable interest to the historical background of syphilis.

In support of their argument, proponents of the first school of thought refer to the "evidence" arising from earlier civilizations. Early Greek and Roman physician-authors, Aules Celsus (25 B.C.–50 A.D.) and Pliny, the Elder (23–79 A.D.), described a disease which may well have been syphilis. Celsus wrote of hard and soft lesions of the mouth, genitalia, tonsils, vulva, and nostrils, and Pliny described painless ulcers which disappeared after several weeks without treatment. He further associated these ulcers with sexual activity. According to some historians, an enlargement of the great blood vessels (aneurysm), nearly always caused by syphilis, was common among early Romans, and only paresis could have produced a Nero, a Caligula, an Augustus, or a Tiberius.

Moreover, it is believed by some authorities that syphilis was present in Biblical times, and Job's affliction is often used as an example of pustular secondary syphilis (Job 2:7).

Further indication that Job's sickness could subsequently have turned into later manifestations of syphilis is found in the passage: "My bones cleaveth to my skin and flesh and I am escaped with the skin of my teeth" (Job 29:4–21). Elsewhere in the Bible (Isaiah 3:16–26) reference is made to the lesions of the genitalia and baldness (alopecia) resulting from the infected daughters of Israel.

The Book of Numbers (31:2–23) describes an epidemic, believed to have been syphilis, that followed sexual promiscuity.

In Deuteronomy (28:27–29) a passage appears which may well have been descriptive of the various stages of syphilis. Congenital syphilis is the only disease known to man which approaches the specifications set forth in the passage: "Visiting the iniquity of the fathers upon the children unto the third and fourth generation" (Exodus 20:5).

Additional evidence of congenital syphilis appears in Joshua (22:17) and Jeremiah (31:29).

According to the second theory, syphilis was unknown in Europe prior to the return of Columbus and his crew from America in 1493. There appears little doubt that a disease (yaws or syphilis) was present among the natives of Hispaniola (West Indies), and that the pilot and several members of the crew were "treated" for a "new exotic" disease upon their return to Barcelona. Within a relatively short period of time, the sailors were spreading the disease among the waterfront prostitutes, who passed it on to others.

Prominent author-physicians such as Ruiz Diaz de Isla (1500–?) and Oviedo (1478–1557) insisted that the disease was new to Europe and that it

*From the Washington State Department of Public Health.

had definitely been brought from the New World. This view seemed supported by the virulence of the disease, by the apparent scarcity of pre-Columbian reference to the disease in European literature, and by pre-Columbian American Indian bones showing marks of late syphilis; pre-Columbian European bones showing such evidence are extremely rare. Rudolph Virchow (1821–1905), however, denied the syphilitic character of the Indian bones and advanced the theory that the damage resulted from the elements and insects.

Whether syphilis existed in Europe prior to 1493 is a problem for medical historians. The answer may lie in the middle of the two schools of thought. Syphilis could have existed but in a much milder form than the virulent type introduced into the populace upon the return of Columbus.

Syphilis — World Traveler

From the waterfronts of Portugal and Spain, syphilis began an uninterrupted worldwide journey. In 1494, ably assisted by the mercenary army of Charles VIII of France, syphilis traveled across Italy to Naples. Throughout the Italian campaign, infected female camp-followers maintained sexual contact between the two opposing camps, spreading syphilis to friends and foes alike.

Following defeat in 1495 in the Naples campaign, the French and Spanish mercenaries disbanded and spread the "red plague," also known as the "great pox," throughout Europe.

Syphilis was reported in Germany, Switzerland, and Greece in 1495. A year later, cases of the disease appeared in Paris and the Netherlands, and records indicate that it was carried from France to England in 1498. Within a half dozen years, syphilis had succeeded in casting its shadow over Europe. The Renaissance was not only a period of marching armies but also a time of exploration. In 1498, Portuguese explorers took syphilis with them to India; Spanish sailors infected Filipinos with "na-na" (syphilis), and in 1505, the disease had appeared in China.

In 1646, John Winthrop (Connecticut) wrote in his diary of the appearance of a "loathsome disease" (lues venera) among the inhabitants of "one of the towns." Within a short time, the disease was transmitted to the Indians. Syphilis, world traveler, had come home to America.

The disease in America was not restricted to any one geographical area. The various races and ethnic groups "moved with the tide of a growing country; syphilis traveled west in wagon trains and in ships." American trading vessels visited many Pacific islands during the 1800s, carrying syphilis with them. The natives of New Zealand, according to one observer, "were helpless against syphilis." "Babies lived for only a short while, and adults wasted away, a curse against the whites on their lips," for introducing the "merlike" (American) disease to the South Seas.

Syphilis — A Name

For nearly 40 years following the return of Columbus to Spain, syphilis masqueraded under many names. In scientific publications, it was known as the great pox. It was also known as the German pox, the Portuguese disease, the Polish illness, the Castilian infection, and the French disease; the Turks, remembering the Crusades, named it the disease of the Christians. However, Morbus Gallicus gradually became the term generally used.

In 1530, an Italian poet, physician, and astronomer (Girolamo Fracastoro) brought an end to name calling with the publication of a poem "Syphilis sive Morbus Gallicus" (Syphilis or the French Disease). This poetical treatise in Latin hexameters told the story of a shepherd named Syphilus who built an altar to his king and worshiped him. The ire of the Sun god was aroused at this sacrilege and he caused a plague to descend upon the land. The disease which destroyed Syphilus was named for its first victim. The poem was widely read and the word syphilis became associated with the disease. It is ironic that Fracastoro should gain lasting fame through his poem and little or no recognition for what is considered the first textbook on communicable disease, "De Contagicone et Contagiosis Morbis" (1546).

Syphilis — The High and Mighty

Of all the diseases known, few made a greater impact on the lives of men or on the course of history.

Some historians feel that Columbus was afflicted with syphilis and died from paresis at the age of 55 in 1506. (Knowledge that he had been infected might account for his failure to log the appearance of the disease among his crew.) Syphilis did not distinguish between the high and the low. The monarch as well as commoner was a victim.

In his frantic desire for a male heir to the throne, Henry VIII (1509–1547), who was infected with syphilis prior to his first marriage, searched industriously for a noninfected wife. When the Church of Rome refused to sanction his divorce from Catherine of Aragon, Henry countered by renouncing Catholicism and establishing the Church of England headed by himself. Despite this drastic move, historians speculate that of his six wives, only Anne of Cleves might possibly have had a negative serology. The progeny of Henry were undoubtedly syphilitic. Mary Tudor (Bloody Mary, 1516–1558), Edward VI (1537–1553), and Elizabeth I (1533–1603) manifested signs of congenital syphilis in various degrees. The deaths of Mary and Edward, attributed to syphilis by many authorities, opened the door to the reign of Elizabeth and an era of English greatness.

Contemporary with Henry, the reign of Francis I of France was a striking example of chaos befalling a nation when its ruler was afflicted with an insanity arising from syphilis. Francis ulitmately ascended the throne only because syphilitic Charles VIII left no heirs.

Syphilis — Early Concepts

Perhaps because the disease had been unknown among some of the population groups, syphilis struck with the power of lightning. As contagious as smallpox, it spread through the ordinary process of living. Patients ran high fevers and experienced intense headaches, bone and joint pains, prostration, and, frequently, early death.

Despite the seriousness of the disease, the view of the populace was light hearted. During the Restoration period, numerous comedies made humorous reference to it. "A pox on you" was a frequently heard expression in all levels of society. Casanova delighted in weaving syphilis into the pattern of his many stories.

In an attempt to relate the events of their time with those of bygone ages, physicians searched fruitlessly through ancient texts. Failure to uncover information about syphilis led to erroneous conclusions often tinged with mysticism.

In 1496, Theodore Ulsenius, City Physician of Nuremberg, issued a handbill, illustrated by Albrecht Dürer, explaining that the syphilis epidemic was due to the conjunction of Jupiter and Saturn in 1484. This document contains the first illustration on the subject of syphilis, appropriately the figure of a soldier. By way of contrasting the ignorance shown through an acceptance of the mystical cause of syphilis, physicians reflected an alertness concerning means of spread.

In 1496, the French Parliament passed a decree that a syphilitic should not leave his home until cured and that infected foreigners should be forced to leave the city within 24 hours.

In 1497, the town council of Aberdeen in Scotland ordered that all night women desist from their vice and venery and work for their support. Later in the same year, the Privy Council ordered all afflicted people into banishment on an island near Leith. Most physicians were well acquainted with syphilis by 1520 and understood its venereal transmission.

Among the earliest drugs used in the treatment of syphilis were purgatives and antitoxins such as theriaca and mithridatium. The insistence that syphilis was a New World disease led physicians in that direction for a cure. The supposition that a cure existed in the New World was based upon the precept that "Divine Providence mercifully provides the antidote or remedy for a disease so inflicted, at the place where the disease originates or among people so inflicted." Of the cures introduced from the New World, quaiacum, or "holy wood," was the most popular. Among the first to recommend holy wood was Nicholas Pol, physician to Charles V (1519–1556), who reported that many Spaniards had been "cured" by the drug. Mercury, which had been used for centuries by the Arabs for scabies, was introduced in 1496 as a treatment for syphilis.

Historians, in describing the indiscriminate use of mercury, point to the ladies of the court who were rarely without their small jeweled "mercury pots" and who, during the course of the day, would frequently retire to privacy for a daub or two of salve.

Unfortunately, no one knew of the risks attached to the continued use of mercury. It was almost as dangerous to the patient as the disease. Yet, despite the agonies associated with overuse, mercury continued as an antisyphilitic for almost four centuries.

Progress in syphilis research during several hundred years was steady, if not spectacular. Ambroise Paré (1517–1590), "Father of French Surgery," introduced the vaginal speculum and observed the indolence of the syphilitic bubo, the induration of the primary syphilitic lesion, and concomitant adenopathy. Fernal (1497–1558) observed that the "syphilitic virus" had to pass through a skin erosion. Fallopius (1563) differentiated between syphilitic and nonsyphilitic condylomata. Morgagni (1682–1722) described syphilis of the viscera, lungs, bones, and the circulatory system. Though syphilis was early recognized as a disease different from gonorrhea, the distinction was twice lost by "experts." First, it was Paracelsus (1493–1541) who, in the 16th century, called syphilis "the French gonorrhea." Later, in the 18th century, an English physician, John Hunter (1728–1793), "proved" that gonorrhea and syphilis were the same disease by inoculating himself with gonorrhea pus and promptly contracting syphilis. The true explanation that the patient happened to have both diseases never occurred to Hunter. So great was Hunter's stature in the medical world that his erroneous conclusions were immediately acclaimed. Venereal disease research then veered along the wrong path for the next half century.

Syphilis — Clinical and Therapeutic Progress

Albert Neisser discovered the organism of gonorrhea in 1879; Augusto Ducrey had demonstrated the organisms of chancroid in 1889, thus clearing several roadblocks which had been impeding progress in the study of syphilis. In 1905, Fritz Schaudin and Paul Erick Hoffman electrified the world with their discovery of the causative agent of syphilis.[*] Hoffman described the treponeme of syphilis as the "pale spirochete" because it required special darkfield illumination to make it visible. Two years before, Elie Metchnikoff and Pierre Roux, while associated with the Pasteur Institute, became the first to inoculate successfully an animal with syphilis.

With the groundwork laid by Jules Bordet and Octave Gengou in 1901, Wassermann, Neisser, and Bruck developed a blood test for the diagnosis of syphilis in 1905. In the intervening 50 years, the Wassermann test has been modified many times. Probably the best known and most widely used modification today is the VDRL (Venereal Disease Research Laboratory test). An additional test (Treponema pallidum immobilization test) lending support to the differential diagnosis was developed in 1949 through the efforts of Nelson and Mayer.

Paul Ehrlich, discoverer of the first specific treatment for syphilis in 1907, followed his numerous efforts to modify an organic compound of arsenic (Atoxyl), and with the 606th combination produced arsenobenzol or Salvarsan. While his "magic bullet" (often called 606) which was to cure syphilis with one injection fell short of the mark, his contribution marked the first hope to millions of infected people. This was the period of therapeutic advancement. In 1917, Wagner von Jauregg introduced fever therapy in the treatment of paresis. In 1921, Sazerac and Levaditi introduced bismuth, a therapy first suggested by Sauton and Robert in 1916.

In time, a growing variety of more effective and less toxic arsenic compounds employed with bismuth became available for the treatment of syphilis, and by the time Dr. John Mahoney of the United States Public Health Service (1943) first reported four syphilis patients treated with penicillin (discovered by Fleming in 1928), the conquest of the disease had already reached a point where most patients could be made rapidly noninfectious and the disease virtually eradicated over a period of a year or two.

---

*In 1837, the Frenchman Donne saw corkscrew-like organisms in matter taken from the initial sores of syphilis. He advanced the hypothesis that they were the cause of syphilis. A few years later, however, he withdrew his hypothesis.

The continued use and evaluation of penicillin and other broad-spectrum antibiotics over the succeeding several decades established therapy other than arsenicals and bismuth as drugs of choice. Especially beneficial were the shorter period of treatment and the higher percentage of cures arising from penicillin therapy.

Syphilis — The Rise and Fall of the Tide

Although Ehrlich's discovery proved effective in the therapeutic management of syphilis, control and public awareness were slow in coming.

The banter associated with syphilis during the Reformation period had disappeared, mention of the disease was but a whisper, the subject in the early part of the twentieth century was taboo. The occasional lone voice seeking to enlighten an ignorant populace was quickly stilled. In 1908, a pamphlet conservatively discussing the venereal disease problem was prepared by the Public Health Service. The Secretary of the Treasury expressed his disapproval of the pamphlet with the statement, "The matter contained in this bulletin is not in keeping with the dignity of the fiscal department of government."

Despite this thinking on the national level, several states moved to cope with the problem. In 1912, California established a law requiring physicians to report venereal disease, and by 1917 other states had adopted similar measures. In World War I, because venereal disease, especially syphilis, cost the Army millions of service days, the problem could no longer be ignored. In 1918, with the passage of the Chamberlain-Kahn Act and the appropriation of several million dollars, the Public Health Service assisted states in carrying out control programs.

Following this heroic beginning, little concerted effort was expended on control for almost two decades. It was not until 1936, with the publication of Surgeon-General Thomas Parran's "Shadow on the Land," that the wall of silence was pierced. In that year, a program of public education was launched and continued in spite of protests. With the passage of the National Venereal Disease Control Act in 1938, which authorized financial assistance to states, venereal disease control assumed a new and significant stature.

With treatment a success, and with momentum gained through case finding activities, man's dream of eradication after centuries of fruitless conflict appeared a certainty. For over a decade, the trend of syphilis was ever downward; from 575,593 cases in 1943 to 122,075 in 1955. In 1956, the dream was shattered with the reporting of an increase over the previous year.

Many factors, including under-reporting and lack of intensive epidemiology and education, undoubtedly contributed to the continued increase of syphilis in the years following 1956. These flaws in control programs appeared as a result of apathy which followed the over-optimism brought about by the effectiveness of antibiotic drugs in the treatment of syphilis and gonorrhea. The result was public apathy and de-emphasis of control programs. Decreased appropriations for the support of control programs followed as a natural consequence. In effect, a program rather than a disease was eradicated.

Today the forces of public health continue to be dedicated to the eradication of syphilis. Aggressive case finding and reporting methods, along with improved public education, have resulted in a stabilization of the incidence of newly reported cases of syphilis during 1974. The next step is to accelerate efforts to decrease the incidence rate until the disease is eradicated.

References

Parran, Thomas: "Shadow on the Land," 1937
Van Wyck, William: "The Sinister Shepherd" (Fracastoro), 1934
Pusey, W. A.: "The History and Epidemiology of Syphilis," 1939
Holcomb, R.C.: "Who Gave the World Syphilis," 1937
"Hieronymus Fracastoro's Syphilis" The Philmar Company, 1911

References

Alford, C. A., Poll, S. S., Cassady, G., Straumfjord, J. U., and Remington, J. S., Jr.: M-fluorescent antibody in diagnosis of congenital syphilis. N. Engl. J. Med. *28:*1086, 1969.

Caldwell, J. R.: The immunologic consequences of infection. *In* Cluff, L. E., and Johnson, J. E. (eds.): Clinical Concepts of Infectious Diseases. Baltimore, Williams and Wilkins Co., 1972.

D'Alessandro, G., and Dardanom, J.: Isolation and purification of the protein antigen of the Reiter treponeme. Am. J. Syph. Gonor. Ven. Dis. *37:*137, 1953.

Deacon, W. E., Falcone, V. H., and Harris, A.: A fluorescent test for treponemal antibodies. Proc. Soc. Exp. Biol. Med. *96:*477, 1957.

Deacon, W. E., Lucas, J. B., and Price, E. V.: Fluorescent treponemal antibody-absorption (FTA-ABS) test for syphilis. J.A.M.A. *198:*624, 1966.

Duncan, W. P., Jenkins, T. W., and Parham, C. E.: Fluorescent treponenal antibody-cerebrospinal fluid (FTA-CSF) test: A provisional technique. Br. J. Vener. Dis. *48:*97, 1972.

Duncan, W. P., Knox, J. M., and Wende, R. D.: The FTA-ABS test in darkfield-positive primary syphilis. J.A.M.A. *228:*859, 1974.

Hunter, E. F., Deacon, W. E., and Meyer, P. E.: An improved FTA test for syphilis. The absorption procedure (FTA-ABS). Public Health Rep. *79:*5, 1964.

Kaufman, R. E., Olansky, D. C., and Wiesner, P. J.: The FTA:ABS (IgM) test for neonatal congenital syphilis: A critical review. J. Am. Ven. Dis. Assoc. *1:*79, 1975.

Kraus, S. J., Haserick, J. R., and Lantz, M. A.: Fluorescent treponemal antibody-absorption test reactions in lupus erythematosus. N. Engl. J. Med. *282:*1287, 1970.

Logan, L. C., and Cox, P. M.: Evaluation of a quantitative automated microhemagglutination assay for antibodies to *Treponema pallidum*. Am. J. Clin. Pathol. *53:*163, 1970.

Moore, M. B., and Knox, J. M.: Sensitivity and specificity in syphilis serology: Clinical implications. South. Med. J. *58:*963, 1965.

Nelson, R. A., Jr., and Mayer, M. M.: Immobilization of *Treponema pallidum* in vitro by antibody produced in syphilitic infection, J. Exp. Med. *89:*369, 1949.

Pangborn, M. C.: A new serologically active phospholipid from beef heart. Proc. Soc. Exp. Biol. Med. *48:*484, 1941.

Rockwell, D. H., et. al.: The Tuskegee study of untreated syphilis. Arch. Intern. Med. *114:*792, 1963.

Chapter 30

DIAGNOSIS AND TREATMENT OF GONORRHEA

Introduction

Gonorrhea is an infectious disease primarily involving the genitourinary tract. The disease is caused by the small gram negative diplococcus *Neisseria gonorrhoeae,* which is an extracellular parasite whose only natural host is man. Transmission is most commonly by some form of sexual contact, and infection usually occurs in the more sexually active age groups. Severe infections involving the eyes can develop in the newborn who become infected during passage through the birth canal.

The number of reported cases of gonorrhea in the United States has increased sharply during the past five years, and it is now alleged that the disease is occurring at "epidemic" proportions. Although better than 900,000 cases were reported during 1974, estimates of the true annual incidence of the disease range up to 2,500,000 cases. Many patients with gonorrhea are treated by nonphysicians or by physicians who do not report the case. The true incidence of the disease in the past and the present remains unknown (Fig. 30–1).

The acute disease is manifested by a purulent urethritis in the male and may or may not be associated with symptoms of urethritis or vaginal discharge in the female (Fig. 30–2). Thirty per cent of females with positive cultures and physical findings consistent with active gonorrhea are asymptomatic. The significance of an infection with gonorrhea lies more in the potential complications following acute infection than in the discomfort of the purulent urethritis. In the male, urethral stricture, chronic prostatitis, and occasionally septic arthritis or tenosynovitis are sequelae if the disease is not recognized and treated promptly.

In women, the complications may be more serious, particularly if the patient is unaware of her infection. Ascending infection involving the uterine tubes and ovaries may result in pelvic inflammatory disease which produces a chronic, debilitating infection that can cause partial or complete obliteration of the patency of the uterine tubes. If the lumen of the uterine tubes is

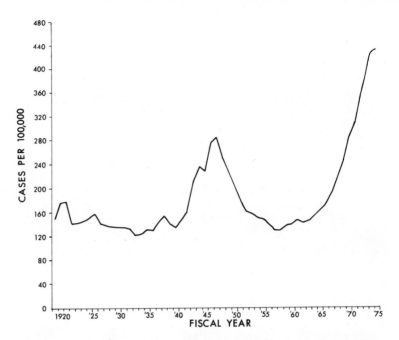

Figure 30–1. Reported cases of gonorrhea in the United States for the fiscal years 1919–1974. (Modified from Center for Disease Control, Morbidity and Mortality Weekly Report, Annual Supplement, July, 1973.)

completely closed, the patient is unable to become pregnant. If infection causes partial obstruction or stenosis of the tubes, there is a possibility that a feritilized ovum may become trapped in a pocket of the mucosal septa, resulting in an ectopic gestation. Rupture, necessitating surgical removal of the tube, may occur. Another complication of gonorrhea, acute suppurative arthritis, is more likely to develop in women; in fact, three of every four cases occur in females.

Recently, several syndromes resulting from acute gonococcal infections have become increasingly apparent owing to renewed interest in case finding and the development of more sensitive techniques for isolation and identification of the causative organism. Among these syndromes are acute gonococcal endocarditis, acute leptomeningitis, and acute pharyngitis, supposedly associated in both males and females with the practice of fellatio. The incidence of gonococcal pharyngitis in those practicing cunnilingus is not significant, presumably owing to the fact that the site of infection in females is considered to be more often in the endocervical canal than in the urethra or Bartholin's glands.

Diagnosis

Culture

The diagnosis of gonorrhea, in contrast to that of syphilis, a condition in which the microorganism cannot be recovered and grown in artificial culture,

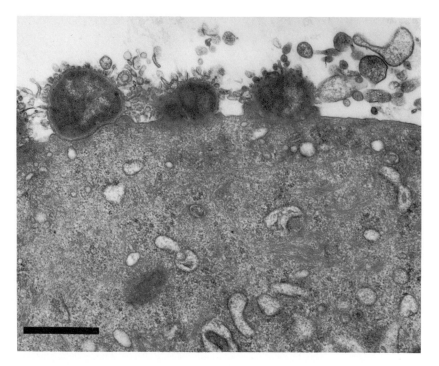

Figure 30–2. Electron micrograph showing gonococci closely attached to the surface of a urethral epithelial cell. The membrane of the host cell appears pushed up around the gonococcus to form cushionlike structures. The bar represents 500 nm (X 46,000). (From Ward, M. E., and Watt, P. J.: Adherence of Neisseria gonorrhoeae to urethral mucosal cells: an electron-microscopic study of human gonorrhea. J. Infect. Dis. 126:601, 1972. The University of Chicago Press, © 1972 by the Journal of Infectious Diseases.)

depends on culture and identification of the microorganism. A significant aid toward improving the isolation of the microorganism has been the development of a selective culture medium which suppresses the growth of contaminating microorganisms that might otherwise overgrow and mask the appearance of *Neisseria gonorrhoeae*. This culture medium has unofficially been given the name of the two men who developed it — James D. Thayer and John E. Martin — and is frequently called Thayer-Martin (TM) medium. The medium is composed of chocolate agar containing a long, carefully compounded list of vitamins and cofactors and was originally made using the antibiotics ristocetin and polymyxin. Several years after the development of the medium, ristocetin was withdrawn from the market because of toxicity to humans, and the antibiotics used in the medium were changed to vancomycin, colistin, and nystatin (VCN). Currently, the terms *Thayer-Martin (TM)* and *VCN* refer to the same culture medium for the selective isolation of both *Neisseria gonorrhoeae* and *Neisseria meningitidis*.

The Venereal Disease Research Laboratory has recently introduced a modification of the VCN medium, adding trimethoprim, a sulfa-like compound found to inhibit certain strains of Proteus that are resistant to vancomycin, colistin, and nystatin. The modified medium is poured into a small prescription bottle and capped under an atmosphere of 10 per cent carbon dioxide. Culture may be taken and placed directly on this medium for transport by messenger or mail to central processing laboratories. This latest modification of selective culture media for *Neisseria gonorrhoeae* is called "Transgrow" and is commercially available for use in clinics and physicians' offices. The medium is complex, and problems in producing it in large quantity have resulted in some irregularity in quality. The medium may be stored in a refrigerator at 4°C until it is used but it is important that it be warmed to either room temperature or preferably 35 to 37°C before inoculation. *N. gonorrhoeae* is very sensitive to cold temperatures and will be killed if inoculated to medium just removed from a refrigerator. (For details of obtaining culture for gonorrhea, see Table 30–1.)

TABLE 30–1. Technique for Culture of Gonorrhea*

I. Obtain Culture Specimen

Women

1. Endocervical canal – the best site to culture
   a. Moisten speculum with warm water; do *not* use any other lubricant.
   b. Remove cervical mucus, preferably with a cotton ball held in ring forceps.
   c. Insert sterile cotton-tipped swab into endocervical canal; move from side to side; allow 10 to 30 seconds for absorption of organisms to the swab.

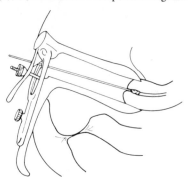

Endocervical Culture Site

2. Anal canal – also called "rectal culture"
   Note: This specimen can easily be obtained without using an anoscope.
   a. Insert sterile cotton-tipped swab approximately one inch into the anal canal. (If the swab is inadvertently pushed into feces, use another swab to obtain specimen.)
   b. Move swab from side to side in the anal canal to sample crypts; allow 10 to 30 seconds for absorption of organisms to the swab.

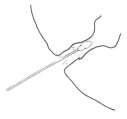

Anal Canal Culture Site

Table continued on the following page

TABLE 30-1. Technique for Culture of Gonorrhea* *(Continued)*

---

3. Urethral or vaginal cultures – indicated when the cervical culture is unsatisfactory; e.g., hysterectomy patients and children.
   a. Urethral
      1. Strip the urethra toward the orifice to express exudate.
      2. Use sterile loop or cotton swab to obtain specimen.
   b. Vaginal
      1. Use speculum to obtain specimen from the posterior vaginal vault, or obtain specimen from the vaginal orifice if the hymen is intact.

Men

1. Urethral culture – indicated when Gram-stain of urethral exudate is not positive, in tests-of-cure, or as test for asymptomatic urethral infection.
   a. Use sterile bacteriologic wire loop to obtain specimen from anterior urethra by gently scraping the mucosa. An alternative to the loop is a sterile synthetic swab (*Calgiswab*) that is easily inserted into the urethra.
2. Anal canal culture – These can be taken in the same manner as for women.

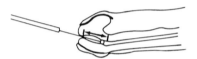

Anterior Urethral Culture

II. Inoculate Thayer-Martin Medium or Transgrow Medium

1. Medium should be at room temperature prior to inoculation.
2. *Do not place* inoculated culture medium in the refrigerator or expose to extreme temperatures.

Thayer-Martin Plates

A. Roll swab directly on Thayer-Martin (TM) medium in a large "Z" pattern.
B. Cross-streak immediately with a sterile wire loop, preferably in the clinic. If not done previously, cross-streaking should be done in the laboratory.

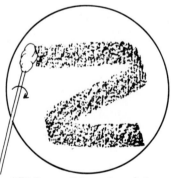

"Z" Pattern Primary Inoculation

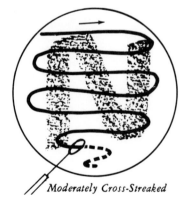

Moderately Cross-Streaked

C. Place culture in a candle jar or CO_2 incubator within 15 minutes. Be sure to relight the candle each time candle jar is reopened.
D. Begin incubation of plates the same day (but the sooner the better) at 35° to 36°C.

TABLE 30-1. Technique for Culture of Gonorrhea* *(Continued)*

Transgrow Bottles

A. Inoculate specimens on the surface of Transgrow medium as follows:

Caution: KEEP NECK OF BOTTLE IN UPRIGHT POSITION TO PREVENT CO_2 LOSS

1. Remove cap of bottle only when ready to inoculate medium.
2. Soak up all excess moisture in bottle with specimen swab and then roll swab from side to side across medium, starting at the bottom of the bottle.
3. Tightly cap the bottle immediately to prevent loss of CO_2.

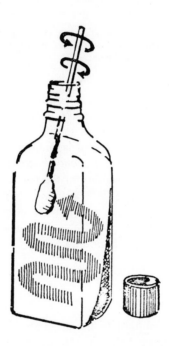

B. When possible, incubate the Transgrow bottle in an upright position at 35°-36°C for 16–18 hours before sending to the laboratory and note this on accompanying request form. Resultant growth usually survives prolonged transport and is ready for identification upon arrival at the laboratory. (If an incubator is not available, store culture at room temperature [25°C or above] for 16–18 hours before subjecting it to prolonged transport and extreme temperatures.)
C. Package the *incubated* Transgrow culture and request form in a suitable container to prevent breakage and immediately transport to a central bacteriologic laboratory by postal service or other convenient means.
D. At the laboratory, preincubated Transgrow bottles will be examined immediately for *Neisseria gonorrhoeae;* other bottles will be incubated at 35°-36°C for 24–48 hours and examined.

Special Considerations

The storage life of Thayer-Martin medium at room temperature is two weeks. Preliminary evaluation indicates storage life of Transgrow medium at room temperature is approximately three months.

Table continued on the following page

TABLE 30-1. Technique for Culture of Gonorrhea* *(Continued)*

General Considerations

Transgrow, a selective medium for the transport and cultivation of *N. gonorrhoeae,* is only recommended when specimens cannot be delivered to the laboratory or incubator on the day they are taken. On the other hand, TM plates are used when there is daily access to a laboratory. Transgrow medium under 10% CO_2 atmosphere in bottles promotes growth of pathogenic *Neisseria* and suppresses contaminating organisms similarly to Thayer-Martin medium in plates. Transgrow medium maintains viability of pathogenic *Neisseria* for more than 48 hours at room temperature. Validity of culture results depends on proper techniques for obtaining, inoculating and handling specimens.

*From the United States Department of Health, Education, and Welfare, Public Health Service, Center for Disease Control, Bureau of State Services, Venereal Disease Branch, Atlanta, Georgia.

Although selective media have made isolation and culture of the gonococcus considerably easier than in the past, there still remains a significant problem in getting individual strains to perform in a reproducible manner in the clinical laboratory. Wide variation in the ability of different strains of *Neisseria gonorrhoeae* to grow on artificial media has led to variability in recovery of the microorganism in different clinical laboratories. In the spring of 1972, a strain of *N. gonorrhoeae* was sent to over 300 federal, state, municipal, and private hospital laboratories as an unknown. The microorganism was properly identified by less than one half of the participating laboratories.

Serologic Tests

In contrast to the diagnosis of syphilis, serologic tests have not been of significant help in the diagnosis of gonorrhea. Hemagglutination and immunofluorescent tests have been developed and are undergoing evaluation. Initial studies have shown that both procedures have suffered from an excessive incidence of both false positive and apparent false negative reactions. A study of three different immunologic parameters, (1) serum immunoglobulins, (2) urethral secretory antibodies, and (3) lymphocytic blastogenic response in patients with first and multiple infections, suggests that all of these combined responses are insufficient for protection from recurrent disease.

Asymptomatic Gonorrhea

As mentioned previously, up to 30 per cent of women who are shown to be culture positive for *Neisseria gonorrhoeae* from the endocervix, vagina, or rectum are asymptomatic and constitute a reservoir of potential disease, either as a further complication to themselves or their sexual partners. Gonorrhea in the male is usually manifested by acute urethritis and occasionally tenosynovitis or arthritis. Asymptomatic infection in the male has not been a recognized source of infection. In a study resulting from the epidemiologic investigation of the sexual partners of women with symptomatic gonorrhea, it was found recently that 40 per cent of asymptomatic males were culture positive for *N. gonorrhoeae*. The microorganisms were recovered more commonly from the anterior urethra by fine calcium alginate swabs than from prostatic secretions.

In a study of over 2600 sexually active soldiers either returned from Vietnam or stationed at a base in the United States, the incidence of urethral carriage of *Neisseria gonorrhoeae* in males was found to be 2.2 per cent. Sixty-eight per cent of this group were asymptomatic (see Table 30–2). Confirming earlier studies, the incidence of resistance to penicillin and tetracyclines was significantly greater in the isolates from soldiers who had returned from Vietnam (see Fig. 30–3). It has now been established that both asymptomatically infected men and asymptomatically infected women constitute a reservoir of *N. gonorrhoeae* and represent a major factor in the current gonorrhea pandemic.

TABLE 30–2. Prevalence of Positive Urethral Cultures for *N. gonorrhoeae* among 2628 Sexually Active Enlisted Men Returned from Vietnam or Stationed at Fort Lewis*

	Vietnam	Fort Lewis	Total
No. examined	1,787	841	2,628
No. infected	45(2.5%)	14(1.7%)	59(2.2%)
Symptomatic	17(0.9%)	2(0.2%)	19(0.7%)
Asymptomatic	28(1.6%)	12(1.4%)	40(1.5%)**

*From Handsfield, H. H., Lipman, T. O., et al.: Asymptomatic gonorrhea in men: Diagnosis, natural course and prevalence. N. Engl. J. Med. *290:*117, 1974.

**Of 40 men who denied symptoms, scant urethral exudate was detected on examination in 15.

Treatment

Since the late 1930s, when sulfa drugs were first used in the chemotherapy of meningitis and gonorrhea, it has been noted that *Neisseria gonorrhoeae* slowly develops resistance to most antimicrobial agents. Although penicillin has been effective against most strains, the increasing number of resistant isolates has made it desirable to continuously monitor the level of resistance in freshly isolated strains (Figs. 30–3 and 30–4).

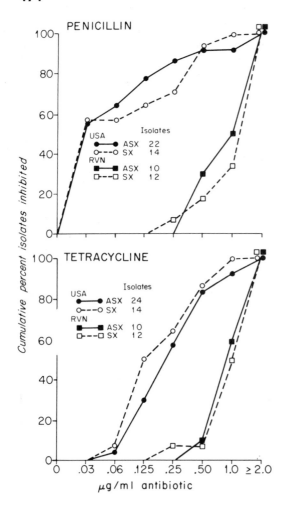

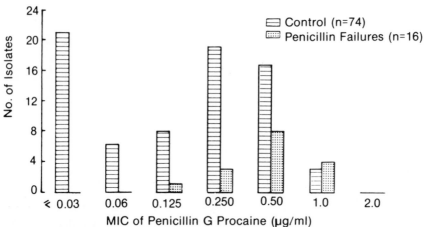

Figure 30–3. Cumulative percentage of gonococcal isolates from asymptomatic (ASX) and symptomatic (SX) infections acquired in the United States (USA) and in Vietnam (RVN) that were inhibited by increasing concentrations of penicillin G and tetracycline hydrochloride. (From Handsfield, H. H., Lipman, T. O. et al.: Asymptomatic gonorrhea in men: Diagnosis, natural course and prevalence. N. Engl. J. Med. *290:*117, 1974. Reprinted by permission of the New England Journal of Medicine.)

Figure 30–4. Distribution of minimal inhibitory concentration (MIC) of penicillin G for *N gonorrhoeae* isolated before treatment from penicillin G treatment failures (failure demonstrated two to seven days after treatment) and from control patients. (From Petersen, A. H. B., Wiesner, P. J., Holmes, K. H., Johnson, C. J., and Turck, M.: Spectinomycin and penicillin G in the treatment of gonorrhea. J.A.M.A. *220:*205, 1972, Copyright 1972, American Medical Association.)

Despite evidence of increasing resistance of *Neisseria gonorrhoeae* to antimicrobial agents, penicillin or the closely related ampicillin appears to be the most effective antibiotic agent against gonorrhea. By administering 1 gm of probenecid orally 30 minutes to one hour prior to giving ampicillin, a higher and more sustained blood level will result, increasing the time the microorganism is exposed to the drug. In Figure 30–5, the cure rate of gonococcal urethritis in males given 3500 mg of ampicillin alone was 71.7 per cent, while the cure rate when the same amount of ampicillin was given with probenicid was 96 per cent. Measurement of the area under the curve for ampicillin with probenecid (224.18 µg per hour) was more than 50 per cent greater than for ampicillin alone (147.35 µg per hour). This means that any gonococcus will be exposed to a significantly higher concentration of ampicillin over a more prolonged period of time.

The introduction of spectinomycin, a new aminoglycoside antibiotic for use solely in the treatment of gonorrhea, provided an additional drug for patients with drug-resistant strains. It is reported that spectinomycin is not effective in the therapy of gonorrheal pharyngitis.

Table 30–3 lists the treatment results obtained during a 21-month gonorrhea therapy monitoring study sponsored by the United States Public Health Service. A total of 1608 men and 1135 women were treated by one of four different therapeutic regimens and then reexamined with cultures for tests of cure 3 to 13 days following treatment. Oral probenecid given 30 minutes before penicillin did not result in a significant improvement in cure rates over probenecid given at the same time as the penicillin. Geographic variation in cure rate occurred and was considered to reflect local strains of resistant gonococci. Penicillin seemed to elicit slightly better results than did ampicillin. The findings of this study have led to recommendations by the Public Health Service's Center for Disease Control for the treatment of gonorrhea. These recommendations for treatment are given in Table 30–4.

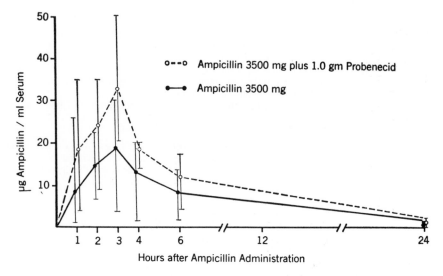

Figure 30–5. Serum values of ampicillin following a single oral dose. (From Kvale, P. A., Keys, T. F., Johnson, D. W., and Holmes, K. K.: Single oral dose ampicillin-probenecid treatment of gonorrhea in the male. J.A.M.A. *215:*1449, 1971. Copyright 1970, American Medical Association.)

TABLE 30–3. Treatment Results from National Gonorrhea Therapy Monitoring Study*

Regimen	Number of Patients Reexamined	Number of Patients Cured (%)
Aqueous procaine penicillin 4.8 mu IM + probenecid 1.0 gm p.o.	1292	1235 (95.7)
Ampicillin 3.5 gms + probenecid 1.0 gm p.o.	614	569 (92.7)
Tetracycline 9.0 gms p.o.	111	107 (96.4)
Spectinomycin 4.0 or 2.0 gms IM	726	690 (95.0)

*From the United States Department of Health, Education, and Welfare, Public Health Service, Center for Disease Control, Atlanta, Georgia.

TABLE 30–4. Gonorrhea — Recommended Treatment Schedules*

Note: Physicians are cautioned to use no less than the recommended dosages of antibiotics.

Uncomplicated Gonococcal Infections in Men and Women

Drug Regimen of Choice

Aqueous procaine penicillin G (APPG) 4.8 million units intramuscularly divided into at least 2 doses and injected at different sites at one visit, together with 1 gm of probenecid by mouth just before the injections.

Alternative Regimens

A. Patients in whom oral therapy is preferred:
   Ampicillin 3.5 gm by mouth, together with 1 gm probenecid by mouth administered at the same time. There is evidence that this regimen may be slightly less effective than the recommended APPG regimen.
B. Patients who are allergic to the penicillins or probenecid (i.e. allergy to penicillin, ampicillin, probenecid, or previous anaphylactic reaction);
   1. Tetracycline hydrochloride, 1.5 gm initially by mouth, followed by 0.5 gm by mouth 4 times per day for 4 days (total dosage 9.5 gm). Other tetracyclines are not more effective than tetracycline hydrochloride. All tetracyclines are ineffective as single-dose therapy.
   2. Spectinomycin hydrochloride, 2 gm intramuscularly in 1 injection.

Treatment of Sexual Partners

Men and women with known recent exposure to gonorrhea should receive the same treatment as those known to have gonorrhea. Male sex partners of persons with gonorrhea must be examined and treated because of the high prevalence of non-symptomatic urethral gonococcal infection in such men.

Follow-up

Follow-up urethral and other appropriate cultures should be obtained from men, and cervical, anal, and other appropriate cultures should be obtained from women, 7 to 14 days after completion of treatment.

Treatment Failures

Most recurrent infection after treatment with the recommended schedules is due to reinfection. True treatment failure after therapy with penicillin, ampicillin, or tetracycline should be treated with 2 gm of spectinomycin intramuscularly.

TABLE 30-4. Gonorrhea — Recommended Treatment Schedules* *(Continued)*

Postgonococcal Urethritis

Tetracycline 0.5 gm 4 times a day by mouth, for at least 7 days.

Pharyngeal Infection

Pharyngeal gonococcal infections may be more difficult to treat than anogenital gonorrhea. Posttreatment cultures are essential follow-up for pharyngeal infection. The schedules of ampicillin and spectinomycin recommended for anogenital gonorrhea are ineffective in pharyngeal gonorrhea. Patients whose infection is not eradicated after treatment with 4.8 million units of APPG plus 1 gm of probenecid may be treated with 9.5 gm of tetracycline in the dosage schedule outlined above (Alternative Regimens).

Syphilis

All patients with gonorrhea should have a serologic test for syphilis at the time of diagnosis. Seronegative patients without clinical signs of syphilis who are receiving the recommended parenteral penicillin schedule need not have follow-up serologic tests for syphilis. Patients treated with ampicillin, spectinomycin, or tetracycline should have a follow-up serologic test after 3 months to detect inadequately treated syphilis

Patients with gonorrhea who also have syphilis should be given additional treatment appropriate to the stage of syphilis.

Not Recommended

Although long-acting forms of penicillin (such as benzathine penicillin G) are effective in syphilotherapy, they have *no* place in the treatment of gonorrhea. Oral penicillin preparations such as penicillin V are not recommended for the treatment of gonococcal infection.

Treatment of Uncomplicated Gonorrhea in Pregnant Patients

A. For women who are not allergic to penicillin:
      Use the regimen of APPG plus probenecid or use ampicillin plus probenecid as defined above.
B. For pregnant patients who are allergic to penicillins (Note: there are several possible alternative regimens, each of which has potential disadvantages):
      1. Erythromycin, 1.5 gm orally, followed by 0.5 gm 4 times a day for 4 days for a total of 9.5 gm. This regimen is safe for mother and fetus, but its efficacy has not been established. Erythromycin estolate should not be used in patients with underlying liver disease.
      2. Cefazolin, 2 gm intramuscularly, with 1 gm of probenecid. Because of the possibility of cross-allergenicity between penicillins and cephalosporins, this regimen should not be used in patients with a history of penicillin anaphylaxis.
      3. Spectinomycin, 2 gm intramuscularly, is an effective dose, but safety for the fetus has not been established.

Contraindicated

Tetracycline should not be used for uncomplicated gonococcal infection in pregnant women because of potential toxic effects for mother and fetus.

Acute Salpingitis (Pelvic Inflammatory Disease)

The diagnosis of acute salpingitis should be considered in women with acute lower abdominal pain and adnexal tenderness on pelvic examination. Since there are no completely reliable clinical criteria on which to distinguish gonococcal from non-gonococcal salpingitis, endocervical cultures for *Neisseria gonorrhoeae* are essential in such patients. Therapy, however, should be initiated immediately, without waiting for the results of the cultures.

A. Hospitalization. It should be strongly considered for women with suspected salpingitis in these situations:
      1. Uncertain diagnosis, where surgical emergencies must be excluded
      2. Suspicion of pelvic abscess
      3. Pregnant patients with salpingitis

Table continued on the following page

TABLE 30–4. Gonorrhea — Recommended Treatment Schedules* *(Continued)*

---

    4. Inability of the patient to follow an outpatient regimen of oral medication, especially because of nausea and vomiting

    5. Failure to respond to outpatient therapy

B. Antimicrobial Agents. Controlled studies of the treatment of acute salpingitis are not available. Initial management must *at least* be adequate for gonococcal salpingitis. These regimens are known to be adequate for the treatment of gonococcal salpingitis:

    1. Outpatients

        a. 1.5 gm tetracycline hydrochloride given as a single oral loading dose, followed by 500 mg taken orally 4 times a day for 10 days.

        b. APPG 4.8 million units intramuscularly, divided into at least 2 doses and injected at different sites at one visit *or* 3.5 gm of oral ampicillin. One gm of oral probenecid is given along with either penicillin or ampicillin, and both are followed by 500 mg of ampicillin taken orally 4 times a day for 10 days.

    2. Hospitalized patients

        a. Aqueous crystalline penicillin G 20 million units given intravenously each day until *clear-cut* improvement occurs, followed by 500 mg of ampicillin taken orally 4 times a day to complete 10 days of therapy. The need for additional or alternative antibiotics for the treatment of nongonococcal salpingitis requires further study. Since it is impossible to distinguish gonococcal from nongonococcal salpingitis clinically, many physicians also use an aminoglycoside in addition to penicillin and/or antibiotics which are effective against *Bacteroides fragilis* as initial therapy.

        b. Tetracycline hydrochloride 500 mg, given intravenously 4 times a day until improvement occurs, followed by 500 mg taken orally 4 times a day to complete 10 days of therapy. This regimen should not be used for pregnant women or for patients with renal failure.

    3. Failure to improve on the recommended regimens does not necessarily indicate the need for stepwise additional antibiotics, but requires reassessment of the possibility of other diagnoses and of the specific microbial etiology.

C. The effect of the removal of an intrauterine device on the response of acute salpingitis to antimicrobial therapy and on the risk of recurrent salpingitis requires further study.

D. *Adequate treatment of women with acute gonococcal salpingitis must include examination and appropriate treatment of their male sex partners because of the high prevalence of nonsymptomatic urethral gonococcal infection in such men. Failure to treat male sex partners is a major cause of recurrent gonococcal salpingitis.*

E. Follow-up of patients with acute salpingitis is essential. All patients should receive repeat pelvic examinations and cultures for *N. gonorrhoeae* after treatment.

Disseminated Gonococcal Infection

A. Equally effective treatment schedule in the arthritis-dermatitis syndrome include:

    1. Aqueous crystalline penicillin G, 10 million units intravenously per day for 3 days or until there is significant clinical improvement. This may be followed with ampicillin, 500 mg 4 times a day orally to complete 7 days of antibiotic treatment.

    2. Ampicillin, 3.5 gm orally, plus probenecid 1 gm, followed by ampicillin, 500 mg 4 times a day orally for at least 7 days.

B. In penicillin- and/or probenecid-allergic patients:

    1. Tetracycline 1.5 gm orally followed by 500 mg 4 times a day orally for at least 7 days. Tetracycline should not be used for complicated gonococcal infection in pregnant women because of potential toxic effects for mother and fetus.

    2. Erythromycin 0.5 gm intravenously every 6 hours for at least 3 days.

C. Additional measures

    1. Hospitalization is indicated in patients who are unreliable, have uncertain diagnosis, or have purulent joint effusions or other complications.

    2. Immobilization of the affected joint(s) appears helpful. Repeated aspirations and saline irrigations appear beneficial, but controlled studies of these procedures have not been performed. Open drainage of joints other than the hip is now generally discouraged in patients with gonococcal arthritis.

TABLE 30-4. Gonorrhea – Recommended Treatment Schedules* *(Continued)*

3. Intra-articular injection of penicillin is unnecessary, since penicillin levels in the synovial fluid of inflamed joints approximate serum levels; furthermore, intra-articular injection per se may produce a toxic synovitis.

D. Meningitis and endocarditis due to the gonococcus require high-dose intravenous penicillin therapy (at least 10 million units per day) for longer periods: usually at least 10 days for meningitis and 3–4 weeks for endocarditis.

Gonococcal Infection in Pediatric Patients

Pediatric patients encompass those from birth to adolescence. When a child is postpubertal and/or over 100 pounds, he or she should be treated with dosage regimens as defined above for adults.

The efficacy of therapeutic regimens for uncomplicated and complicated gonococcal infections of childhood is unproven at present.

With gonococcal infection in children, the possibility of child abuse must be considered.

Prevention of Neonatal Infection

All pregnant women should have endocervical cultures examined for gonococci as an integral part of prenatal care.

Prevention of Gonococcal Ophthalmia

A. One percent silver nitrate (do not irrigate with saline, as this may reduce efficacy).
B. Ophthalmic ointments containing tetracycline, erythromycin, or neomycin are also probably effective.
C. *Not Recommended:* Bacitracin ointment (not effective) and penicillin drops (sensitizing).

Management of Infants Born to Mothers with Gonococcal Infection

Orogastric and rectal cultures should be taken from all patients. Blood cultures should be taken if septicemia is suspected. Aqueous crystalline penicillin G, 50,000 units/kg/day should be administered in 2 daily doses intravenously if cultures or Gram-stained smears reveal gonococci. The duration of therapy should be determined by clinical response. In suspected septicemia, an aminoglycoside should also be given.

Neonatal Disease

A. Gonococcal ophthalmia: Patient should be hospitalized. Antimicrobial agents: Aqueous crystalline penicillin G 50,000 units/kg/day in 2 or 3 doses intravenously for 7 days *plus* frequent saline irrigations and instillation of penicillin, tetracycline, or chloramphenicol eyedrops.
B. Complicated infection: Arthritis and septicemia should be treated by hospitalization and administration of aqueous crystalline penicillin G 75,000–100,000 units/kg/day in 4 doses or procaine penicillin G 75,000–100,000 units/kg/day in 2 doses for 7 days. Meningitis should be treated with aqueous crystalline penicillin G 100,000 units/kg/day, divided into 2 or 3 intravenous doses a day and continued for at least 10 days.

Childhood Disease

Gonococcal ophthalmia should be treated with hospitalization and by the administration of aqueous crystalline penicillin G intravenously 75,000–100,000 units/kg/day in 4 doses or procaine penicillin G intramuscularly 75,000–100,000 units/kg/day in 2 doses for 7 days *plus* saline irrigations and instillation of penicillin, tetracycline, or chloramphenicol eyedrops. Topical antibiotics *alone* are *not* recommended in therapy of gonococcal ophthalmitis. The source of the infection must be identified.

Uncomplicated vulvovaginitis and urethritis usually do not require hospitalization. Both may be treated at one visit with APPG 75,000–100,000 units/kg intramuscularly and probenecid 25 mg/kg by mouth. Topical and systemic estrogen therapy are of no benefit in vulvovaginitis. All patients should have follow-up cultures, and the source of infection should be identified, examined, and treated.

Table continued on the following page

TABLE 30-4. Gonorrhea — Recommended Treatment Schedules* *(Continued)*

Infection complicated by peritonitis or arthritis should be treated by hospitalization and administration of aqueous crystalline penicillin G intravenously 75,000–100,000 units/kg/day in 4 doses or procaine penicillin G 75,000–100,000 units/kg/day intramuscularly in 2 doses for 7 days.

Treatment of patients with allergy to penicillin: Patients under 6 years of age should be treated with erythromycin 40 mg/kg/day in 4 doses by mouth for 7 days for uncomplicated disease. Complicated disease should be treated with cephalothin 60–80 mg/kg/day in 4 doses intravenously for 7 days. Patients older than 6 may be treated with an oral regimen of tetracycline 25 mg/kg as an initial dose followed by 40–60 mg/kg/day in 4 doses for 7 days or an intravenous regimen of tetracycline 15–20 mg/kg/day in 4 doses for 7 days.

*From the United States Department of Health, Education, and Welfare, Public Health Service, Center for Disease Control, Atlanta, Georgia, 1974.

Historical Notes*

Unlike syphilis, which was melodramatic in its European appearance as well as in its spread and chronological progression, gonorrhea has infected man from time immemorial. One of the earliest descriptions of clinical gonorrhea appears in an Egyptian papyrus dating 3500 B.C., which prescribes plant extract to soothe painful micturition.

Translations from Mesopotamian tablets provide evidence that a discharge from the urethra described by Assyrian physicians was probably gonorrhea. A disease described in the Book of Leviticus as a "running issue" bears a similarity to gonorrhea. Moses, who may well have been the first public health officer, enjoined the strictest sanitary measures both for persons having an "issue" and for all persons who came into contact with him or articles he had used.

Early Romans translated "issue" into "fluxum feminis" (impure semen) thought by many historians to signify a gonorrheal discharge. Hippocrates, (377–450 B.C.) clearly defined the mode of transmission when he listed "excesses of the pleasure of Venus." Galen (130–210 A.D.), who gave the disease a name (gonos, seed: rhoia, flow), erroneously assumed the discharge to be an involuntary loss of semen.

Artistic representations uncovered on walls in the ruins of Pompeii associate Pompeian prostitutes with the genitourinary infections prevalent at the time.

Medical historians have identified descriptions of the extensive existence of the disease in writings of the Chinese, Arabs, and Hindus.

The recommendations of Hippocrates for the cure of "strangury" (painful urination) associated with gonorrhea were suppuration and free flow of pus.

Many early physicians recommended surgery to relieve gonorrhea. Many ascribed it to an accumulation of pus in the urinary tract or to an ulceration produced by overheated urine. Several physicians, Rhazes (850–923) and

*From the Washington State Department of Public Health.

Avicenna (980–1037) recommended the employment of sounds "to relieve strangury," Avenzoar (1094–1162) recommended injections of sea water and vinegar. John of Gaddesden (1280–1361), an early advocate of prophylaxis, stressed in simple terms the use of cold water mixed either with vinegar or with one's own urine.

During the periods of exploration and discovery, gonorrhea traveled much the same course as syphilis. Among primitive groups, gonorrhea and syphilis were Hunterian* in their appearance; the "civilized" diseases usually traveled together. This is a rarity today.

In 1787, gonorrhea was introduced into Samoa by the crews of French ships. Tahiti and the Marquesas had been the first islands to receive the full impact of the discoverers and traders. By the year 1800, it was a rare country that remained untouched by gonorrhea.

For years the mistaken belief that gonorrhea and syphilis were one and the same disease hampered medical knowledge. In 1879, marking the first significant milestone, Albert Neisser put an end to ignorance with his discovery of the gonorrhea organism.

Janet, in 1892, first proposed the use of potassium solutions in the treatment of the disease and the organic silver salts were introduced early in the 20th century. Despite these advancements, therapy was long and tedious and quite often ineffective.

Throughout the years, the "Great Sterilizer" continued to exact a tragic toll from millions of infected persons. Immediately prior to World War II, at a time of desperate need, it was discovered that gonorrheal infections yielded remarkably to treatment with sulfanilamide and related compounds. Subsequently, and at a time when it appeared the gonococcus was resisting the sulfanilamides, penicillin became the drug of choice. Yet despite effective therapy over the past several decades, gonorrhea is still very much with us. Because a short incubation period and great prevalence contribute to its spread, control measures have not materially reduced the problem. In addition, there is no natural or acquired immunity. Each year, in most areas of the United States, gonorrhea ranks first among reportable communicable diseases.

References

Goldston, Iago: "Progress in Medicine," 1940
Lodge, Henry Cabot: "History of Nations," 1920

References

Amies, C. R.: Development of resistance of gonococci to penicillin — An eight year study. Can. Med. Assoc. J. *96:*33, 1967.
Cooke, C. L., Owen, D. S., Irby, R., and Toone, E.: Gonococcal arthritis — A survey of 54 cases. J.A.M.A. *217:*204, 1971.

---

*John Hunter, English physician who erroneously assumed gonorrhea and syphilis to be one disease rather than two.

Kearns, D. H., Seibert, G. B., O'Reilly, R., Lee, L., and Logan, L.: Paradox of the immune response to uncomplicated gonococcal urethritis. N. Engl. J. Med. *289:*1170, 1973.

Kvale, P. A., Keyes, T. F., Johnson, D. W., et al.: Single oral dose ampicillin-probenecid treatment of gonorrhea in the male. J.A.M.A. *215:*9, 1971.

Logan, L. D., Cox, P., and Norins, L. C.: Reactivity of two gonococcal antigens in an automated microhemagglutination procedure. Appl. Microbiol. *20:*907, 1970.

Martin, J. E., Billings, T. E., et al.: Primary isolation of N. gonorrhoeae with a new commercial medium. Public Health Rep. *82:*361, 1971.

Pederson, A. H. B., Wiesner, P. J., et. al.: Spectinomycin and penicillin G in the treatment of gonorrhea. J.A.M.A. *220:*205, 1972.

Sayeed, Z. A., Bhadwin, U., et. al.: Gonococcal meningitis. A review. J.A.M.A. *219:*1730, 1972.

Welch, B. G., and O'Reilly, R. J.: An indirect fluorescent-antibody technique for study of uncomplicated gonorrhea. J. Infect. Dis. *127:*69, 1973.

Wiesner, P. J., Tronca, E., et. al.: Clinical spectrum of pharyngeal gonococcal infection. N. Engl. J. Med. *288:*181, 1973.

VI

INTESTINAL TRACT INFECTION

INFECTIOUS DIARRHEA

Introduction

Diarrheal disease still ranks high as a major cause of illness and death among infants and young children, especially in developing nations. Although the incidence of diarrheal disease is highest in tropical countries, geography is not the most important aspect, as the incidence is also excessive in Alaska. Socioeconomic factors as manifested by clean drinking water, proper sewage disposal, and availability of balanced food supplies are more significant determinants.

In 1900, the diarrheal disease death rate in New York City was 5603 per 100,000 infants. Today in the United States it is less than 60 per 100,000 infants. Although there has been a dramatic decrease in the number of deaths from diarrheal disease in the past 70 years, occasional outbreaks still occur. Clinically, such outbreaks may be characterized by a sudden onset and fulminating course, resulting in death of the child within a few hours. This chapter describes a number of the more common infectious agents associated with gastrointestinal infection and compares the pathogenesis of their diseases.

Bacterial Diarrhea

Bacteria usually cause disease in the gastrointestinal tract by one of two mechanisms: (1) colonization and growth within the gastrointestinal tract, where the microorganisms may invade the tissues of the host or secrete exotoxins, or (2) secretion of an exotoxin which may be preformed in food and then ingested by the host. This latter mechanism is more properly called "intoxication." Examples of the first group of diseases are salmonella enteritis, bacillary dysentery, and cholera; examples of the second group include botulism and staphylococcal and clostridial food poisoning. This chapter deals with the pathogenic mechanisms of the first group when the replicating microorganism interacts within the host to cause disease.

In the following discussion, the terms *dysentery* and *diarrhea* are used to distinguish between two distinct clinical syndromes. The term *dysentery* refers to abdominal cramps, tenesmus, and pus and blood in the stool. These are symptoms and findings associated with bacterial invasion of the intestine, usually the colon, resulting from epithelial necrosis with focal mucosal ulceration and an acute inflammatory response as manifested by the presence of red blood cells and large numbers of neutrophils in the stool. Bacillary dysentery is produced by gram negative bacteria of the genus Shigella. In contrast, the *diarrhea* syndrome refers to a profuse watery discharge usually from the small intestine. This syndrome does not produce histopathologic changes in the mucosa or submucosa of the small or large intestine, and inflammatory cells are not present in the diarrheal stool. In the diarrhea syndrome, the primary disease results from the rapid, profuse secretion of fluid across the mucosal surface of the small intestine in response to a specific toxin (enterotoxin) secreted by the infecting microorganism. Examples of agents causing the diarrhea syndrome are *Vibrio cholerae* and toxigenic infection from enteropathogenic *Escherichia coli*.

In this discussion, the term *enterotoxin* refers to specific toxins secreted by several different bacteria. Inasmuch as the toxin is secreted by a living organism, it might more properly be referred to as an exotoxin; however, since it acts at a specific site in the intestine, the term *enterotoxin* has been applied. Enterotoxins are to be distinguished from *endotoxin,* the lipopolysaccharide found in the cell walls of many gram negative bacteria. A brief summary of the characteristic distinguishing features of the four most common causes of bacterial enteric disease are listed in Table 31–1.

Salmonellosis

The most ubiquitous group of microorganisms that cause bacterial diarrhea is the salmonella. The widespread dissemination of these microorganisms reflects a vicious cycle in the food processing industry, particularly in egg and poultry production. Poultry growers use high-protein additives as food supplements. These are obtained from slaughter house by-products and mixed with feed grains. Many of the by-products are derived from swine and other animals having a high incidence of infection with salmonellae. Unfortunately, it is not economically feasible to sterilize the additives before

TABLE 31-1. Characteristics of Enteropathogenic Bacterial Infections*

	Diarrhea**/ Dysentery†	Site of Disease	Mode of Interaction	Enterotoxin	Extraintestinal Manifestations
Salmonella *Salmonella typhi*	0/±	Small intestine	Penetrates mucosal cells, carried throughout body by macrophages	0 (?)	Fever-bacteremia
Salmonella enteritidis var. typhimurium	−/±	Small intestine Large intestine (?)	Penetrates mucosal cells Septicemia	0 (?)	Fever, focal infection
Shigella *Shigella dysenteriae* *Shigella flexneri* *Shigella boydii* *Shigella sonnei*	+/+ 0/+	Large intestine	Penetrates mucosal cells. Bacteria multiply within and kill epithelial cells; cause ulceration, acute inflammatory reaction	+††	Seizures: meningismus
Cholera *Vibrio cholerae*	+/0	Small intestine	Bacteria attach to mucosal cells; rarely penetrate; multiply on epithelial cell surface. Induce disease by producing enterotoxin	+	Dehydration, shock Hypokalemic nephropathy
Enteropathogenic *Escherichia coli*	+/0 0/+	Small or large intestine	Depending on strain, may cause dysentery or diarrhea syndromes. Individual strains may cause one or other syndrome but not both	+	Dehydration, shock

*Adapted from Grady, G. F., and Keusch, G. T.: Pathogenesis of bacterial diarrheas. N. Engl. J. Med. 285:831, 1971; and Savage, D. C.: Survival on mucosal epithelia, epithelial penetration and growth in tissues of pathogenic bacteria. *In* Smith, H., and Pearce, J. H. (eds.): Microbial Pathogenicity in Man and Animals. New York, Cambridge University Press, 1972.

**Diarrhea – profuse, watery diarrhea – no inflammatory cells.

†Dysentery – abdominal cramps, tenesmus, pus, blood in stools.

††*Shigella dysenteriae* I only.

feeding them to chickens, turkeys, and other poultry. Once ingested, the salmonellae proliferate within the bird's gastrointestinal tract. Varying numbers of salmonellae remain in the region of the cloacae contaminating the surface of eggs and remaining on the bird, after evisceration and dressing. The incidence of salmonella isolated from 50-pound cans of pooled, frozen eggs has been found on occasion to be greater than 50 per cent. Thus, the high incidence of availability of salmonellae in our food supply suggests that although a total of more than 26,900 isolates of salmonella were recorded from humans in 1973, the exposure and probably the true incidence of the disease must have been considerably greater. The possibility that most of the population in the United States has had mild clinical or subclinical disease, and therefore has been actively immunized by salmonella early in life, is suggested by Figure 31–1 in which the rate of isolation of salmonellae from humans is plotted against age. The large number of isolates from children under 10 with a uniformly low incidence after age 10 would indicate a rather high proportion of immune persons, particularly in view of the potential, widespread exposure.

The classification of the Salmonella species has only recently been simplified, a situation made necessary following the description of more than 1800 different serotypes. When the different Salmonella species are grouped according to host preference (e.g., those whose natural host is man, those adapted primarily to animals, and those capable of inducing disease in both), three prototype species are formed — *Salmonella typhi, Salmonella cholerae-suis,* and *Salmonella enteritidis* (Table 31–2). The first two species consist of a single serotype each, while better than 1800 different serotypes of *S. enteritidis* have been described. Each of the large number of individual serotypes listed under *S. enteritidis* is designated by a name following the postscript *var* (variety) after the proper name *Salmonella enteritidis,* e.g., *Salmonella enteritidis* var. *typhimurium, Salmonella enteritidis* var. *derby,* etc. (see Table 31–2). Although the thought of having to deal with 1800 separate serotypes, and therefore different names, is overwhelming, it is comforting to learn that approximately 95 to 98 per cent of the strains

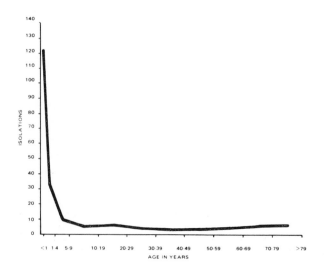

Figure **31–1.** Rate of human isolations, by age group, United States, 1973. (From Current Population Reports, Series P25, No. 490, September, 1973.)

causing disease in man occur in less than 40 serotypes. A list of the 10 most commonly isolated serotypes from both humans and animals in the United States in 1971 is given in Table 31-3. The similarity of serotypes between human and animal isolates illustrates the pattern of spread between man and his food supply.

TABLE 31-2. Relation of Salmonella Species and Representative Serotypes to Human Disease*

Species	Representative Serotype†	Natural Host	Human Disease
Salmonella choleraesuis		Animal (swine)	Septicemia and arteritis
Salmonella typhi		Man	Enteric (typhoid) fever
Salmonella enteritidis	paratyphi A schottmuelleri**	Man	Enteric fever or gastroenteritis
	pullorum	Animal (fowl)	None
	dublin	Animal (cattle)	Gastroenteritis
	typhimurium		Gastroenteritis, septicemia or focal infection
	derby enteritidis heidelberg and hundreds of related serotypes	Man and many animals	Gastroenteritis

*From Grady, G. F., and Keusch, G. T.: Pathogenesis of bacterial diarrheas. N. Engl. J. Med. *285:*831, 1971.
**Current name for paratyphi B.
†Or serotypes

Epidemiologic Notes and Reports*

Between March and May 1972, 17 infections of *Salmonella agona* were detected in residents of a northeast Arkansas town. Four of these persons were hospitalized with symptoms of severe gastroenteritis including nausea, diarrhea, fever, and abdominal cramps. The 13 remaining persons were asymptomatic. Five infected persons were detected through the routine

*This epidemiologic investigation of *Salmonella agona* in Arkansas was reported in the United States Public Health Service Publication Morbidity and Mortality Weekly Report for January 27, 1973. It serves to illustrate the means of dissemination of new strains of salmonella and how antigenic specificity of salmonella permit highly specific epidemiologic studies.

TABLE 31–3. 10 Most Frequently Isolated Serotypes From
Human and Nonhuman Sources*

Human			Nonhuman		
Serotype	Number	Per Cent	Serotype	Number	Per Cent
typhimurium	8607	32	typhimurium	345	23
newport	2058	8	senftenberg	87	6
enteritidis	1461	6	newport	65	4
infantis	1376	5	oranienburg	55	4
saint-paul	1198	5	litchfield	48	3
heidelberg	1155	4	infantis	45	3
agona	864	3	saint-paul	45	3
typhi	680	3	anatum	39	3
derby	558	2	heidelberg	36	2
javiana	549	2	montevideo	32	2
Total	18,506	70	Total	797	53
Total (all serotypes)	26,693	100	Total (all serotypes)	1498	100

*Adapted from Center for Disease Control, Salmonella Surveillance Report, Annual Summary, 1973.

salmonellosis screening program required by Arkansas state law for food handlers, and the remaining were detected during the subsequent investigation and by routine follow-up of contacts of infected persons.

Epidemiologic investigation revealed that the only common association of all infected persons was patronage of a local drive-in restaurant (Table 31–4). Analysis of food-specific attack rates for infected persons and 50 non-infected patrons and employees of Restaurant A showed that the infection rate was significantly higher in persons eating cole slaw and onions (Table 31–5).

TABLE 31–4. Incidence of S. agona Infections, by Restaurant
Patronage, Arkansas — May 1972*

	Exposed			Not Exposed		
Restaurant	Infected	Non-Infected	Attack Rate (Per Cent)	Infected	Non-Infected	Attack Rate (Per Cent)
A	17	50	25	0	23	0**
B	6	16	27	11	57	16
C	5	39	11	12	34	26
D	1	8	11	15	65	19
E	6	20	23	11	43	20
F	3	21	13	14	52	21

*From Center for Disease Control, Morbidity and Mortality Weekly Report, Vol. 22, No. 4, 1973.
**$p = 0.004$ (Fishers exact test)

TABLE 31-5. Food-Specific Attack Rates, Restaurant A,
Arkansas — May 1972*

Food Item	Ate			Did Not Eat		
	Infected	Non-Infected	Attack Rate (Per Cent)	Infected	Non-Infected	Attack Rate (Per Cent)
Slaw	15	29	34	2	21	9**
Hamburgers	14	42	25	3	8	27
Hot Dogs	7	18	28	10	32	24
Chili Dogs	9	17	35	8	33	20
Coney Dogs	9	16	36	8	19	30
Chicken	11	24	32	6	27	18
Onions†	10	16	39	2	20	9
French Fries	17	45	28	0	5	0

*From Center for Disease Control, Morbidity and Mortality Weekly Report, Vol. 22, No. 4, 1973.
**$p < 0.05$
†Interviewees were asked to add this item to the questionnaire, but not everyone did so.

Investigation of Restaurant A revealed marginal sanitary conditions and numerous errors in food handling procedures. The only work table present in the restaurant was used to cut up chicken and catfish as well as cabbage, onions, and lettuce. Employees also ate at this table during their lunch breaks. Of the environmental and food samples collected, *Salmonella agona* was isolated from the table top, knives, meat slicer, sink, fresh-frozen catfish, fresh chicken parts, and lettuce. From the food-specific attack rates and the culture results, it was apparent that cross-contamination occurred from either raw chicken or catfish to food items which were eaten raw.

Further investigation revealed that the chicken was the source of infection for the restaurant and came from a large Mississippi poultry operation. *Salmonella agona* was recovered from the slaughterhouse and from offal at the rendering plant. The organism was not recovered from the hatchery, breeder, or broiler flocks nor from the complete feed or various feed ingredients. However, one or two deliveries of feed ingredients were made weekly, and samples were collected more than two months after the clinical cases occurred. Peruvian fishmeal made up 8 per cent of the complete feed ration for the broiler flocks in this operation.

The Food and Drug Administration, which is responsible for monitoring imported fishmeal for salmonella contamination, isolated *Salmonella agona* from Peruvian fishmeal on two occasions in 1970 and from Puerto Rican fishmeal on two occasions in 1971–72. Domestically produced fishmeal which is also monitored for salmonella contamination has never been found positive for this serotype.

Editorial Note. Prior to 1971, *Salmonella agona* was reported from humans only six times in this country, but during 1971 and 1972, the number reported markedly increased (Fig. 31–2). In the last quarter of 1972, it ranked ninth in the list of most commonly reported serotypes.

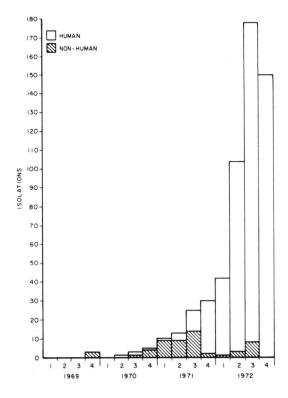

Figure 31–2. Isolations of *Salmonella agona* by quarter, United States, 1969 to 1972. December, 1972 data not included. (From Morbidity and Mortality Weekly Report, January 27, 1973.)

Twenty-seven states have reported isolation of *S. agona,* but the majority have been from Pennsylvania, Arkansas, Michigan, Wisconsin, Maryland, and Illinois.

The same increases in and epidemiologic associations of *Salmonella agona* have been observed in several other countries. The first isolations in Israel and the Netherlands were from Peruvian fishmeal in 1969. In a short period of time, this serotype was recovered from poultry or other animals whose feeds are generally supplemented with fishmeal, and eventually from humans. The first isolation of *S. agona* in England was in 1970 from "imported fishmeal," and the organism was soon commonly cultured from food animals and meat products. Human cases were reported with increasing frequency in 1971, and at the present time, *S. agona* is the seventh most common serotype isolated from humans in the United States. From the international data and the epidemiologic evidence of this investigation, Peruvian fishmeal is probably the original vehicle for the occurrence of *S. agona* infection in widely scattered parts of the world since 1969.

Types of Infection from Salmonella

In man, infection from different species of Salmonella is usually seen in one of three forms: (1) enteric fever, such as typhoid or paratyphoid fever, (2) gastroenteritis, the most common form of salmonella disease, and (3) extraintestinal focal infections such as osteomyelitis, pleural empyemas, and, with the more widespread use of reconstructive vascular surgery, local infection at sites of peripheral vascular grafts or prostheses.

Enteric Fever. Typhoid fever represents the classic enteric infection, spread by contaminated food or polluted water supplies. In contrast to salmonella gastroenteritis, *Salmonella typhi* causes gastrointestinal symptoms only late in the course of the disease, usually after prolonged fever, bacteremia, and finally localization in the submucosal lymphoid tissue of the small intestine. The microorganism is an example of a facultative intracellular parasite, surviving well within macrophages and requiring cell-mediated immunity for control. Chronic foci of infection in the biliary tree of carriers may be related in part to intracellular persistence of the microorganism in macrophages. In addition to protection of the bacteria from humoral defense mechanisms, intracellular residence within macrophages makes eradication by antibiotics more difficult, although the intestinal-biliary recirculation of ampicillin probably contributes to the effectiveness of this drug in the treatment of carriers. Several serotypes of *Salmonella enteritidis,* e.g., *paratyphi A* and *schottmuelleri,* may also cause a clinical syndrome of enteric fever similar to *S. typhi.* Unlike salmonella gastroenteritis, enteric fever is a prolonged, generalized, usually serious infection and requires specific therapy for proper control. Fortunately, the incidence of typhoid fever in the United States has been falling steadily over the past few decades (Fig. 31–3*A*). By contrast, either through greater availability of the microorganism in processed foods or greater awareness by the physician, coupled with improved laboratory capabilities, there has been a steady increase in *Salmonella enteritidis* infections during the past few years (Fig. 31–3*B*). There were 426 cases of typhoid fever in the United States in 1974.

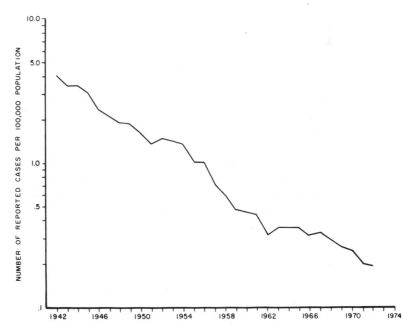

Figure 31–3. *A,* Typhoid fever. Reported case rates, United States, 1942 to 1972. (From Center for Disease Control, Morbidity and Mortality Weekly Annual Summary, 1972.)

Illustration continued on the following page

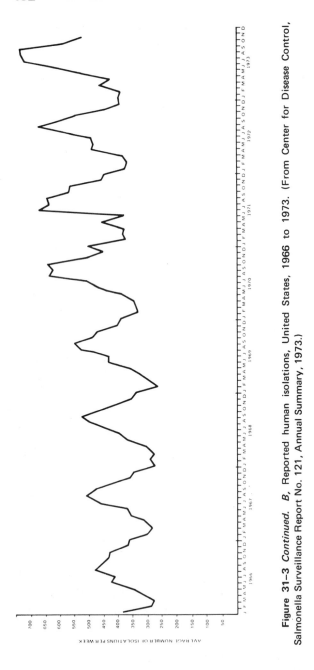

Figure 31–3 *Continued.* *B,* Reported human isolations, United States, 1966 to 1973. (From Center for Disease Control, Salmonella Surveillance Report No. 121, Annual Summary, 1973.)

Gastroenteritis. Gastroenteritis resulting from the various serotypes of *Salmonella enteritidis* may vary from a mild to a severe infection and may occasionally be associated with bacteremia, or bacteruria. In mild cases, prudent withholding of antibiotics does not appear to slow the clinical recovery and will result in a more rapid clearing of the microorganism from the stool. The decision to withhold antibiotics depends on the severity of the illness in the individual patient and the presence of underlying disease that could impair host defense mechanisms, such as cancer, immunologic defects, or occlusive vascular disease, e.g., sickle cell disease.

Signs and symptoms of salmonella gastroenteritis vary widely but are usually manifested by abdominal cramps, pain, and diarrhea which sometimes becomes bloody. The microorganisms invade focal areas of the small and large intestine where they are ingested by neutrophils in the lamina propria (Fig. 31–4). The exact site of infection with these microorganisms in humans, whether the small or large intestine, is not clear, possibly because they represent a wide and diverse group. It is known that different serotypes of *Salmonella enteritidis* may incite a significant acute inflammatory response with large numbers of neutrophils and red blood cells in the stool, suggesting mucosal ulceration.

Extraintestinal Infection. Extraintestinal infections with salmonella are frequently associated with other chronic disease or an identifiable defect in host defenses. Patients with sickle cell disease are thought to be more susceptible to infection with salmonella, and patients with metastatic cancer appear to be more prone to develop extraintestinal infections than the otherwise normal population. The increased incidence of salmonella disease in patients with cancer may be in part related to localization of microorganisms in foci of ischemic necrosis within the tumor.

A variety of different serotypes of *Salmonella enteritidis* have been found in association with infections of peripheral vascular grafts. Grafts of the abdominal aorta and femoral arterial bypasses will frequently yield salmonella

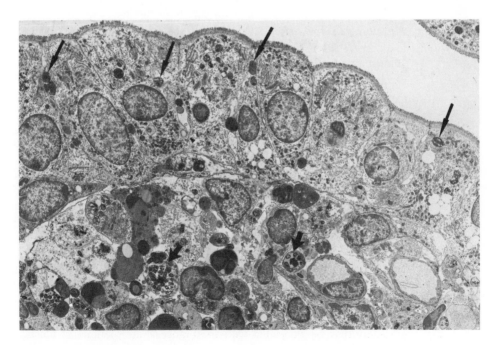

Figure 31–4. Salmonella gastroenteritis. Cytoplasmic dense bodies (thin arrows) are readily identified. Bacteria are absent from epithelium. In contrast, many phagocytosed bacteria (thick arrows) are present in neutrophils and macrophages in the lamina propria. (X 2500.) (From Takeuchi, A., and Sprinz, H.: Electron-microscope studies of experimental Salmonella infection in the preconditioned guinea pig. Am. J. Pathol. *51:*137, 1967.)

if they become infected. The reasons for this predilection of salmonella for blood vessels are not clear but may reflect a continuing intake of the microorganisms from various food sources with a resulting low-level intestinal colonization and periodic subclinical bacteremia. The possibility of preferential attachment of salmonella to endothelial cells should be considered. Two serotypes, *Salmonella choleraesuis* and *S. enteritidis* var. *typhimurium,* are most commonly involved. The presence of foreign bodies in the vascular system, as in other parts of the body, predisposes to colonization by smaller numbers of microorganisms than otherwise might be needed.

Shigellosis

Members of the genus Shigella, in contrast to those of Salmonella, are essentially restricted to man as a natural host. Although the disease has been found in subhuman primates, man is the natural reservoir as well as the main mode of dissemination. Shigellosis, or bacillary dysentery, is transmitted by the fecal-oral route, primarily by hand-to-mouth contact, but also by food handlers and insect vectors, e.g. flies, in areas of food preparation and serving. The prevalence of outdoor latrines and the density of flies can be related directly to the incidence of the disease. The availability of water for frequent washing of hands is of significant importance in controlling outbreaks. In the susceptible person, as few as 200 bacilli are said to be capable of causing dysentery. Because of the problem of teaching adequate sanitary precautions to mentally retarded children, both shigellosis and hepatitis are endemic in institutions for their care. Reflecting both the mode of fecal-oral transmission and perhaps some element of local immunization, two thirds of the isolations studied at the Center for Disease Control in Atlanta, Georgia, came from children under 10 years of age (Table 31–6). The incidence of bacillary dysentery in older age groups is similar to that of salmonellosis.

Four species of Shigella have been described: *Shigella dysenteriae,* with 10 subtypes; *Shigella boydii,* rarely seen; *Shigella flexneri,* with six subtypes; and *Shigella sonnei,* having a single type. For reasons that are not apparent, the incidence of various species has varied in different parts of the world over cycles of several years. For many years, *S. flexneri* was the most common species isolated in the United States, but for the past few years, *S. sonnei* has been dominant (Fig. 31–5). Recently, the appearance of the very virulent *S. dysenteriae* type I (Shiga's bacillus) from an endemic focus in Central America has produced several outbreaks of severe disease in the southwestern United States.

Infections from shigella differ from those of salmonella in that tissue invasion is usually limited to the lining of epithelial cells and possibly the submucosa. Rarely do the microorganisms penetrate beyond the submucosa. Extraintestinal infections with shigella seldom occur. Severe cases of dysentery may be associated with focal mucosal destruction and ulceration but do not extend beyond the intestinal tract. Shigellae have rarely been found in blood cultures. The limited exposure of shigella to deep structures in the body may account for the minimal amounts of circulating antibody found in convalescent patients.

TABLE 31-6. Shigellosis Cases by Age Group and Sex*

Age (Years)	Male	Female	Unknown	Total	Per Cent	Cumulative Per Cent	Number of Reported Isolations/ Million Population
Under 1	324	285	11	620	5	5	186
1–4	2589	2285	11	4885	39	44	352
5–9	1339	1333	2	2674	22	66	143
10–19	780	896	3	1679	14	79	41
20–29	468	907	–	1375	11	90	42
30–39	284	405	2	691	6	96	30
40–49	96	117	–	213	2	98	9
50–59	41	81	–	122	1	99	6
60–69	21	57	–	78	1	99	5
70–79	23	41	–	64	1	100	7
80 or over	11	16	–	27	0.5	100	6
Subtotal	5976	6423	29	12428			
Child (unspec)	49	41	1	91			
Adult (unspec)	20	58	–	78			
Unknown	2054	2141	76	4271			
TOTAL	8099	8663	106	16868			
Per Cent	48	52					

*Adapted from Center for Disease Control, Shigella Surveillance Report No. 35, November, 1974.

Episomal Drug Resistance

In 1955, a woman returned to Japan from Hong Kong, ill with an infection from a strain of Shigella that was resistant to several commonly used and previously effective antimicrobial agents. Over the next few years, additional outbreaks of shigella dysentery appeared that were resistant to multiple antimicrobial agents. A combination of findings suggested that the multiple antibiotic resistance patterns seen in different episodes could not be explained only on the basis of spontaneous mutation of the microorganisms with development of resistance to individual drugs. Both drug-sensitive and drug-resistant strains of Shigella could be isolated from a single outbreak. The same patient might excrete both resistant and sensitive microorganisms. It was also found that the administration of a single antimicrobial agent, e.g., sulfonamide, to a patient harboring drug-sensitive shigella, could promptly induce the appearance of strains resistant to four different antimicrobial agents, including drugs not previously used on that patient or in that outbreak. It was then noted that patients harboring drug-resistant mutants of shigella also harbored *Escherichia coli* or other strains of bacteria which were resistant to the same drugs. In contrast to the clinical findings, the

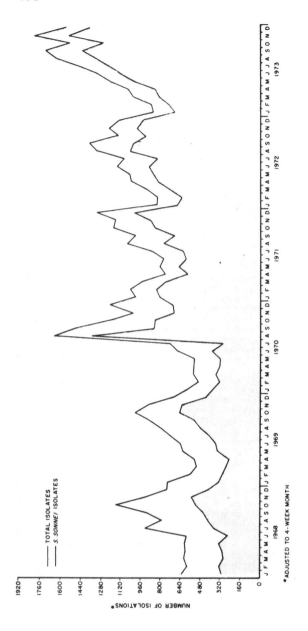

Figure 31–5. Reported isolations of shigella in the United States. (From Center for Disease Control, Shigella Surveillance Report No. 35, November, 1974.)

development of multiple drug resistance by bacteria in vitro from mutation occurred very slowly by repeated subcultures of microorganisms to graded concentrations of single drugs. Taken all together, the findings suggested that resistance to multiple antibiotics was being transferred by a genetic mechanism.

Such a mechanism has been established and is now known to function by means of sexual conjugation (Fig. 31–6). Sexual conjugation of bacteria may result in the transfer of *episomes*, also called *resistance transfer factors*. Episomes are nonchromosomal packets of genetic material that may control resistance of host organisms to one or more antibiotics. The finding that the

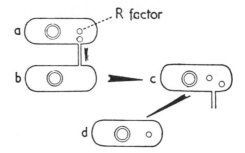

Figure 31–6. Transfer of drug resistance by conjugation (cytoplasmic R factor). (From Crofton, J.: Some principles in the chemotherapy of bacterial infections. Br. Med. J. *2:*209, 1969.)

transfer of episomes was not restricted to bacteria of the same species or genus but could also occur between bacteria of widely varying characteristics was sobering. The possibility existed that the development of antibiotic resistance by transfer factors might rapidly make existing antibiotics obsolete and quickly outdate new antibiotics. Several prospective studies since that time have shown that a more significant factor in developing resistant strains of bacteria to antimicrobial agents has been the appearance of local "hospital" strains, not associated with transfer factors, that are disseminated by interpersonal transfer. Although it is now known that episomal transfer of antibacterial resistance is a constant and potential danger in clinical medicine, it has not developed into the serious problem that was initially feared. The reasons are not completely clear. It is known that episomal transfer is not frequent in the absence of an antimicrobial agent exerting selective pressure and that once acquired, there is a trend for the bacterium to lose the transfer factor after several generations.

Antibiotic resistance of shigella to ampicillin has been increasing steadily in the United States. Currently, 85 to 90 per cent of recent isolates have been reported to be resistant to ampicillin. Depending on the severity of the disease, the patient may clear the microorganism from the gastrointestinal tract more quickly if antibiotics are not used in therapy. One exception to this is infection with *Shigella dysenteriae* type I. Disease from this microorganism is usually associated with a significant morbidity and mortality. The recent outbreak of antibiotic-resistant strains of this microorganism in Central America has made the prompt recovery of the microorganism for identification and susceptibility testing even more important.

Shigella Enterotoxin

Although most species of Shigella are not known to secrete enterotoxins, *Shigella dysenteriae* type I has long been considered to secrete a neurotoxin. The term *neurotoxin* has been used because of the appearance of symptoms which include motor ataxia in rabbits and meningismus in humans. Similarities between a recently described enterotoxin from *S. dysenteriae* and the well-studied enterotoxin from *Vibrio cholerae* suggest that the shigella enterotoxin is primarily directed against capillary endothelial cells, and that the symptoms previously thought to result from primary action on the neurons can be better explained on the basis of focal ischemia in the brain and peripheral nerves because of capillary damage. Isolation of toxin-producing, nonepithelial-penetrating and non–toxin-producing, epithelial-penetrating mutants has suggested that virulence of shigella is better correlated with epithelial penetration than enterotoxin production. Although enterotoxin from shigella can cause considerable fluid accumulation in experimental animal models, the mode of secretion is apparently different from cholera (see below).

Cholera

Cholera is a disease only of man. Man, and his contaminated water supply, are the only major reservoirs of infection. Cholera is an ancient disease, having been known for thousands of years; epidemics consistent with cholera were described in Sanskrit writings. The disease has been endemic in Asia for centuries and is most prevalent along the great rivers of the Indian subcontinent. During the nineteenth century, several epidemics of cholera appeared in the Western World, each claiming large numbers of lives. In 1849, during one of these epidemics, John Snow, a perceptive English physician, became convinced that the disease was being spread by the drinking water in London. To stop the use of drinking water from one well in an area of high infection, Snow removed the handle of the Broad Street water pump, succeeded in reducing the number of new cases, and thereby helped establish the means of spread of the disease.

Although there has been very little cholera in most of the Western World since 1900, the reappearance of a pandemic in the Philippines in 1958 and its subsequent spread to Asia and the Middle East during the next 14 years are constant reminders that the disease is still with us. During the massive population shifts resulting from the Pakistani-Indian War in 1971, thousands of deaths were due to cholera. An outbreak in Italy and an epidemic in Portugal occurred in 1973. A single case was seen in Texas in August, 1973, in a man who had not traveled out of the United States nor had known contact with foreign travelers. With the increased availability of air travel, the disease can be spread throughout the world "as far and as fast as man can fly."

Clinical Disease

Clinically, the patient developing cholera first notices a slight fullness in the abdomen and loss of appetite. His hands and feet become cold, and he may vomit. Shortly thereafter he begins to have large numbers of liquid stools, first brown and then almost clear, which contain small amounts of mucus and are classically described as "rice water" stools. If fluids are not restored by oral or intravenous therapy, death from severe dehydration and hypovolemic shock occurs within hours or a few days (Fig. 31–7). In severe cases, a stool volume of up to 24 liters per day may occur. In the acute disease, between 50 and 75 per cent of patients will die unless proper fluid therapy can be given.

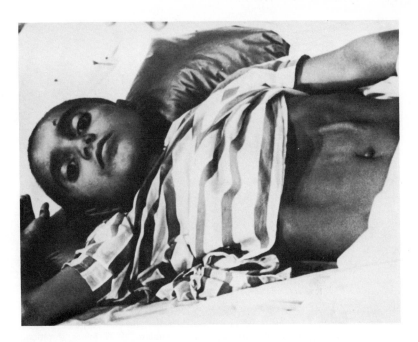

Figure 31–7. A child with severe cholera. Note markedly diminished turgor of abdominal skin which remains elevated after being released by the examiner's hand. Note also apathetic expression and sunken eyes. (From Barua, D., and Burrows, W. (eds.): Cholera. Philadelphia, W. B. Saunders Co., 1974.)

Pathophysiology of Cholera

In contrast to the causative organisms of salmonellosis and shigellosis, *Vibrio cholerae* does not penetrate the epithelial surface of the gastro-intestinal tract to incite an inflammatory response but elicits its effects through the secretion of a potent enterotoxin. The microorganism first colonizes the small intestine starting at the duodenum and progressing to the ileum. It then secretes an enterotoxin which results in a massive outpouring of isotonic fluid from the mucosal surface of the small intestine. Grossly, the bowel may be slightly edematous, but histologically it appears normal (Fig. 31–8). Although occasional inflammatory cells can be seen, there is no significant cellular response, either within the mucosa or in the intestinal lumen.

Recent studies have provided a great deal of information on the mode of action of the toxin. Since the toxin is essentially "outside" the body, it first must bind to the mucosal cell surface. Cholera enterotoxin, in contrast to other known enterotoxins, binds preferentially to gangliosides in the cell membrane. Once binding has occurred, the effect will last for 20 to 24 hours and is not reversible. After a 15- to 60-minute latent period following binding, an increase of adenyl cyclase, the enzyme catalyzing the trans-formation of ATP to AMP, begins to appear in the mucosal cells. The increase in adenyl cyclase is then followed by a marked increase in cyclic-AMP. The increased cyclic-AMP brings about the active secretion of chloride and

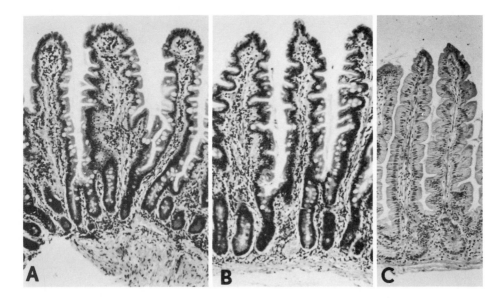

Figure 31–8. Three jejunal biopsies. All hemotoxylin and eosin (X 200.). *A,* Small bowel biopsy from a 32-year-old Pakistani male with acute cholera of 38 hours' duration. Patient had received intravenous fluids for 24 hours. The epithelium is intact and the goblet cells, especially towards the tips of the villi, have discharged their mucus. A moderate inflammatory infiltrate composed of lymphocytes, monocytes, and plasma cells is present in the lamina propria. The subepithelial capillaries are hyperemic. *B,* Small bowel biopsy of a 28-year-old asymptomatic Pakistani male who served as a control. Biopsies *A* and *B* are almost identical. A similar degree of inflammatory infiltration is present in the lamina propria of both of these biopsies. (Pakistani biopsies courtesy of the Department of Experimental Pathology, Walter Reed Army Institute of Research.) *C,* Small bowel biopsy from a 30-year-old asymptomatic North American male. Very few inflammatory cells are present in the lamina propria of this biopsy. The villi are shorter in length, indicating that the biopsy was taken more distally than the Pakistani biopsies. (From Barua, D., and Burrows, W. (eds.): Cholera. Philadelphia, W. B. Saunders Co., 1974.)

bicarbonate ions from the mucosal cells into the intestinal lumen, taking along a large volume of water (Fig. 31–9). The bound toxin does not block or prevent reabsorption of sodium and water by the small intestine or the colon. In the acute phase, the secretion of water from the small intestinal mucosal cells is greater than the capacity of the colon to absorb the loss. In mild cases, fluid balance can be achieved and water reabsorption facilitated by the use of prepackaged envelopes of electrolytes containing glucose, bicarbonate, and potassium (see Table 31–7). Inclusion of 2 to 5 per cent glucose promotes sodium, electrolyte, and water reabsorption in both the small intestine and colon (Fig. 31–10). These solutions can be given orally or by nasal drip and have been very effective in maintaining hydration in the patient when intravenous fluids are not available.

Cholera is a self-limited disease, provided the patient does not die from dehydration or shock before recovery. Although the causative organism is susceptible to tetracycline, the irreversible binding of the toxin to the epithelial surface of the mucosal cell results in little or no evidence of clinical effect from administration of the antibiotic for at least the first 24 to 36 hours after onset of diarrhea. Although antibiotics and large volumes of

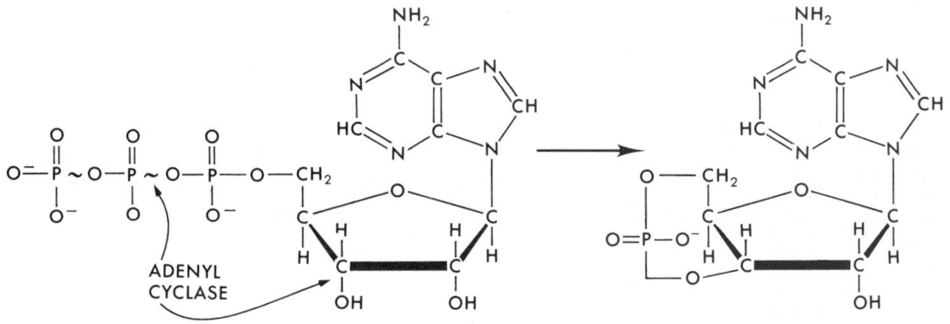

Figure 31–9. Cholera. Specific effect of the cholera toxin is exerted through the enzyme adenyl cyclase. The enzyme converts the cell's primary energy-carrier, adenosine triphosphate (ATP), into cyclic-AMP; the higher AMP level causes the intestine wall to secrete chloride (and with it water) into the intestine. The coincident decrease in the absorption of sodium (and with it water) enhances the fluid loss.

TABLE 31–7. Oral Solution Formula*

	Drinking Water (gm/L)		Drinking Water (mEq/L or mmol/L)
Glucose	20.0	Glucose	110
Sodium chloride	4.2	Sodium	120
Sodium bicarbonate	4.0	Chloride	97
Potassium chloride	1.8	Potassium	25
		Bicarbonate	48

*From Malin, D. R., and Cash, R. A.: Oral therapy for cholera. *In* Barua, D., and Burrows, W.: Cholera. Philadelphia, W. B. Saunders Co., 1974.

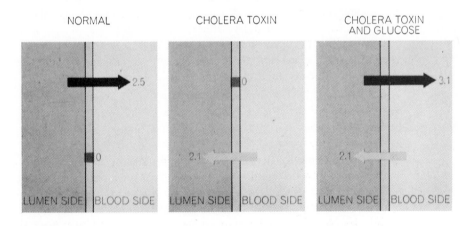

Figure 31–10. Cholera. Net ion flow across intestinal tissue is given in microequivalents per square centimeter per hour. The normal flow of sodium ion (top) and chloride ion (bottom) is reversed (center) if cholera toxin is added to fluid. Adding glucose on lumen side helps restore balance (right). (From Cholera, by N. Hirschhorn and W. B. Greenough, III. Sci. Am. *225:*15, 1971. Copyright © 1971 by Scientific American, Inc. All rights reserved.)

intravenous fluids are readily available in medical centers in this country, in most areas of the world where cholera occurs, supplies of these agents may be rapidly exhausted during an epidemic. In many outbreaks, packets of glucose, bicarbonate, and potassium (see Table 31–7) may be the only therapy available. Oral therapy has been found to be very effective in replacing fluid loss, provided the patient has not already progressed to hypovolemic shock.

Immunity to Cholera

Immunity to cholera is complex. The body produces both circulating vibriocidal immunoglobulins and local secretory IgA to the bacteria and antibodies to the enterotoxin. It is now clear that circulating antibodies can readily cross the mucosa and enter the gastrointestinal tract, but it is likely that these antibodies do not survive enzymatic digestion. In the small intestine, secretory IgA develops soon after antigenic stimulus and is thought to function by preventing attachment of the vibrios to the small intestinal mucosa. Although secretory IgA is resistant to enzymatic digestion, it persists for relatively short periods of time, and frequent administration of oral vaccines is required for maintenance of a protective effect.

The role of antitoxic antibodies is not yet clear. To be effective, these antibodies would have to intercept the enterotoxin before binding to the mucosal cell membrane, and clearly a large amount of enterotoxin might overcome a limited amount of antitoxin waiting in the intestinal lumen.

Extensive clinical trials using oral and parenteral forms of vaccines are currently in progress. Preliminary results indicate that previous diarrhea caused by infection with *Vibrio cholerae* will prevent diarrhea after second challenge with the homologous microorganism 4 to 12 months later. A whole cell vaccine, given either parenterally or orally, provided significant protection against excretion of the microorganisms and lowered the incidence and severity of diarrhea. Interestingly, the vaccine was most effective when administered parenterally. A partially purified toxoid vaccine also provided some protection. Immunity, either naturally acquired or vaccine-induced, appeared to be directed against the vibrio rather than against the toxin. Currently, cholera vaccines are less effective than previous illness in preventing subsequent disease.

Noncholera Vibrios

In addition to the several well-defined serotypes of *Vibrio cholerae* associated with the diarrhea syndrome, a number of similar microorganisms, termed *noncholera vibrios* or *nonagglutinating vibrios,* have been described which also secrete enterotoxin and produce a similar clinical syndrome in humans. Studies of these microorganisms reveal that although they are similar in many ways to *V. cholerae* they differ in certain antigenic characteristics and do not agglutinate in specific antisera. Many of the noncholera vibrios secrete enterotoxin and produce the diarrhea syndrome. (See Case Presentation at end of chapter.)

Vibrio Parahaemolyticus

Another related microorganism currently achieving increasing recognition as an agent of bacterial diarrhea is *Vibrio parahaemolyticus*. The disease caused by this microorganism may be sudden in onset and is associated with marked diarrhea. Usually, the symptoms and duration of the infection are not as severe as those of cholera. *V. parahaemolyticus* prefers salty environments and normally is found in sea water or tidal flats. For many years it has been the most common cause of food poisoning in Japan, where it is usually transmitted by "sashimi" (raw fish). Although previously not recognized in this country, within the last several years *V. parahaemolyticus* has been found to be the cause of several outbreaks of food poisoning. Most recognized outbreaks have occurred along the east coast of the United States and involved steamed crabs. Other shellfish have also been found to contain the microorganism, and its survival on frozen shrimp has been described. Determination of the true incidence of *V. parahaemolyticus* as a cause of food poisoning in the United States is difficult, as recovery of the microorganism depends on the use of special types of culture media not always available in laboratories. As clinical laboratories become more aware of the microorganism and the need for special culture media, we can expect to identify increasing numbers of cases. Although no well-defined enterotoxin has been described for this microorganism, the signs and symptoms strongly suggest that its ability to cause disease depends on such a toxin.

Enteropathogenic Escherichia coli

For many years, veterinarians have known that certain strains of *Escherichia coli* were associated with severe diarrhea in piglets and calves. Frequently, entire litters of piglets would die within a few hours to several days from a profuse, watery diarrhea.

In 1945 and 1947, a number of outbreaks of lethal diarrhea in infants occurred in England, Mexico, and Scotland. Several of these outbreaks were associated with *Escherichia coli* serotypes (O111:B4 and O55:B5) which were able to cause diarrhea more readily in infants than other *E. coli* serotypes. In the years following these outbreaks, additional serotypes were described which also are capable of causing severe diarrhea. Most outbreaks of diarrhea from enteropathogenic *E. coli* in humans are found to be due to 12 to 15 different serotypes.

Diarrhea Syndrome

Classically, the disease is seen in newborn infants in hospital nurseries and has a clinical picture of a sudden onset of severe, watery diarrhea leading to dehydration and shock; a high mortality rate accompanies the disease. During 1960 and 1961 in Chicago, more than 1300 cases of gastroenteritis occurred in infants and young children, with 77 deaths. The highest attack rate was in newborn infants, who also had the highest death rate (16 per cent). Breast-fed infants are less likely to be involved than are those given an artificial diet, and the incidence of the disease is much higher in urban hospital nurseries than in rural communities. Diarrhea results from colonization of the small intestine by enteropathogenic strains of *Escherichia coli.* Enterotoxin secretion by the microorganism results in a diarrhea syndrome similar to that seen in cholera.

Episomal Transmission of Toxin Production. Recently, it has been found that the ability of enteropathogenic strains of *Escherichia coli* to produce enterotoxin is determined by an episome which can be transmitted from one strain of *E. coli* to another by sexual conjugation. This may explain in part the not uncommon finding of *E. coli* serotypes associated with diarrheal disease that do not belong to previously described enteropathogenic serotypes. Episomal coding of enterotoxin production is, therefore, similar to antimicrobial resistance transfer factor episomes. The loss of an enterotoxin-producing episome explains the previous paradox that certain isolates of *E. coli,* known to be the same serotypes as diarrhea-producing strains, could be isolated from patients without any symptoms of the diarrhea syndrome. The finding that transferable episomes mediate enterotoxin production suggests that diarrhea-producing serotypes have the ability to accept the episome and maintain it in order to produce enterotoxin. There is also the uncomfortable possibility that the episome might be passed to any strain of *E. coli* or similar gram negative bacterium, thus creating large numbers of enterotoxin-producing bacteria. One explanation that has been offered for the association of enterotoxin-producing strains with a relatively small number of *E. coli* serotypes is that these serotypes are more receptive to episomal transfer than others. Increased receptiveness to episomal transfer in enteropathogenic *E. coli* would also explain the relatively high incidence of multiple antibiotic resistance in enteropathogenic *E. coli.* Multiple antibiotic resistance is a well-known therapeutic problem with this group of micro-organisms and presumably results from episomes coding for antimicrobial inactivating eyzymes.

Dysentery Syndrome

Although the classic disease syndrome associated with enteropathogenic *Escherichia coli* is enterotoxin-induced diarrhea in infants, within the past few years a number of well-studied outbreaks of dysentery caused by *E. coli* in both infants and adults have been described. These outbreaks are similar to those caused by shigella, and the symptoms involved include severe abdominal cramping with bloody diarrhea. In these outbreaks, the isolated *E. coli* strains have the ability to penetrate and replicate within epithelial cells to cause focal epithelial necrosis, characteristics not possessed by enterotoxin-producing strains (Fig. 31–11). Therefore, *E. coli* may cause disease resembling either cholera or bacillary dysentery. The procedures necessary to demonstrate enterotoxin production and epithelial invasion are not readily available to most clinical laboratories, and distinguishing these characteristics in strains isolated from outbreaks of diarrhea is slow and time consuming. Several new approaches to assay enterotoxin have recently been described, and hopefully simple assay procedures will be more readily available for general use in the near future. The ability to identify enterotoxin production by an uncomplicated assay will expand our understanding of bacterial related diarrheal disease.

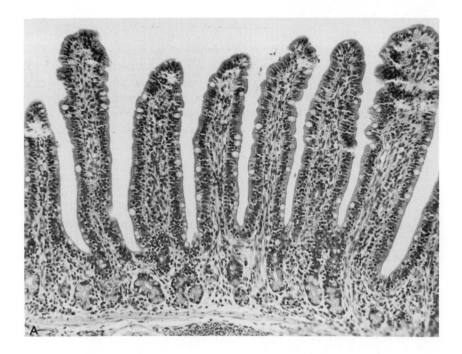

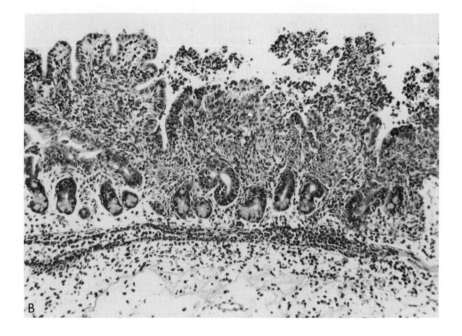

Figure 31–11. *A,* Effects of enterotoxin producing strains of *Escherichia coli* on rabbit ileum. (X 170.) Section of ligated small bowel loop seven hours after inoculation with enterotoxin-producing organisms shows normal morphology. *B,* Effect of epithelial-penetrating strains of *E. coli* on rabbit ileum. Section of ligated loop seven hours after inoculation with penetrating organisms shows marked mucosal disarray, with necrosis, ulceration, and intense acute inflammatory reaction. (From DuPont, H. L., Formal, S. B., Hornick, R. B., et al.: Pathogenesis of Escherichia coli diarrhea. N. Engl. J. Med. *285:*1, 1971. Reprinted by permission from The New England Journal of Medicine.)

Traveler's Diarrhea

"Traveler's diarrhea," well-known to those persons visiting other countries, can often be a serious medical problem. Numerous efforts to identify specific microorganisms in an attempt to explain the transitory diarrhea and abdominal cramping characterizing this disease have recovered known agents in less than 10 to 15 per cent of cases. Recently, a study of a large group of American students on a three-week visit to Mexico revealed that 30 per cent developed clinical symptoms of diarrhea during the trip. Cultures of both sick and asymptomatic students recovered enterotoxin-producing strains of *Escherichia coli* in 72 per cent of the sick and 15 per cent of the nonsick students. The high incidence of toxicogenic *E. coli* associated with "traveler's diarrhea" has not been recognized previously, since enterotoxin-producing strains of *E. coli* cannot be differentiated from the nontoxicogenic strains by standard cultural characteristics. It is becoming increasingly apparent, however, that the importance of diarrhea-producing strains of *E. coli* acquired by travelers has been underestimated in the absence of biologic assays to detect enterotoxin.

Yersinia enterocolitica

Yersinia enterocolitica is a gram negative bacillus that may cause severe enterocolitis and occasionally death. The disease has been reported more frequently in Scandinavia and other European countries than in the United States. The geographic preference for Western Europe may in part represent a lack of familiarity of cultural and identification characteristics of the microorganism by many clinical laboratories in the United States. Even so, increasing numbers of isolates of *Y. enterocolitica* are being reported in this country. Symptoms include fever, diarrhea, and severe abdominal pain. Infection with *Y. enterocolitica* in occasional patients has been recognized only following surgery for suspected appendicitis or on culture of mesenteric lymph nodes. The site or mode of infection has not yet been defined. Of particular interest is the association of erythema nodosum in 20 to 25 per cent of cases and the appearance of arthritis and occasionally Reiter's syndrome. The relationship between infection with *Y. enterocolitica* and these associated diseases is not clear at this time.

Acute Infectious Nonbacterial Gastroenteritis

Acute infectious nonbacterial gastroenteritis is a common infectious disease of the gastrointestinal tract. It is one of the most frequent causes of illness in our society, second only to the common cold. Acute infectious nonbacterial gastroenteritis probably accounts for most of the nonspecific episodes of vomiting and diarrhea seen in this country as well as in other parts of the world, particularly the Tropics. It is surprising that so little information about the origin and pathogenesis has been available until recently.

Acute infectious nonbacterial gastroenteritis is a self-limited disease, is usually benign, and occurs most frequently from September to March. Symptoms last from 24 to 48 hours and include combinations of diarrhea, nausea, vomiting, low-grade fever, abdominal cramps, headache, and malaise. Clinical features may vary from one patient to another, with vomiting more prominent in some and diarrhea more frequent in others. Treatment is generally unnecessary, and serious sequelae have not been described.

In the absence of definable bacterial agents, the disease has long been considered to be of viral origin. Intensive efforts to recover viruses have yielded little positive information. In several studies of patients with relatively severe gastroenteritis, up to 14 per cent were found to harbor viruses in the stool, while recovery of similar viruses from an asymptomatic group of controls could be shown in 10 per cent. Not all efforts to recover viruses in gastrointestinal ingestions have provided such discouraging results. A study in Mexico City yielded the recovery of viral agents from 34 per cent of patients with acute diarrheal disease, while only 6 per cent of controls harbored similar viruses. The significance of such studies is dependent on the ability and sensitivity of viral recovery systems currently available. Viruses that have been shown to be implicated in gastroenteritis include adenoviruses, coxsackieviruses, polioviruses and members of the echovirus group.

Although currently available viral recovery techniques have not yielded a consistent agent or group of agents to explain the syndrome of acute infectious nonbacterial gastroenteritis, a number of filterable infectious agents have been described and shown to be capable of causing the disease in volunteers. The use of human volunteers in the study of disease lacking a well-characterized etiologic agent makes possible three important elements: (1) a source of infectious material, (2) an experimental host, and (3) the opportunity to study the clinical course and pathogenetic developments of this disease under controlled conditions.

Norwalk Agent

At least three infectious agents producing the syndrome of acute infectious nonbacterial gastroenteritis have been described since 1945. The most intensively studied agent was derived from an outbreak of "winter vomiting disease" that occurred in Norwalk, Ohio, in October, 1968. The Norwalk agent was recovered during an outbreak of illness at an elementary school, where about half of the students became ill. Attempts to identify known bacterial or viral agents or filterable enterotoxins were unsuccessful. Three serial passages with stool filtrates from sick patients were made through human volunteers, with a resulting attack rate of 67 per cent. The disease was characterized by an incubation period of 16 to 48 hours, with symptoms lasting from 24 to 48 hours. Symptoms included low-grade fever and combinations of diarrhea, vomiting, abdominal cramps, malaise, and headache. Manifestations of the disease varied from one volunteer to another; vomiting was seen in some, and diarrhea in others (Fig. 31–12). Immunity to the agent, as shown by subsequent challenge of previously infected

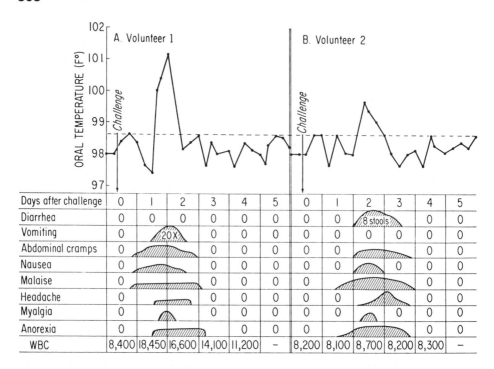

Days after challenge	0	1	2	3	4	5	0	1	2	3	4	5
Diarrhea	0	0	0	0	0	0	0	0	8 stools	0	0	
Vomiting	0	20X	0	0	0		0	0	0	0	0	
Abdominal cramps	0		0	0	0		0	0		0	0	
Nausea	0		0	0	0		0	0		0	0	
Malaise	0		0	0	0		0			0	0	
Headache	0		0	0	0		0	0		0	0	
Myalgia	0		0	0	0		0	0		0	0	
Anorexia	0			0	0	0				0	0	
WBC	8,400	18,450	16,600	14,100	11,200	–	8,200	8,100	8,700	8,200	8,300	–

Figure 31–12. Response of two volunteers to oral administration of stool filtrate derived from a volunteer who received original Norwalk rectal-swab specimen. The height of the shaded curve is roughly proportional to the severity of the sign or symptom. (From Dolin, R., Blacklow, N. R., DuPont, H., et al.: Transmission of acute infectious nonbacterial gastroenteritis to volunteers by oral administration of stool filtrates. J. Infect. Dis. *123:*307, 1971.)

volunteers, was present for periods of 6 to 14 weeks. Physical characteristics of the agent indicate it to be small, probably less than 36 mμ in size, ether stable, and both acid and heat stable. Man is probably the only natural host, as no animal models of the disease are known. The high rate of susceptibility to the disease in volunteers and community outbreaks suggest little widespread immunity (see Table 31–8).

TABLE 31–8. Biological Properties of Norwalk Agent*

Diameter	< 66 mμ, probably < 36 mμ
Ether-stable	Yes; lacks lipid coat
Acid-stable	Yes; resists pH 2.7 for 3 hr.
Heat-stable	Yes; resists 60°C for 30 min.
Homologous immunity	Yes; present at least 6 to 14 weeks after initial infection
Species specificity	Pathogenicity restricted to man
Widespread immunity	Probably absent

*From Blacklow, N. R., et al.: Acute infectious nonbacterial gastroenteritis: Etiology and pathogenesis. Ann. Intern. Med. 76:993, 1972.

Attempts have been made to isolate and grow the Norwalk agent in a human fetal intestinal organ culture system. Although volunteers have become ill from ingestion of supernatants from such cultures, results have been inconstant. Further use of this method as an in vitro culture system is under investigation.

Morphologic and Functional Abnormalities

The histopathologic changes of the mucosal architecture at the duodenal-jejunal junction of patients with acute infectious nonbacterial gastroenteritis have been studied by biopsy in a group of volunteers given the Norwalk agent. Abnormalities were found in all patients by 12 to 48 hours following challenge. The mucosal villi became shortened, the crypts hypertrophied, and the interstitial tissue of the villi became more cellular, containing both mononuclear cells and segmented neutrophils. Abnormal changes persisted for several days but had cleared by six to eight weeks after the acute illness (Fig. 31–13). In contrast to the abnormal findings in the small intestinal mucosa, biopsies of the rectosigmoid colon from patients ill with the disease appeared normal. This suggests that the disease has a preferential localization to the small intestine, at least the region of the duodenal-jejunal junction, where the biopsies were obtained. Electron microscopy of mucosal biopsies taken from the small intestine have shown particles consistent with viruses. Immune electron micrographs of fecal material from acutely ill patients have been reported to show viral bodies after incubation with convalescent serum.

Functional abnormalities of the small intestine found during the acute and convalescent phases of this disease include an abnormal D-xylose absorption, both in patients with acute clinical disease and in patients challenged with Norwalk agent but remaining asymptomatic (Fig. 31–14). Lactose absorption studies suggest that intestinal lactase deficiency also occurs transiently during the acute disease. Malabsorption of fat developed both in patients with clinical illness and in those without symptoms. Fat malabsorption cleared within six days after infection.

In summary, the current evidence would suggest that the common clinical syndrome of acute infectious nonbacterial gastroenteritis as typified by the Norwalk agent is probably due to a small-sized, ether-stable virus. Considerable information has been gained by studies on volunteers, using stool filtrates from clinically ill patients. Further information will have to await a reproducible means of recovering the agent and the development of practical techniques to culture it in vitro.

Inflammatory Cells in Stool as a Guide to Type of Infection

During the foregoing discussion, it has been stressed that infections in the gastrointestinal tract result from either the parasite invading the host, usually with an appropriate neutrophilic or mononuclear cell inflammatory reaction,

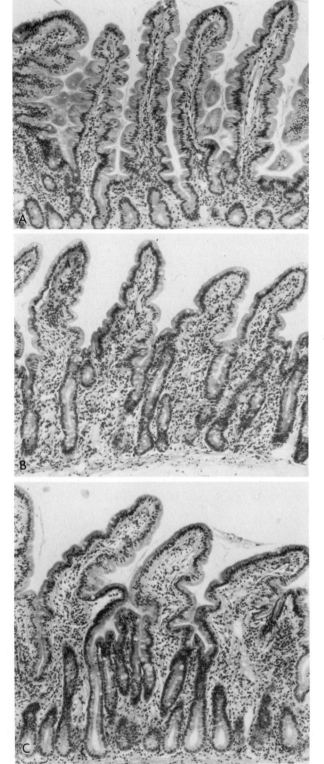

Figure 31–13. Biopsies of the small intestine before and after oral ingestion of Norwalk agent. Before ingestion (*A*), villi are tall, and the cellularity of the lamina propria is normal. Two days after ingestion (*B*), the villi are shortened, the crypts are hypertrophied and contain increased numbers of mitoses, and the cellularity of the lamina propria is increased. Six days after ingestion (*C*), shortened villi, hypertrophied crypts, and increased mitoses persist. (Hematoxylin and eosin stain, × 100.) (From Schreiber, D. S., Blacklow, N. L., and Trier, J. S.: The mucosal lesion of the proximal small intestine in acute infectious nonbacterial gastroenteritis. N. Engl. J. Med. *288:*1318, 1973. Reprinted by permission from The New England Journal of Medicine.)

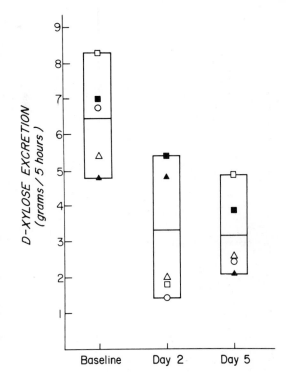

Figure 31–14. D-Xylose excretion after intraduodenal instillation of 25 gm of D-xylose before and after ingestion of Norwalk agent. Each of the five volunteers is represented by a different symbol. (From Schreiber, D. S., Blacklow, N. L., and Trier, J. S.: The mucosal lesion of the proximal small intestine in acute infectious nonbacterial gastroenteritis. N. Engl. J. Med. *288:*1318, 1973. Reprinted by permission from The New England Journal of Medicine.)

or the action of an enterotoxin causing loss of body water through increased activity of cyclic-AMP.

Understanding the pathogenesis of these diseases has led to a simple, rapid, and reasonably specific test for the type of bacterial gastrointestinal infection in any patient. The test consists of making a stained smear of the stool or diarrhea contents and looking for the presence or absence of inflammatory cells. If inflammatory cells are present, the type, e.g., neutrophils or mononuclear cells, may be helpful in determining the kind of gastrointestinal infection. Typhoid fever is associated with a large number of mononuclear inflammatory cells. Shigella bacillary dysentery results in stool smears showing 80 to 90 per cent neutrophils, due to the acute inflammatory reaction following mucosal penetration. Cholera and enterotoxigenic *Escherichia coli* are characterized by the absence of inflammatory cells (Table 31–9) inasmuch as little or no inflammatory response occurs to metabolic enterotoxin.

CASE PRESENTATION*

On November 12, 1974, four days after her arrival in Acapulco, Mexico, a 37-year-old Massachusetts woman developed a mild diarrheal illness. Her illness lasted two days, and she was asymptomatic upon her arrival in the

*From Center for Disease Control, Morbidity and Mortality Weekly Report, Vol. 23, No. 48, 1974.

TABLE 31–9. Diseases Associated with Fecal Leukocytes*

Disease	Number of Patients	Number with Fecal Leukocytes	Predominant Cell Type (Acute Illness)
Shigellosis	44	44	Polymorphonuclear (mean, 84%)
Salmonellosis	11	9	Polymorphonuclear (mean, 75%)
Typhoid fever**	8	8	Mononuclear (mean, 95%)
Invasive *Escherichia coli* colitis**	4	4	Polymorphonuclear (mean, 85%)
Ulcerative colitis	2	2	Polymorphonuclear (mean, 88%) and eosinophils (mean, 8%)
"Allergic" diarrhea	1	1	Mononuclear (mean, 95%)

*From Harris, J. C., DuPont, H. L., and Hornick, R. B.: Fecal leukocytes in diarrheal illness. Ann. Intern. Med. 76:697, 1972.
**Experimentally induced.

United States on November 14. On November 17, she had the onset of severe diarrhea, with up to 30 greenish, watery bowel movements a day, vomiting, and abdominal cramps. She was hospitalized that day; physical examination was normal except for tachycardia. She was treated with oral fluids and tetracycline and was asymptomatic after three days.

A stool specimen was obtained for culture on the day of admission. On November 21, the hospital laboratory reported the isolation of an organism with biochemical characteristics compatible with *Vibrio cholerae.* At the state reference laboratory the organism was identified as a non-cholera vibrio when it failed to agglutinate in cholera antisera. The isolate was confirmed as a non-cholera vibrio at the Center for Disease Control.

This patient's most recent illness was very likely caused by a non-cholera vibrio, an organism biochemically similar to *Vibrio cholerae,* but lacking the O-subgroup 1 antigen and thus failing to agglutinate in specific antisera.

These organisms can produce a severe diarrheal illness indistinguishable from cholera that is probably mediated by an enterotoxin very similar to that of *V. cholerae.*

This patient may have acquired her infection in Acapulco or Massachusetts. The extent to which this organism is present in American coastal waters is unknown. Non-cholera vibrio enteritis was recently reported in an American who had traveled to New Orleans.

References

Books

Barua, D., and Burrows, W.: Cholera. Philadelphia, W. B. Saunders Co., 1974.

Davis, B. D., Dulbecco, R., Eisen, H. N., Ginsberg, H. S., and Wood, W. B., Jr.: Microbiology. 2nd ed. Hagerstown, Maryland, Harper and Row, 1973.

Dremery, V., Rosival, L., and Watanabe, T.: Bacterial Plasmids and Antibiotic Resistance. Berlin, Springer-Verlag, 1972.

Smith, H., and Pearce, J. H.: Microbial Pathogenicity in Man and Animals. Cambridge, Cambridge University Press, 1972.

Original Articles

Blacklow, N. R., Dolin, R., Fedson, D. S., et al.: Acute infectious nonbacterial gastroenteritis: Etiology and pathogenesis. Ann. Intern. Med. *76:*993, 1008, 1972.

Carpenter, C. C. J.: Cholera and other enterotoxin-related diarrheal disease. J. Infect. Dis. *126:*551, 1972.

Cash, R. P., Masic, S. I., Libonati, J. P., Craig, J. P., Pierce, N. F., and Hornick, R. B.: Response of man to infection with *Vibrio cholerae.* II. Protection from illness afforded by previous disease and vaccine. J. Infect. Dis. *130:*325, 1974.

Drachman, R. H.: Acute infectious gastroenteritis. Pediatr. Clin. North Am. *21:*3, 1974.

DuPont, H. L., et al.: Pathogenesis of *Escherichia coli* diarrhea. N. Engl. J. Med. *285:*1, 1971.

Flores, J., Grady, G. F., McIven, J., Witkim, P., Beckman, B., and Sharp, G. W. G.: Comparison of the effects of enterotoxin of *Shigella dysenteriae* and *Vibrio cholerae* on the admylate cyclase system of the rabbit intestine. J. Infect. Dis. *130:*374, 1974.

Freter, R.: Intestinal immunity. Studies of the mechanism of action of intestinal antibody in experimental cholera. Tex. Rep. Biol. Med. *27* (Suppl):299, 1969.

Gardner, P., and Smith, D. H.: Studies on the epidemiology of resistance (R) factors. Ann. Intern. Med. *71:*1, 1969.

Gorbach, S. L., Kean, B. H., Evans, D. G., Evans, D. J., and Bessudo, D.: Traveler's diarrhea and toxigenic Escherichia coli. N. Engl. J. Med. *292:*933, 1975.

Grady, G. F., and Keusch, G. T.: Pathogenesis of bacterial diarrheas. N. Engl. J. Med. *285:*831, 891, 1971.

Gutman, L. T., Ottesen, E. A., et al.: An inter-familial outbreak of *Yersinia enterocolitica* enteritis. N. Engl. J. Med. *288:*1372, 1973.

Harris, J. C., DuPont, H. L., and Hornick, R. B.: Fecal leukocytes in diarrheal illness. Ann. Intern. Med. *76:*697, 1972.

Schreiber, D. S., Blacklow, N. R., and Trier, J. S.: The mucosal lesion of the proximal small intestine in acute infectious nonbacterial gastroenteritis. N. Engl. J. Med. *288:*1318, 1973.

South, M. A.: Enteropathogenic *Escherichia coli* disease: New developments and perspective. J. Pediatr. *79:*1, 1971.

Chapter 32

VIRAL HEPATITIS

Introduction

The term *viral hepatitis* refers to two highly communicable diseases — viral hepatitis, type A, and viral hepatitis, type B — which together constitute the major infectious cause of hepatitis in the United States. Both diseases are also referred to by a series of terms which are somewhat descriptive of their epidemiologic behavior. *Viral hepatitis, type A*, has been called acute epidemic hepatitis, infective hepatitis, short incubation hepatitis, and infectious (epidemic) hepatitis. Synonyms for *viral hepatitis, type B*, include serum hepatitis, homologous serum jaundice, and long incubation hepatitis. Until late in the 1930s, many medical authorities regarded these two illnesses as noninfectious. During World War II, investigations of outbreaks of hepatitis among military personnel stationed in the Middle East and North Africa, as well as among recipients of yellow fever vaccine, established the infectious nature of these two viral diseases. Types A and B viral hepatitis are regarded as distinct entities because of differences in certain laboratory, clinical, and epidemiologic features (see Table 32–1).

Viral Hepatitis, Type A

Epidemiology

The major mode of transmission of hepatitis is by the fecal-oral route through person-to-person spread or by way of food and water. For this reason, the epidemiology of type A viral hepatitis frequently resembles that of poliomyelitis. Person-to-person transmission occurs among people who live under unsanitary conditions and among those who are unable to apply rules

TABLE 32-1. Pertinent Comparisons between Viral Hepatitis Type A and Viral Hepatitis Type B

Marker	Type A	Type B
Synonym	Infectious hepatitis	Serum hepatitis
Principal sources	Food, water	Blood products
Major mode of transportation	Fecal-oral	Parenteral injection
Viral particles	Large (40 nm) Small (20 nm)	Dane particle (40 nm) Small (20 nm) Tubular (20 nm)
Viral nucleic acid (and polymerase)	Enterovirus (?)	RNA (?) (DNA polymerase)
Viral antigen	Fecal antigen Liver antigen	HB_S-surface antigen HB_C-core antigen
Clinical onset	Acute	Gradual
Incubation period	15–50 days (Av. 30)	50–180 days (Av. 60)
Increased IgM	Marked	Moderate
Prevention by gamma globulin	Effective	Poor

of sanitation to their daily lives. As a result, infections with type A hepatitis are endemic in nursery schools, institutions for the mentally retarded, and primitive societies, all consisting of populations which live in an environment favoring a high risk of fecal contamination. In the United States, food-borne transmission usually results from accidental breakdown of sanitary safeguards established to protect food sources. Fecal contamination of oysters, orange juice, and prepared cold cuts and sandwich meats has caused sharp outbreaks of type A viral hepatitis. Like poliomyelitis, water-borne epidemics usually occur in late summer and early autumn. Occasionally, outbreaks occur in other seasons. Water-borne spread also results from fecal contamination of drinking water.

As in poliomyelitis, viral hepatitis has a high attack rate among children where the level of sanitation is poor. Viral hepatitis usually occurs as a mild, subclinical illness in children, so that the actual number of cases is not appreciated. In countries with poor sanitation, the incidence of hepatitis A in adults is low because infection occurs in childhood, leaving an immune older population. As the level of sanitation of a country improves, the risk of childhood infections falls, and susceptibility to infection with type A hepatitis virus is retained past childhood into adult life. If the susceptible adult becomes infected, overt clinical disease results, since adults usually show the full clinical picture. These epidemiologic features explain in part the high incidence of viral hepatitis among American and British troops in the Mediterranean during World War II. Presumably, these soldiers did not have viral hepatitis as children because they were raised in countries with high sanitary levels; therefore, they were susceptible to infection during their sojourn in lands where type A hepatitis was endemic.

Type A viral hepatitis can be transmitted by injection of contaminated blood products, but this is not a common route. The finding of an inordinate amount of viral hepatitis among homosexuals suggests that the virus might be transmitted as a venereal infection. Type A hepatitis is generally limited to man, but accidental infection of chimpanzees and experimental infection of marmosets have been reported.

Causative Agent

Present knowledge pertaining to the properties of hepatitis A virus has been gained by epidemiologic studies. This virus seems to be exceptionally hardy and apparently survives heating at 56°C for 30 minutes, exposure to 10 per cent ether at 4°C for 20 hours, and storage at -10° to -20°C for at least one and one half years. Infectivity is destroyed by boiling for 15 minutes in water, heating at 180°C for one hour, and autoclaving at 121°C (15 pounds pressure). Exposure to chlorine, one part per million, for 30 minutes in water also destroys infectivity if solid wastes are absent.

From time to time, investigators claim discovery of viruslike agents which they have obtained from hepatitis patients and assume may be the agent of type A hepatitis. Most of these claims have not been substantiated by other investigators, and in some instances the discoverers have themselves been unable to consistently reproduce their findings. Of late, electron microscopy has revealed small (20 nm) particles and larger (40 nm) viruslike particles in fecal samples from patients with type A hepatitis. The particles are aggregated by serum from patients who recently recovered from the illness. More recently, Dienhardt, also Hilleman, produced hepatitis in marmosets by experimental infection with a virus associated with type A hepatitis in man. Physical, chemical, and morphologic dimensions of the agent suggest that it may be an enterovirus. Serum and liver extracts from infected marmosets serve as complement-fixation antigen and as an antigen for immune adherence. Immune adherence is an immunologically specific in vitro reaction between normal human erythrocytes and an antigen that has been sensitized with antibody and complement. The immune adherence test for hepatitis type A depends on red cell clumping and is said to be more sensitive than complement-fixation. Preliminary data relative to the frequency of hepatitis A antibody in small groups suggest a greater than 60 per cent susceptibility to this agent in the United States.

Clinical Disease

The clinical picture of viral hepatitis, type A, particularly in adults, has two stages: a preicteric stage and an icteric stage (Fig. 32–1). The preicteric stage begins 15 to 50 days (average, 30 days) after exposure and is accompanied by fever, abdominal discomfort, nausea, and anorexia. Nausea may be so severe as to cause a pronounced distaste for food and, in smokers,

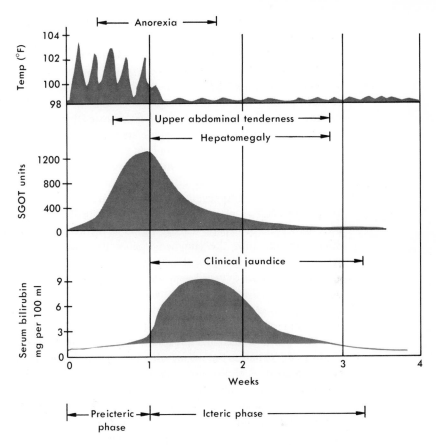

Figure 32–1. Schematic representation of course of type A hepatitis. (After Havens, W. P., Jr., and Paul: In Horsfall, F. L., Jr., and Tamm, I. (eds.): Viral and Rickettsial Infections of Man. 4th ed. Philadelphia, J. B. Lippincott Co., 1965.

loss of desire for tobacco. The initial symptoms increase progressively in intensity during the first four to six days. By the end of the preicteric stage, the patient may complain also of headache and myalgia. Some variation is seen. In certain patients, the onset is so severe as to be marked by fever, true shaking chills, and prostration, thereby suggesting the possible diagnosis of bacteremia. In other patients, the symptoms may be so mild as to be almost unnoticed. Subclinical disease is common among children, in whom the illness may be undetected unless liver function tests are done.

There are few specific physical findings in patients with type A hepatitis. The preicteric stage may be marked by nothing more than tenderness in the right upper quadrant and a slightly enlarged liver. Laboratory tests performed during the preicteric stage reveal evidence of increasing disease of the liver parenchyma. The best indexes are the alkaline phosphatase and serum glutamic-oxaloacetic transaminase (SGOT) levels. The alkaline phosphatase rises above normal levels during the preicteric stage but does not show as great an elevation as does the SGOT. The typical findings of viral hepatitis are a marked increase in SGOT and a slight to moderate increase in alkaline phosphatase. Leukopenia is common. Atypical lymphocytes are occasionally seen. Serum IgM levels may be increased. None of these findings is pathognomonic for type A hepatitis, and consequently other diagnoses should be considered. For example, a moderate increase in the level of alkaline phosphatase and SGOT also occurs with infectious mononucleosis and cytomegalovirus mononucleosis. Serologic tests for these two illnesses should be performed to rule out these diagnoses.

The end of the preicteric stage is indicated by the onset of jaundice. Jaundice is the hallmark of the icteric stage and occurs in two of every three adults with type A hepatitis but only in one or two of every 10 children. It is probably the lack of jaundice which successfully masks hepatitis in children, enabling them to serve as efficient transmitters of the infection among susceptible persons. Appearance of jaundice is associated with an increase in the serum alkaline phosphatase and serum bilirubin levels, but neither of these indicators of hepatic damage shows as marked an elevation as does the SGOT. By the time the jaundice reaches its peak, some improvement is evident clinically; the patient will have a sense of well-being which seems incongruous to the outward appearance. Even as the jaundice deepens, there may be a gradual return of appetite and a reduction of nausea and vomiting. The prognosis is good and, in otherwise normal persons, fatalities occur with a frequency of one to three per one thousand. The disease is more severe in postmenopausal women and in patients who have chronic liver disease.

In a few patients, the degree of jaundice may be so intense and the level of serum alkaline phosphatase may rise so high as to lend confusion to the diagnostic process. The high levels indicate a disproportionate amount of bile duct obstruction and are probably the basis for the term *catarrhal jaundice,* which was once applied to the disease now known as type A hepatitis. If surgery is performed with the goal of relieving the assumed biliary tract disease, the stress of surgery will be added to the stress of the hepatitis and may result in a fatal outcome.

In 90 per cent of patients with type A hepatitis, recovery, as measured by laboratory findings, is complete within three months. However, approximately 5 per cent of patients show a recurrence of liver disease of a much milder form within six months. Recovery from the recurrent illness is usually complete, but in a few patients more chronic forms of hepatitis may develop.

Immune Response

Natural exposure as a child appears to protect against reinfection in later life. However, in the absence of identification of the agent responsible for type A hepatitis, the data indicating long-lasting immunity are chiefly epidemiologic. The most direct evidence for this is found in Krugman's observations in the Willowbrook State Home for mentally retarded children of New York State. Studies in that institution showed that recovery from type A hepatitis protected against experimental reinfection in approximately 95 per cent of the patients. However, the explanation for second attacks in 5 per cent of the patients is not clear, but the fact that second attacks do occur suggests that recovery from type A hepatitis may not be as solid as initially conceived. If so, the long-lasting immunity that is seen following childhood infection may result from repeated subclinical infections later in life. Resolution of the question awaits studies using the newly developed specific tests for this type of viral hepatitis.

Prevention

Sanitation

The objective of such sanitary procedures as careful disposition of excreta and hand-washing is to reduce the risk of transmission of the infectious agent by the fecal-oral route. With person-to-person spread, this is not easily accomplished, since the virus probably appears in stools during the last half of the incubation period and persists for up to two weeks after the onset of symptoms. Moreover, the occurrence of subclinical disease increases the problem of identifying individuals who are carrying the virus. With food or water spread, control is best handled by the citizens' support of public health officials in their efforts to maintain a high level of sanitation in the community.

Passive Immunization

Immune serum globulin (ISG) gives highly effective protection against clinical manifestations of type A hepatitis, but its effectiveness depends on the dosage and timing relative to exposure. When given in proper dosage (see Table 32–2) before or within one to two weeks after exposure, it prevents illness in 80 to 90 per cent of those exposed. However, because immune serum globulin may not suppress inapparent or subclinical infections, its administration may be followed by long-lasting natural immunity. Immune serum globulin should be given as soon as possible after a known exposure, but its prophylactic value decreases with time. Its use more than six weeks after exposure is not recommended.

TABLE 32–2. Guidelines for ISG Prophylaxis against
Viral Hepatitis, Type A*

Person's Weight (lb)	ISG Dose (ml)**
50	0.5
50–100	1.0
100+	2.0

*From Center for Disease Control, Morbidity and Mortality Weekly Report, Vol. 21, p. 194, 1972.
**Intramuscular injection.

Since close personal contact is important to the spread of type A hepatitis, immune serum globulin is recommended for all permanent and temporary household contacts who have not already had the disease. Contact at school is usually not an important means of spread, and routine administration of immune serum globulin is not recommended unless epidemiologic evidence clearly shows a school outbreak. During epidemics in institutions such as prisons and homes for mentally retarded, immune serum globulin can limit spread of the disease. When type A hepatitis is endemic in such institutions, immune serum globulin is given in higher doses. Travelers to foreign countries in which type A hepatitis is endemic may also require higher doses of immune serum globulin. On the other hand, its routine administration is not recommended for hospital personnel. Rapid advances in identifying hepatitis A virus promise development of procedures for active immunization against this disease.

Viral Hepatitis, Type B

Epidemiology

The principal means of transmission of type B hepatitis is via parenteral routes (see Table 32–1). The agent is transmitted by blood transfusion and by use of contaminated syringes or instruments. Evidence that type B hepatitis virus occurs in blood was gained during efforts to develop an attenuated yellow fever vaccine for military personnel in World War II. Human serum was added to the freshly developed vaccine to stabilize the viral particle. Several batches of vaccine were stabilized with some human serum which was later shown to contain hepatitis virus. The occurrence of jaundice in recipients of the contaminated yellow fever vaccine prompted studies which quickly showed the infectious nature of the associated hepatitis. This realization led to recognition retrospectively of other outbreaks of jaundice in diabetic clinics where syringes and needles used for giving insulin were occasionally contaminated by hepatitis virus. Hepatitis, type B, virus has been found in all blood fractions other than gamma globulin; blood plasma and Cohen Fraction/VIII, which is used for therapy of hemophilia, have frequently been vehicles for the virus. Populations at risk include both patients who receive contaminated blood products at the hands of medical personnel and physicians or nurses who acquire the infection by either inadvertently injecting themselves or accidentally being stuck with contaminated needles while administering contaminated materials. In addition, drug addicts who share syringes with one another form another population at risk. Hospital personnel in dialysis and transplantation units, clinical laboratories, and blood banks are at high risk of serious exposure to type B hepatitis.

The agents causing viral hepatitis, type B, can be transmitted by nonparenteral means, but this type of transmission occurs with markedly lower frequency than parenteral transmission. Nonparenteral spread appears to require intimate contact between the donor and recipient, and venereal transmission by asymptomatic hosts has been suspected on the basis of certain epidemiologic data.

Causative Agent

The term *hepatitis B virus* (HBV) is reserved for the as yet unidentified agent that causes serum hepatitis. Epidemiologic studies indicate that this agent, like that which causes type A viral hepatitis, is resistant to environmental conditions which inactivate most viruses and bacteria. Type B hepatitis virus survived storage at room temperature for six months and at −10 to −20°C for four and one half years. The agent will survive a temperature of 60°C for four hours but is inactivated if held at this temperature for 10 hours. It resists many common disinfectants but is inactivated by chlorine 10,000 ppm for 10 minutes. Materials contaminated by type B hepatitis virus can be sterilized by heat or steam sterilization in the same manner as that previously described for type A hepatitis virus.

Krugman found that boiling sera containing type A or type B viral hepatitis agents for one minute destroyed their infectivity but not their antigenicity. Exploiting these physical characteristics of the particles, he prepared inactivated viral suspensions which were successfully used to immunize children against infection with type B viral hepatitis. His observations offer the first promise for an effective vaccine against viral hepatitis. Krugman has also estimated that there are 10^{12} to 10^{14} infectious particles in the blood of carriers of type B hepatitis virus, basing this estimate on his studies of the transmission of the disease in experimental infections. Although the hepatitis type B virus has not been found, DNA polymerase activity has been detected in the serum of patients with heptatis B infections before and during the increase in serum glutamic-oxaloacetic transaminase (SGOT) levels.

Three particles have been seen by electron microscopy in sera from patients with type B viral hepatitis. The largest is the Dane particle. This spherical particle (42 nm in diameter) is made up of a core which is 28 nm in diameter, a shell which is 2 nm in thickness, and an outer coat which is 7 nm in thickness. Dane particles which lack a core look like small doughnuts. The outer coat is associated with a distinctive surface antigen which has also been found on the small 20-nm particles and on 20-nm tubular particles which appear in the serum of patients with type B hepatitis. A distinctive antigen has also been associated with the core of the Dane particle. Particles associated with type B hepatitis are not rich in nucleic acids and for a time were believed to actually lack nucleic acids. Further studies have shown that these particles contain 5 per cent ribonucleic acid. In contrast, polioviruses, which are 15 to 30 nm in diameter, contain 20 to 25 per cent ribonucleic acid. One interpretation of this finding is that the virus of type B hepatitis is unlike other viruses. The possibility has been raised that hepatitis is caused by a novel class of subviral particles known as viroids. *Viroids* are defined as replicating RNA molecules which lack protein coats and are represented by the agent of potato spindle tuber disease. According to this suggestion, the three particles presently associated with type B viral hepatitis would not be components of the infectious agent for this disease. Another possibility is that hepatitis type B virus may be a multicomponent virus in which separated portions of the virus genome are found in individual virus-like particles. Infection would require that at least one of each type of particle enter the cell in order that viral replication may occur.

Clinical Disease

The clinical pictures of type B hepatitis and type A hepatitis are similar in many respects, and differentiation between the two illnesses frequently cannot be made. In general, type B viral hepatitis is more severe, more chronic, and affects somewhat older persons than does type A viral hepatitis. A major clinical difference between the two illnesses is in their onset. While the onset of type A hepatitis is abrupt and stormy, the onset of type B hepatitis is usually insidious. In some patients, the onset of jaundice may be preceded by a period of variable duration characterized by anorexia, fatigue, fever, and chills. In other patients, the presenting symptoms are urticaria, arthralgia, arthritis, and angioneurotic edema. These phenomena are considered indicative of a hypersensitivity reaction or a serum sickness–like illness because of associated findings of vasculitis. The average incubation period for serum hepatitis is 60 days, ranging from 45 to 180 days. Actually, the length of the incubation period is difficult to assess because the circumstances of exposure may be forgotten by the time symptoms appear.

The clinical course of type B hepatitis consists of two major phases: a preicteric and an icteric stage. While the onset of type B hepatitis may be insidious in some patients, the preicteric stage, which lasts from 5 to 8 days, suggests a systemic disease. In patients thus affected, the illness is characterized by fever and chills and gastrointestinal symptoms such as nausea and abdominal discomfort. The icteric stage, which lasts from two to six weeks, is characterized by jaundice and dark urine. Jaundice increases to a maximum by 14 days and then disappears over a variable period. As the jaundice deepens, the fever falls sharply and subjective complaints such as malaise, weakness, and arthralgia decrease. Hepatomegaly occurs in about 70 per cent of patients during the icteric stage and persists after jaundice disappears. Splenomegaly reportedly is seen in one third of adults. In children, the duration of the illness is not as long, and hepatosplenomegaly is the rule.

The severity of type B hepatitis is variable. Mild attacks may be asymptomatic and associated with a transient increase in liver enzymes. In adults, jaundice usually lasts one to four weeks and is then followed by a progressive recovery. In children, jaundice is usually absent, and recovery is more rapid. Occasionally, the illness is prolonged, and jaundice is cholestatic in character. The onset is rapid, and jaundice is deep and associated with itching. Hepatomegaly may be noticed. A fulminant clinical picture occasionally occurs in which changes in cerebral function are accompanied by massive hepatic necrosis. Hepatic encephalopathy is an ominous sign, and if deep coma results, the prognosis is poor. Complete recovery from type B hepatitis may not occur, leading to the development of a chronic form of hepatitis.

Clinical laboratory findings in type B hepatitis are indicative of hepatocellular injury and show marked elevation of SGOT levels comparable to those seen in type A hepatitis. However, SGOT levels remain elevated for a longer time in type B hepatitis. In otherwise healthy persons, IgM levels are also increased but to a lesser extent than in type A hepatitis.

Antigens Associated with Type B Hepatitis

Two major antigens have been associated with type B viral hepatitis particles. Since they are easily confused, they are designated below, along with their abbreviations:

Hepatitis B surface antigen: HB_s-Ag
Hepatitis B core antigen: HB_c-Ag
Antibody to HB_s-Ag: anti-HB_s
Antibody to HB_c-Ag: anti-HB_c

A definitive diagnosis of type B viral hepatitis is made by demonstrating the presence of a specific antigen which was initially called the Australian antigen, later the hepatitis-associated antigen, and, more recently, the hepatitis B surface antigen. Discovery of the HB_s-Ag by Blumberg resulted from his studies of genetic polymorphism in man. Blumberg was testing human sera for isoprecipitins, using two-dimensional immunodiffusion-in-agar, and in the course of his studies he tested sera from patients with hemophilia against other sera collected from people from many different countries. His choice of hemophiliac sera was based on the reasoning that hemophiliacs receive multiple transfusions as part of the therapy for their disease and therefore have the greatest opportunity for producing antibodies against foreign serum proteins. Two of the hemophiliac sera formed precipitin lines with serum from an Australian aborigine. Further studies showed that sera from some hemophiliacs who had received multiple transfusions could also react with sera from patients with viral hepatitis, type B.

The HB_s-Ag has been associated with the small 20-nm particle found in sera of patients with type B viral hepatitis and appears on the surface of the Dane particle and the tubular particle (see Table 32–3). The antigen is composed of three polypeptides of 26, 32, and 64 times 10^3 daltons. On immunoelectrophoresis and DEAE (diethylaminoethyl)-cellulose chromatography, HB_s-Ag shows the physical and chemical properties of a beta-globulin. Its properties are consistent with those belonging to the infectious agent as they are defined by various epidemiologic studies. Further studies have shown at least two antigen subgroups based on differences detected between subtype-specific determinants in agar-gel diffusion.

At least seven different tests can identify HB_s-Ag. The most sensitive method is that of radioimmunoassay, which is 10,000 to 100,000 times more sensitive than either immunoelectrophoresis or immunodiffusion, the earliest tests employed. Counterimmunoelectrophoresis has been used by many clinical laboratories because it requires little equipment and provides rapid results, in contrast with radioimmunoassay which is slower and requires more expensive equipment. Reverse passive hemagglutination, which is not quite as sensitive as radioimmunoassay but is more sensitive than immunodiffusion and counterimmunoelectrophoresis, offers high sensitivity and low cost. Complement-fixation has not been highly satisfactory because sera from

TABLE 32-3. Surface Antigen (HB$_S$-Ag) Associated with
Type B Viral Hepatitis

Site: Found on 20-nm particles and surface of Dane particle

Composition: Lipoprotein

Peptides: 26,000, 32,000, 64,000 daltons

Immunoelectrophoresis: Behaves as gamma globulin

DEAE-cellulose chromatography: Elutes after IgG

Physical and chemical characteristics
  Resists: Freezing and thawing, heating at 56°C for 18 hours, heating at 60° for one
  hour, ether, sodium desoxycholate
  Inactivated by detergent, heating at 85 to 100°C

Antigenic determinants
  Group-specific determinant: a
  Subtype-specific determinants: d or r

Subgroups
  D (d + r–)a
  Y (r + d–)a

Identification tests (by decreasing sensitivity)
  Radioimmunoassay
  Reverse passive hemagglutination
  Electron microscopy
  Complement-fixation
  Latex agglutination
  Counterimmunoelectrophoresis
  Immunodiffusion

---

patients with type B hepatitis frequently show anticomplementary activity due, in part, to the presence of circulating antigen-antibody complexes.

Blood obtained from type B hepatitis patients is infectious several days before the onset of symptoms and for approximately three weeks thereafter. During the same interval, HB$_S$-Ag is found in association with the various particles. Seven to 12 days after HB$_S$-Ag appears, antigen-antibody complexes develop and are most likely associated with the hypersensitivity-like reactions and vasculitis observed at the onset of symptoms, e.g., arthralgia and skin rash. Antigen-antibody complexes may be associated with anticomplementary activity of serum obtained from patients with hepatitis.

A unique antigen has also been associated with the core of the Dane particle and is designated as the hepatitis B core antigen (HB$_C$-Ag). This antigen has been detected in infected liver homogenates and in Dane-rich, HB$_S$-Ag positive serum samples which were treated with detergent to disrupt Dane particles. HB$_C$-Ag can be detected by immune electron microscopy, fluorescent antibody techniques, radioimmunoassay, and complement-fixation, using antibody against the core antigen (anti-HB$_C$). Anti-HB$_C$

correlates well with the period of HB$_s$-Ag in the serum and disappears with recovery from acute illness. Anti-HB$_c$ persists in the serum of chronic HB$_s$-Ag carriers and may be an indicator of persistent hepatitis B virus replication.

HB$_s$-Ag can be found in most body tissues and, along with HB$_c$-Ag, has been revealed in hepatic cells of patients with hepatitis by use of fluorescent antibody methods. Eighty-five per cent of patients with acute hepatitis show HB$_s$-Ag for 1 to 13 weeks, and in 5 per cent, HB$_s$-Ag persisted for 13 weeks to 6 months. HB$_s$-Ag antigenemia has been observed in asymptomatic carriers; in one patient, the antigen was found in serum collected over a 20-year interval. HB$_s$-Ag also occurs in 1 per cent of hospital and clinic personnel. Persistent finding of the antigen in the blood of patients with chronic hepatitis has also been described, but the significance of the association is unclear, since the incidence of the antigen in such patients also appears to be related to the carrier rate in the general population.

Persistence of antigen is associated, in part, with impaired activity of thymus-dependent lymphocytes. That T cells play a role in recovery from acute hepatitis is suggested by the observation that T-lymphocyte function as measured by phytohemagglutinin-induced lymphocyte transformation was significantly higher in patients with acute hepatitis who eventually cleared the HB$_s$-Ag than in those who showed persistence of antigen or chronic hepatitis. HB$_s$-Ag also persists in patients with decreased T-cell function, e.g., in leukemia, lymphoma, and advanced renal disease. Humoral immune phenomena may not appreciably influence the course of hepatitis type B infection. For example, patients with agammaglobulinemia who lack the capacity for antibody production still develop acute and chronic forms of hepatitis. Liver damage may not appear in patients with high levels of HB$_s$-Ag and the absence of antibody. In addition, immunoglobulin levels and B-cell functions of patients with chronic hepatitis do not differ significantly, whether or not antigenemia is present.

Prevention

Exposure to materials containing HB$_s$-Ag can have several possible effects. In most patients, one of the common clinical pictures of acute hepatitis will occur, and in better than 80 per cent of these patients, antibody will appear. Although infection usually confers immunity, reinfection does occur at a low rate. It is not clear whether reinfection is due to contact with a virus which differs antigenically from the original strain, or whether reinfection results because the challenge dose overwhelmed the level of immunity. However, in most patients with previous exposure, contact with HB$_s$-Ag will have no discernible effect.

Prevention of type B hepatitis rests squarely on the avoidance of the use of contaminated blood products. Passive immunization with current preparations of gamma globulin is ineffective, and active immunization is presently not available. Transmission of type B hepatitis in the hospital can be reduced by disposing of syringes and needles with care and by avoiding the use of HB$_s$-Ag contaminated blood products. At present, blood for transfusion should be obtained from nonpaid volunteer donors, among whom the level of HB_s-Ag positive blood is less than 0.5 per cent. In contrast, blood from paid professional donors may show a HB_s-Ag positive reaction in 10 to 15 per cent of samples. Carriers of HB_s-Ag must not be accepted as blood donors. In addition, type B hepatitis can be transmitted by nonparenteral means; however, there are no obvious methods for preventing transmission that occurs via venereal and other nonparenteral routes.

Demonstration of HB_s-Ag in the serum of a patient or an apparently healthy person has certain public health as well as clinical implications. Since HB_s-Ag usually does not persist in the serum of a patient with type B hepatitis, its demonstration for more than three months after the onset of the acute illness suggests that the patient may become a chronic carrier of the antigen who may or may not have associated liver disease. The extent to which chronic carriers are a source of infection to others is not clear, but for practical purposes they should be considered infectious. Control measures should be taken with respect to the possibility of transmitting type B hepatitis through blood or blood-contaminated secretions. Since HB_s-Ag has also been found in all secretions and excretions from patients with type B hepatitis, some degree of infection control should be taken to prevent transmission to others, at least during the acute stage of the illness, by nonpercutaneous routes. At present, the risk of medical and nursing personnel infecting patients by nonparenteral routes seems to be small.

References

Books

Bedson, S., Downie, A. W., MacCallum, F. O., and Stuart-Harris, C. H.: Virus and Rickettsial Diseases of Man. London, Edward Arnold Ltd., 1967.

Horsfall, F. L., Jr., and Tamm, I.: Viral and Rickettsial Infections of Man. 4th ed. Philadelphia, J. B. Lippincott Co., 1965.

Original Articles

Blumberg, B. S., and Riddell, N. M.: Inherited antigenic differences in human serum beta lipo proteins. A second antiserum. J. Clin. Invest. *42:*867, 1963.

Bryan, J. A., Carr, H. E., and Gregg, M. B.: An outbreak of non-parenterally transmitted hepatitis B. J.A.M.A. *223:*229, 1973.

Byrne, E. B.: Viral hepatitis: An occupational hazard of medical personnel. J.A.M.A. *195:*362, 1966.

Cross, G. F., Waugh, M., and Ferris, A. A.: Virus-like particles associated with a faecal antigen from hepatitis patients and with Australia antigen. Aust. J. Exp. Biol. Med. Sci. *49:*1, 1971.

Dienhardt, F., Holmes, A. W., Capps, R. B., and Popper, H.: Studies on the transmission of human viral hepatitis to Marmoset monkeys. I. Transmission of disease, serial passages, and description of liver lesions. J. Exp. Med. *125:*673, 1966.

Gocke, D. J., and Kavey, N. B.: Hepatitis antigen: Correlation with disease and infectivity of blood-donors. Lancet *1:*1055, 1969.

Havens, W. P., Jr.: Etiology and epidemiology of viral hepatitis. J.A.M.A. *165:*1091, 1957.

Krugman, S., Giles, J. P., and Hammond, J.: Infectious hepatitis. J.A.M.A. *200:*365, 1967.

Krugman, S., Hoofnagle, J. H., Gerety, R. J., Kaplan, P. M., and Gerin, J. L.: Viral hepatitis B, DNA polymerase, and antibody to HB core antigen. N. Engl. J. Med. *290:*1331, 1974.

Krugman, S., and Giles, J. P.: Viral hepatitis. J.A.M.A. *212:*1019, 1970.

Krugman, S., Friedman, H., and Lattimer, C.: Viral heptatitis, type A. Identification by specific complement-fixation and immune adherence tests. N. Engl. J. Med. *292:*1141, 1975.

MacCallum, F. O. (ed.): Viral hepatitis. Br. Med. Bull. *28:* 1972.

Morbidity and Mortality Weekly Report *21:*194, 1972; *23:*125, 1974.

Prince, A. M., Hargrove, R. L., Szmuness, W., Cherubin, C. E., Fontana, V. J., and Jeffries, G. H.: Immunologic distinction between infectious and serum hepatitis. N. Engl. J. Med. *282:*987, 1970.

Provost, P. J., Wolanski, B. S., Miller, W. J., Ittensohn, O. L., McAleer, W. J., and Hilleman, M. R.: Physical, chemical and morphologic dimensions of human hepatitis A virus strain CR326. Proc. Soc. Exp. Biol. Med. *148:*532, 1975.

Ruddy, S. J., Johnson, R. F., Mosley, J. W., Atwatch, J. B., Rossettie, M. A., and Hart, J. C.: An epidemic of clam-associated hepatitis. J.A.M.A. *200:*649, 1969.

Sabesin, S. M., and Koff, R. S.: Pathogenesis of experimental viral hepatitis. N. Engl. J. Med. *290:*944, 966, 1074.

VII

CENTRAL NERVOUS SYSTEM INFECTION

Chapter 33

CENTRAL NERVOUS SYSTEM INFECTION: GENERAL CONSIDERATIONS

Classification, Pathogenesis, and Etiology

Acute Bacterial Infections

Acute bacterial infections of the central nervous system can be divided into either focal abscesses or diffuse inflammatory processes, mainly involving the leptomeninges (see Table 33–1). Abscess or meningeal inflammation may result from (1) direct invasion of nervous tissue or the subarachnoid space by bacteria, or (2) "metastatic" seeding of the central nervous system by microorganisms from the bloodstream.

Brain abscesses often develop in conjunction with traumatic head injury or from direct extension of bacterial infections of contiguous or adjacent anatomic tissues or spaces; examples include osteomyelitis of the skull or a vertebral body, acute mastoiditis, sinusitis, and wound infections following neurosurgical or orthopedic surgical procedures involving the spinal column.

Previous head trauma, particularly if associated with loss of consciousness, can be of great diagnostic importance in evaluating a patient with possible central nervous system infection. A fracture line through the petrous portion of the temporal bone allegedly never heals, providing a permanent means whereby bacteria residing in the middle ear or mastoid cells can reach the subarachnoid space. Fractures involving the cribriform plate represent

531

TABLE 33–1. Classification of Infections of the Central Nervous System

Type of Infection and Specific Examples		Pathogenesis	Most Frequent Causative Microorganisms	Chapter References
Acute bacterial infections	Abscesses: Brain Epidural Subdural	Metastatic* (lung, intestinal tract, skin, paranasal sinuses) or direct invasion (trauma or ENT, neuro-orthopedic surgery)	Peptostreptococci Bacteroides sp. Staphylococci Group A or D streptococci	7, 13, 31 7, 31 7, 37 7, 13, 14, 36
	Meningitis: Infants (2 months)	Metastatic (intestinal tract) or direct invasion (birth canal)	*Escherichia coli* Group B streptococci	7, 31 7, 13
	Children (2 months to 5 years)	Metastatic (oropharynx); rarely direct invasion	*Haemophilus influenzae*, type b *Streptococcus pneumoniae* *Neisseria meningitidis*	21 7, 20 34
	Adults	Metastatic (oropharynx); rarely direct invasion	*Streptococcus pneumoniae* *Neisseria meningitidis* (*Haemophilus influenzae*, occasionally in adults),	20 34
	All ages	Direct invasion secondary to head trauma (old or recent), congenital neuromalformations, neurodiagnostic procedures, and neuro-orthopedic surgery	Staphylococci Group A streptococci *Streptococcus pneumoniae* *Pseudomonas aeruginosa*	7, 13, 20, 36, 37
Granulomatous meningitis	Tuberculous meningitis	Metastatic (lung)	*Mycobacterium tuberculosis*	23, 24, 25
	Cryptococcal meningitis	Metastatic (lung)	*Cryptococcus neoformans*	43
Acute viral infections	"Aseptic" meningitis	Metastatic (intestinal tract or oropharynx)	Enteroviruses Mumps virus	35
	Viral encephalitis	Metastatic (intestinal tract) or arthropod vector feeding	Mumps virus Herpes virus Enteroviruses Arboviruses	35

*The term *metastatic* is commonly employed to denote hematogenous spread of microorganisms to the central nervous system, i.e., in association with bacteremia, fungemia, or viremia.

another source for bacterial invasion from the paranasal sinuses. Patients with such fractures usually have a history of excessively "watery" nasal discharges owing to intermittent or continuous drainage of cerebrospinal fluid into the nasal cavities.

Invasion of the central nervous system by microorganisms secondary to bacteremia from primary infection of other organ systems is probably the most common basis for acute bacterial infections. Primary infections of the skin, lung, and intestinal tract–biliary system are the most frequent sources of bacteremia resulting in meningitis, epidural or subdural abscesses of the spinal cord, or brain abscesses.

A wide variety of microorganisms are implicated in acute bacterial infections of the nervous system (see Table 33–1). The specific types of bacteria commonly encountered, however, depend on the type of infection, the pathogenesis of the infection, and the age of the patient. Age of the host becomes an important determinant in terms of serum levels of opsonizing bactericidal antibody. This type of immune response is thought to be a major defense mechanism in the majority of patients with acute bacterial infections of the nervous system. Microorganisms that most often cause brain, epidural, or spinal abscesses are peptostreptococci (anaerobic or microaerophilic streptococci), Bacteroides sp., *Staphylococcus aureus* or *Staphylococcus epidermidis,* and Lancefield Group A or D streptococci. In premature or newborn infants less than two months of age, meningitis may develop in association with colonization of the intestinal tract by certain microorganisms, e.g., *Escherichia coli.* Rarely, infection may result from direct invasion of bacteria secondary to trauma and contamination of wounds by bacteria indigenous to the birth canal. *Escherichia coli* and Lancefield Group B streptococci are the most important causative agents of meningitis in newborn infants. Of the *E. coli* strains associated with meningitis in infants, most have been shown to possess an envelope or capsular antigen designated as K1. Opsonizing antibody for K1 antigen is an IgG_2 immunoglobulin. This particular class of antibody passes through the placenta only during the last stages of a full-term gestation. If an infant is born prematurely, there is less likelihood that he/she will have passively acquired a protective level of maternal *E. coli* K1 antibody. The number of cases of meningitis due to *E. coli* K1 in newborns appears to be a direct reflection of prematurity. Both *E. coli* and Group B streptococci, the latter being common members of the microbial flora of the birth canal, can colonize the newborn intestinal tract or skin. Bacteremia resulting from such colonization in the absence of a sufficient level of opsonizing antibody may cause central nervous system infection. It is also possible for either microorganism to invade the subarachnoid space directly because of infection of the skin associated with trauma during delivery.

In children more than two months of age and up to approximately five years of age, meningitis almost always results from "metastatic" or hematogenous spread of microorganisms colonizing the oropharynx. The three microorganisms most often causing meningitis in patients of this age range are *Haemophilus influenzae,* type b, *Streptococcus pneumoniae,* and *Neisseria meningitidis.*

In most adult patients, meningitis is also the result of dissemination of microorganisms colonizing the oropharynx. The microorganisms of special significance in adults are *Streptococcus pneumoniae* and *Neisseria meningitidis.* In some adults, especially those over the age of 65 years, *Haemophilus influenzae* infections may occasionally be observed because some of these individuals have lost adequate bactericidal opsonizing antibody for type b strains.

In any patient, irrespective of age, microorganisms may reach the subarachnoid space by direct invasion and cause meningeal inflammation. Specific clinical settings include trauma to the head, congenital malformations of the central nervous system such as spina bifida, neurodiagnostic procedures such as pneumoencephalography or lumbar puncture, spinal anesthesia, and surgical procedures involving the central or peripheral nervous system or contiguous bone or other adjacent tissues. The most common microorganisms causing meningitis by direct invasion are *Staphylococcus aureus* or *Staphylococcus epidermidis,* Group A streptococci, *Streptococcus pneumoniae,* and miscellaneous gram negative bacteria including *Pseudomonas aeruginosa* and occasional strains of Enterobacteriaceae.

Granulomatous Meningitis

This type of meningitis is characterized by a subacute clinical course that is usually progressive, although it may be remittent, with definite remissions and relapses. The major histopathologic changes are those characteristic of granuloma formation, i.e., accumulation of lymphocytes and mononuclear cell-derived histiocytes, and epithelioid and multinucleated giant cells. *Mycobacterium tuberculosis* and *Cryptococcus neoformans* are the most common causes of granulomatous meningitis. Infection of the central nervous system by either microorganism usually occurs in the course of hematogenous dissemination of infection originating in the lungs as a result of inhalation of infectious aerosols. Dissemination of the microorganisms to the central nervous system may be so intense that meningitis may be the first clinical manifestation of tuberculosis or cryptococcal disease. Chest roentgenograms in such instances may show little or no evidence of underlying infection. Rarely, a previously silent granuloma, e.g., a tuberculoma, which had developed many years earlier in conjunction with hematogenous dissemination, may break down and allow multiplying microorganisms to reach the leptomeninges by direct local extension. In such instances, chest roentgenograms may not reveal any evidence of active pulmonary disease.

Acute Viral Infections

Acute central nervous system infections of viral origin are usually designated as "aseptic" meningitis or encephalitis, the latter being characterized by altered cerebral function. Either form of infection usually represents spread of viruses from the intestinal tract and oropharynx or, rarely, viremia induced by feeding of an arthropod vector. Viruses commonly causing "aseptic" meningitis and encephalitis are listed in Table 33–1. These and other viruses, together with the pathogenesis and epidemiologic features of viral meningitis and encephalitis, are discussed in detail in Chapter 35.

Clinical Aspects

Manifestations of Meningitis

The major clinical expressions of meningeal inflammation include fever, headache, nuchal rigidity, and altered central nervous system function. Temperature elevations may be extremely high, on occasion reaching levels of 106°F or even greater for short periods of time (see Chap. 8). The headache is usually generalized, is more severe than the patient has previously experienced, and is persistent. Resistance to dorsiflexion of the head is caused by cervical and upper thoracic paraspinal muscle spasm secondary to meningeal inflammation. It is usually an early and pathognomonic clinical finding of acute meningitis. True nuchal rigidity indicative of meningeal infection per se should be carefully distinguished from meningismus, i.e., painful or difficult dorsiflexion or rotation of the head. Meningismus may be caused by inflammation and spasm of posterior cervical or shoulder girdle musculature secondary to acute pharyngitis-tonsillitis, especially peritonsillar abscess, and acutely inflamed posterior or anterior cervical lymph nodes.

The course of bacterial meningitis can be extremely variable, undoubtedly reflecting the immune status of the infected host and the virulence of the specific strain of infecting microorganism. In some patients one or two days may be required for meningitis to become fully developed. In others, it may follow a fulminating course, with only a few hours elapsing between onset of headache and death. It is the extraordinarily rapid course of meningococcal meningitis, its propensity to occur in endemic or epidemic form, and its often high mortality rate that account in large part for the fact that meningitis evokes strong emotional responses on the part of both laymen and physicians.

Major variations in the expected or typical clinical presentation of bacterial meningitis may be encountered in very young or old patients. Newborns often exhibit nothing more than extreme irritability and "failure to thrive." Fever may be of low order or even absent in newborns and neonates, as well as in very elderly patients. Nuchal rigidity may not be demonstrable in the very young. Bulging of the fontanel due to increased intracranial pressure is a common finding in infants.

Confusing Differential Diagnostic Situations

Focal abscesses often masquerade as noninfectious disorders. They are not infrequently mistaken for neoplastic processes. The clinical presentation and course of a solitary cerebral abscess, for example, may be extremely difficult to distinguish from a neoplastic lesion. In both neoplasm and abscess, increased intracranial pressure often accounts for the most conspicuous neurologic signs; the cerebrospinal fluid may be entirely normal, except for the fact that it is under increased pressure.

The principal manifestations of epidural or subdural spinal abscesses usually are the result of spinal cord compression. These manifestations often simulate those associated with several noninfectious disease processes, including Guillian-Barré syndrome, spinal cord tumor, meningioma, and a herniated nucleus pulposus. Cerebrospinal fluid changes also may be similar to those seen in noninfectious disease processes, viz., little or no pleocytosis, elevated protein content, and normal glucose level. A very low opening or closing cerebrospinal fluid pressure suggesting blockage of the subarachnoid space may be the first clue to the correct diagnosis. Emergency myelography is often essential to confirm spinal cord compression and identify the precise site of blockage in the subarachnoid space. When infection or abscess formation impinges on or occurs within the spinal canal, the spinal cord must be decompressed by appropriate neurosurgical means within 24 hours or less, if return of normal neurologic function is to be expected.

Neoplastic metastases involving the meninges may produce a clinical picture simulating granulomatous meningitis. The cerebrospinal fluid abnormalities may be identical to those characterizing tuberculous or cryptococcal meningitis.

Cerebrospinal Fluid Abnormalities

Examination of cerebrospinal fluid secured by lumbar puncture may be an invaluable adjunct in evaluating patients with suspected infection of the central nervous system. Lumbar puncture is essential for obtaining cerebrospinal fluid and promptly recognizing the occurrence of acute bacterial or viral meningitis or granulomatous meningitis (see Table 33–1).

In patients with brain abscess, examination of the cerebrospinal fluid is often of little help diagnostically. Furthermore, because increased intracranial pressure may occur, lumbar puncture may be contraindicated. Removal of even small amounts of cerebrospinal fluid, i.e., 3 to 4 ml, from the lumbar subarachnoid space may result in downward displacement of the brain into the foramen magnum, with squeezing of the cerebellar peduncles against the lower medulla and consequent cardio–respiratory center failure. Sudden removal of cerebrospinal fluid under increased pressure also may cause shifting of the brain, with transtentorial herniation of portions of the cerebral hemispheres into the posterior fossa. Transtentorial or foraminal herniation of the brain constitutes an extreme emergency and requires rapid neurosurgical decompression in order to save the patient. For the above reasons and also in light of substantial improvements in neurodiagnostic procedures, especially those of a noninvasive type, lumbar puncture should be reserved primarily for those patients in whom examination of cerebrospinal fluid, including smear and culture, is clearly required for confirming a provisional diagnosis of acute or granulomatous meningitis.

The expected cerebrospinal fluid abnormalities associated with each of the main types of meningitis are shown in Table 33–2. Special points deserve emphasis. The cerebrospinal fluid changes in bacterial meningitis are modified to a surprisingly small degree by previous administration of antimicrobial therapy. Thus, failure to find bacteria on the Gram stain of the centrifuged fluid sediment or to isolate bacteria from cerebrospinal fluid that is grossly abnormal is not readily explained on the basis of a patient previously receiving antimicrobial drugs. Cerebrospinal fluid containing relatively large numbers of segmented neutrophils and revealing a negative smear and culture for bacteria is commonly associated with acute bacterial meningitis due to *Neisseria meningitidis*. Failure to demonstrate acid-fast bacilli in cerebrospinal fluid specimens similarly reflects the small number of microorganisms present per unit volume. It should be remembered that India ink used for demonstration of *Cryptococcus neoformans* yeast cells with their large capsules may on occasion contain endogenous contaminating yeast cells. The Pelican brand of India ink contains sufficient phenol to inhibit proliferation of contaminating yeasts and is the preferable preparation for negative stains. (see Chap. 10).

TABLE 33-2. Cerebrospinal Fluid Abnormalities Associated with Meningitis

Type of Meningitis	Predominant Cell Type	Cerebrospinal Fluid Findings			Result of Culture
		Glucose	*Protein*	*Stained Smear*	
Bacterial	Segmented neutrophils	Very low (< 5–20 mg%)	Elevated	Usually positive*	Usually positive*
Tuberculous	Mononuclear cells (neutrophils early)	Low (20–40 mg%)	Elevated	Usually negative	Usually negative
Fungal	Mononuclear cells	Low (20–40 mg%)	Elevated	Often positive	Usually positive
Viral ("aseptic")	Mononuclear cells	Normal (65–70 mg%)	Slightly elevated early	Negative	Negative

*A major exception is bacterial meningitis caused by *Neisseria meningitidis* in which the Gram stain of cerebrospinal fluid sediment often fails to reveal microorganisms, and cultures may be negative for growth.

The cerebrospinal fluid changes associated with tuberculous, fungal, and viral meningitis are frequently overlapping, and it may be difficult to separate one from the other. This is especially true in those patients with viral meningitis and a slightly depressed cerebrospinal fluid glucose (see Chap. 35) or in patients with very early tuberculous meningitis in whom the glucose has not yet reached a very low level. In each of these three forms of meningitis, viz., tuberculous, fungal, and viral, cerebrospinal fluid collected very early in the course of illness may contain a preponderance of segmented neutrophils and consequently be thought to reflect bacterial meningitis. Should the proper diagnosis and appropriate therapy be delayed, the end result can be disastrous. In most instances, the clinical findings, chest roentgenogram, epidemiologic data, and other aspects of the evaluation of the patient give the physician a good idea as to which one of these three forms of meningitis is present.

Some of the recently developed diagnostic methods for detection of bacterial antigens or cellular constituents are discussed elsewhere (see especially Chaps. 9 and 10) and are becoming valuable adjuncts in examination of cerebrospinal fluid specimens. Counterimmunoelectrophoresis has been successfully employed in the diagnosis of meningitis due most commonly to 3 microorganisms, viz., *Streptococcus pneumoniae, Neisseria meningitidis,* and *Haemophilus influenzae,* type b. There are some suggestions that detection of fungal constituents and metabolic products in cerebrospinal fluid by means of gas chromatography may be diagnostically useful. The procedure is as reported for detection of circulating yeast cell products in systemic disease due to *Candida albicans* (see Chaps. 9 and 43). *Cryptococcus neoformans* antigen can be detected by several different immunologic procedures. Monitoring the level of this antigen not only in the cerebrospinal fluid but also in the serum is helpful in evaluating therapy.

Therapy

Urgency of Specific Antimicrobial Therapy

The major concern in approaching the problem of acute bacterial meningitis is rapid diagnosis and institution of effective antimicrobial therapy. The overriding objective of therapy is to suppress and eliminate the infection as rapidly as possible in hopes of minimizing the occurrence of additional nervous tissue damage. The obvious sequelae of meningitis, such as gross neurologic deficits, are not so important as the more subtle and later appearing personality and behavioral problems that may seriously impair the patient's chances of assuming or resuming a responsible role in society.

There is no reason why more than 30 to 60 minutes should elapse between the time a physician takes on responsibility for a patient with suspected meningitis and the time specific antimicrobial therapy is underway. A situation precluding lumbar puncture and confirmation of the provisional diagnosis of bacterial meningitis should be no reason for withholding antimicrobial therapy anymore than the inability to secure a blood glucose level should delay insulin therapy in a patient with suspected diabetic acidosis or coma. Vigorous antimicrobial therapy must be started and continued while the patient is transported to a facility where lumbar puncture and appropriate examination of cerebrospinal fluid can be carried out.

General Approach to Antimicrobial Therapy

Prior to the time when *Neisseria meningitidis* isolates developed resistance to sulfonamides (see Chap. 34) it was common practice to use a different type of antimicrobial therapeutic regimen for each of the common forms of acute bacterial meningitis (see Table 33-1). Meningococcal meningitis was treated with one of the sulfonamide derivatives; crystalline penicillin G was employed for pneumococcal infections, and chloramphenicol with or without a sulfonamide derivative was used for patients with infection due to *Haemophilus influenzae.*

The introduction of ampicillin, a semisynthetic derivative of penicillin, in the early 1960s, represented a major step forward in the therapy of meningitis. Each of the common etiologic agents causing meningitis in young children or adults (see Table 33–1) was found to be highly susceptible to ampicillin. Each has remained so until recently. Comparative clinical studies revealed that ampicillin in large doses gives therapeutic results equivalent to, if not better than, those obtained with other antimicrobial therapeutic regimens.

Representative data supporting this viewpoint are shown in Table 33–3. The relatively large proportion of cases of infection due to *Haemophilus influenzae* reflects the large number of children in this study. In each group, even those in whom the cause of the meningitis was undetermined (and probably represented *Neisseria meningitidis* infection), the outcome in the ampicillin-treated groups of patients was equal if not superior to that of the groups treated with another antimicrobial agent or combination of agents. For the past decade, therefore, the conventional approach to patients of all ages, except for neonates less than two months of age (see Table 33–1), has been to initiate therapy using very high doses of intravenous ampicillin. Ampicillin is a relatively nontoxic drug, thereby permitting large doses to be employed and assuring high serum levels and satisfactory levels of antibacterial activity in the cerebrospinal fluid. Measurement of such levels is useful in monitoring the effectiveness of therapy for meningitis (see Chap. 45).

TABLE 33–3. Comparative Therapeutic Results of Ampicillin Versus Penicillin or Penicillin Plus Chloramphenicol in Bacterial Meningitis*

Etiology	Antimicrobial Therapy	No. of Patients	Mortality (Per Cent)
Streptococcus pneumoniae	Penicillin	42	29
	Ampicillin	41	22
Neisseria meningitidis	Penicillin	77	9
	Ampicillin	56	5
Haemophilus influenzae (type b)	Chloramphenicol	107	9
	Ampicillin	66	6
Unknown	Penicillin and chloramphenicol	35	6
	Ampicillin	29	0

*Data from study reported by Mathies, A. W., Jr., et al.: Experience with ampicillin in bacterial meningitis. Antimicrob. Agents Chemother. *5:*610, 1965.

Specific Therapeutic Problems

Restrictive Blood-Brain Barrier

The blood-brain barrier and the blood–cerebrospinal fluid barrier restrict penetration of most antimicrobial drugs into the brain and cerebrospinal fluid. Drug concentrations in these two nervous system compartments of clinically well human volunteers and experimental animals are approximately 1/200 to 1/500 those in serum. Inflammation involving the central nervous system materially enhances drug penetration. Even with inflammatory changes of an intensity characterizing acute bacterial meningitis, passage of antimicrobial agents is still hindered because of the restrictive nature of the blood-brain barrier and blood–cerebrospinal fluid barrier. Thus, the physician faces a significant problem in achieving essential therapeutic levels of antimicrobial activity within the nervous system.

Unfortunately, the advantage of relatively good penetration of the sulfonamide derivatives into the nervous system can no longer be realized in the treatment of meningococcal infections owing to the high incidence of sulfonamide-resistance exhibited by most strains of meningococci currently causing acute meningococcal infection. Chloramphenicol is of special interest because of its unique capacity to concentrate in brain tissue. For this reason, it is an invaluable antimicrobial adjunct in the treatment of central nervous system infections. The penicillin-class drugs, with the exception of ampicillin, vary tremendously in their capacity to penetrate the blood-brain barrier, even when present in the blood in high levels. High levels of penicillin G in cerebrospinal fluid and brain tissue can be achieved with a reasonable degree of success, providing massive doses of the crystalline form are injected every two hours by the intravenous or intramuscular routes. It is much more difficult to achieve comparable levels with the semisynthetic penicillinase-resistant penicillin derivatives, especially the cephalosporin derivatives, e.g., cephalothin and cephaloridine. The latter two drugs should not be used for the treatment of central nervous system infections except under very special circumstances. The aminoglycosides, i.e., streptomycin and gentamicin, penetrate to such a low degree that they cannot be used unless injected intrathecally.

The blood-brain barrier also restricts the transport of antibody and complement components from the intravascular compartment to the central nervous system. Opsonizing antibody with or without C3 represents an important host defense mechanism in combating bacterial infections. Low levels of opsonizing antibody in the blood may be one reason for the initial development of meningitis and may account for a very poor prognosis in a high proportion of patients, especially older adults.

Antimicrobial Drug Antagonism

Despite attempts to improve the survival rate of patients with pneumococcal meningitis, approximately 30 per cent of affected adults die of the disease. In 1951 an attempt was made to improve the therapy of this disease by treating patients with massive doses of penicillin in combination with one of the tetracyclines, chlortetracycline. A mortality rate of 79 per cent was observed in the 14 patients receiving this antimicrobial drug combination, whereas patients treated with massive doses of penicillin alone had a mortality rate of only 30 per cent, a rate in line with that in most medical centers at the time this study was reported. Because of the excessive mortality rate, the study was terminated and has never been repeated. It stands as the singular example of clinically significant antagonism between antimicrobial agents (see Chap. 44). The usual explanation given for the less favorable response in patients receiving both drugs in contrast to penicillin alone is that chlortetracycline exerts a bacteriostatic effect on the otherwise rapidly multiplying pneumococci and thereby prevents or impairs the bactericidal activity of penicillin. Whether or not this is the correct interpretation is not known. This classic study serves as a warning that the use of more than one antimicrobial drug may have an adverse rather than a beneficial effect.

Antimicrobial Drug Resistance

As already mentioned in this chapter, during the past 15 years meningococcal isolates have shown increasing resistance to the bacteriostatic action of sulfonamide derivatives. This is true of virtually all Group C strains, which account for the majority of sporadic cases of meningococcal meningitis in both civilian and military populations. A high proportion of Group B strains also exhibit sulfonamide resistance. In the last two or three years, epidemic outbreaks of sulfonamide-resistant strains of Group A meningococci have been reported in Africa and South America. Therefore, patients with suspected meningococcal meningitis can no longer be treated with sulfon-amide derivatives and should be treated with high doses of crystalline penicillin G or ampicillin.

Within the past two years, *Haemophilus influenzae* has shown a propensity for developing resistance to ampicillin, the drug formerly relied upon entirely for treatment of infection by this microorganism. Recent surveys have suggested that up to 10 per cent of strains of *H. influenzae,* type b may be moderately or markedly resistant to ampicillin. For this reason, most physicians advise instituting ampicillin plus chloramphenicol therapy in young children or older adults in whom *H. influenzae,* type b may be the etiologic agent of meningitis. Revision of the antimicrobial drug program can be made once the antimicrobial susceptibility of the *H. influenzae* isolate has been determined. At the present time, there is no clinical evidence that ampicillin and chloramphenicol are antagonistic.

Alternate Antimicrobial Drug Therapy for Patients with Allergy to Penicillin-Class Drugs

In patients who are anaphylactically sensitized to penicillin-class drugs and in whom penicillin G cannot be used, chloramphenicol can be employed as an alternate drug with essentially equivalent results. As discussed elsewhere (see Chaps. 44 and 46), it is the unpredictable hematologic toxicity of chloramphenicol that accounts in large part for it being viewed as an "alternate" antimicrobial agent.

CASE PRESENTATION

An 18-year-old white male high-school student was brought by police ambulance to the emergency room of a suburban community hospital on the evening of March 7, 1971. The patient was acutely agitated and incoherent. According to the patient's parents, he had complained that morning at breakfast of diffuse muscular aching, malaise, and anorexia. He had vomited his breakfast soon after eating and declined to go to school. Because of a very severe headache that was unresponsive to aspirin, and a rise in temperature to 104°F during the early afternoon of March 7, a physician was consulted and examined the patient in his home. The physician could find no physical abnormalities and prescribed medication for nausea. During the next several hours, the patient became extremely agitated, began to mutter in an incoherent fashion, and was totally disorientated. There was no history of previous sinus or middle-ear disease or surgery. The patient had never been rendered unconscious or sustained a head injury of any type. No other members of the family had been ill.

Brief physical examination in the emergency room revealed a temperature of 100.8°F (estimated axillary recording) and a blood pressure of 150/60 mm Hg. The patient was flailing about in a violent manner, rendering anything more than an abbreviated examination impossible. The neck was stiff, and even a small degree of dorsiflexion was impossible. There was, however, no evidence of a positive Kernig's sign or pyramidal tract plantar reflexes. A few 1- to 3-mm petechial skin lesions were observed over the thighs and in each antecubital fossa. The lungs appeared clear; the heart seemed to be of normal size and no murmurs were heard.

Immediate lumbar puncture was performed, with the patient securely restrained. The cerebrospinal fluid appeared moderately cloudy and contained 15,000 leukocytes per cubic millimeter, of which 94 per cent were segmented neutrophils. The cerebrospinal fluid glucose was less than 5 mg per 100 ml, and a simultaneous blood glucose was 194 mg per 100 ml. Direct Gram smear on the centrifuged cerebrospinal fluid sediment failed to reveal bacteria. Culture of the specimen failed to show growth after 72 hours. Counterimmunoelectrophoresis of the cerebrospinal fluid gave a sharp line of precipitation with Group C meningococcal antiserum within a period of two hours (see Fig. 33–1).

This patient exhibited typical manifestations of meningococcal inflammation, viz., fever, headache, altered sensorium and cerebral function, vomiting, and stiff neck. It is important to note that he had no predisposition for meningeal inflammation based on the absence of past signs or history of middle-ear disease or skull fracture. Note how fast the disease progressed, a particular feature of meningococcal infection. The few petechial skin lesions noted in the emergency room, together with the time of year and the age of the patient, suggested that *Neisseria meningitidis* was the most likely cause of the bacterial meningitis. The absence of bacteria on the Gram-stained smear of the cerebrospinal fluid and the inability to isolate *N. meningitidis* from the cloudy spinal fluid further point to a diagnosis of meningococcal infection as opposed to disease caused by *Streptococcus pneumoniae* (see above).

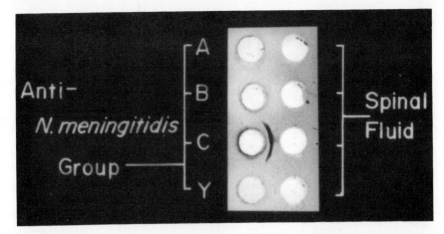

Figure 33-1. The result observed in counterimmunoelectrophoresis using cerebrospinal fluid collected from the patient in Case Presentation 1 four hours after hospitalizaton. Note the band of immune precipitation between the well containing Group C meningococcal antiserum and the opposing well containing the patient's cerebrospinal fluid. This finding is indicative of the presence of Group C meningococcal polysaccharide in the patient's cerebrospinal fluid. No bands of immune precipitation were observed when the same sample of cerebrospinal fluid was simultaneously tested using antisera to a multiplicity of pneumococcal serotypes or antiserum to *Haemophilus influenzae,* type b.

A specific definitive diagnosis was provided within hours after admission to the hospital by means of counterimmunoelectrophoresis, which demonstrated Group C meningococcal polysaccharide in the spinal fluid (Fig. 33–1 and see Chap. 10). Although blood cultures were not taken, it is probable that they would have been positive in view of the petechial eruption and thus would have provided bacteriologic confirmation of the disease. Another approach to diagnosis could have been aspiration of the skin lesions under aseptic conditions, smearing the tissue fluid, and then Gram staining it. Presence of gram negative coccal bacilli on the smear either within neutrophils or free in the interstitial fluid would have provided strong evidence of infection with neisseria. While the lesions and such a positive smear would suggest *N. meningitidis,* it should be kept in mind that septicemia due to *Neisseria gonorrhoeae* does occur, and skin lesions in this type of infection may simulate those due to meningococcal bacteremia.

References

Adair, C. V., Gauld, R. L., and Smadel, J. E.: Aseptic meningitis, a disease of diverse etiology: clinical and etiologic studies on 854 cases. Ann. Intern. Med. *39:*675, 1953.

Alexander, C. E., Sanborn, W. R., Cherriere, G., Crocker, W. H., Ewald, P. E., and Kay, C. R.: Sulfadiazine-resistant group A Neisseria meningitidis. Science *161:*1019, 1968.

Amundson, S., Braude, A. I., and Davis, C. E.: Rapid diagnosis of infection by gas-liquid chromatography: Analysis of sugars in normal and infected cerebrospinal fluid. Appl. Microbiol. *28:*298, 1974.

Barrett, F. F., Eardley, W. A., Yow, M. D., and Leverett, H. A.: Ampicillin in the treatment of acute suppurative meningitis. J. Pediatr. *69:*343, 1966.

Coonrod, J. D., and Rytel, M. W.: Determination of etiology of bacterial meningitis by counterimmunoelectrophoresis. Lancet *1:*1154, 1972.

Dalton, H. P., and Allison, M. J.: Modification of laboratory results by partial treatment of bacterial meningitis. Am. J. Clin. Pathol. *49:*410, 1968.

Edwards, E. A., Muehl, P. M., and Peckinpaugh, R. O.: Diagnosis of bacterial meningitis by counterimmunoelectrophoresis. J. Lab. Clin. Med. *80:*449, 1972.

Feigin, R. D., Richmond, D., Hosler, M. W., and Shakelford, P. G.: Reassessment of the role of bactericidal antibody in *Hemophilus influenzae* infection. Am. J. Med. Sci. *262:*338, 1972.

Fisher, L. S., Chow, A. W., Yoshikawa, T. T., and Guze, L. B.: Cephalothin and cephaloridine therapy for bacterial meningitis. An evaluation. Ann. Intern. Med. *82:*689, 1975.

Fothergill, L. D., and Wright, J.: Influenzal meningitis. The relation of age incidence to the bactericidal power of blood against the causal organism. J. Immunol. *24:*273, 1933.

Goodman, J. S., Kaufman, L., and Koening, M. G.: Diagnosis of cryptococcal meningitis. Value of immunologic detection of cryptococcal antigen. N. Engl. J. Med. *285:*434, 1971.

Heineman, H. S., and Braude, A. I.: Anaerobic infection of the brain. Observations on eighteen consecutive cases of brain abscess. Am. J. Med. *35:*682, 1963.

Jarvis, C. W., and Saxena, K. M.: Does prior antibiotic treatment hamper the diagnosis of acute bacterial meningitis? An analysis of a series of 135 childhood cases. Clin. Pediatr. *11:*201, 1972.

Khan, W., Ross, S., Rodriquez, W., Controni, G., and Saz, A. K.: *Haemophilus influenzae* type B resistant to ampicillin. A report of two cases. J.A.M.A. *229:*298, 1974.

Kislak, J. W., Marcuse, D. J., and Hass, W. K.: Staphylococcal meningitis following pneumoencephalography. Ann. Intern. Med. *57:*128, 1962.

Kubik, C. S., and Adams, R. D.: Subdural empyema. Brain *66:*18, 1943.

Leedom, J. M., Ivler, D., Mathies, A. W., Jr., Thrupp, L. D., Portnoy, B., and Wehrle, P. F.: Importance of sulfadiazine resistance in meningococcal disease in civilians. N. Engl. J. Med. *273:*1395, 1965.

Lepper, M. H., and Dowling, H. F.: Treatment of pneumococcic meningitis with penicillin compared with penicillin plus aureomycin. Arch. Intern. Med. *88:*489, 1951.

Levin, S., Nelson, K. E., Spies, H. W., and Lepper, M. H.: Pneumococcal meningitis: the problem of the unseen cerebrospinal fluid leak. Am. J. Med. Sci. *264:*319, 1972.

Mathies, A. W., Jr., Leedom, J. M., Thrupp, L. D., Ivler, D., Portnoy, B., and Wehrle, P. F.: Experience with ampicillin in bacterial meningitis – 1965. Antimicrob. Agents Chemother. *5:*610, 1965.

McCracken, G. H., Jr., Sarff, L. D., Glode, M. P., Mize, S. G., Schiffer, M. S., Robbins, J. B., Gotschlich, E. C., Orskov, I., and Orskov, F.: Relation between *Escherichia coli* K1 capsular polysaccharide antigen and clinical outcome in neonatal meningitis. Lancet *2:*246, 1974.

Millar, J. W., Seiss, E. E., Feldman, H. A., Silverman, C., and Frank, P.: In vivo and in vitro resistance to sulfadiazine in strains of Neisseria meningitidis, J.A.M.A. *186:*139, 1963.

Norden, C. W., Callerame, M. L., and Baum, J.: *Haemophilus influenzae* meningitis in an adult. A study of bactericidal antibodies and immunoglobulins. N. Engl. J. Med. *282:*190, 1970.

Petito, F., and Plum, F.: The lumbar puncture. (Editorial.) New Engl. J. Med. *290:*225, 1974.

Robbins, J. B., Schneerson, R., Argaman, M., and Handzel, Z. T.: Haemophilus influenzae type b: disease and immunity in humans. Ann. Intern. Med. *78:*259, 1973.

Rogers, D. E., and McDermott, W.: Neoplastic involvement of the meninges with low cerebrospinal fluid glucose concentrations simulating tuberculous meningitis. Am. Rev. Tubercl. *69:*1029, 1954.

Samson, D. S., and Clark, K.: A current review of brain abscess. Am. J. Med. *54:*201, 1973.

Smith, H. V., and Villum, R. L.: The diagnosis of tuberculous meningitis. Br. Med. Bull. *10:*140, 1954.

Tomeh, M. O., Starr, S. E., McGowan, J. E., Jr., Terry, P. M., and Nahmias, A. J.: Ampicillin-resistant Haemophilus influenzae type b infection. J.A.M.A. *229:*295, 1974.

Westenfelder, G. O., and Paterson, P. Y.: Life-threatening infection: Alternate drugs when penicillin cannot be given. J.A.M.A. *210:*845, 1969.

Wilfert, C. M.: Mumps meningoencephalitis with low cerebrospinal fluid glucose, prolonged pleocytosis and elevation of protein. N. Engl. J. Med. *280:*855, 1969.

Yu, J. S., and Grauaug, A.: Purulent meningitis in the neonatal period. Arch. Dis. Child. *38:*391, 1963.

Chapter 34

NEISSERIA MENINGITIDIS AND MENINGOCOCCAL DISEASE

Introduction

Neisseria meningitidis is a gram negative coccus found among the indigenous microbiota of the upper respiratory tract of man (see Chap. 7). It should be distinguished from other species of the family Neisseriaceae that constitute part of the normal oropharyngeal flora but have little pathogenic potential (see Chap. 7). The other important disease-producing member of the family Neisseriaceae, *Neisseria gonorrhoeae,* is discussed in detail in Chapter 30.

Neisseria meningitidis, or the meningococcus, has been historically associated with worldwide epidemic outbreaks of leptomeningeal inflammation for centuries. Ever since "cerebrospinal fever" was recognized as an often fatal and communicable disease in the early 1800s, occurrence of even a solitary case of "spinal meningitis" has invariably evoked anxiety sometimes approaching panic among both medical personnel and laymen. Probably no other microorganism rivals the capacity of *N. meningitidis* to produce fulminating illness and death within a matter of a few hours. Outbreaks of meningococcal disease have all too frequently posed serious medical and epidemiologic problems for large numbers of susceptible persons living in close proximity to each other, e.g., young recruits entering military training or children in boarding schools.

Neisseria meningitidis also is well known to cause a nonmeningeal form of disease, acute meningococcal septicemia. Meningococcemia may progress to septic shock with intravascular clotting, irreversible circulatory failure, and a characteristic high mortality rate (see Chap. 27). In addition to meningitis and septic shock, *N. meningitidis,* like *N. gonorrhoeae,* has been implicated in a variety of clinical syndromes involving inflammation of different organ systems, especially serous membranes, e.g., pericarditis and polyarthritis.

Basic Microbiology

Morphology and Cultural Characteristics

Neisseria meningitidis is a gram negative, nonmotile, nonsporulating, round or oval, small coccus. The bacterial cells usually exist as pairs, their opposing surfaces flattened or indented, giving them the appearance of "biscuit shaped" diplococci. Meningococci grow on suitable media as convex, smooth, and glistening colonies measuring 1 to 5 mm in diameter. Colonies may have a mucoid appearance if a large amount of capsular polysaccharide material is synthesized.

In contrast to the less fastidious commonly occurring indigenous strains of the family Neisseriaceae, such as *Neisseria catarrhalis,* meningococci and gonococci require enriched complex media. Such media must have been treated, or specially prepared, in order to reduce or eliminate a variety of "toxic" components which inhibit growth of meningococci. Some of these growth inhibitory factors have been identified, e.g., heavy metals and fatty acids. Other toxic components remain unknown except for the fact that they are relatively heat labile. Blood agar plates prepared by heating sheep blood in molten agar at 80 to 90°C and referred to as "chocolate agar" because of their brown color are used by most clinical microbiology laboratories for the isolation and propagation of *Neisseria meningitidis* strains. The medium devised by Mueller and Hinton is particularly good as a basic culture medium, appears to be free of injurious components, and is widely used for cultivating *N. meningitidis.* Selective culture medium patterned after that developed by Thayer and Martin and containing polymyxin and other antimicrobial agents that inhibit overgrowth of contaminants is often used to isolate *N. meningitidis* from heterogeneous bacterial populations. Thayer-Martin type medium is especially useful in epidemiologic studies to detect persons harboring *N. meningitidis* in their oropharynx or nasopharynx, the so-called meningococcal carriers (see Chap. 30 for more details of Thayer-Martin type medium).

Neisseria meningitidis strains are aerobic and prefer a humid environment at a temperature of 37°C for optimal growth; isolation and growth are also enhanced by a concentration of 5 to 10 per cent carbon dioxide. The nasopharynx allegedly provides a significantly more humid environment with a higher carbon dioxide content than the oropharynx, but whether this explains why *N. meningitidis* preferentially colonizes the nasopharyngeal region of the upper respiratory tract is dubious at best. Selective adherence of *N. meningitidis* to specific receptor substances synthesized by nasopharyngeal mucosa, a characteristic analogous to that already described for Group A streptococci and other microorganisms infecting the respiratory tract (see Chaps. 3, 7, and 13), seems more likely. The fact that *N. meningitidis* preferentially infects the nasopharynx is of practical moment. The nasopharynx is the best site to culture if one wishes to determine whether a person is infected with *N. meningitidis*. Culture of this anatomic area requires special swabs consisting of cotton-tipped thin wires, which can be passed through the nose, or cotton-tipped bent wires, which are passed through the mouth and permit the cotton tip to come in contact with the nasopharyngeal mucosa behind and above the soft palate and uvula.

Identification

Speciation of the family Neisseriaceae is important for establishing a definite diagnosis of meningococcal or gonococcal disease or, rarely, infection caused by another Neisseria species. Accurate differentiation of *Neisseria meningitidis* from *Neisseria gonorrhoeae* may be of medicolegal significance. Identification procedures usually depend on biochemical and serologic (immunologic) tests. Many *N. meningitidis* isolates, however, possess insufficient amounts of group-specific antigen to permit recognition by reaction with corresponding antisera. Furthermore, all other Neisseria species, including *N. gonorrhoeae,* usually lack specific antigens that would allow identification by immunologic means. Biochemical tests, therefore, are especially important. Not infrequently, final distinction between *N. meningitidis* and *N. gonorrhoeae* rests on specific sugar fermentation patterns.

Biochemical Tests

Neisseria meningitidis oxidizes glucose and maltose, whereas *Neisseria gonorrhoeae* oxidizes only glucose. Some of the Neisseria species less frequently associated with disease, e.g., *Neisseria sicca,* oxidize glucose, maltose, and sucrose, while other species, including *Neisseria catarrhalis* and *Neisseria flavescens,* fail to utilize any of these three carbohydrates as a source of energy.

Of special note is *Neisseria lactamicus,* which utilizes glucose and maltose and thereby appears to be similar to *N. meningitidis. N. lactamicus,* in contrast to *N. meningitidis,* oxidizes lactose and can be readily separated in this manner. Occasionally, this distinction can be of clinical importance, since *N. lactamicus* reportedly can cause significant infectious disease. Since many laboratories may not investigate lactose utilization owing to time-honored identification based on other sugar fermentation tests, the physician should be aware of *N. lactamicus* and the means of distinguishing it from *N. meningitidis.*

Neisseria meningitidis, like *Neisseria gonorrhoeae,* produces indol oxidase. Colonies flooded with a solution of dimethyl- or tetramethylparaphenylenediamine give a positive oxidase test, i.e., they turn pink or dark blue, depending on which reagent is employed. A positive oxidase test is often cited as a useful means for identifying *N. meningitidis* and *N. gonorrhoeae.* However, nonpathogenic neisseria as well as other bacterial species that colonize the upper respiratory tract also may give a positive oxidase reaction. Therefore, the test is of questionable reliability when used alone for identification of *N. meningitidis* in oropharyngeal or nasopharyngeal cultures.

Antigenic Specificity

Most strains of *Neisseria meningitidis* that cause clinical disease elaborate antigenic capsular polysaccharides. Just as described for *Streptococcus pneumoniae, Haemophilus influenzae,* and *Klebsiella pneumoniae* (see Chaps. 20 and 21), encapsulated *N. meningitidis* isolates give a quellung reaction or form specific precipitates when mixed with appropriate antisera.

Three major serotypes of *Neisseria meningitidis* have been recognized for decades: Groups A, B, and C. Each has been the subject of extensive clinical, immunologic, and epidemiologic studies. Group A strains historically have been responsible for worldwide epidemic outbreaks involving large numbers of individuals and occurring with a cyclic periodicity not unlike that of influenza virus serotypes. Therefore, Group A *N. meningitidis* was considered for decades to be an epidemic serotype. In contrast, Groups B and C *N. meningitidis* tended to cause solitary cases of sporadic disease or limited outbreaks of meningococcal disease during the interepidemic periods when Group A strains were not prevalent. Group B and C strains were designated endemic serotypes of *N. meningitidis.*

Since World War II, but especially since the early 1960s, a progressive shift in the relative importance of these three serotypes has occurred. Around 1963, Group B strains began to replace those of Group A as the cause of most cases of meningococcal disease. Since 1967, however, Group C strains have been responsible for proportionately more cases than Group B strains and are currently replacing Group B as the most important serotype. Epidemics of Group A disease still occur in various parts of the world, e.g., South America and Africa, but such epidemics have become less extensive and less frequent than during earlier decades of this century.

Emergence of sulfonamide-resistant strains of Group B *Neisseria meningitidis* in 1963, together with the increasing importance of this and other non–Group A serotypes in outbreaks of disease particularly affecting the military forces of the United States, has led to a marked escalation in meningococcal disease research. New thrusts in both clinical and laboratory investigation have identified the following new serotypes: Groups D, X, Y, Z, 29-E, and 135. Many of these newer Groups, especially Y, seem to be of considerable clinical significance and have caused small outbreaks of *N. meningitidis* disease. One wonders whether another shift is in progress, Group Y becoming dominant over Group C.

Antigenic and Virulence Factors

There are several antigenic or toxic constituents of *Neisseria meningitidis* that are important in the pathogenesis of meningococcal disease and retrospective diagnosis of *N. meningitidis* infection based on detection of a rising titer of antibodies. The three constituents which are discussed here briefly are (1) group-specific capsular polysaccharide, (2) lipopolysaccharide-endotoxin cell wall complex, and (3) genus (Neisseria)-specific protein.

As illustrated schematically in Figure 34–1, the outer coating of the meningococcal cell wall consists of group-specific capsular polysaccharide. The polysaccharide capsule is a major virulence factor. It enables meningococci to resist phagocytosis by segmented neutrophils. Resistance to phagocytosis allows *Neisseria meningitidis* to multiply extracellularly until the infected host produces antibodies that specifically react with capsular polysaccharide antigen and abrogate its antiphagocytic property.

Group C and A capsular polysaccharides induce specific antibodies of either IgG or IgM. These antibodies exert a bactericidal effect on *Neisseria meningitidis* in two ways. In the first mechanism, IgG and perhaps IgM act as opsonizing antibodies and in concert with complement (heat-labile serum factor) augment phagocytosis of *N. meningitidis* by segmented neutrophils. Once ingested, the microorganisms are broken down by lysosomal enzymes discharged into the phagolysosomal vacuole (see Chap. 3). Whether these antibodies enhance phagocytosis by other phagocytic cells such as circulating monocytes and extravascular macrophages is not known.

The second mechanism accounting for bactericidal activity involves in vitro binding of either IgG or IgM to *Neisseria meningitidis,* activation of the complement cascade, and focal lysis of the bacterial cell wall and membrane by terminal complement components C8 and C9 (see Chap. 3). It is not known whether C8 and C9 can be activated only via the classic sequence or whether the C3 "bypass" pathway is a possible mechanism for activation of these enzymes. The type of bactericidal activity that is described here for *N. meningitidis* is identical to the antibody-mediated complement-dependent bacteriolysis known to occur with virtually all gram negative bacteria (see Chap. 3). Recent observations indicate that Group C polysaccharide also may induce secretory IgA antibody and that this type of antibody can block bacteriolysis by IgG or IgM antibodies plus complement. If antibody-mediated complement-dependent bacteriolysis occurs to any significant degree

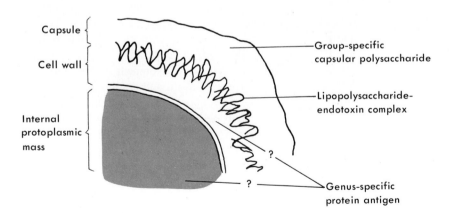

Figure 34–1. Major antigenic and virulence constituents of *Neisseria meningitidis.*

in vivo (a point that is not clear and deserves attention), secretory IgA antibodies might retard eradication of *N. meningitidis* from the oropharynx or nasopharynx by interfering with IgG or IgM bacteriolytic activity. Persistence of *N. meningitidis* in the nasopharynx for days or even weeks is well documented and is a feature of the so-called chronic meningococcal carrier state.

Group C or A capsular polysaccharides can be prepared in reasonably defined form and used to coat erythrocytes. Erythrocytes coated with these polysaccharides are agglutinated by sera containing specific antibodies for the corresponding *Neisseria meningitidis* serotype. This is the basis for the hemagglutination test, a relatively simple method for assessing the immune status of individuals with respect to *N. meningitidis* infection. It is curious that clinical meningococcal disease elicits hemagglutinating activity that is due almost entirely to IgM–type antibodies, whereas the hemagglutinins called forth by meningococcal polysaccharide vaccines may be either IgM or IgG antibodies.

Group B capsular polysaccharide is relatively nonimmunogenic. Injection of reasonably good preparations of Group B polysaccharide elicits little or no antibody. Even after full recovery from Group B *Neisseria meningitidis* infection, the host's polysaccharide hemagglutinating antibody titers are low; bactericidal activity usually does not reach high levels. Two theories have been proposed to explain the relative lack of immunogenicity of Group B polysaccharide antigen. Chemically, the polysaccharide consists largely of neuraminic acid that is very similar or even identical to neuraminic acid residues on mammalian host cell membranes. The polysaccharide may therefore be recognized as "self" rather than "foreign" by an infected host that is immunologically unresponsive or "tolerant" of his own neuraminic acid determinants. Failure to recognize the capsular polysaccharide as foreign results in failure to produce antibody. The second possibility is that neuraminidase enzyme concentrations in host tissue fluids and cells are such as to result in rapid degradation of Group B polysaccharide. In this case, breakdown of the antigen is so fast that critical antigenic determinants never impinge on critical receptor sites of immunocompetent lymphoid cells. The net result is failure to trigger antibody production.

A significant portion of the meningococcal cell wall consists of the lipopolysaccharide-endotoxin complex (see Fig. 34–1). This macromolecular complex is physically associated with the capsular polysaccharide. The lipopolysaccharide-endotoxin complex and capsular polysaccharide are released into the extracellular environment during log phase growth of *Neisseria meningitidis* or with death and autolysis of meningococci, either in vitro or in vivo. The toxic lipopolysaccharide-endotoxin complex accounts for the "toxicity" and lethality of *N. meningitidis* cultures and culture filtrates when they are injected into experimental animals. Endotoxin derived from *N. meningitidis* has been used extensively in studies of mammalian tissue injury caused by gram negative bacillary endotoxins in general. From countless studies, especially those focusing on the local or general Shwartzman reaction in animal model systems, a great deal has been learned about the biologic activities of endotoxin as they translate to tissue damage. Many of the physiologic and immunohistopathologic events elicited by injection of endotoxin into experimental animals are commonly observed in patients developing septic shock during the course of disease due to *N. meningitidis* or other gram negative bacteria. These events include the following: activation of the clotting cascade with extensive deposition of fibrin, particularly in glomerular arterioles but also in small vessels of other tissues; hemorrhage of the adrenal glands and hemorrhagic necrosis of other organ systems; altered peripheral vascular resistance and circulatory collapse, and death. Although definitive proof is still lacking, it is widely believed that the lipopolysaccharide-endotoxin complex of *N. meningitidis* causes all of these events in the infected patient and is directly responsible for the fulminating course and high mortality rate so often associated with meningococcemia.

Group C meningococci, more than do all other serotypes of *Neisseria meningitidis,* literally "shed" their capsular polysaccharide and associated lipopolysaccharide-endotoxin complex during growth in vitro or in vivo. Therefore, detection and quantitation of capsular polysaccharide in blood and cerebrospinal fluid can be used to monitor the amount of lipopolysaccharide-endotoxin complex released during meningococcal infections. Determination of titers of capsular polysaccharide, using specific antibody reagents, provides a means of assessing the severity of infection in individual patients. Such information can have considerable diagnostic and prognostic import. Such knowledge also allows one to follow the outcome of treatment discussed later in this chapter.

A third constituent of *Neisseria meningitidis* is the genus-specific protein antigen. As indicated in Figure 34–1, it is uncertain whether this antigen is part of the cell wall or is located within the internal protoplasmic mass of the bacterial cell. The antigen has specificity only for the Neisseria genus. A complement-fixation test can be used to screen large numbers of individuals for antibodies induced by *N. meningitidis, Neisseria gonorrhoeae,* or other Neisseria species. Positive results of screening tests would dictate need for more discriminatory group-specific hemagglutinating antibody tests, which would offer a more detailed study of *N. meningitidis* infections.

Clinical Disease

Pathogenesis

Meningococcal Carrier State and Host Immune Responses

Neisseria meningitidis only infects man. Infection is acquired through inhalation of infectious aerosols of respiratory secretions derived from humans carrying *N. meningitidis* in their nasopharynx or oropharynx. Colonization of the upper respiratory tract of a new host by *N. meningitidis* is usually followed by the circulating bactericidal and hemagglutinating antibodies within 7 to 10 days. These immune responses do not appear to interact with or eliminate *N. meningitidis* residing within the nasopharynx or oropharynx, since the meningococcal carrier state persists for many weeks or months in the face of high titers of serum bactericidal activity. Susceptibility or resistance to clinical meningococcal disease is determined by the absence or presence of serum bactericidal activity. Circulating bactericidal antibody appears to prevent any meningococci that invade the bloodstream from the nasopharynx or oropharynx from multiplying and disseminating to other tissues, particularly the central nervous system. There is good evidence derived from meningococcal vaccine field trials (see below) that bactericidal antibody also may decrease the likelihood of *N. meningitidis* infection, as represented by asymptomatic carriage of this microorganism within the nasopharynx or oropharynx. It is not known whether immunity to clinical disease ascribed to bactericidal activity results from augmented phagocytosis and accelerated intracellular digestion of *N. meningitidis* or actual lysis of the microorganisms, as occurs in such striking fashion in vitro. Perhaps both mechanisms are important for maximum resistance. It also is uncertain whether immunity is due solely to bactericidal antibody or whether cell-mediated immune functions of the host contribute to some extent, particularly with respect to the degree and durability of the immune state.

From the foregoing, it appears clear that the issue as to whether clinical disease will or will not develop in a given individual following colonization of his nasopharynx or oropharynx is decided within a short period of time, 10 days or less. Very recent data pertaining to this point have been secured from a study of military recruits at San Diego Naval Base.* This study involved 2870 men in 42 Navy companies or Marine platoons. Nasopharyngeal cultures were obtained from each recruit at approximately two-week intervals during his period of training. The overall mean carrier rate for nasopharyngeal colonization by *Neisseria meningitidis* was 35.4 per cent. Carrier rates within individual companies and platoons were observed to fluctuate widely at different times during the investigation, ranging from a low of 1 per cent to a maximum of 74 per cent. It is of interest that the greatest carrier rate of 74 per cent occurred in one company on the very day a recruit from this company was hospitalized with acute meningococcal disease. Despite the wide variation in meningococcal nasopharyngeal carrier rate, in only six companies or platoons was more than one case of clinical meningococcal disease reported. This finding supports earlier epidemiologic data indicating that no direct relationship exists at any point in time between carrier rates and the incidence of meningococcal disease.

The most interesting finding from the San Diego project is uncovered in retrospective study of the 36 cases of meningococcal disease that occurred among recruits undergoing fortnightly culturing. Twenty-two of these 36 cases were cultured seven days or less before onset of disease and

---

*Edwards, E. A., Devine, L. F., and Ward, H. W.: Immunologic investigations of meningococcal disease. III. Group C meningococcal carrier status and disease occurrence. (Manuscript in preparation.) This study provides beautiful redocumentation of the lack of any direct relationship between nasopharyngeal carrier rates of *Neisseria meningitidis* and incidence of clinical disease due to this microorganism. The investigation is unique in revealing that *N. meningitidis* colonizes the nasopharynx for only an extraordinarily brief period before clinical manifestations of illness occur in those rare individuals destined to develop acute meningococcal disease. One cannot help but wonder whether this finding concerning the pathogenesis of disease caused by *N. meningitidis* does not also apply to the sequence of events underlying other diseases in which carriage of pathogenic microorganisms in the upper respiratory tract is believed to be a vital factor, e.g., infections with *Streptococcus pneumoniae* and *Haemophilus influenzae*.

hospitalization. Only 5 of the 22 men had a positive culture for *Neisseria meningitidis* during this period. Especially noteworthy is the fact that 4 of the 22 men had negative throat cultures one day before they became ill and entered the hospital. The findings demonstrate an extremely brief period of colonization by *N. meningitidis* before explosive development of disease in a very small proportion of those individuals acquiring *N. meningitidis* infection of their upper respiratory tract.

Enigma of Host Resistance

The specific reason why colonization of the respiratory tract by *Neisseria meningitidis* progresses directly to acute meningococcal disease in an occasional individual, whereas it does not do so in the great majority of others who are seemingly at comparable risk, is unknown. An answer to this perplexing question has not been found in comparative studies of *N. meningitidis* strains isolated from the blood and strains isolated from the oropharynx of asymptomatic carriers. In other words, such obvious differences as the amount of capsular polysaccharide or the amount and biologic activity of lipopolysaccharide-endotoxin complex have not been uncovered.

Host defense factors may well be a more rewarding area for study. Cell-mediated immune mechanisms have received virtually no attention and deserve detailed study. It also seems clear that bactericidal antibodies can be elicited by antigenic stimuli other than *Neisseria meningitidis*. For example, sera of adults not infrequently contain relatively high titers of bactericidal antibody reactive with Group A capsular polysaccharide despite the fact that these individuals have resided in geographic areas where Group A *N. meningitidis* has not been detected for years. Microorganisms with antigenic constituents that cross-react with capsular polysaccharides of *N. meningitidis* could provide an explanation for this finding. For example, the envelope or capsular antigen of *Escherichia coli* designated as serotype K1 is chemically similar to Group B polysaccharide of *N. meningitidis*. Low titers of meningococcal bactericidal antibody induced by cross-reacting antigens of other microorganisms but below the threshold of detection by conventional tests might increase rapidly in response to colonization of the nasopharynx or oropharynx by *N. meningitidis*. Rise in antibody titer might prevent bloodstream invasion by these microorganisms, thereby preventing clinical disease.

Clinical Aspects of Meningococcal Disease

The most frequent forms of *Neisseria meningitidis* infection are meningococcemia, which may follow a fulminating course and progress rapidly to septic shock (Waterhouse-Friedericksen syndrome), and meningitis. Features of both *N. meningitidis* septicemia and meningitis occur in some patients at the outset of infection. Meningitis may be associated with extensive inflammation of brain tissue causing deep coma lasting for several days; in such cases the disease is often designated as a *meningoencephalopathy*. These different clinical forms of disease have already been referred to briefly in

Chapters 27 and 33; detailed descriptions can be found in standard textbooks of medicine.

Three aspects of clinical disease emphasized here are (1) diagnostic problems associated with the cutaneous manifestations of meningococcemia, (2) relationships between concentrations of capsular polysaccharide in the serum and cerebrospinal fluid and clinical course and outcome of disease, and (3) unusual manifestations of meningococcal disease pertaining to the pulmonary system and inflammation of serous membranes.

Cutaneous Lesions

Meningococcal septicemia is usually accompanied by cutaneous lesions that have a definite petechial or frankly purpuric nature (Figs. 34–2 and 34–3). The cutaneous lesions generally have a centrifugal, i.e., peripheral, distribution and are most apt to occur initially over the volar surfaces of the wrists and forearms, on the palms or over the lower legs or ankles, and over the soles (Fig. 34–4). Meningococcal skin lesions, however, may spare the palmar or plantar surfaces (see Fig. 34–2) and may first be noted in large numbers on the trunk. Furthermore, the lesions may not have a hemorrhagic component, at least during their early evolution, in which case they may be indistinguishable from typical macules or papules. Lesions of meningo-coccemia that appear in atypical locations and lack any petechial or purpuric appearance may be confused with the cutaneous lesions or exanthemas of a number of other diseases. Erroneous diagnosis and inappropriate therapy can have fatal consequences. The diseases that are most likely to be confused with *Neisseria meningitidis* septicemia on the basis of incorrect recognition of skin lesions include Rocky Mountain spotted fever, rubeola, rubella, secondary

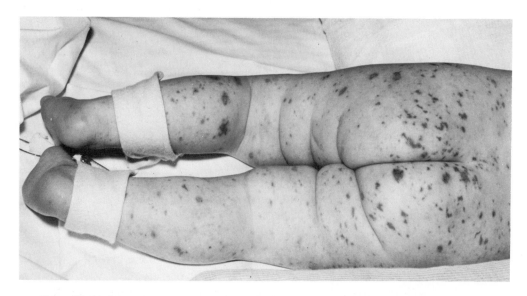

Figure 34–2. Representative cutaneous eruption of acute meningococcemia in a young child with meningococcal meningitis. (From Bell, W. E., and McCormick, W. F.: Neurologic Infections in Children. Philadelphia, W. B. Saunders Co., 1975.)

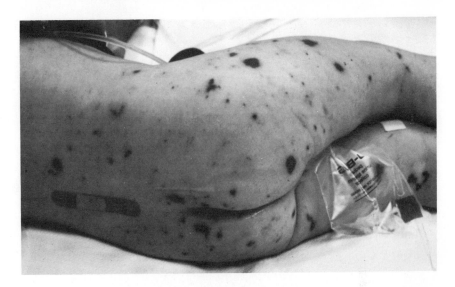

Figure 34–3. More extensive purpuric skin lesions characteristic of acute meningococce-mia in a child with meningococcal meningitis and septic shock. Systemic hypotension is also present and there is laboratory evidence of disseminated intravascular coagulation (see Chap. 27). (From Bell, W. E., and McCormick, W. F.: Neurologic Infections in Children. Philadelphia, W. B. Saunders Co., 1975.)

syphilis and, rarely, acute bacterial endocarditis due to gram positive coccal bacteria and cutaneous eruptions associated with penicillin allergy or serum sickness.

The usual "rules" concerning the differential diagnosis of these cutaneous eruptions place a great deal of emphasis on whether the lesions blanch on pressure, occur on the palms and soles, or have a centrifugal or centripetal distribution. There are enough exceptions to the rules as to lead to serious diagnostic uncertainty. If doubt exists, it is best to incise a representative lesion under aseptic conditions, permitting two or three drops of tissue fluid to be expressed for the preparation of a smear for Gram staining and culturing. The presence of segmented neutrophils and gram negative cocci or diplococci within these phagocytic cells or lying free in the tissue fluid is highly suggestive or even pathognomonic of *Neisseria meningitidis* infection. The fluid from the incised lesion is best cultured by placing one or two drops directly onto chocolate agar at the bedside; streaking of the plate should be done as soon as feasible. Isolation of *N. meningitidis* from the tissue fluid provides a definitive diagnosis of meningococcemia. Culture of skin lesions sometimes yields the microorganism when blood cultures remain sterile. This is another good reason for smearing and culturing any cutaneous lesion(s) thought to result from *N. meningitidis* infection.

Meningococcal Antigenemia and Patterns of Disease

Reference already has been made (see above) to the value of detecting and quantitating capsular polysaccharide in blood and cerebrospinal fluid for the purpose of diagnosis and prognosis. The results of a study illustrating this point are shown in Table 34–1.

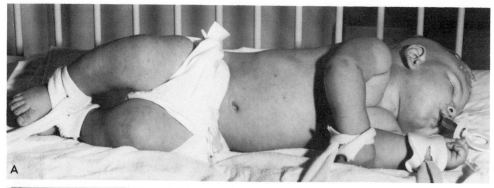

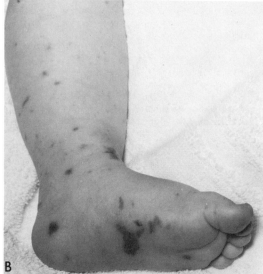

Figure 34–4. The cutaneous lesions in this infant with meningitis due to *Neisseria meningitidis* have a peripheral distribution; those occurring on the ankles and plantar surfaces have a frankly purpuric appearance. (From Bell, W. E., and McCormick, W. F.: Neurologic Infections in Children. Philadelphia, W. B. Saunders Co., 1975.)

TABLE 34–1. Group C *Neisseria meningitidis* Capsular Polysaccharide Antigen in Body Fluids of Military Recruits with Meningococcal Disease as Detected by Counterimmunoelectrophoresis*

Body Fluid	Clinical Disease	Group C Polysaccharide		Mortality
		Present	*Amount (µg/ml)*	
Serum	Meningococcemia	1/33	0.04	0/33
	Meningococcemia – fulminant type	13/13	0.02–1.25	1/13
	Meningitis or meningoencephalopathy	11/41	0.02–0.16	2/41
Cerebrospinal fluid	Meningitis	17/32	0.02–1.25	0/32
	Encephalopathy	9/9	0.32–20.0	2/9

*Adapted from Hoffman, T. A., and Edwards, E. A.: Group-specific polysaccharide antigen and humoral antibody response in disease due to Neisseria meningitidis. J. Infect. Dis. *126:*636, 1972.

A definitive diagnosis of meningococcal disease was made by isolation of Group C *Neisseria meningitidis* from 71 of the 87 military recruits in this study; clinical features of illness, together with a diagnostic rise of Group C bactericidal or hemagglutinating antibody, were used as diagnostic criteria in the remaining 16 patients. Blood serum and cerebrospinal fluid were collected at the time of hospitalization as well as on subsequent days in some cases. The fluids were tested for Group C capsular polysaccharide with counter-immunoelectrophoresis and a highly specific Group C antiserum.

Antigenemia was demonstrable in only 1 of the 33 patients with relatively benign meningococcemia; the concentration of antigen was low in this one patient, i.e., 0.04 μg per ml. None of the 33 patients died. In contrast, all 13 patients with fulminating meningococcemia had antigenemia; concentrations of antigen ranged from 0.02 to 1.25 μg per ml. One of the 13 patients died. Among 41 patients with a clinical picture of meningitis or meningoencephalopathy, 11 had antigenemia. The concentrations of antigen in the sera of these patients ranged from 0.02 to 1.16 μg per ml. Two of these patients died. A clearer relationship between presence of antigen in body fluid and clinical pattern of disease becomes apparent when one considers whether or not antigen was present in the cerebrospinal fluid of the patients with nervous system disease. Slightly more than half of the 32 patients with meningitis had antigen in their cerebrospinal fluid; concentrations ranged from 0.02 to 1.25 μg per ml. No deaths occurred among this group of patients. In contrast, all nine patients with meningoencephalopathy had antigen in their cerebrospinal fluid, and the concentration of antigen ranged from 0.32 to 20.0 μg per ml. Two of these nine patients died; both deaths occurred in individuals who had very high concentrations of antigen in their cerebrospinal fluid.

The conspicuously low mortality rate among military recruits with fulminating meningococcemia and meningitis-meningoencephalopathy (see Table 34–1) in contrast to the higher mortality rates invariably observed among civilian populations deserves comment. There are several factors to consider. All of the military cases were young recruits who had been in excellent physical condition prior to onset of illness. Disease was reported very soon after onset, literally within hours. Early recognition of illness in turn led to prompt hospitalization and rapid institution of antimicrobial therapy, as evidenced by the relatively small proportion of cases that progressed to a fulminating form of meningococcemia. Heparin therapy was employed in some of these cases in an effort to prevent occurrence or retard further development of already evident disseminated intravascular coagulation. There are no compelling reasons to believe that heparin therapy per se was responsible for the low mortality rate that was observed (Table 34–1) vis-à-vis the more important factor of prompt institution of effective antimicrobial drugs very soon after onset of disease.

Unusual Clinical Presentations of Meningococcal Disease

It is obvious from what has been emphasized in Chapter 33 and this chapter that *Neisseria meningitidis* has a special propensity for infecting respiratory and nervous system tissues. It is of interest to note that following intravenous injection into chick embryos, *N. meningitidis* localizes preferentially within these organ systems. It is likely that the basis for this "tissue tropism" lies in the fact that these tissues possess receptor sites that facilitate *N. meningitidis*–host cell interaction and binding (see Chaps. 3, 7, 13, and 41).

Perhaps as many as one fourth of patients presenting with meningococcemia or evidence of meningitis have evidence of pulmonary infection, e.g., pneumonia or pleural inflammation. Recent studies have called attention to *Neisseria meningitidis* as a primary cause of acute bacterial pneumonia, occuring without other manifestations of meningococcal disease. Patients with this condition have physical signs of pulmonary consolidation and a density in the chest roentgenogram, and *N. meningitidis* may be the only pathogen isolated from sputum or lower respiratory tract secretions obtained by translaryngeal aspiration.

Neisseria meningitidis closely resembles *Neisseria gonorrhoeae* with respect to eliciting inflammation involving serous membranes and joint tissues. Pleuritis, pericarditis, and migratory polyarthritis may be dominant features of clinical disease associated with infection by either Neisseria species. Fluids aspirated from sites of inflammation for diagnostic purposes may not be purulent, may contain predominantly mononuclear cells, may fail to have demonstrable microorganisms on Gram stain, and may remain sterile on culture. In such instances, the clinical picture may be remarkably similar to that of acute rheumatic fever and serum sickness. Absence of meningococci in joint, pleural, and pericardial fluids has led to the suggestion that the inflammation has an immunologic rather than a primary infectious basis. A diagnosis of meningococcal infection is based on finding a greater than fourfold rise in hemagglutinating or bactericidal antibody specifically reactive with *N. meningitidis*. Cultures of the nasopharynx or oropharynx of some patients may reveal that they are meningococcal carriers and may provide additional support for the diagnosis of *N. meningitidis* infection. Termination of the meningococcal carrier state, either spontaneously or following appropriate antimicrobial therapy (see below), not infrequently is associated with prompt disappearance of inflammation of serous and synovial membranes and adjacent joint tissues.

Therapy

Reference already has been made to the emergence of sulfonamide-resistant strains of Groups C, B, and A meningococci since 1963 (see above and Chap. 33). So far, no strain of *Neisseria meningitidis* has been shown to exhibit resistance to a penicillin-class drug or chloramphenicol. Ampicillin or crystalline penicillin given in large doses by vein is the recommended therapeutic regimen for patients with meningococcemia or meningitis. Chloramphenicol therapy can be used for those few individuals in whom hypersensitivity to penicillin precludes use of this class of antimicrobial drugs (see Chap. 33).

Debate continues as to the most appropriate therapeutic approach to septic shock associated with fulminating meningococcemia. This syndrome was initially described by Waterhouse and Friedericksen and is characterized by irreversible circulatory failure and hemorrhage involving the adrenal glands as well as other organs. Both Waterhouse and Friedericksen carefully noted in their papers published more than 50 years ago that this syndrome may occur in patients in the absence of any hemorrhagic changes involving the adrenal glands. Nevertheless, the idea that adrenal gland injury, more specifically adrenal cortical failure, accounts for fulminating meningococcemia has dominated therapeutic thinking for decades despite pointed evidence to the contrary. It is abundantly clear that septic shock accompanying meningococcemia is not due solely to adrenal cortical dysfunction and resulting insufficient output of endogenous corticosteroid hormones. Concentrations of these hormones in the blood and urine of patients with septicemia due to *Neisseria meningitidis* and other gram negative as well as gram positive microorganisms are invariably high. Indeed, despite the fact that adrenal cortical extracts and corticosteroid preparations of ever greater potency have been widely employed for over four decades as adjuncts to therapy of meningococcal disease, the mortality rate among civilian populations has remained at a distressingly high level. It seems clear that administration of corticosteroids as "replacement therapy" has no rational basis. Double-blind studies using moderately large doses of hydrocortisone or dexamethasone, a preparation with 25-fold more biologic activity, have failed to reveal any significant beneficial results (see discussion of the septic shock syndrome in Chap. 27). Whether massive doses of corticosteroids, equivalent to 6 or 10 gm of hydrocortisone per day as now used in a few medical centers, will stabilize the peripheral circulation and increase contractility of cardiac myofibers and offer a beneficial effect remains in doubt.

The use of heparin to counteract intravascular clotting in patients with meningococcal septicemia is another unsettled issue. Early institution of heparin may be a key factor in the treatment of meningococcal septicemia based on favorable experience with relatively few military recruits with fulminating meningococcemia who received heparin therapy *before* onset of irreversible circulatory changes because elevated concentrations of *Neisseria meningitidis* polysaccharide were found in their circulation (see Table 34–1 and related text discussion). More studies focusing on very early heparin therapy or brief courses given routinely are needed.

Prophylaxis

Antimicrobial Prophylaxis

Based on studies involving military personnel during World War II, sulfonamide derivatives have a remarkable capacity to eliminate rapidly *Neisseria meningitidis* from the nasophayrnx or oropharynx. As little as 1.0 or 2.0 gm of sulfadiazine is able to eradicate *N. meningitidis* from the nasopharynx or oropharynx within 24 to 72 hours. Prior to 1963, when all strains of meningococci could be presumed to be susceptible to sulfonamide drugs, these antimicrobial agents were widely used to terminate *N. meningitidis* carriage among military personnel and proved strikingly successful in preventing outbreaks of meningococcal disease. However, rapid emergence of sulfonamide-resistant strains of first Group B and then Group C *N. meningitidis* led to the discontinuation of routine sulfonamide prophylaxis on a wide scale at many military bases by 1969 or 1970. It is of considerable interest that sulfonamide-susceptible strains of *N. meningitidis* are now again being found with increasing frequency in the nasopharyngeal and oropharyngeal cultures of military recruits. If the trend continues, it will not be long before sulfonamide derivatives can once again be used for prophylaxis and treatment.

Even though all meningococcal isolates have remained highly susceptible to penicillin, massive doses of penicillin-class drugs do not eliminate the meningococcal carrier state. Studies from several laboratories indicate that for any antimicrobial drug to terminate meningococcal carriage, the drug must be present in the oropharyngeal secretions in a concentration which exceeds that required to inhibit growth of *Neisseria meningitidis* in vitro. Sulfonamide derivatives are readily secreted by the parotid and accessory salivary glands, whereas penicillin and virtually all other antimicrobial drugs are not. Rifampin is an exception and resembles sulfonamide drugs in that it is found in high concentration in the oral secretions. At present, rifampin is the only reliable means of eliminating the carrier state. However, there are two drawbacks to the use of rifampin. Treatment for more than several days results in emergence of rifampin-resistant strains of *N. meningitidis* in a small proportion of patients, and rifampin is currently licensed only for treatment of tuberculosis in the United States.

Vaccines

Preparation of essentially nontoxic immunogenic vaccines of Group C capsular polysaccharide of *Neisseria meningitidis* and subsequent field trials demonstrating the efficacy of such vaccines in induction of group-specific immunity represent a major achievement in the control of meningococcal disease among members of the United States military forces. For example, in one field trial, in members of platoons at five recruit training centers who received a single injection of 50 μg of Group C polysaccharide vaccine, acquisition of Group C *N. meningitidis* infection of the oropharynx was reduced two- to threefold, and only one instance of clinical disease caused by Group C *N. meningitidis* was reported; this represents an attack rate of 0.07 (number of cases per 1000 recruits over the eight-week study period). In contrast, there were 38 instances of clinical meningococcal disease among nonvaccinated recruits in the same platoons, representing an attack rate of 0.7 (cases per 1000 per eight weeks).

Encouraging progress has also been reported concerning development of Group A polysaccharide vaccines. For reasons previously discussed, Group B capsular polysaccharide is relatively nonimmunogenic. All efforts to produce efficacious vaccines for this serotype of *Neisseria meningitidis* have so far proved unsuccessful.

References

Artenstein, M. S., Gold, R., Zimmerly, J. G., Wyle, F. A., Schneider, H., and Harkins, C.: Prevention of meningococcal disease by group C polysaccharide vaccine. N. Engl. J. Med. *282:*417, 1970.

Beam, W. E., Newberg, N. R., Devine, L. F., Pierce, W. E., and Davies, J. A.: The effect of rifampin on the nasopharyngeal carriage of Neisseria meningitidis in a military population. J. Infect. Dis. *124:*39, 1971.

Devine, L. F., Johnson, D. P., Hagerman, C. R., Pierce, W. E., Rhode, S. L., Peckinpaugh, R. O.: Rifampin: Levels in serum and saliva and effect on the meningococcal carrier state. J.A.M.A. *214:*1055, 1970.

Devine, L. F., Johnson, D. P., Rhode, S. L., Hagerman, C. R., Pierce, W. E., and Peckinpaugh, R. O.: Rifampin: Effect of two-day treatment on the meningococcal carrier state and the relationship to the levels of drug in sera and saliva. Am. J. Med. Sci. *26:*79, 1971.

Devine, L. F., Pierce, W. E., Floyd, T. M., Rhode, S. L., Edwards, E. A., Siess, E. E., and Peckinpaugh, R. O.: Evaluation of group C meningococcal polysaccharide vaccine in marine recruits, San Diego, Calif. Am. J. Epidemiol. *92:*25, 1970.

Edwards, E. A., and Devine, L. F.: A genus specific complement fixation antigen from Neisseria meningitidis. Proc. Soc. Exp. Biol. Med. *128:*1168, 1968.

Edwards, E. A., and Driscoll, W. S.: Group-specific hemagglutination test for Neisseria meningitidis antibodies. Proc. Soc. Exp. Biol. Med. *126:*876, 1967.

Edwards, E. A.: Immunologic investigations of meningococcal disease. I. Group-specific Neisseria meningitidis antigens present in the serum of patients with fulminant meningococcemia. J. Immunol. *106:*314, 1971.

Edwards, E. A.: Immunologic investigations of meningococcal disease. II. Some characteristics of Group C antigen of Neisseria meningitidis in the sera of patients with fulminant meningococcemia. J. Infect. Dis. *129:*538, 1974.

Goldschneider, I., Gotschlich, E. C., and Artenstein, M. S.: Human immunity to the meningococcus. I. The role of humoral antibodies. J. Exp. Med. *129:*1307, 1969.

Gotschlich, E. C., Goldschneider, I., and Artenstein, M. S.: Human immunity to the meningococcus. IV. Immunogenicity of Group A and Group C meningococcal polysaccharides in human volunteers. J. Exp. Med. *129:*1367, 1969.

Gotschlich, E. C., Goldschneider, I., and Artenstein, M. S.: Human immunity to the meningococcus. V. The effect of immunization with meningococcal Group C polysaccharide on the carrier state. J. Exp. Med. *129:*1385, 1969.

Hoffman, T. A., and Edwards, E. A.: Group-specific polysaccharide antigen and humoral antibody response in disease due to Neisseria meningitidis. J. Infect. Dis. *126:*636, 1972.

Jacobs, S. A., and Norden, C. W. Pneumonia caused by Neisseria meningitidis. J.A.M.A. *227:*67, 1974.

Munford, R. S., Vasconcelos, Z. J. S., Phillips, C. J., Gelli, D. S., Gorman, G. W., Risi, J. B. N., and Feldman, R. A.: Eradication of carriage of Neisseria meningitidis in families: A study in Brazil. J. Infect. Dis. *129:*644, 1974.

Putsch, R. W., Hamilton, J. D., and Wolinsky, E.: Neisseria meningitidis, a respiratory pathogen? J. Infect. Dis. *121:*48, 1970.

Smilack, J. D.: Group-Y meningococcal disease. Twelve cases at an army training center. Ann. Intern. Med. *81:*740, 1974.

Swanson, J., and Goldschneider, I.: The serum bactericidal system: Ultrastructural changes in Neisseria meningitidis exposed to normal rat serum. J. Exp. Med. *129:*51, 1969.

Winkelstein, A., Songster, C. L., Caras, T. C., Berman, H. H., and West, W. L.: Fulminant meningococcemia and disseminated intravascular coagulation. Arch. Intern. Med. *124:*55, 1969.

Zollinger, W. D., Kasper, D. L., Veltri, B. J., Artenstein, M. S.: Isolation and characterization of a native cell wall complex from Neisseria meningitidis. Infect. Immun. *6:*835, 1972.

Chapter 35

VIRAL MENINGITIS AND ENCEPHALITIS

Introduction

Viral diseases of the central nervous system are divided into specific categories, e.g., meningitis and encephalitis, on the basis of clinical symptoms and signs reflecting involvement of a specific anatomic area. With the virtual elimination of paralytic poliomyelitis in the United States, meningitis and encephalitis remain as the most common forms of viral central nervous system infection. All neurotropic viruses (except rabies) can cause both of these syndromes, but certain viruses are much more frequently associated with one syndrome than the other. By definition, *viral meningitis* results when the inflammatory process is limited primarily to the coverings of the brain and spinal cord, and is associated with stiff neck, headache, and lethargy. By contrast, the term *encephalitis* is used when the inflammatory process clearly has extended to or primarily involves parenchymal brain tissue with clinical signs and symptoms of cerebral dysfunction, e.g., altered consciousness, abnormal mentation and behavior, or seizures. Although there are some cases which do not fall clearly into one or the other category, most do. The distinction between meningitis and encephalitis is also useful because of the different prognosis associated with each form of viral infection; the prognosis is favorable in meningitis, but significant mortality and appreciable morbidity accompany encephalitis.

Viral Meningitis

Viral meningitis was recognized as a distinct clinical syndrome called *aseptic meningitis* long before the diverse viral causes were known. Wallgren's description of aseptic meningitis, even though written in 1925, is valid today. It is a disease characterized by the acute onset of meningeal symptoms accompanied by a bacteriologically sterile mononuclear inflammatory response in the cerebrospinal fluid. The disease is usually of short duration and is benign and relatively devoid of serious or persistent secondary complications. Although diseases such as leptospirosis and meningeal tuberculosis can present illness which initially are identical to aseptic meningitis, the term is generally used as a synonym for viral meningitis.

Epidemiology

Viral meningitis occurs occasionally during the course of many viral or presumed viral infections. Specific viruses etiologically associated with viral meningitis are listed in Table 35–1. Mumps virus, coxsackievirus B, echovirus, and coxsackievirus A are the most frequent causes of viral meningitis in the United States. In long-term studies of the same population group, the relative incidence of disease due to different viruses varies widely from year to year. There is seasonal variation as well. Enteroviral infections occur primarily in the late summer and early fall. Mumps occurs year round but has a peak incidence in the winter and spring. Although viral meningitis is seen in all age groups, it is most common in children and young adults, and its incidence decreases markedly with advancing age.

TABLE 35–1. Viruses Associated with Central Nervous System Infection*

	Meningitis	Encephalitis
	Coxsackie B	Mumps
	Echo	Herpes simplex
	Mumps	Arboviruses
	Coxsackie A	Polio
	Polio	Coxsackie B

*Approximate order of frequency.
Data from cases studied between 1958 and 1963 in the continental United States and Hawaii by Buescher, E. L., Artenstein, M. S., and Olson, L. and reported in Res. Publ. Assoc. Res. Nerv. Ment. Dis. *44:*147, 1968.

The frequency with which a specific agent can be identified as a cause of aseptic meningitis depends on the thoroughness with which laboratory studies are pursued. In one series, an agent was identified, using standard virologic and serologic techniques, in 75 per cent of cases. In contrast, of cases reported annually to the Center for Disease Control as being aseptic meningitis, a specific agent is identified in less than 25 per cent. Since the seasonal distribution of cases of aseptic meningitis of unknown origin corresponds to that of the group of known causes, it is likely that most of the unknown cases are due to the same group of viruses.

Pathogenesis

The portal of entrance of the virus into the body varies with the particular agent; the gastrointestinal tract is the site for enteroviruses, the respiratory tract for mumps, and other viruses enter at the point of their usual site of infection. Invasion of the central nervous system in most instances is thought to occur from the bloodstream during viremia. Experimental studies demonstrating retrograde movement of certain neurotropic viruses within peripheral nerve axoplasm (discussed in Chapter 6 in connection with slow virus diseases) have shown another mechanism whereby certain viruses may be transported to central nervous system tissues.

Diagnosis

Clinical Signs and Symptoms

The onset of viral meningitis is usually gradual with a few days of fever, malaise, anorexia, and perhaps sore throat and myalgia preceding the development of evidence of meningeal inflammation, i.e., stiff neck, severe headache and lethargy. Fever, mild to moderate nuchal rigidity and characteristic lethargy are usually the only physical findings. The exanthems that may be seen with some enteroviral infections are found in only a small proportion of patients infected with these viruses, primarily children less than 3 years of age. About one-half the patients with mumps meningitis have parotitis. When it occurs, parotitis usually, but not always, precedes the central nervous system disease.

Laboratory Examination

Laboratory studies are of limited value. The peripheral leukocyte count is usually normal or moderately elevated. In mumps infection, with or without obvious parotitis, the serum amylase may be raised, in the latter case indicating some involvement of the pancreas. To help exclude other diseases which may simulate viral meningitis, a chest film, urinalysis, tuberculin test, and serologic tests for syphilis and deep fungal infections are useful.

The following findings on lumbar puncture, in combination with the characteristic clinical picture, are sufficient to establish the diagnosis of viral meningitis. The opening cerebrospinal fluid pressure is usually slightly increased. The number of leukocytes per cubic millimeter of cerebrospinal fluid is almost always increased, i.e., exhibits pleocytosis. In most instances, the total leukocyte count is in the low hundreds, e.g., 100 to 300 cells per cubic millimeter. Leukocyte counts in this range may or may not render the cerebrospinal fluid somewhat opalescent or faintly turbid. The important point is that cerebrospinal fluid which appears clear is consistent with the diagnosis of viral meningitis. Cerebrospinal fluid cell counts above 1000 are unusual in viral meningitis, although higher counts have been reported in some infections due to echovirus, type 9. The majority of the leukocytes are mononuclear cells. Rarely, polymorphonuclear cells predominate, particularly during the first 24 hours of the illness. The protein content is normal or moderately elevated but rarely over 150 mg per 100 ml; glucose concentration is typically normal. In about 10 per cent of patients with mumps meningitis, and very rarely in those with other viral meningitides, lowered glucose concentrations may be observed. Gram stains of cerebrospinal fluid reveal no bacteria, and cultures for nonviral agents remain sterile.

Specific Diagnosis

The following specimens should be obtained in an attempt to identify a specific agent in a case of viral meningitis: (1) Acute and convalescent serums. To demonstrate a diagnostic fourfold rise in antibody titer, the timing of the first specimen is critical. It must be obtained during the first few days of the illness. The second specimen is obtained 10 to 14 days later. (2) Cerebrospinal fluid for viral isolation studies, if the specimen can be obtained within the first day or two of clinical illness. Recoverable virus usually disappears quickly from the cerebrospinal fluid, but enteroviruses in particular are readily isolated from this source. (3) Throat and rectal swabs for viral isolation, particularly if an enterovirus is suspected. Carriage of enteroviruses is more prolonged in these sites than in the cerebrospinal fluid. If a viral isolate is obtained, systemic infection should be confirmed by demonstrating a fourfold or greater rise in antibody titer to the virus in question.

In the absence of a viral isolate, enteroviral infection is difficult to establish by serologic means because there are more than 60 serologically distinct enteroviruses, and most laboratories usually perform tests which will detect only a few types, e.g., the three poliovirus serotypes and six coxsackievirus B serotypes. Demonstration of an increase in specific antibodies is the primary means of establishing a diagnosis of mumps and a number of other viral diseases.

Differential Diagnosis

All the causes of cerebrospinal fluid pleocytosis must be considered at least briefly in the differential diagnosis of viral meningitis. Leptospirosis is an uncommon disease in the United States, but when it occurs it is frequently accompanied by meningitis. Severe myalgia, gastrointestinal symptoms, marked conjunctival injection, jaundice, and abnormalities in the urinary sediment are common in disease due to *Leptospira icterohaemorrhagiae* and are less frequent in infections due to other Leptospira species.* These

---

*According to the 8th edition of Bergey's Manual of Determinative Bacteriology, all leptospires have been placed in one species, *Leptospira interrogans.* We are using the older terminology here because the clinical manifestations do vary among diseases caused by the formerly recognized species.

infections may be manifest clinically only as aseptic meningitis. A history of contact with rodents, including pet hamsters, or contact with stagnant water contaminated by rodent excreta might suggest aseptic meningitis of leptospiral origin. This diagnosis can be established by serologic tests. Bacterial endocarditis is frequently accompanied by central nervous system complications and should be considered in any patient with cerebrospinal fluid pleocytosis.

Those conditions, however, which can closely mimic viral meningitis and are most important to rule in or out because they are treatable with specific antimicrobial therapy include the granulomatous meningitides due to *Mycobacterium tuberculosis, Cryptococcus neoformans,* and other deep fungi; bacterial meningitis partially treated with antimicrobial agents, and a variety of localized suppurative infections in the immediate vicinity of the meninges, e.g., epidural or subdural abscess, vertebral osteomyelitis, etc. (see Chap. 33).

Course and Treatment

Treatment of viral meningitis is symptomatic. The fever and other symptoms usually resolve within a few days to a week, and most patients appear clinically well within 10 days to 2 weeks. Complications, often of a subtle nature, e.g., muscle tightness or objective weakness of specific muscle groups, and persisting for weeks or months, may be demonstrable in a small number of patients who are followed closely and examined thoroughly at frequent intervals. Rarely, viral meningitis may result in death, sharply contradicting its supposedly "benign" character.

Abnormalities in the cerebrospinal fluid usually reach their peak or maximum values early in the course of the disease, i.e., within three to four days, and then return slowly toward normal range. The lumbar puncture ordinarily need not be repeated if the patient's clinical course is satisfactory. Repetitive lumbar punctures and cerebrospinal fluid examinations may lead to unwarranted concern unless the physician is aware of the fact that elevated protein levels and abnormal numbers of cells in the cerebrospinal fluid can persist for several weeks, long after the patient appears clinically well.

Encephalitis

Encephalitis is a localized or diffuse inflammatory process involving brain tissue. Patients with encephalitis usually but not necessarily have all of the clinical manifestations and cerebrospinal fluid abnormalities characterizing viral meningitis and, in addition, exhibit evidence of cerebral dysfunction, i.e., changes in personality, localizing neurologic signs, and alterations in level of consciousness. Unlike viral meningitis, encephalitis is a serious disease with significant mortality and appreciable morbidity, especially when measured in regard to long-term neurologic sequelae.

Because a specific etiologic agent can be identified in only about 30 per cent of reported cases of encephalitis in the United States, only a general estimate can be made of the precise role of different viruses as causative agents. The most important viruses known to be involved are mumps, *Herpesvirus hominis,* types 1 and 2 (herpes simplex virus), and the arbovirus subgroup of togaviruses.

Pathogenesis

In meningitis, invasion of central nervous system tissues by the majority of the causative viruses occurs principally from the bloodstream. Centripetal spread toward or into the central nervous system via the peripheral nerves and ganglions has been convincingly demonstrated in laboratory animals with only two viruses that cause encephalitis in man, viz., rabies and herpes simplex viruses.

Studies in mice after ophthalmic inoculation of herpes simplex virus suggest that the spread of the virus occurs along axonal cylinders into the central nervous system. In similar fashion, spread of herpes simplex virus via the olfactory tract system of mice is comparatively unrestricted and culminates in brain tissue invasion and the development of acute herpetic encephalitis. This observation may have special meaning for man in light of the frequency with which *Herpesvirus hominis,* type 1, infects upper respiratory tract tissues, specifically the oropharynx. In addition, some evidence suggests that acute herpetic encephalitis in very young children may be temporally related to the initial acquisition of *Herpesvirus hominis,* type 1, infection; primary infection is usually manifest clinically as acute gingivostomatitis (see Chap. 12).

In both experimental and human rabies, considerable evidence suggests that the virus causing this condition reaches the central nervous system target via either the bloodstream or the peripheral nerve pathways.

Pathology

Gross examination of the brain in patients with total encephalitis reveals meningeal thickening and often cerebral swelling and petechial hemorrhages. Depending on the particular virus, either gray matter, white matter or both may be affected. Histopathologic changes seen during acute or early phases of encephalitis include neuronal necrosis accompanied by a perivascular accumulation of lymphocytes, plasma cells, macrophages, and occasionally neutrophils. As the process continues, degenerating neurons are removed by macrophages (neuronophagia), and reparative responses are seen, viz., proliferation of microglia and astrocytes. Intranuclear inclusion bodies may be seen in encephalitis due to *Herpesvirus hominis,* types 1 and 2, as well as in other herpesvirus encephalitides. Although some pathologic features are more frequent in particular infections, such as the marked temporal lobe necrosis or cavitation seen in severe herpes simplex, the pathologic changes are not distinctive enough to permit a specific diagnosis. Etiologic diagnosis requires isolation of the causative virus or diagnostic serologic findings.

Diagnosis

Clinical Signs and Symptoms

Although the onset may be acute or gradual, severe cases of encephalitis tend to have a more abrupt onset. Headache is the most frequent symptom. It is typically severe and bursting, often with maximum intensity retro-orbitally, and is aggravated by eye movements. Fever in the 102° to 104°F range is usual. Malaise, nausea, vomiting, and anorexia may occur. Convulsions are frequent, particularly in the more severe cases.

Physical examination almost always reveals disturbances of consciousness. Tremor, cranial nerve weakness, and pathologic reflexes are frequent. Psychiatric disturbances, marked memory loss, and auditory or visual hallucinations are often described with herpes simplex encephalitis, reflecting the propensity of this virus to involve specific areas and centers within the brain.

Laboratory Examination

Routine laboratory studies frequently reveal a peripheral leukocytosis. The cellular and protein abnormalities of the cerebrospinal fluid vary with the particular virus and the individual case. The range of abnormalities is similar to that observed in viral meningitis, although low cell counts, i.e., 10 to 50 cells per cubic millimeter, are apt to be more frequent. Rarely, the initial cerebrospinal fluid examination reveals no abnormalities. In such cases, examination of a second specimen of fluid collected 24 to 36 hours later almost always reveals pleocytosis or increased protein concentration. If the cerebral cortex rather than the cerebellum is involved, the electroencephalogram is abnormal. When focal or lateralizing neurologic signs are present, such studies as brain scan and carotid arteriography should be done to exclude a space-occupying lesion. This is especially important in cases of herpes simplex encephalitis in which focal necrosis, especially of the temporal lobe, may produce a mass lesion on brain scans. In recent years, biopsy of the brain has been used to obtain histopathologic and virologic evidence supportive of a specific etiologic diagnosis. This procedure is a prerequisite if herpes simplex encephalitis is suspected and antiviral therapy is contemplated. Biopsy of the brain is not associated with the production of serious clinical neurologic deficits.

Specific Diagnosis

Isolation of a virus from the cerebrospinal fluid or from the tissue provides a definitive diagnosis. However, mumps virus and togaviruses can be isolated from the cerebrospinal fluid of only a small percentage of patients, even when the specimen is obtained early in the course of disease and subjected to optimal laboratory studies. Herpes simplex virus is almost never isolated from cerebrospinal fluid of adults with acute encephalitis. A fourfold rise in serum antibody titer against a specific reference or laboratory strain of virus usually is accepted as evidence that a particular virus is responsible for the concurrent infection and the encephalitis. Caution must be observed in attributing encephalitis to herpes simplex viral infection solely on the basis of antibody titer rise. Most individuals in excellent health have antibody against this virus, and its titer may be observed to rise with recurrent mucocutaneous lesions or sometimes without any recognizable stimulus.

Differential Diagnosis

The differential diagnosis of encephalitis includes the diseases mentioned in the discussion of viral meningitis. In addition, because of the deeper cortical involvement and frequent localizing neurologic signs, other intracranial lesions which may cause cerebrospinal fluid pleocytosis must be considered. These include subdural empyema and effusion, primary and secondary brain neoplasms, brain abscess, and vascular disease, e.g., hemorrhage or infarcts. Correlation of the clinical signs, temporal course of the illness, and the special diagnostic neurologic studies mentioned will allow differentiation of these diverse processes.

Clinical Characteristics of Specific Encephalitides

Mumps

Mumps is a frequent cause not only of viral meningitis but also of encephalitis. The encephalitis, which may occur with or without parotitis, is usually mild, and neurologic residua and death are rare.

Herpes Simplex

In contrast, herpes simplex encephalitis usually follows a moderate to very severe course and is associated with significant mortality. In the newborn infant, herpes simplex encephalitis is usually due to infection with type 2 virus acquired during parturition. Infection of the brain is part of a disseminated disease. In the older child or adult, encephalitis occurs due to infection with type 1 virus. Disease is localized to the nervous system; other organs are not involved. The incidence of herpes simplex encephalitis has little or no seasonal variation. The disease may involve any area of the brain, but the orbital region of the frontal lobe and the inferior and medial portions of the temporal lobe are most apt to show inflammation and injury.

Togaviruses (Arbovirus Subgroups)

Current virologic nomenclature is based on the physical and chemical properties of the virion rather than on epidemiologic features of the disease. For this reason most but not all of the large group of viruses which at one time traditionally constituted the arbovirus group are now called togaviruses. The togavirus group also includes other agents, such as rubella virus, which are quite different epidemiologically from arboviruses.

The arbovirus subgroups of togaviruses take their name from their mode of transmission; i.e., all multiply in arthropods without producing apparent ill effect in the host. The arthropod vector, be it a mosquito or tick, becomes infected by ingesting the blood of a vertebrate host during the viremic phase of infection. During the next several days, the infected arthropod may transmit the disease by biting a new susceptible host. Epidemiologic studies of the arboviruses associated with encephalitis demonstrate that the incidence of inapparent infection with these agents far exceeds that of infection with clinical manifestations of central nervous system disease.

All North American arbovirus encephalitides occur during the summer and early fall, when their arthropod vectors are most prevalent. Nevertheless, each etiologically specific form of encephalitis has its own geographic and clinical characteristics. Six arbovirus encephalitides which occur in the United States are Eastern, Western, and Venezuelan equine, St. Louis and California encephalitis, and Colorado tick fever. Some of their features are listed in Table 35–2.

TABLE 35–2. Some Characteristics of American Arbovirus Encephalitides

	Mosquito-borne				Tick-borne
	Western Equine	Eastern Equine	St. Louis	California	Colorado Tick Fever
Geographical distribution	West	East, South	Central, West	Central, Southwest	West
Age group usually affected	Infants and adults > 50	Children	Adults > 50	Children	Children
Mortality (per cent)	5–15	60–75	2–11	1	1 of 4 reported cases
Incidence of serious sequelae	Infants–moderate Others–low	90%	Low	Low	

California encephalitis merits special mention. This disease has been widely recognized only in recent years. The number of cases reported annually does not show the marked variation seen with most of the arbovirus encephalitides. At present, the California group of viruses appears to be the leading cause of arbovirus encephalitis in the United States. Despite its name, California encephalitis occurs throughout the country, most of the cases having been reported from the north central region of the United States. This encephalitis occurs almost exclusively in children. The acute illness is often severe, with coma and convulsions, but the prognosis for total recovery is excellent.

Course and Treatment

The length of the acute illness in viral encephalitis varies from a few days to several weeks. Typically, the convalescence is prolonged, with slow return of neurologic function. There are two major prognostic factors in encephalitis – the severity of the acute neurologic illness and the etiologic agent. Certain agents (e.g., Eastern equine encephalitis and herpes simplex viruses) cause encephalitis of high morbidity and high mortality. On the other hand, California encephalitis viral infection usually has a good prognosis, even in the face of severe acute illness.

The basic treatment of encephalitis is supportive. Three drugs which exert an antiviral effect in vitro on DNA viruses are currently under clinical investigation. Two of these agents are pyrimidine nucleosides, viz., 5-iodo-2′-deoxyuridine (idoxuridine, IUDR) and 1-beta-D-arabinofuranosyl-cytosine (cytosine arabinoside, Ara-C). Both have been used in therapeutic trials of treatment of severe DNA viral infections, including herpes simplex encephalitis. Investigators reporting effects of treatment of herpes simplex encephalitis have not included control patients with comparable degrees of illness. For this reason, and also because of the variable course that the disease may assume in a given patient, the results to date are difficult to evaluate. Overall, the drugs do not appear to be consistently or remarkably effective.

An important factor in therapy is achieving certain levels of IUDR within the target tissue, i.e., brain, following parenteral administration of the drug. These levels must be capable of exerting a therapeutically significant effect on the virus at that site. Reaching these levels has proved to be the major limiting factor in recent and carefully designed studies of IUDR in the treatment of herpes simplex encephalitis experimentally induced in marmosets by intracerebral or parenteral injection of the virus. Even though the drug was started four hours before infection and given in a dose and by a route considered to be optimal, and even though replication of virus was suppressed in tissues other than the brain, the IUDR-treated marmosets fared no better than the untreated control animals, at least as judged by the clinical and histopathologic criteria which were employed. To further complicate matters, both IUDR and cytosine arabinoside are demonstrably cytotoxic and immunosuppressive when used in doses required to achieve serum levels with antiviral activity.

A third drug, the purine nucleoside 9-beta-D-arabinofuranosyladenine (vidarabine, Ara-A), has been used less widely. Experimental antiviral and clinical pharmacologic studies suggest that this drug may be more effective and is less toxic than IUDR or cytosine arabinoside. Clinical investigation is currently in preliminary stages.

The use of corticosteroids in the treatment of encephalitis is contro-versial. Their use is detrimental in systemic or disseminated herpes simplex viral infections in experimental animals. A few patients have been reported to improve after corticosteroid treatment. It is not clear whether the beneficial effect observed should be attributed to a reduction in cerebral edema or to another unknown mechanism. Cerebral edema can be treated by other medical means such as osmotic diuretics or by surgical decompression.

CASE PRESENTATION 1

A nine-year-old male had been well until three days before admission to the hospital in early September. At that time he complained of malaise and intermittent ill-defined abdominal pain. Temperatures ranging from 99° to 101°F were noted. On the day of hospital admission, he complained of severe headache and had one episode of vomiting. There were no complaints suggestive of middle ear or sinus infection. There was no history of recent exposure to recognized infectious diseases. Other members of the family were well.

On physical examination, the patient was noted to be irritable and restless, but he answered questions appropriately. His temperature was 103°F rectally; his pulse was 124 per minute, and respirations were 20 per minute. There was mild nuchal rigidity. Physical and neurologic examinations otherwise were normal.

Laboratory studies revealed a peripheral leukocyte count of 11,000 per cubic millimeter with 73 per cent segmented neutrophils. Lumbar puncture revealed clear cerebrospinal fluid and an opening pressure of 120 mm of water (normal = < 180). Microscopic examination of the cerebrospinal fluid revealed 156 cells per cubic millimeter (normal = < 5 mononuclear cells per cubic millimeter) of which 57 per cent were mononuclear cells and 43 per cent were neutrophils. Protein content of the cerebrospinal fluid was 76 mg per 100 ml (normal = < 45) and glucose 65 mg per 100 ml (normal = 60 to 80). A Gram stain of the centrifuged sediment failed to show any stainable microorganisms. Bacterial and mycobacterial cultures of the cerebrospinal fluid were later reported as negative for growth, as were blood cultures. Chest roentgenogram was normal. A skin test with intermediate strength tuberculin (5 IU of PPD) was negative.

No specific treatment was given. The patient felt better the day after admission, but fever over 100°F persisted for two additional days. By the fifth hospital day the patient was afebrile and asymptomatic. No virus was isolated from the sample of cerebrospinal fluid collected on the first hospital day. Throat and rectal viral cultures yielded a virus subsequently identified as coxsackievirus B5. Serum taken on the day of admission had no demonstrable neutralizing antibody to coxsackievirus B5, but serum drawn at the time of an outpatient visit 12 days later had an antibody titer of 1:256 against the throat-rectal viral isolate. Single rectal swabs from the patient's clinically well parents and 7-year-old sister were taken at that time. Coxsackievirus B5 was isolated from the sister's specimen but not from the specimens of the parents.

This patient's brief, self-limited illness is typical of viral meningitis. It appeared during the late summer, the peak period for enteroviral infections and the time when occurrence of viral meningitis in general is most common. Although cerebrospinal fluid was collected quite early in the clinical illness, no virus was grown. The isolation of a coxsackievirus from the patient's gastrointestinal tract and concomitant rise in antibody titer to this agent enable one to make a diagnosis of systemic coxsackievirus B infection with the presumption that the meningitis was due to the same agent. The ratio of inapparent to clinically apparent enteroviral infections is very high, and asymptomatic shedding of virus by members of family of patients with enteroviral disease is frequent, as illustrated in the case presented.

CASE PRESENTATION 2

A 21-year-old previously healthy male student was hospitalized in early December after complaining of malaise, headache, and low-grade fever for several days. Friends who brought him to the hospital had noticed that he had experienced some difficulty speaking and was exhibiting peculiar behavior.

Physical examination at the time of admission to the hospital was within normal limits except for the presence of fever. During the next few days, the patient was intermittently confused and complained of recent memory loss. On the fourth hospital day, he was noted to have a stiff neck and a fever of 104°F. His mental status deteriorated, and he became semiconscious.

At the time of admission, a lumbar puncture revealed an opening pressure of 300 mm of water and slightly cloudy cerebrospinal fluid containing 500 cells per cubic millimeter, of which all were mononuclear cells. The cerebrospinal fluid glucose was 68 mg per 100 ml and the protein was 98 mg per 100 ml. Attempts to isolate a virus from cerebrospinal fluid, throat, urine, and stool specimens were unsuccessful.

Over the next 10 days, the patient became more alert, and his temperature dropped to 101 to 102°F, at which time he was transferred to another hospital.

On admission to the second hospital, the patient had a temperature of 101°F. The general physical examination was unremarkable except for neurologic findings. The patient was totally disoriented and unstable. He had a profound receptive aphasia (inability to understand speech) and was unable to repeat words and phrases or to follow commands. He demonstrated agnosia (could not recognize common objects) and had speech perseveration in the form of persistence of one reply in response to various questions. He exhibited marked oralism, placing any available object in his mouth. A repeat lumbar puncture revealed an opening pressure of 160 mm of water. The cerebrospinal fluid contained 32 mononuclear cells per cubic millimeter, glucose was 66 mg per 100 ml, and protein was 161 mg per 100 ml. Complement-fixing antibodies against herpes simplex virus were present in a single serum specimen at a dilution of 1:2560.

Over the next two weeks the patient's temperature returned to normal. During the six weeks of his hospital stay his mental status improved slowly but incompletely. The oralism disappeared; the receptive aphasia and agnosia improved. Perseveration persisted. At the time of discharge from the hospital, the patient had learned his first name, but recent memory remained very poor.

The virologic diagnosis in this case can only be presumptive because it rests solely on a very high serum antibody level against herpes simplex virus rather than on a demonstrated rise in antibody titer. Isolation of virus from cerebrospinal fluid or a brain biopsy specimen would have been better. Low serum titers (e.g., 1:8 to 1:32) of herpes simplex viral antibody are frequently found in normal individuals. The titer of antibody in this patient, viz., 1:2560, is distinctly unusual and strongly suggestive of recent, antecedent infection due to herpes simplex virus.

The patient's clinical course is typical of severe herpes simplex encephalitis. His illness was heralded by mild malaise and headache and progressed rapidly to semicoma and high fever. The acute phase of his illness, including the high fever, lasted several weeks. Slow improvement in his neurologic status will probably occur over the following months, although he is likely to have severe residual impairment. It has been estimated that 70 per cent of individuals who have severe herpes simplex encephalitis, usually defined as the presence of semicoma or coma during the acute stage, either die or have significant neurologic impairment if they survive.

References

Review Articles

Hammon, W. M., and Ho, M.: Viral encephalitis. DM pp. 1–47, February, 1973.

Horstmann, D. M., and Yamada, N.: Enterovirus infections of the central nervous system. Res. Publ. Assoc. Res. Nerv. Ment. Dis. *44:*236, 1968.

Johnson, R. T., and Mims, C. A.: Pathogenesis of viral infections of the nervous system. N. Engl. J. Med. *278:*23, 84, 1968.

Johnson, R. T., Olson, L. C., and Buescher, E. L.: Herpes simplex virus infections of the nervous system. Problems in laboratory diagnosis. Arch. Neurol. *18:*260, 1968.

Luby, J. P., Johnson, M. T., and Jones, S. R.: Antiviral chemotherapy. Annu. Rev. Med. *25:*251, 1974.

Miller, J. R., and Harter, J. H.: Acute viral encephalitis. Med. Clin. North Am. *56:*1393, 1972.

Rosenthal, M. S.: Viral infections of the central nervous system. Med. Clin. North Am. *58:*593, 1974.

Original Articles

Balfour, H. H., Siem, R. A., Bauer, H., and Quie, P. G.: California arbovirus (LaCrosse) infections. I. Clinical and laboratory findings in 66 children with meningo-encephalitis. Pediatrics *52:*680, 1973.

Boston Interhospital Virus Study Group and the NIAID–sponsored Cooperative Antiviral Clinical Study: Failure of high dose 5-iodo-2'-deoxyuridine in the therapy of herpes simplex virus encephalitis. N. Engl. J. Med. *292:*599, 1975.

Buescher, E. L., Artenstein, M. S., and Olson, L.: Central nervous system infections of viral origin: The changing pattern. Res. Publ. Assoc. Res. Nerv. Ment. Dis. *44:*147, 1968.

Drachman, D. A., and Adams, R. D.: Herpes simplex and acute inclusion body encephalitis. Arch. Neurol. *7:*61, 1962.

Knotts, F. B., Cook, M. L., and Stevens, J. G.: Pathogenesis of herpetic encephalitis in mice after ophthalmic inoculation. J. Infect. Dis. *130:*16, 1974.

Lepow, M. L., Carver, D. H., Wright, H. T., Jr., Woods, W. A., and Robbins, F. C.: A clinical, epidemiologic and laboratory investigation of aseptic meningitis during the four-year period, 1955–1958. I. Observations concerning etiology and epidemiology. N. Engl. J. Med. *266:*1181, 1962.

Lepow, M. L., Coyne, N., Thompson, L. B., Carver, D. H., and Robbins, F. C.: A clinical, epidemiologic and laboratory investigation of aseptic meningitis during the four-year period, 1955–1958. II. The clinical disease and its sequelae. N. Engl. J. Med. *266:*1188, 1962.

Levitt, L. P., Rich, T. A., Kinde, S. W., Lewis, A. L., Gates, E. H., and Bond, J. O.: Central nervous system mumps. A review of 64 cases. Neurology *20:*829, 1970.

Olson, L. C., Buescher, E. L., Artenstein, M. S., and Parkman, P. D.: Herpesvirus infections of the human central nervous system. N. Engl. J. Med. *277:*1271, 1967.

Sköldenberg, B.: On the role of viruses in acute infectious diseases of the central nervous system. Scand. J. Infect. Dis. *3* (Suppl. 3):1, 1972.

Wallgren, A.: Une nouvelle maladie infectieuse due systeme nerveux central? Acta Paediatr. *4:*158, 1924–1925.

VIII

CUTANEOUS INFECTIONS

Chapter 36

PYODERMA

Introduction

Types of Organisms and Lesions

Group A streptococci, staphylococci, and *Corynebacterium diphtheriae* are the most common bacteria involved in skin infections. Any of these microorganisms may appear alone or in combination. Several M-type streptococci are particularly prone to invade the skin. Most instances of pyoderma result from secondary invasion of existing lesions such as burns and traumatic or surgical wounds, as well as scabies and similar skin lesions. Whether streptococci and staphylococci can invade intact normal skin is uncertain. However, some investigators believe that certain strains of both strepotococci and staphylococci with distinctive biologic features indeed can produce impetigo de novo, especially in the newborn and children. Although differentiation of streptococcal and staphylococcal origin of impetigo cannot always be made on clinical grounds, the condition can be divided on clinical and bacteriologic features into two types: (1) a bullous type with thin, amber, varnish-like crusts due to staphylococci, and (2) a vesicular type with thick crusts due to streptococci.

Incidence

Pyoderma occurs most commonly in children of preschool age and is seen especially during the summer months in the southern United States and during or near the end of rainy seasons in the Tropics. At these times, children are most likely to experience minor trauma and insect bites on their extremities which predispose to secondary invasion. Lower economic groups, most of whom live in crowded conditions, and rural populations are at greater risk. In one study of preschool children in rural Mississippi, 92 per cent had skin lesions sometime or another over a 13-week period during the summer. Group A streptococci were isolated in serial cultures from 77 per cent of this group.

Under certain circumstances pyoderma can affect older age groups. For instance, a survey of United States troops in the Mekong Delta of South Vietnam in the late 1960s revealed a high incidence of disabling bacterial skin infections which presented as ecthymatous lesions surrounded by erythema and induration, located on the lower extremities. Group A streptococci were recovered from 90 per cent of these specific lesions, and from 60 per cent of all skin lesions. *Staphylococcus aureus* was also recovered from 50 to 70 per cent of the skin lesions. Vietnamese children in the same geographic area also had a high incidence of skin lesions from which Group A streptococci could be recovered, whereas Vietnamese military personnel rarely had pyoderma but commonly did have *S. aureus* furunculosis. Perhaps frequent streptococcal skin infections in childhood conferred immunity to streptococcal infections. Immunity to staphylococcal infections is much less solid.

Transmission and Source

The major source of skin-infecting microorganisms appears to be other infected skin lesions rather than the respiratory tract. The latter, however, may at times serve as a reservoir. The normal skin on rare occasion may be a source for staphylococci, which can survive for some time. However, only a few strains of Group A streptococci can persist on normal skin for more than a few hours.

Transmission of microorganisms from one person to another can occur by direct skin-to-skin contact. Fomites occasionally may be responsible for spread of bacteria but probably do not play a major role in epidemics except in schools and military barracks. Insect vectors play a major role in the indirect transmission of microorganisms under certain circumstances. A small gnatlike fly (Hippelates) is attracted to and feeds on open skin lesions and can carry viable streptococci and staphylococci for some hours. Hippelates is a major vector in Trinidad and probably in other tropical regions.

Impetigo

Impetigo (Fig. 36–1), a form of pyoderma, is a superficial infection of the skin due to either Group A streptococci or hemolytic staphylococci. It occurs

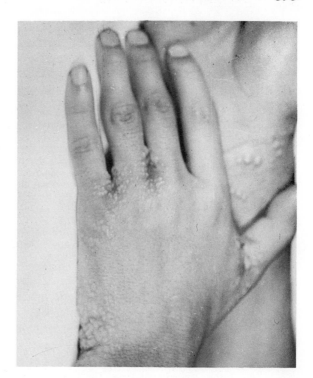

Figure 36–1. Impetigo. (Courtesy of Dr. Samuel M. Bluefarb.)

almost exclusively in children during warm weather. Why children but not adults are susceptible is unclear. Possible explanations include greater exposure to minor trauma which sets the stage for infection, greater personal contact conducive to spread from person to person, or increasing immunity with age following repeated exposure to streptococci and staphylococci.

Impetigo most commonly begins on the extremities. The lesions may itch intensely. The disease is readily spread to other areas of the body by scratching. Some instances of impetigo, especially in epidemic settings, appear to result from primary invasion of the superficial cutaneous layers of the skin by certain strains of Group A streptococci which secrete an agent capable of dissolving the intercellular cement of basal epithelial cells. However, it is practically impossible to be certain that the microorganisms did not gain entrance through some minor breach of the skin's integrity.

The characteristics of streptococcal and staphylococcal impetiginous lesions sometimes permit their differentiation, at least in the early stages (see Table 36–1).

Streptococcal Impetigo

The initial lesion of streptococcal impetigo is a tiny papule. A vesicle filled with serous fluid and a few leukocytes rapidly forms and is surrounded by a narrow rim of erythema. The blisters are flat, with a diameter of 2 to 3 mm. The clear fluid of such a vesicle usually yields a pure culture of Group A

TABLE 36–1. Comparison of Streptococcal and Staphylococcal Impetigo*

	Streptococcal	Staphylococcal
Vesicular stage	Ephemeral — often missed	Persistent bullae
Crusted stage	Thick, "stuck-on," amber colored, and persistent	Varnish-like, white or gray colored, more transient
Bacteriology	Usually Group A streptococci; sometimes Group C or G; staphylococci of various phage types may also be present	Usually phage type 71 staphylococci

*From Wannamaker, L. W.: Differences between streptococcal infections of the throat and of the skin. N. Engl. J. Med. *282:*23, 78, 1970.

streptococci. However, the vesicles are transient and may be missed if the patient is not seen early in the course of the disease. They rapidly become pustular. The serous fluid infects by direct extension to other areas, where new vesicles form. These soon break, and the surface becomes covered by a thick, hard, brownish, "candy" crust which is characteristic of streptococcal impetigo. Although the final lesions may be as large as 30 cm in diameter, they remain discrete. The lesions may later become secondarily infected by staphylococci which are present on normal skin.

Impetiginous lesions rarely, if ever, are accompanied by fever or constitutional symptoms or signs. Subepithelial tissues are not involved. Even untreated lesions rarely, if ever, leave permanent scars, although skin discolorations may persist for some time. The bacteriologic findings, complications, and treatment of streptococcal impetigo are similar to those of pyoderma and are discussed in the next section.

Staphylococcal Impetigo

Staphylococcal impetigo is characterized by persistent bullous lesions which subsequently form thin, varnish-like crusts which may be white or gray in color. The bullous form of impetigo usually yields pure cultures of phage type 71 staphylococci, or closely related strains. Phage type 71 strains have several unusual features. They can inhibit the growth of *Corynebacterium diphtheriae* on the surface of blood agar, produce large amounts of hyaluronidase, and in broth culture produce an extracellular substance that is bactericidal for Group A streptococci. This may account for the infrequency of isolation of Group A streptococci in patients with bullous impetigo.

Streptococcal Skin Infections

As noted in the introductory section, most streptococcal skin infections represent secondary invasion of existing lesions (see Table 36–2).

TABLE 36-2. Streptococcal Skin Infections

Secondary invasion of skin lesions

Erysipelas

Pyoderma
  Impetigo (contagiosa)
  Sycosis barbae
  "Scrum pox"
  Occupational

Lymphangitis

Secondary Infections

Invasion of surgical or open traumatic wounds in children or adults by Group A streptococci can result in serious infections which have systemic symptoms requiring prompt treatment. Cutaneous burns can support rapid proliferation of hemolytic streptococci. Burns so infected are characterized by diffuse inflammation with marked edema, weeping, and exudate. Systemic symptoms may be severe. Lesions of atopic eczema in infants, herpes simplex in adults, and scabies in any age group may become secondarily infected by hemolytic streptococci. In these instances, systemic symptoms are unusual. *Intertrigo* is an erythematous and weeping dermatitis that occurs in skin in areas where two folds are in constant contact; the lesions of this condition also may become secondarily infected by streptococci.

Erysipelas

Erysipelas (St. Anthony's fire) presents a unique clinical picture which has been recognized for 2000 years. This serious infection, which can follow unnoticed minor abrasion or complicate surgical wounds in any age group, is caused by hemolytic streptococci, usually Group A and only rarely Group C. It may begin anywhere on the body as a minute lesion which spreads marginally for four to six days. The full-blown lesion is characterized by a red, brawny thickening of the skin. On palpation, the margins present a peculiar hard induration, while all of the diseased skin has a rubbery consistency related to edema and inflammatory infiltration. Erysipelas of the face (Fig. 36-2) usually begins near the external nares and may spread over both cheeks in a butterfly distribution. In other areas, the lesion may be round or irregularly oval. Lesions on the trunk may become very large and be rapidly fatal. Occasionally, small blisters from which streptococci may be cultured appear on the edges of spreading lesions. Since septicemia is common, blood cultures should be obtained. Fever and systemic symptoms are present consistently. Histologically, extensive inflammation involves the superficial lymphatic vessels, which are filled with fibrin, leukocytes, and chains of streptococci. Perilymphatic tissues are edematous. The peculiar evolution of the lesion reflects a progressively diffuse involvement of the lymphatics.

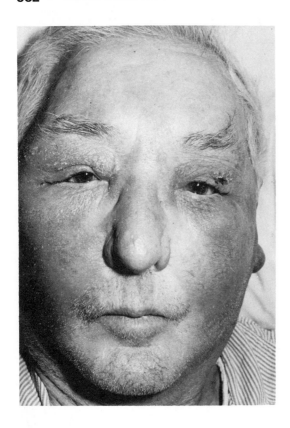

Figure 36–2. Erysipelas. (Courtesy of Dr. Samuel M. Bluefarb.)

Erysipelas used to carry a high mortality and was one of the most serious complications of surgical or traumatic wounds. Although the disease has been recognized for two milleniums, its incidence recently has decreased dramatically, presumably because penicillin is used promptly whenever streptococcal infections of wounds are suspected. Penicillin is the drug of choice.

Pyoderma

Pyoderma as a diagnostic term includes impetigo. However, many other lesions can become secondarily infected by hemolytic streptococci. Invasion of the skin by streptococci usually follows some break in the integrity of the skin caused by minor trauma such as abrasions or insect bites (Fig. 36–3). A number of other lesions, including scabies (Fig. 36–4), chronic eczema, herpes, and exfoliative dermatitis also are readily invaded by hemolytic streptococci. Crowding, poor socioeconomic conditions, and lack of general cleanliness all undoubtedly contribute to the spread of streptococcal skin infections. Pyodermic lesions, as are those of impetigo, frequently are covered by brownish or amber crusts representing dried seroexudate.

Poststreptococcal and staphylococcal skin infections may occur under several special circumstances. Sycosis barbae used to be common among males frequenting barber shops of questionable cleanliness. Outbreaks of

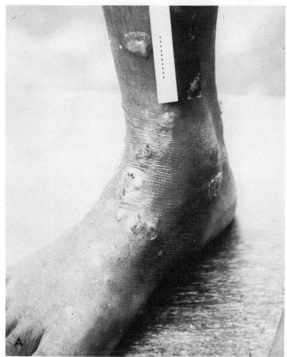

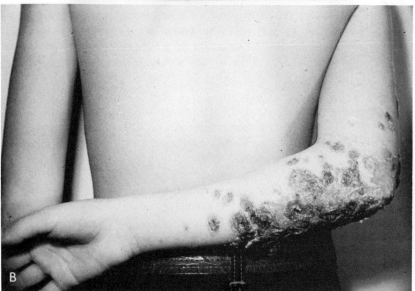

Figure 36-3. *A* and *B,* Pyoderma. (*A* courtesy of Dr. Elizabeth V. Potter; *B,* courtesy of Dr. Samuel M. Bluefarb.)

streptococcal impetigo among schoolboys playing rugby have been labeled "scrum pox" by the British. Similar outbreaks have been described among American football players. A form of impetigo called "horse pox" is highly contagious in both stablemen and horses. Another occupational form of

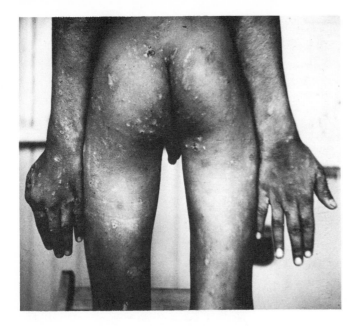

Figure 36–4.   Infected scabies. (Courtesy of Dr. Elizabeth V. Potter.)

streptococcal skin infection occurs on the fingers of women who wash sausage skins. Whether these infections result from particularly virulent microorganisms or environmental effects on the host is not known. These particular special instances of infections no longer are common problems. However, physicians should remain alert to new circumstances that might promote spread of streptococcal skin infections.

Although not strictly a skin disease, *lymphangitis* is conveniently considered here. Hemolytic streptococci, usually Group A, rarely Group C or G, enter the lymphatics through small, often inapparent breaks in the skin of the hand or foot. Once the microorganisms have gained entrance, one or more red streaks corresponding to lymphatic channels rapidly extend up the extremity. Very soon, the inguinal or axillary lymph nodes are involved. Fever, systemic symptoms, and bacteremia develop rapidly. The disease may be very serious, but its course is short. Penicillin should be administered by intramuscular injection as soon as possible.

Recurrent tropical lymphangitis is associated with repeated attacks of streptococcal invasion of the lymphatics of the legs, with enlargement of the inguinal and other satellite nodes. Streptococci gain entrance through a variety of minor lesions or fungal infections. Each acute attack is followed by further increase in skin thickness and induration secondary to lymphatic obstruction. Resultant skin ulcers may be the site for further secondary streptococcal infections. Permanent cutaneous thickening, or a form of elephantiasis, may follow repeated attacks.

Bacteriology

Impetiginous vesicles and pyodermic lesions that produce thick crusts initially yield pure cultures of Group A streptococci. Later, cultures may yield staphylococci as well as streptococci. Under such circumstances, staphylococci of a variety of phage types are recovered, suggesting secondary invasion, in contrast to specific phage type staphylococci recovered from bullous impetigo (discussed in the next section). When crusts are present, they should be removed carefully with saline-moistened swabs before attempts to obtain culture material are made.

Group A streptococci recovered from impetiginous and pyodermic lesions differ in several significant respects from strains responsible for pharyngitis. M serotypes of strains responsible for skin lesions represent for the most part recently established M types. For instance, all M types above 48 were first and predominantly isolated from skin lesions. With rare exception, pharyngeal M strains do not cause pyoderma. Group A streptococci recovered from skin lesions usually fall into a few T-agglutination types, often complex in that a single strain may contain several T types. Several of these strains also are nephritogenic.

The basis for the ability of certain streptococci to infect the pharynx and not the skin and for other strains to have the opposite propensity is not known. Several but not all skin strains may have such unusual features as a high content of the lipid cell wall membranes and a tendency to hemolyze slowly on blood agar surfaces and to grow as satellite colonies. A number of differences between streptococcal pharyngeal and skin infections are listed in Table 36–3.

Immunology

The serum anti–streptolysin O titer for some years has been the standard serum antibody for detection of Group A streptococcal infections antecedent to acute rheumatic fever and acute glomerulonephritis. Serum anti–streptolysin O titers increase significantly in 80 per cent of pharyngeal infections; however, their response to streptococcal skin infections is nonexistent to weak. Fortunately, serum anti-hyaluronidase and anti-DNAse B titers usually increase in response to streptococcal skin infections.

Streptococci responsible for pharyngitis induce serum antibodies specific to the strain's M protein. These antibodies are protective against further infections by the same M serotype. For instance, second attacks of pharyngitis due to type 12 streptococci have not been observed. Streptococci associated with pyoderma likewise induce M–type specific antibodies. Although the observation periods are not yet long enough, strains responsible for skin lesions do appear to induce long-lasting immunity.

Nonsuppurative Complications

As in the case of pharyngeal infections, only some streptococcal M types recovered from skin infections are nephritogenic, especially M types 49, 55, and 57. Large epidemics of impetigo or pyoderma have been reported without any case of acute nephritis. A given population prone to skin lesions is subject to exposure to a number of different nephritogenic strains of streptococci. Thus, second attacks of acute nephritis are more common following streptococcal pyoderma than after streptococcal pharyngitis, in

TABLE 36–3. General Features of Streptococcal Infections at Different Sites*

Feature	Streptococcal Pharyngitis and Tonsillitis	Streptococcal Impetigo and Pyoderma
Clinical		
Erythema	Usually present and generalized	Often minimal and localized to immediate area around lesion
Vesicular stage	Absent	Typical of early lesion but transient
Pustular stage	Patchy exudate – sometimes confluent	Usually discrete; flora often mixed
Crusted stage	Absent	Frequent and characteristic
Local pain	Common – may be intense	Usually absent
Systemic reaction	Fever, headache, and malaise occur commonly	Unusual
Regional adenitis	Common	Less common, but adenopathy frequently seen
Deep-seated cellulitis	May occur	Occurs perhaps less commonly
Bacteremia	Rare	May be relatively more frequent
Scarlatiniform rash	Sometimes present	Rare
Course	Typically acute, except in infants	Often chronic; lesions may become ecthymatous
Laboratory		
Leukocytosis	Usually present	Often absent
Bacteriology	Group A streptococci usually predominate	Often contain large numbers of staphylococci
Serologic types of Group A streptococci	Many different types	Few types predominate
Anti-streptolysin O response	Common	Uncommon
Epidemiology		
Seasonal occurrence	Winter and spring	Late summer and early fall
Common-source epidemics	May occur	Not described
Geographic distribution	More common in temperate or cold climates	Common in hot or tropical climates
Age	Young school-age children	Children of preschool age
Sex	Equal	Equal
Transmission	Direct spread from human reservoirs, particularly nasal carriers	Unknown: may be insects

TABLE 36–3. General Features of Streptococcal Infections at Different Sites *(Continued)*

Feature	Streptococcal Pharyngitis and Tonsillitis	Streptococcal Impetigo and Pyoderma
Carrier state	Common in pharynx of many populations	Unusual on skin, except in certain situations
Preceding trauma	Not present	May predispose to natural or experimental infection
Preceding viral infection	Uncommon	Uncommon
Complications		
Acute nephritis	Occurs; partially preventable (50 per cent)	Occurs; preventability unknown
Acute rheumatic fever	Occurs; preventable	Does not occur
Treatment		
Local	Not important	Removal of crusts and scrubbing with hexachlorophene soap
Systemic	Single injection of intramuscular benzathine penicillin or oral penicillin for 10 days	May not be necessary; extensive lesions may require intramuscular benzathine penicillin

*From Wannamaker, L. W.: Differences between streptococcal infections of the throat and the skin. N. Engl. J. Med. *282:*23, 78, 1970.

which M type 12 streptococci account for most instances of acute glomerulonephritis.

Unlike pharyngeal infections, streptococcal skin infections are not followed by rheumatic fever, erythema nodosum, or chorea.

Treatment and Prevention

Streptococcal skin infections respond readily to penicillin therapy. Injection of long-acting benzathine penicillin or penicillin by mouth for 10 days is recommended. Although group A streptococci are inevitably eradicated by penicillin, the skin lesions may persist for some time, and penicillin-resistant staphylococci may emerge and flourish. Although local treatment alone of pyoderma hardly ever will eradicate Group A streptococci, removal of crusts and scrubbing the affected areas with soap may help to speed recovery.

Prophylaxis of streptococcal pyoderma, especially among poor populations in rural tropical areas, presents a very difficult and complex problem. Covering all skin surfaces and avoiding contact with others is easily recommended but impossible from the practical aspect, since children are the usual victims. Nevertheless, simple measures of cleanliness, if practiced faithfully by all neighboring families, should help to reduce the incidence.

Administration of penicillin to all individuals with pyoderma in a reasonably small and closed population can eradicate the disease, at least temporarily. However, if circumstances make continuation of abrasions and insect bites likely, recurrence of streptococcal invasion can be expected. Treatment of large populations with penicillin on a mass scale seems impractical.

Nevertheless, when a predisposing condition is known and is one which can be controlled, prevention is possible. For example, a major epidemic of acute nephritis in Trinidad was associated with an explosive epidemic of scabies. The scabetic lesions soon were invaded by nephritogenic M type 55 streptococci, which were spread from lesion to lesion by Hippelates flies. The epidemic was brought under control by measures which were successful in containing the spread of scabies.

Staphylococcal Skin Infections

All skin lesions which are subject to invasion by hemolytic streptococci similarly are susceptible to colonization and infection by staphylococci, either alone or in association with streptococci or *Corynebacterium diphtheriae*. Since staphylococci are normal inhabitants of the skin, infections due to those microorganisms are not unexpected. In addition to pyoderma and impetigo, staphylococci are associated with several other characteristic infections of the skin (see Table 36–4).

TABLE 36–4. Staphylococcal Skin Infections

Pyoderma
    Impetigo contagiosa

Folliculitis
    Sycosis barbae
    Hidradenitis suppurativa
    Pustular acne vulgaris

Carbuncle

Pemphigus neonatorum or toxic epidermal necrolysis
    (Ritter's disease)

Staphylococci are by far the most common microorganisms responsible for suppuration of the skin. Fifty to 80 per cent of serious hospital-acquired staphylococcal infections are due to coagulase positive microorganisms. Thirty to 70 per cent of these infections are due to the epidemic phage type 80/81 microorganisms which are resistant to penicillins.

Pyoderma and Impetigo

As previously stated, pyoderma and wound infections may be associated with many different strains and phage types of staphylococci.

Folliculitis

Folliculitis (Fig. 36–5) is a simple infection of hair follicles by staphylococci, often of the *Staphylococcus albus* variety. The infection usually follows obstruction of a hair follicle. The surrounding tissue is not involved. Recurrent folliculitis of the beard area is called *sycosis barbae.*

Furunculosis

A more extensive and invasive staphylococcal infection of obstructed hair follicles or sebaceous glands with some involvement of subcutaneous tissues is called a *furuncle* or *boil.* When the lesions are multiple, the condition is called *furunculosis.* Furuncles sometimes can appear in crops and then clear for months or years before recurring. Perhaps transient immunologic deficiencies of the host are responsible for recurrent crops.

Furuncles most commonly occur on the face, neck, forearms, axillae, back, groin, and legs. Local itching and mild pain are soon followed by progressive local swelling and erythema. The overlying skin becomes thinned, tense, and very tender. Spontaneous or surgical drainage generally affords prompt relief. The pus is usually creamy yellow. Most furuncles that reach the abscess stage are due to coagulase positive *Staphylococcus aureus.*

Staphylococcal invasion of axillary sweat glands results in a deep-seated infection called *hidradenitis suppurativa* (Fig. 36–6). This infection is stubbornly resistant to treatment and frequently recurs.

Furuncles usually are not accompanied by fever and general symptoms. However, when they are located on the face, staphylococci may enter venous

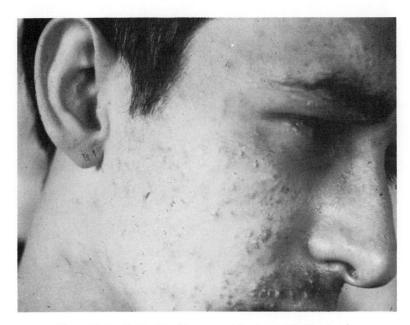

Figure 36–5. Folliculitis. (Courtesy of Dr. Samuel M. Bluefarb.)

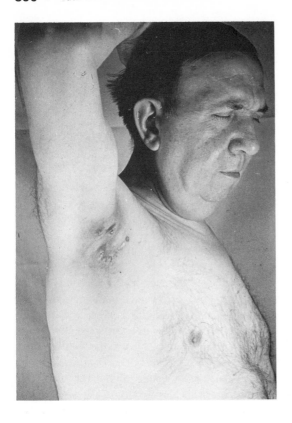

Figure 36-6. Hidradenitis suppurativa. (Courtesy of Dr. Samuel M. Bluefarb.)

sinuses which drain into the skull, resulting in sinus thrombosis and brain abscess.

Recurrent boils may be difficult to manage. The patient should be instructed to avoid oils, dust, and trauma to the affected areas, and to use only mild soaps and cool water when washing. When infections recur frequently, tyrothricin cream or bacitracin ointment should be applied to the skin daily. These measures are particularly important in diabetic patients. Clean clothes and proper disposal of dressings are essential. A vacation in a cool, dry climate can be helpful by decreasing environmental factors that can contribute to obstruction of sweat glands, hair follicles, and sebaceous glands.

Carbuncle

Carbuncles (Fig. 36-7) occur in the thick, relatively inelastic and fibrous skin of the nape of the neck and the upper back. The lesion usually begins with an infection of an obstructed hair follicle. The thickness and impermeability of the overlying skin lead to lateral extension and loculation of the infection. The large, indurated lesion is red, very tender, and painful, and usually has multiple ineffective drainage sites. The patient holds his head rigidly. Carbuncles often are associated with fever, extreme pain, prostration, and leukocytosis. Elderly patients may be critically ill. Bacteremia is not uncommon. Any patient with a large boil or carbuncle and fever should have serial blood cultures performed.

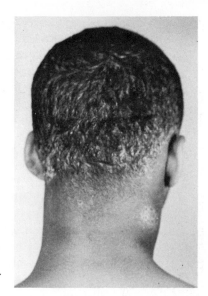

Figure 36–7. Carbuncle. (Courtesy of Dr. Samuel M. Bluefarb.)

Boils or carbuncles, when seen prior to abscess formation, may be aborted by oral administration of penicillin. Treatment should be maintained for 10 days. Lincomycin or cephalothin may be used in patients sensitive to penicillin. If bacteremia is present, maximum doses should be used. Prior to drainage, hot packs may yield some relief of pain, but should not be used after drainage occurs. The involved part should be kept at rest and the patient should stay in bed when the infection is severe. Surgical drainage usually is necessary. The skin around a draining sinus should be protected from discharging pus with a thick layer of penicillin or tyrothricin cream.

Pemphigus Neonatorum or Toxic Epidermal Necrolysis (Ritter's Disease)

Bullous response to staphylococcal skin infection in the newborn can develop in two forms. Impetigo of the newborn, or pemphigus neonatorum, begins on the fourth to tenth day of life, usually on the face or extremities and in the upper diaper area. Easily ruptured bullae on a slightly erythematous base are characteristic. They usually spread rapidly over the body. Staphylococci are introduced into a nursery by carriers among the staff, and group 2 phage (especially type 71) staphylococci are particularly virulent in the newborn.

Toxic epidermal necrolysis, or Ritter's disease, is also known as dermatitis exfoliativa neonatorum, or the "scalded child" syndrome. It is an acute reaction of the skin to hemoltyic staphylococcal infections. The disease begins suddenly, with perioral erythema and crusting. These symptoms are followed within 24 to 48 hours by a tender, generalized skin erythema which spreads over the face and then the rest of the body and is associated with fever from 101 to 104°F and systemic symptoms. The epidermis is quickly separated by fluid in poorly circumscribed areas of various sizes. The bullae are flaccid and are easily wiped off by light rubbing, as is the erythematous skin in nonblistered areas. At first the denuded areas are moist and merge to give the skin a scalded appearance. The denuded areas dry quickly so that in a few days the skin becomes scaly. The skin returns to normal in 7 to 10 days. However, the disease may be fatal in less than 36 horus. Bacteremia is relatively common. Blood cultures should be obtained from all patients.

Toxic epidermal necrolysis is most common in the newborn but does occur in older children up to the age of 10 years. It is very rare in adults but has been described in patients with deficiency of cell-mediated immunity.

The best way to control an outbreak of this serious disease in a nursery is to admit all subsequent newborn to a nursery set up in a remote area and staffed by entirely different personnel. A much less preferred technique is to treat all newborn admissions with appropriate antibiotics until the carriers among the staff are detected.

Loosened areas of the skin should be debrided. A 1:10,000 solution of benzalkonium may be used to clean the skin. Bacitracin ointment should also be applied. The infant should be kept in an incubator so that temperature and humidity may be kept within comfortable ranges. Penicillin should be used for susceptible microorganisms.

Skin Infections Due to Corynebacterium diphtheriae

Cutaneous diphtheria occurs primarily in the Tropics, although it has been observed in temperate regions. *Corynebacterium diphtheriae* apparently is unable to penetrate normal skin. Thus, as will streptococcal and staphylococcal skin infections, *C. diphtheriae* usually is a secondary invader of existing skin lesions such as abrasions, burns, or pyoderma. Cutaneous diphtheria usually involves the lower extremities but may appear anywhere on the body surface. The scrotum is a common site.

Some instances of cutaneous diphtheria present fairly characteristic features. The typical lesion is a round or oval, "punched out" ulcer with a diameter of 0.5 to 3 cm. The edges are rolled, bluish, tender, and sharply demarcated. The ulcer is covered with a gray to gray-yellow membrane, or sometimes by a crust. These can be stripped off. Some pain may be present at first, but the development of local anesthesia is a strong clinical clue for the diagnosis of cutaneous diphtheria. Healing is from the periphery and is slow. Scarring is common. Toxic manifestations such as myocarditis or peripheral neuritis may develop. However, their incidence is low enough to suggest that diphtheria toxin is either poorly formed or absorbed from skin lesions. More commonly, *Corynebacterium diphtheriae* may be recovered from pyodermic lesions which do not have the characteristics described above.

In one study of school children with a high incidence of pyoderma, at least half of *Corynebacterium diphtheriae* strains isolated from skin lesions were toxigenic. However, none of the 70 children with toxigenic *C. diphtheriae* had evidence of toxicity. Subsequent study of serum antitoxin levels revealed high and protective levels in the children who had had toxigenic *C. diphtheriae* in their skin lesions. Several months after the increase in the incidence of toxigenic *C. diphtheriae* in skin lesions, a significant increase of symptomatic nasopharyngeal diphtheria occurred in other members of the school-age population.

Use of diphtheria antitoxin has not modified the course or incidence of toxicity due to skin diphtheria. Nevertheless, if a diphtheritic membrane is present, 20,000 to 40,000 units of antitoxin should be administered. In the absence of a membrane, however, antitoxin is not necessary, even when toxic *Corynebacterium diphtheriae* microorganisms are secondary invaders of pyoderma, since cardiac myopathy and peripheral neuropathy are extremely rare in association with skin diphtheria.

CASE PRESENTATION

A seven-year-old boy living in a rural area outside Birmingham, Alabama, was observed by his mother to have puffy eyes one morning in late August. On questioning, she learned that the boy had noted very dark urine the day before. She took her son to a physician, who observed pitting edema of the ankles, a blood pressure of 130/85 mm Hg, 3+ protein, and many erythrocytes in the urine. He also noted several small scabs on both legs, and a normal pharynx. He cultured the pharynx and one of the lesions on the right leg, after removing the scab with a gauze square soaked in sterile saline. The physician arranged for his office nurse to ask parents in the community to observe their children for skin sores and dark urine. Three days later the nurse reported that at least nine children had open skin sores, and that 3 of 18 urines she tested by dipstick had protein and blood. Meanwhile, the throat culture from the patient revealed no streptococci. Cultures of skin lesions from eight of the nine children with open sores were positive for beta-hemolytic streptococci. Seven cultures also demonstrated coagulase-positive staphylococci. The nurse requested that the laboratory test the staphylococci for penicillin sensitivity. All strains were sensitive.

The physician and the nurse, who obviously had good rapport with the community, obtained further cultures, urinalyses, and blood for serum anti–streptolysin O and anti-hyaluronidase titers as well as blood urea nitrogen and serum creatinine levels. Before results were obtained from the laboratory, three more children were found to have proteinuria and hematuria on dipstick tests. At this point, the physician decided to administer 1,200,000 units of procaine penicillin intramuscularly to all children in families with either abnormal urine or positive cultures in one or more siblings.

Shortly after the two days required for this program, the physician received a report that the serum anti–streptolysin O titers were in the normal range, and that serums for the anti–hyaluronidase titer tests had been sent out to another laboratory. The results would be available within one week. Subsequently, three more children developed edema and dark urine. Two required hospitalization for acute circulatory congestion.

Reevaluation of the children of the affected families two weeks after penicillin injections revealed almost the same incidence of skin sores as was present before penicillin therapy. None of the repeat skin lesion cultures demonstrated streptococci, but 80 per cent contained staphylococci which now were resistant to penicillin. On careful follow-up examination of family members, no other members developed abnormal urine, despite continued appearance of skin lesions throughout September.

The initial patient and all other children who subsequently developed edema, hematuria, or abnormal urine had normal urines by the last week of October. At this time, the physician finally received a report that the serum anti-hyaluronidase titers were greatly increased.

The circumstances described in this hypothetical situation represent a level of community medicine not yet available except on a research basis. Indeed, very similar observations have been made in the course of epidemiologic studies. However, techniques necessary for such studies should eventually be available to communities as they develop effective medical care delivery systems. The described hypothetical delivery system, although not ideal, represents a distinct advance which can become reality only when sufficient competent paramedical personnel become available.

The initiation of penicillin prophylaxis therapy was quite appropriate, despite the risk of penicillin allergy. Fortunately, no anaphylactic reactions occurred. If they had, the physician and his nurse were well prepared, for they always had available epinephrine, prednisone, and antihistaminic agents.

The fact that the incidence of skin lesions did not decrease after penicillin injections and disappearance of streptococci was not surprising, for streptococci are not the cause of skin lesions. Furthermore, although penicillin eradicated streptococci, penicillin-resistant staphylococci rapidly emerged. Thus, the incidence of staphylococci in the skin lesions increased. However, in the particular population involved, adverse conditions developed from this evolution of penicillin-resistant staphylococci.

References

Books

Swartz, M. N., and Weinberg, A. N.: Bacterial diseases with cutaneous involvement. *In* Fitzpatrick, T. B., et al. (eds.): Dermatology in General Medicine. New York, McGraw-Hill Book Co., 1971.

Vaughn, V. C., III, and McKay, R. J.: Nelson Textbook of Pediatrics. 10th ed. Philadelphia, W. B. Saunders Co., 1975.

Symposium Volume

Dillon, H. C., and Wannamaker, L. W.: Skin infections and acute glomerulonephritis: Report of a symposium. Milit. Med. *136:*122, 1971.

Review Article

Wannamaker, L. W.: Streptococcal infections of the throat and of the skin. N. Engl. J. Med. *282:*23, 78, 1970.

Original Articles

Bray, J. P., Burt, E. G., Potter, E. V., Poon-King, T., and Earle, D. P.: Epidemic diphtheria and skin infections in Trinidad. J. Infect. Dis. *126:*24, 1972.

Melish, M. E., and Glasgow, A.: The staphylococcal scalded-skin syndrome. N. Engl. J. Med. *282:*1114, 1970.

Parker, M. T., Tomlinson, A. J. H., and Williams, R. E. O.: Impetigo contagiosa: The association of certain types of Staphylococcus aureus and of Streptococcus pyogenes with superficial skin lesions. J. Hyg. (Camb.) *53:*458, 1955.

Potter, E. V., Ortiz, J. S., Sharrett, A. R., Burt, E. G., Bray, J. P., Finklea, J. F., Poon-King, T., and Earle, D. P.: Changing types of nephritogenic streptococci in Trinidad. J. Clin. Invest. *50:*1197, 1971.

Svartman, M., Potter, E. V., Poon-King, T., and Earle, D. P.: Streptococcal infection of scabetic lesions related to acute glomerulonephritis in Trinidad. J. Clin. Lab. Med. *81:*183, 1973.

Chapter 37

STAPHYLOCOCCI

Introduction

Staphylococci are among the most important bacteria which may cause disease in man. They are normal inhabitants of the upper respiratory tract, skin, or intestinal tract of man, and are particularly prone to produce infection when some factor has lowered host resistance, e.g., an antecedent viral infection. The fact that staphylococci are members of the indigenous microbial flora creates special problems in prevention and treatment of staphylococcal disease. These microorganisms also are noteworthy for the production of large numbers of exotoxins and other substances, some of which may play an important role in their capacity to cause disease.

Classification

Staphylococci are nonmotile, gram positive, and catalase-positive cocci, approximately 0.5 to 1.5 microns in diameter. These cells are able to divide in more than one plane, and as a result the cells form irregular masses resembling bunches of grapes. The name *Staphylococcus* is derived from the Greek word *staphule*, meaning cluster of grapes.

Only two of the three species in the genus Staphylococcus, *Staphylococcus aureus* and *Staphylococcus epidermidis*, are of medical importance. These two species differ in variety of characteristics (see Table 37–1). The difference of greatest importance in medicine is their relative capacity to produce disease. *S. aureus* is the pathogenic species; *S. epidermidis* seldom produces progressive infection in man.

TABLE 37–1. Differential Characteristics of Species of Staphylococcus*

Characteristic	aureus	epidermidis
Coagulases	+	–
Mannitol		
Acid aerobically	+	d
Acid anaerobically	+	–
Alpha toxin	+	–
Heat-resistant endonucleases	+	–
Biotin for growth	–	+
Cell wall		
Ribitol	+	–
Glycerol	–	+
Protein A	+	–

*Modified from Baird-Parker, A. C.: Classification and identification of staphylococci and their resistance to chemical and physical agents. *In* Cohen, J. O. (ed.): The Staphylococci. New York, John Wiley and Sons, 1972.
+ = most (90 per cent or more) strains positive.
– = most (90 per cent or more) strains negative.
d = some strains positive, some negative.

Growth and Microscopic Appearance

Staphylococci are aerobes and facultative anaerobes. They grow very well on ordinary media and the colonies are fairly large, smooth, and glistening after 24 to 48 hours of incubation on agar plates. Colonies of *Staphylococcus aureus* are usually pigmented. This pigmentation may vary from light yellow to a deep orange or a lemon yellow color and is caused by the presence of carotenoid pigments which are elaborated by the microorganism. Colonies of *Staphylococcus epidermidis* are white, since this species does not produce carotenoid pigments. Because S. aureus produces hemolysins, the colonies are usually surrounded by a variable zone of beta-type hemolysis on blood agar plates. The colonies of *S. aureus* and *S. epidermidis* on blood agar plates are much larger than those of Streptococcus, Neisseria, or Haemophilus species. An experienced observer can usually recognize staphylococcal colonies on sight.

Other staphylococcal colony forms, i.e., rough colonies, also may be found. Of particular importance in medical microbiology are small colony variants (G forms, dwarf forms) that may appear on plates inoculated with material from infected tissue. These form very minute colonies which may be overlooked or may be confused with colonies of streptococci or the hemophilic bacteria.

Soft forms (L-form variants) have been isolated from an occasional patient with staphylococcal osteomyelitis. Although such variants may appear in chronic lesions, they do not appear to be able to initiate infection or disease. Staphylococcal cells grow over a wide range of temperature, from 5 to 46°C. The optimum temperature for growth lies somewhere between 30 and 37°C. Two other cultural growth characteristics are of importance. Most strains of *Staphylococcus aureus* grow in high concentrations of sodium chloride (10 to 15 per cent) and are resistant to the action of bile salts since they grow well in concentrations of bile as high as 40 per cent.

Habitat

Staphylococcus aureus and *Staphylococcus epidermidis* are members of the indigenous microbial flora of man. Thus, many persons are asymptomatic carriers of staphylococci and may serve as a source of infection for themselves as well as other people. This situation is analogous to that seen in infections with *Streptococcus pyogenes*, *Streptococcus pneumoniae*, *Haemophilus influenzae*, and *Neisseria meningitidis*. Epidemics of staphylococcal disease may occur, especially when so-called epidemic types of *S. aureus* are involved, but they are seen only in hospitals or other institutions. For the most part, staphylococcal disease occurs sporadically, since it is usually a disease of carriers.

In contrast to the other microorganisms mentioned above, which are carried primarily in the upper respiratory tract of man, *Staphylococcus aureus* and *Staphylococcus epidermidis* are also found in other regions of the body. Skin is frequently inhabited, and staphylococci are commonly found in the following areas: umbilicus, axilla, perineum, face, hands, and hair.

In the upper respiratory tract, staphylococci appear in large numbers in the oropharynx and nasopharynx. However, they are more common and occur in even greater numbers in the anterior nares. The colonization of the anterior nares by *Staphylococcus aureus* provides a convenient source for colonization of the skin.

Staphylococci may also be found in the gastrointestinal tract. They do not commonly produce gastrointestinal disease but may under certain circumstances when the normal microbial flora is suppressed in persons being given broad-spectrum antibiotics. Under these conditions, antibiotic-resistant staphylococci may develop, multiply, and produce disease; for example, pseudomembranous enterocolitis is caused by uninhibited growth of antibody-resistant, enterotoxin-producing strains of *Staphylococcus aureus* in the gut. This is an extremely serious and frequently fatal situation.

It is estimated that from 20 to 75 per cent of all persons at any given time harbor *Staphylococcus aureus*. Asymptomatic staphylococcal carriers can be divided into several types: *persistent carriers,* those who harbor a specific type of *S. aureus* for prolonged periods; *occasional carriers,* those who sporadically harbor pathogenic staphylococci; *intermittent* or *transient carriers,* those who harbor one staphylococcal type for a certain period and then harbor a different type; and *noncarriers,* those who never, or only rarely, carry virulent *S. aureus* strains.

A number of factors may be involved in the maintenance of the carrier state, but the most important is the immune state of the host. Those persons with efficient immune mechanisms handle staphylococci more readily and are less apt to be persistent carriers. Symptomatic carriers are those people who are suffering from overt staphylococcal disease.

Dissemination

Figure 37–1 shows the epidemiologic cycle of staphylococci in the hospital and in the community. Staphylococci harbored by either asymptomatic carriers or a person with disease can be disseminated in a number of ways to other persons or to the environment. Staphylococci may be expelled from the upper respiratory tract during the act of sneezing. Inanimate objects and even the dust on the floors and walls of rooms may be contaminated in this manner. These then may serve as sources of infection for persons whose resistance is lowered. Staphylococci can also be transmitted to others from the upper respiratory tract by the hands of an asymptomatic carrier. Hands are readily contaminated by staphylococci which occupy the anterior nares, and *Staphylococcus aureus,* therefore, can be transmitted directly to others. Hospital personnel such as physicians, nurses, and nurse's aids are particularly apt to spread staphylococci in this manner. The asymptomatic carrier can also transmit staphylococci to his own skin and clothing by sneezing or by his contaminated hands.

A number of studies have been made of the spread of strains of *Staphylococcus aureus* in nurseries for the newborn. The upper respiratory tract of newborn infants and the skin become colonized with staphylococci within a few hours after birth. Diseases such as impetigo, conjunctivitis, infection of the umbilical stump, and even pneumonia and septicemia may develop. The staphylococcus strain acquired may originate from another colonized infant in the nursery or from carriers among the nurses or other hospital personnel. The major mode of transmission to the newborn appears to be by the hands of the nurses who handle the infants. Fomites such as diapers, undershirts, sheets, and blankets, if heavily contaminated with staphylococci, may also serve as vectors, but the hands of attendants are by far the most common and important means of transmission.

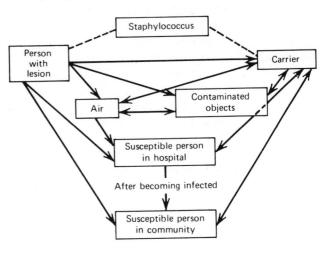

Figure 37–1. Epidemiologic cycle of staphylococci in the hospital and in the community. (From Nahmias, A. J., and Schulman, J. A.: Epidemiologic aspects and control methods. *In* Cohen, J. O. (ed.): The Staphylococci. New York, John Wiley and Sons, 1972.)

Staphylococcal disease occurs more frequently in patients in hospitals than in persons in a nonhospital population. The major reason for this higher incidence is that staphylococcal infection occurs primarily in persons with lowered host resistance. Asymptomatic carriers of pathogenic staphylococci will not develop staphylococcal disease while their resistance to this microorganism is high; if there is a reduction in either local or systemic resistance, however, resident staphylococci may produce either local or systemic disease. Table 37–2 shows the factors which are known to predispose to disease by *Staphylococcus aureus*. This list readily explains why *S. aureus* infections are more common in hospital patients.

TABLE 37–2. Factors Predisposing to *Staphylococcus aureus* Infection*

Injury to normal skin, e.g., traumatic abrasions and wounds, surgical incisions, burns, primary skin diseases

Prior viral infections, e.g., influenza, measles

Leukocyte defects
    Decreased numbers of leukocytes, e.g., congenital or acquired leukopenia, immunosuppressive drugs
    Defects in chemotaxis
    Defects in phagocytosis or facilitation of this process by serum opsonins or other serum factors
    Defects in intracellular killing, e.g., chronic granulomatous disease

Deficiencies in humoral immunity

Presence of foreign bodies, e.g., intravenous catheters, sutures, prosthetic cardiac valves

Prior prophylactic or therapeutic use of antibiotics to which the infecting *S. aureus* is not susceptible

Miscellaneous illnesses with less well-understood defects in host resistance, e.g., diabetes mellitus, alcoholism, mucoviscidosis, coronary artery disease, various malignant tumors, uremia

*From Schulman, J. A., and Nahmias, A. J.: Staphylococcal infections: Clinical Aspects. *In* Cohen, J. O. (ed.): The Staphylococci. New York, John Wiley and Sons, 1972.

Pathogenesis

Staphylococci may produce disease in almost every organ and tissue of the body. The skin is particularly prone to infection, and it is estimated that staphylococcal skin infections are probably one of the most common of all infectious disease processes. For example, it has been estimated that over 1.5 million cases of furunculosis occur in the United States each year. The spread of staphylococcal infection within the body and the major organs and tissues in which infection occurs are shown in Figure 37–2. This figure demonstrates that *Staphylococcus aureus* infections may spread by extension to contiguous tissues, or by way of lymphatics and then blood. Metastatic lesions are produced in a wide variety of tissues.

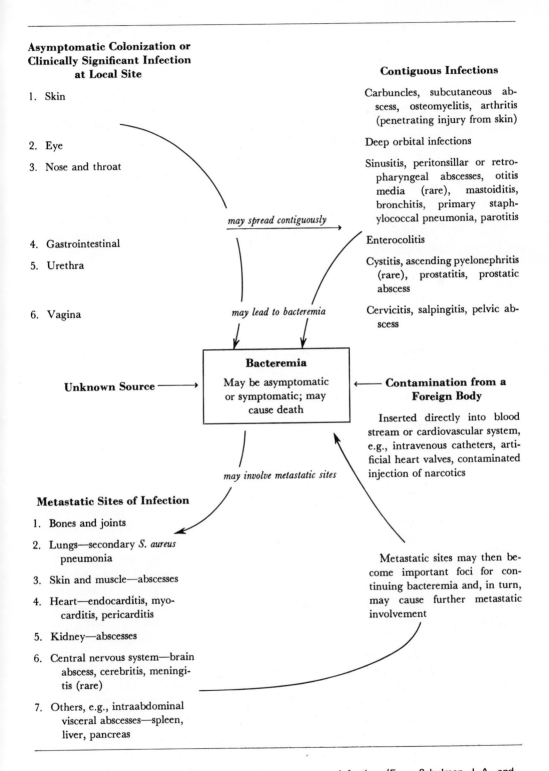

Figure 37–2. Pathogenic sequence of *Staphylococcus aureus* infection. (From Schulman, J. A., and Nahmias, A. J.: Staphylococcal infections: clinical aspects. *In* Cohen, J. O. (ed.): The Staphylococci. New York, John Wiley and Sons, 1972.)

The disease process is initially localized wherever *Staphylococcus aureus* lesions occur. There is an acute inflammatory response and an accumulation of enormous numbers of segmented neutrophils. Lesions tend to be walled off owing to the deposition of fibrin. Subsequently, central necrosis appears, and an abscess is formed which may be either small or large. Thus, staphylococcal infections are characterized by abscess formation. Dissemination as outlined in Figure 37–2 may occur from an initial abscess. It should be reemphasized that staphylococcal disease for the most part occurs only in those persons whose defense mechanisms have been compromised.

The enormous influence of foreign bodies on resistance to staphylococcal infection has been dramatically shown by Elek and Conan. These investigators found that it was necessary to inject 5×10^6 viable *Staphylococcus aureus* cells into the skin of human volunteers in order to produce infection and disease. However, as few as 100 viable *S. aureus* cells were required if the microorganisms were impregnated on a silk suture and tied into the skin. It is no wonder that cardiac prostheses, indwelling venous catheters, and other foreign bodies are so frequently colonized by staphylococci, even *Staphylococcus epidermidis.*

Virulence Factors

Probably no other bacterium produces as many extracellular toxins, hemolysins, enzymes, and cellular components, all of which at one time or another have been thought to be responsible for virulence; as does *Staphylococcus aureus.* Table 37–3 shows a partial list of these substances. At the present time, we cannot state that any one or combination of these factors accounts for the virulence of *S. aureus.* Probably many of them play some role in the pathogenesis of staphylococcal disease, but it is more likely that no one of them is essential for pathogenicity.

Some of these substances are, however, of more than passing interest. Coagulase, a protein which has the capacity to cause the clotting of plasma, has been held by some to be mainly responsible for the virulence of these microorganisms. There is a high correlation between the presence of coagulase in a strain and virulence because most strains isolated from infectious processes in human beings are coagulase positive (see Table 37–1). Because of this high correlation, a simple procedure has been developed for detecting the presence of coagulase, and this method is used to support the claim that a particular strain isolated from the infectious process is pathogenic.

The hemolysins of *Staphylococcus aureus* are of interest, and the alpha hemolysin (toxin) is particularly so. This was the first staphylococcal hemolysin to be investigated. It is a protein and not only hemolyzes red cells but also kills rabbits when injected intravenously in sufficient amount (lethal action). If injected into the skin of rabbits or guinea pigs, alpha toxin also produces acute inflammation and necrosis (dermonecrotic action). Upon sheep blood agar plates, colonies of *S. aureus* are surrounded by a large zone of beta-type hemolysis. The student should not confuse this with the beta hemolysis produced by the streptococci. This type of hemolysis merely refers to the complete clearing of the medium due to the lysing of all the red cells.

TABLE 37-3. Virulence Factors ?

Enzymes	Hemolysins
Coagulase	Alpha toxin
Hyaluronidase	Beta toxin
Phosphatase	Delta toxin
DNAase	Gamma toxin
Penicillinase	
Proteases	
Lipases	
Lysozyme	
Lactic dehydrogenase	

Enterotoxins   Leukocidin   Exfoliatin

Cellular Antigens

Polysaccharide A
Polysaccharide 263
Protein A
Protein B
Antigen D
Capsular antigen (SSA, SPA)
Teichoic acids

The beta-hemolytic streptococci produce beta hemolysins, and the alpha hemolysin of the staphylococci produces beta-type hemolysis.

A great deal of research has been done to determine whether alpha hemolysin may be responsible for the pathogenicity of *Staphylococcus aureus*. It seems rather clear that while it may play a role in the pathogenesis of staphylococcal disease (since it may be responsible for some of the extensive necrosis which occurs), it is not a major factor in disease production. Experimental work demonstrates that antitoxin directed against alpha hemolysin has no protective effect against staphylococcal infection even though the toxin can be effectively neutralized in this manner. None of the other hemolysins appears to play an important role in the pathogenicity of this microorganism.

The enterotoxins deserve special mention. There is no question that they are responsibile for a syndrome known as *staphylococcal food poisoning*. There are four enterotoxins, and each one differs antigenically from the other. Staphylococcal food poisoning occurs when food, particularly cold meats, pastry, or milk, becomes contaminated with an enterotoxin-producing strain of *Staphylococcus aureus*. If such food is left at room temperature, the staphylococci will multiply rapidly and produce toxin which is excreted into the food; when the food is ingested, acute gastroenteritis results. Initial symptoms are usually noted two to five hours after the ingestion of the contaminated food and include the rather sudden onset of diarrhea and vomiting. The toxin apparently is absorbed and acts upon the central nervous system. The vomiting and diarrhea may be severe and last for several hours. Not infrequently, there are marked malaise and sometimes prostration. Normally, the acute phase is self-limited and lasts no longer than 24 hours. Rarely, prostration and dehydration are severe enough to require hospitalization.

Staphylococcus aureus is the most common cause of food poisoning in the Western World. The disease frequently occurs in epidemics which are due to the ingestion of contaminated food by large groups of people. (An example of such an epidemic is given at the end of this chapter.) The disease can also occur sporadically and be limited to members of a household.

Food is usually contaminated by a diseased or asymptomatic carrier. A person with a staphylococcal lesion on the hand may infect food directly. Food may also be contaminated by the hands of a noninfected person if he is carrying an enterotoxin-producing strain of staphylococci on the skin. In addition, food may be contaminated by an asymptomatic carrier of staphylococci in the oropharynx or nasopharynx through sneezing. Regardless of the manner in which the food is contaminated, all staphylococcal food poisoning cases have one characteristic in common. Following contamination with staphylococci, there must be a period of several hours in which the food is maintained at a temperature high enough to permit multiplication of staphylococci and the production of a sufficient amount of enterotoxin. Therefore, staphylococcal food poisoning can best be prevented by refrigerating prepared foods at all times. It is worth pointing out that ham is a very common source of staphylococcal enterotoxin. Because of the method of using a high salt concentration for curing ham, the meat does not readily support bacterial growth. As noted previously, however, staphylococci grow readily in high concentrations of sodium chloride. Therefore, ham is an excellent medium for the growth of these microorganisms, and it is wise to avoid ingestion of ham and other food preserved in this manner when it cannot be ascertained that the food has been carefully kept at refrigerator temperatures until serving time.

Recently, a toxin produced by *Staphylococcus aureus* phage type 2 strain has been described which causes marked exfoliation of the skin of infants, producing the so-called scalded-skin syndrome. This toxic principle has been named *exfoliatin* and apparently selectively destroys cells of the stratum granulosum of the epidermis, sparing other cells. (For a more detailed discussion of this condition, see Chap. 36).

All of the cellular antigens of *Staphylococcus aureus* are of interest but apparently do not bear a large relationship to virulence since they are not antiphagocytic. One possible exception to this statement must be noted — the capsular antigens which have been found in certain strains of *S. aureus.* Apparently, certain strains of *S. aureus,* when cultivated under appropriate circumstances, will produce definite capsules. These capsules are antiphagocytic, and antibody against the capsular material serves as opsonin. Three antigenic types of specific capsular polysaccharides have so far been detected. The exact role of capsular antigens in the virulence of these strains for man has not been ascertained. It is clear, however, that in experimental animals they do act as antiphagocytic factors and that the antiphagocytic action can be neutralized by the use of specific antibody.

Penicillinase plays an important role in the resistance of many staphylococcal strains to penicillin. Resistant strains appear rather rapidly in some patients after the initiation of therapy. It is possible to show in vitro that penicillinase is an adaptive enzyme inducible by penicillin. It is much less clear whether an adaptive enzyme is formed in response to the presence of penicillin in patients receiving therapy. Frequently, the penicillinase-producing staphylococci isolated from patients receiving penicillin therapy are of a different phage type than that of the original infecting strain. This suggests that the penicillin acts as a selective agent and permits the growth of penicillinase-resistant staphylococci already present in the patient.

However, penicillinase-producing strains of staphylococci can be found in the absence of known exposure to penicillin. Such strains were isolated from human beings in 1950 at a time when and in a region where penicillin had never been introduced and used by man. These strains may have been induced to produce penicillinase by contact with *Penicillium notatum* and, therefore, penicillin in nature.

Immunity

There is little information not only on the role of the various antigens in enzymes and substances produced by *Staphylococcus aureus* in the genesis of staphylococcal disease but also on the host factors which specifically operate against staphylococcal infection. *S. aureus* is an extracellular parasite and therefore is ordinarily killed following phagocytosis. Most human beings, particularly adults, have fairly high levels of circulating antibody to staphylococcal cells. Such persons are highly resistant to infection, and it can be inferred that one or more of the antibodies to staphylococcal cells function as opsonin to promote phagocytosis. However, only in the case of those few staphylococcal strains which produce capsules can the antigen responsible for the opsonizing antibody be specifically identified. In these instances, anticapsular antibody is protective because of its opsonizing activity. With the nonencapsulated strains, any one or conceivably a number of the staphylococcal cell wall antigens could be responsible for inducing opsonizing antibody.

Laboratory Diagnosis

The definitive diagnosis of staphylococcal disease can be made only by isolation and identification of the species of Staphylococcus involved. Material such as sputum or purulent discharge from an infected wound can be plated on appropriate media, particularly blood agar. The somewhat large size and the pigmentation of colonies of *Staphylococcus aureus* and the presence of a zone of beta hemolysis usually make the recognition of staphylococci on the plate fairly easy. Once the identification of a staphylococcus has been made, the problem that remains is primarily one of differentiating between *S. aureus* and *Staphylococcus epidermidis*. *S. aureus* frequently shows little pigmentation. The most important differential characteristic is the demonstration of coagulase production. There is a high correlation between production of coagulase and pathogenicity. Strains of *S. epidermidis* seldom if ever produce coagulase. Table 37–1 shows the major differential characteristics between *S. aureus* and *S. epidermidis*.

Coagulase-positive strains can be differentiated into groups and types by bacteriophage typing. Coagulase-negative strains cannot be phage typed. Bacteriophage typing is not necessary for identification of staphylococci but is very useful when one wishes to determine the source of infection. Many strains of *Staphylococcus aureus* are susceptible to more than one phage and, depending upon their phage susceptibility pattern, they can be placed in a phage group and then typed. Bacteriophage typing is particularly useful when investigating epidemics of staphylococcal disease in hospitals. The source of such hosptial infections can frequently be traced to a diseased patient or a carrier among the hospital personnel.

Using the teichoic acid antigens, staphylococcal antibody in the serum of patients can readily be identified. This is a particularly useful test for determining whether *Staphylococcus epidermidis* or *Staphylococcus aureus* is the cause of staphylococcal endocarditis.

Prevention

No specific prevention for staphylococcal disease is available. Human beings, particularly adults, are highly resistant to staphylococcal infections. Presumably, exposure to these microorganisms during infancy and childhood builds up high levels of antibodies and therefore resistance to infection. Immunization with products of the staphylococci, while producing some increase in resistance in experimental animals, has not been particularly useful in man. It can be speculated that most adult human beings are already about as resistant to staphylococcal infection as they can become. This is supported by the fact that staphylococcal disease occurs only under those conditions in which host-acquired immunity or natural resistance has been appreciably lowered. Certainly, no specific immunizing antigen that is highly effective can be isolated from strains of staphylococci. The one exception, as mentioned previously, is the capsular material from the three types of encapsulated staphylococci. The role of these encapsulated strains in the production of disease in human beings is not clear, however.

Spread of pathogenic strains of staphylococci in the nursery has been prevented by artificially colonizing newborn infants with a staphylococcal strain of very low virulence. Such colonization of the skin or upper respiratory tract will significantly interfere with subsequent colonization by more pathogenic strains, thus reducing the incidence of staphylococcal disease in this group. The same principle has been applied to the prevention of recurrent furunculosis following antibiotic treatment in older persons. After the population of the staphylococcal strain has been reduced to a minimum by antibiotic therapy, the upper respiratory tract and skin on the patient is artificially colonized with a culture of an appropriate strain of reduced virulence. The furuncles usually do not recur as long as the staphylococcal strain of low virulence persists.

Staphylococcal Gastroenteritis (Food Poisoning), A Typical Epidemic*

On July 26–27, 1973, approximately 725 incoming freshmen, 475 parents, and 150 faculty and administration staff attended summer pre-registration activities at a large state university in Johnson City, Tennessee. On July 27, several hours after a box lunch was served between 12:00 and 1:00 p.m., an estimated 300 persons experienced the onset of vomiting and diarrhea, and 84 were subsequently admitted to the nearby community hospital emergency room. Two adults and one student had documented hypotension responsive to intravenous fluids. All but four patients were released the same evening.

From the 725 students who registered, a sample of 198 students (27 per cent) and their families was randomly chosen for a telephone survey; 22 students and 45 parents with gastrointestinal symptoms were identified. For those eating the box lunch, the attack rate was 27.5 per cent for students and 50.6 per cent for parents. For those not eating the box lunch, the attack rate was 0 per cent. Symptoms included nausea (76 per cent), cramps (71 per cent), diarrhea (67 per cent), vomiting (44 per cent), chills (25 per cent), fever (25 per cent), and collapse (9 per cent). The incubation period in 98 per cent of cases was between 1 and 10 hours; the median was 4.5 hours. Those whose symptoms included nausea and vomiting tended to have shorter incubation periods than those with diarrhea. Forty per cent of those ill sought medical attention. The median duration of illness was 5 hours for students and 7.5 hours for parents. Of the 150 faculty given free tickets to the box lunch, 84 ate the lunch and 47.7 per cent of those became ill.

Food-specific attack rates implicated macaroni salad. Chicken could not be excluded as a vehicle of transmission because all but one of the individuals ate chicken. No other foods were significantly associated with illness.

The macaroni was cooked and rinsed on July 25 and refrigerated overnight. On July 26, between 10 a.m. and 2 p.m., celery, fresh green peppers, onions, and canned red peppers were hand sliced, chopped mechanically, and hand mixed with the macaroni and commercial dressing that did not contain egg. The salad was placed into 30-lb closed plastic containers in a walk-in cooler overnight. At 6:00 a.m. on July 27, it was taken out of storage, and from 6:30 a.m. to 12:20 p.m. individual portions were served into Styrofoam boxes, which were transported in large groups to eating areas. The lunches were kept at room temperature during this time.

Examination of portions of macaroni salad from unused trays left at room temperature until 7–8 p.m. revealed 10^4 to 10^5 coagulase-positive staphylococci per gram and 10^6 to 10^9 enterococci per gram. The chicken contained small numbers of coagulase-positive staphylococci. The staphylococci isolated from these foods were nontypable on bacteriophage testing.

---

*This report of staphylococcal gastroenteritis is taken from the Center for Disease Control, Morbidity and Mortality Weekly Report, Vol. 22, No. 34, 1973.

Twenty-four kitchen workers were interviewed, and culture specimens from anterior nares, back of wrist, and rectum were obtained on August 2. Four workers had nontypable staphylococci isolated from wrists or nares. Antibiotic sensitivity testing of nontypable organisms from two workers and the macaroni salad revealed all to be sensitive. One of these workers was directly involved in the preparation and serving of the macaroni salad.

The remaining macaroni salad available for direct enterotoxin assay was culture negative and Gram stain negative for staphylococci; however, it contained type C staphylococcal enterotoxin.

References

Book

Elek, S. D.: *Staphylococcus pyogenes* and Its Relation to Disease. Baltimore, Williams and Wilkins, 1959.

Symposium Volume

Cohen, J. O. (ed.): The Staphylococci. New York, John Wiley and Sons, 1972.

Review Articles

Abramson, C.: Staphylococcal Enzymes. *In* Cohen, J. O. (ed.): The Staphylococci. New York, John Wiley and Sons, 1972.

Bergdoll, M. S.: The enterotoxins. *In* Cohen, J. O. (ed.): The Staphylococci. New York, John Wiley and Sons, 1972.

Ekstedt, R. D.: Immunity to the staphylococci. *In* Cohen, J. O. (ed.): The Staphylococci. New York, John Wiley and Sons, 1972.

Jeljaszewicz, J.: Toxins (hemolysins). *In* Cohen, J. O. (ed.): The Staphylococci. New York, John Wiley and Sons, 1972.

Kagan, B. M.: L-Forms. *In* Cohen, J. O. (ed.): The Staphylococci. New York, John Wiley and Sons, 1972.

Nahmias, A. J., and Schulman, J. A.: Epidemiologic aspects and control methods. *In* Cohen, J. O. (ed.): The Staphylococci. New York, John Wiley and Sons, 1972.

Schulman, J. A., and Nahmias, A. J.: Staphylococcal infections: Clinical aspects. *In* Cohen, J. O. (ed.): The Staphylococci. New York, John Wiley and Sons, 1972.

Shinefield, H. R., Ribble, J. C., Boris, M., and Eichenwald, H. F.: Bacterial interference. *In* Cohen, J. O. (ed.): The Staphylococci. New York, John Wiley and Sons, 1972.

Wiley, B. B.: Capsules and pseudocapsules of *Staphylococcus aureus*. *In* Cohen, J. O. (ed.): The Staphylococci. New York, John Wiley and Sons, 1972.

Original Articles

Crowder, J. G., and White, A.: Teichoic acid antibodies in staphylococcal and nonstaphylococcal endocarditis. Ann. Intern. Med. *77:*87, 1972.

Elek, S. D., and Conan, P. E.: The virulence of Staphylococcus pyogenes for man. A study of the problems of wound infection. Br. J. Exp. Pathol. *38:*573, 1957.

Gonzaga, A. J., Mortimer, E. A., Wolinsky, E., and Rammelkamp, C. H.: Transmission of staphylococci by fomites. J.A.M.A. *188:*711, 1964.

Melish, E. M., Glasgow, A. L., and Turner, M. D.: The staphylococci scalded-skin syndrome: Isolation and partial characterization of the exfoliative agent. J. Infect. Dis. *125:*129, 1972.

Mortimer, E. A., Lipsitz, P. J., Wolinsky, E., Gonzaga, A. J., and Rammelkamp, C. H.: Transmission of staphylococci between newborns. Am. J. Dis. Child. *104:*289, 1962.

Shinefield, H. R., Ribble, J. C., Boris, M., and Eichenwald, H. F.: Bacterial interference: Its effect on nursery-acquired infection with Staphylococcus aureus. I. Preliminary observations on artificial colonization of newborns. Am. J. Dis. Child. *105:*636, 1963.

Strauss, W. E., Maibach, H. I., and Shinefield, H. R.: Bacterial interference treatment of recurrent furunculosis. J.A.M.A. *208:*863, 1969.

Watanakunakorn, C., and Blake, C.: Pathogenicity of stable L-phase variants of Staphylococcus aureus: Failure to colonize normal and oxamide-induced hydronephrotic renal medulla of rats. Infect. Immun. *9:*766, 1974.

Wolinsky, E., Lipsitz, P. J., Mortimer, E. A., and Rammelkamp, C. H.: Acquisition of staphylococci by newborns, direct versus indirect transmission. Lancet *2:*620, 1960.

IX

ADDITIONAL LOCAL AND SYSTEMIC INFECTIONS

Chapter 38

ANAEROBIC BACTERIAL DISEASE: GENERAL CONSIDERATIONS

Introduction

Anaerobic bacteria outnumber aerobic and facultative anaerobic bacteria in the colon by 300 to 1000 to 1. They also outnumber aerobic and facultative anaerobic bacteria in the mouth, vagina, and other sites in the body, although not always at the same ratio. It is surprising that despite the predominance of anaerobic bacteria in the indigenous flora relatively little has been written of anaerobic bacterial infections until the last five or six years. Perhaps one of the more significant restrictions has been the technical difficulty encountered in the isolation and identification of anaerobic bacteria. The recent development and general application of improved procedures for the recovery and classification of anaerobic bacteria have shown anaerobes to be more widely involved with disease at all sites in the body than had previously been recognized. In the future, widespread application of more sensitive procedures to culture specimens will result in the increased isolation and identification of large numbers of anaerobic bacteria, and improved recovery of anaerobic bacteria can be expected to result in a realignment of our present concepts of the incidence and significance of anaerobic bacterial infections.

Factors Associated with Anaerobic Infection

Oxidation-Reduction Potential (Eh)

Disease from anaerobic bacteria may be defined in a broad sense as tissue disease and/or severe systemic intoxications due to microorganisms growing in a reduced oxidation-reduction potential. The oxidation-reduction potential (Eh), like the hydrogen ion concentration (pH), can be measured and expressed in terms of defined units. An oxidation is defined as a reaction in which electrons are lost, while a reaction in which electrons are gained is called a reduction. Any compound has a tendency to be oxidized and can be thought of as possessing a corresponding pressure of electrons available for donation. If a solution of such a compound is arranged to form a half cell in a circuit with a different half cell of known potential, a potential difference is set up whose magnitude is related to the oxidizing (or reducing) power of the compound and can be expressed in volts. Oxidation-reduction potential is expressed by the positive or negative electrical potential across a calomel half cell and can be measured in either in vivo or in vitro culture systems. The oxidation-reduction potential at any site in the body is usually but not necessarily related to the distance of that site from oxygen-carrying red blood cells and the integrity of the vascular capillary network. The Eh of the blood depends on the oxygen saturation of hemoglobin in red blood cells and to a lesser but significant extent on dissolved oxygen content in the serum. The Eh in most tissues in the body varies between +0.126 and +0.246, depending on blood supply and whether the measurement is taken near sites of high (arterial) or low (venous) oxygen saturation. Anaerobes will not grow at these levels. For example, the highest Eh recorded for germination of *Clostridium tetani* is +0.110v, while clostridial spores usually need an Eh less than −0.100v for germination and growth. The majority of anaerobic bacteria require an Eh of −0.100 to −0.250 for growth in vitro. The oxidation-reduction potential of normal tissue will therefore prevent growth of anaerobic bacteria unless blood flow is reduced and the Eh falls.

Those parts of the body removed from an active capillary perfusion, such as the lumen of the colon and the vagina, have large populations of anaerobic bacteria. Other regions where anaerobic bacteria are found in high concentration include the nasal sinuses, tonsillar crypts, and other parts of the body where the microorganisms are kept warm and moist and are protected from levels of oxygen that would inhibit or prevent growth.

Effect of Tissue Injury on Eh

Inasmuch as anaerobic bacteria are present in well-defined sites throughout the body, conditions predisposing to disease can in part be predicted. Any injury which produces interruption of the capillary blood flow, with a resulting decrease in tissue Eh at that site, predisposes to anaerobic bacterial replication and, in the case of clostridia, toxin production. Injury may result from surgery, trauma, arteriosclerosis, or growth of a malignant tumor with ischemic necrosis. The importance of the reduction of blood flow and its subsequent effect on the decrease in the tissue Eh have been illustrated by experimental clostridial infections in animals. Production of vascular spasm and ischemia by injection of epiniphrine, together with a suspension of *Clostridium perfringens,* into the hind leg of a guinea pig reduces by 1000-fold the number of microorganisms required to initiate infection.

Variability of Bacterial Anaerobic Requirements

Some anaerobic bacteria are more fastidious than others in the need for a low oxidation-reduction potential. *Clostridium perfringens,* the micro-organism most frequently associated with gas gangrene, will grow with only a slight reduction of oxygen tension, 70 to 80 mm of Hg (normal ± 150 mm Hg), while *Clostridium tetani* has been reported to be intolerant of oxygen concentrations greater than 2 mm Hg.* This variation of oxygen sensitivity suggests that the number and types of microorganisms isolated by the clinical laboratory depend on the method of collection of the specimen, protection of the specimen from exposure to air or oxygenated mediums, and the speed of delivery of the culture to the laboratory. Table 38–1 lists the oxygen tolerance of different strains of anaerobic bacteria found in association with dental plaque and shows that some microorganisms are much more tolerant of oxygen than others. The number of species of anaerobic bacteria isolated by the laboratory, therefore, reflects the effort expended to maintain anaerobiasis.

TABLE 38–1. Oxygen Sensitivity of Various Anaerobic Bacteria*

Species	Oxygen in Gas Atmosphere (Per Cent)					
	0.1	*0.5*	*1.0*	*3.0*	*6.0*	*10*
Treponema macrodentium	++**	0				
Treponema denticola	++	0				
Butyrivibrio fibrisolvens	++	+	0			
Clostridium haemolyticum	++	++	0	0		
Clostridium novyi type A	++	++	++	0		
Bacteroides oralis	++	++	++	++	+, V	0
Bacteroides melaninogenicus	++	++	++	++, V	+, V	0
Fusobacterium nucleatum	++	++	++	++	++	0
Bacteroides fragilis	++	++	++	++	+, V	0
Vibrio fetus	+	++	++	++	++	++

*Adapted from Loesche, W. J.: Oxygen sensitivity of various anaerobic bacteria. Appl. Microbiol. *18:*723, 1969.
**Symbols: ++, growth; +, slight growth; V, growth varied with strain or length of incubation (or both); 0, no growth.

---

*Partial pressures and per cent content of oxygen are other measures of expressing anaerobiasis but do not have the same significance as the Eh equivalent.

Most species of anaerobic bacteria must have certain conditions necessary for growth before they can cause disease. Frequently, these conditions can be produced more rapidly in company with other anaerobic or facultative anaerobic bacteria. Facultative anaerobic bacteria are those bacteria that can grow in either the presence or absence of oxygen. In vitro experiments have shown that dilute suspensions of anaerobic bacteria, incapable of growth when widely dispersed in a fresh broth culture medium, demonstrate rapid growth when centrifuged to concentrate the microorganisms in a smaller volume of medium. The change from a stationary to a rapidly growing bacterial population is thought to be due to the ability of bacteria to reduce the immediate microenvironment by metabolism of residual oxygen, thus making rapid growth possible. This same principle of rapid utilization and depletion of available oxygen facilitates the development of anaerobic disease. Facultative anaerobic bacteria, e.g., *Escherichia coli* or *Klebsiella pneumoniae,* will metabolize and use available oxygen, thereby reducing the Eh of the in vivo microenvironment to a level where strict anaerobic bacteria can grow. With reduction of the tissue Eh, the anaerobes start to grow, producing necrosis, toxins, or other virulence factors. The ability of microcolonies of mixed bacteria to reduce the Eh of their immediate environment helps to explain what is otherwise the confusing finding that large numbers of anaerobic bacteria can be cultured from the mouth, nasal sinuses, and lower respiratory tract — areas that might usually be considered unlikely sites for colonization with anaerobic bacteria. Recognition that the normal indigenous microflora generally contains many species of bacteria should be taken into consideration when planning antimicrobial therapy. It should also be remembered that isolation of one or more bacterial species from any site does not necessarily establish the isolated microorganism(s) as the infectious agent(s). In many instances, the assignment of pathogenicity to bacterial isolates becomes a highly subjective interpretation. As mentioned previously, isolation of *Propionibacterium acnes* from a blood culture is rarely associated with disease (see Chap. 7).

Cultivation and Identification of Anaerobic Bacteria

Anaerobic bacteria have one cardinal requirement for growth — a low oxidation-reduction potential. The critical factors necessary for a low Eh are not clearly understood. It is known that peroxides formed during metabolism may be toxic and are usually inactivated by catalase, an enzyme that many anaerobes lack. Exposure to oxygen may be fatal to a large number of anaerobes. However, exposure to oxygen is not the only factor involved, since it is known that oxygen can be bubbled through a culture medium containing growing anaerobes if a low oxidation-reduction potential is maintained by strong chemical reducing agents. The presence of the enzyme superoxide dismutase in aerobic and facultative anaerobic bacteria but not in anaerobic bacteria also plays a role. Superoxide (O_2^-) is a highly reactive compound produced when oxygen is reduced by a single electron, and it may be generated during the normal catalytic action of a number of enzymes.

Superoxide dismutase catalyzes the conversion of two molecules of super-oxide to one molecule of oxygen and one molecule of hydrogen peroxide. The absence of superoxide dismutase from obligate anaerobic bacteria would appear to confer obvious survival advantages.

Most anaerobic bacteria grow more slowly in culture than do facultative anaerobic bacteria and usually require 48 hours for colony formation. This means that the isolation, separation, and complete characterization of individual species may take from 3 to 10 days or longer.

Collection of Specimens

For the optimal recovery of anaerobic bacteria, cultures should be taken in a manner which minimizes exposure to air. When cultures for anaerobes are to be obtained, oxygen-free tubes and vials should be used (Fig. 38–1). A variety of methods for culture taking are available, but most are based on an atmosphere free of oxygen and incorporation of a reducing agent to diminish the effect of residual air. Direct smears for Gram stains should be made when the culture is taken in order to correlate the bacterial forms present with bacteria isolated by culture.

Methods for Culture

One of the earliest methods used to make an anaerobic environment was to place a handful of oat seeds in a dish of water, close the container tightly, and wait until the oat seeds germinated, utilizing all available oxygen, and produced small amounts of carbon dioxide. The period of time necessary to achieve anaerobiasis precluded the study of any microorganisms except those with well-developed spores. Non–spore-forming anaerobic bacteria would perish long before the oxygen was utilized by the seeds. Considerable progress has been made since that time, however. Many of the more current useful techniques have been borrowed from veterinary microbiologists who developed sensitive methods for studying the complex anaerobic microbial flora of the cow's rumen.

The standard procedure for isolation of anaerobic bacteria in many clinical laboratories includes the use of a Brewer jar to obtain anaerobiasis. Culture plates are placed in a container, either a plastic or glass jar, and hydrogen is added either by evacuation and replacement with a mixture of 80 per cent N_2, 10 per cent CO_2, and 10 per cent H_2, or by a disposable H_2-CO_2 generating system. This latter system consists of a metal foil envelope activated by adding water to sodium borohydride to generate hydrogen and a tablet of citric acid and sodium bicarbonate to make CO_2 (Gas-Pak) (Fig. 38–2). Five to ten per cent CO_2 is added to stimulate the growth of anaerobes. Hydrogen reacts in the presence of a catalyst with atmospheric oxygen to form H_2O. In the past, the catalyst was a coil of platinum that required heating by an electrical element for activation. Enthusiasm for the use of this chamber was dampened when breaks in the

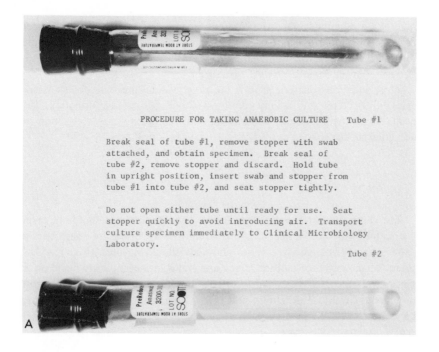

PROCEDURE FOR TAKING ANAEROBIC CULTURE   Tube #1

Break seal of tube #1, remove stopper with swab
attached, and obtain specimen. Break seal of
tube #2, remove stopper and discard. Hold tube
in upright position, insert swab and stopper from
tube #1 into tube #2, and seat stopper tightly.

Do not open either tube until ready for use. Seat
stopper quickly to avoid introducing air. Transport
culture specimen immediately to Clinical Microbiology
Laboratory.

Tube #2

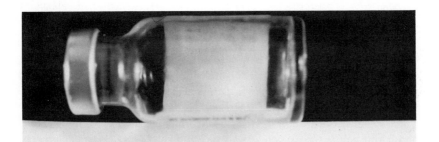

USE OF OXYGEN-FREE TRANSPORT VIALS FOR
ANAEROBIC BACTERIAL CULTURE

Use sterile needle and syringe to aspirate
specimen. Expel all air from needle and
syringe prior to inoculation into vial.
Inject specimen through rubber stopper.
Send immediately to Clinical Microbiology
Laboratory.

Figure 38–1. *A,* Collection kits for obtaining specimens for anaerobic culture.
Directions are attached. Each tube contains an oxygen-free atmosphere and a small
quantity of a reducing agent. A smear for a Gram stain should be made with a second
swab to correlate the bacterial forms present with subsequent isolates. *B,* Oxygen-free
transport vial for anaerobic culture of pleural, peritoneal, or other fluids.

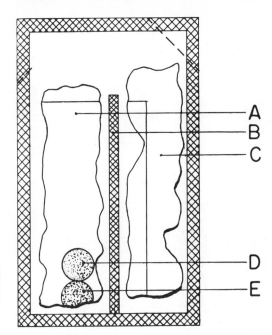

Figure 38–2. Cutout view of the hydrogen–carbon dioxide generator. *A*, filter; *B,* heat seal; *C,* water added to this side; *D,* CO_2 tablet; *E,* H_2 tablet. Gas Pak. (From Brewer, J. H., and Allgeier, D. L.: Safe self-contained carbon dioxide–hydrogen anaerobic system. Appl. Microbiol. *14:*985, 1966.)

safety screen occasionally resulted in explosions. Currently, most anaerobic jars contain catalysts of palladinized alumina pellets that do not need to be heated and require less than 10 per cent hydrogen to convert remaining atmospheric oxygen to water (see Fig. 38–3).

One of the more recent methods facilitating work with anaerobic bacteria utilizes small cannulas that carry a slowly moving stream of oxygen-free gas. When culture tubes containing anaerobic bacteria are opened for transfer or staining, the cannula is placed in the tube and prevents the entry of atmospheric oxygen (Fig. 38–4). This method is frequently called the "VPI System," referring to the Virginia Polytechnic Institute, where it was developed for clinical laboratories. Another technique for working with anaerobic bacteria in the absence of oxygen is the use of an anaerobic "glove box," a closed chamber of plastic film with transfer ports in which cultures can be handled in a completely controlled, oxygen-free atmosphere. These chambers may be heated and serve as both an incubator and a work area (Fig. 38–5).

Culture Media for Anaerobes

Most culture media for anaerobic bacteria require components not found in standard media. Reducing agents may be necessary to keep the Eh in the −0.010v range or less. Anaerobic culture media contain an indicator showing when the Eh of the media is above a certain level. The most commonly used indicator is resazurin, which is colorless when reduced and pink when oxidized. Recovery of different bacterial species may be enhanced if different additives are incorporated, such as bile for the stimulation of growth of

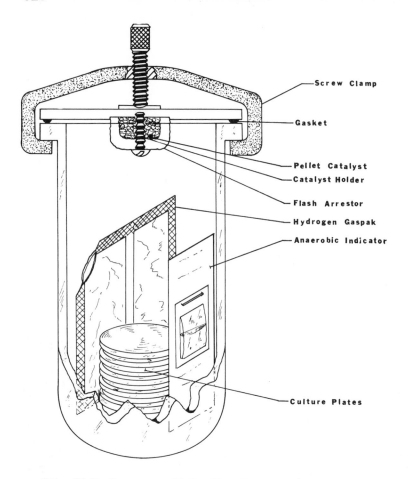

Screw Clamp

Gasket

Pellet Catalyst

Catalyst Holder

Flash Arrestor

Hydrogen Gaspak

Anaerobic Indicator

Culture Plates

Figure 38–3. Brewer anaerobic jar. (From Brewer, J. H., and Allgeier, D. L.: Safe self-contained carbon dioxide–hydrogen anaerobic system. Appl. Microbiol. *14:*985, 1966.)

Bacteroides fragilis or hemin and menadione (vitamin K) for the growth of *Bacteroides melaninogenicus.*

The best results for the isolation and identification of anaerobic bacteria are reportedly obtained by the use of pre-reduced, anaerobically sterilized culture mediums. These are prepared under an oxygen-free gas, reducing exposure to air or oxygen during preparation. Culture mediums exposed to air and oxygen during preparation may form "toxic peroxides" which will inhibit growth of fastidious microorganisms. One such microorganism, *Clostridium haemolyticum,* is said not to be able to grow on a blood agar plate exposed to atmospheric air for more than three hours.

Identification of different species of anaerobic bacteria has been facilitated by the use of gas chromatography for the detection and semiquantitation of volatile fatty acids produced by different bacterial species. Propionibacteria will produce propionic acid; lactobacilli, lactic acid; butyrobacteria, butyric acid; etc. (see Chap. 10). Production of volatile acids by anaerobic bacteria in the intestine is one of the mechanisms that

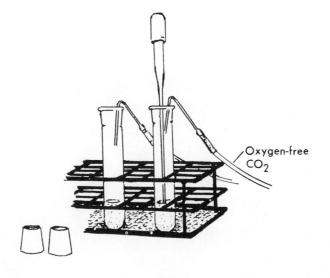

A

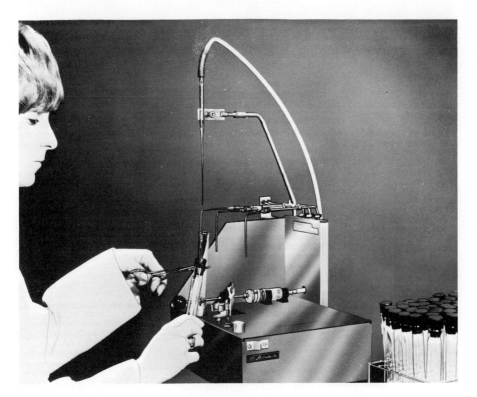

B

Figure 38–4. *A,* Simple transfer of anaerobic culture. (From Holdeman, L. V., and Moore, W. E. C. (eds.): Anaerobe Laboratory Manual. 3rd Ed. Blacksburg, Virginia, Virginia Polytechnic Institute and State University Anaerobe Laboratory, 1975. Drawing by Dr. W. E. C. Moore.) *B,* Virginia Polytechnic Institute anaerobic culture system. (Courtesy of Bellco Glass, Inc., 340 Edrudo Rd., Vineland, New Jersey, 08360.)

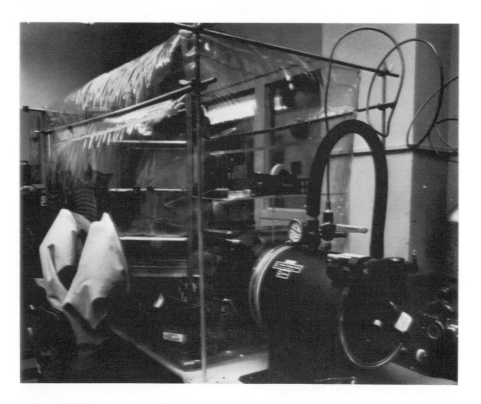

Figure 38–5. Anaerobic glove box system. (From Dowell, V. R., Jr., and Hawkins, T. M.: Laboratory Methods in Anaerobic Bacteriology. CDC Laboratory Manual. Washington, D.C., United States Government Printing Offices, 1974.)

experimentally retards colonization of *Salmonella typhimurium* in the colon of animals and presumably of humans as well. The strong and offensive odor often associated with anaerobic disease is in part related to the release of volatile fatty acids and the formation of strongly aromatic amines, e.g., cadaverine and putrescine, by proteolytic enzymes.

It is evident from the foregoing discussion that several points should be kept clearly in mind when taking cultures for the purpose of establishing disease due to anaerobic bacteria. First, the culture should be collected and transported to the laboratory in a manner which excludes or minimizes exposure of the specimen to air. Second, the slow growth and special media needed for anaerobic bacteria and the unique growth requirements of these bacteria are frequently reflected in a prolonged time for species identification and the reporting of results to the physician. Third, the extra effort necessary for identification of anaerobic bacteria results in an increased cost for processing the culture. The return for this effort is justified, however, if specific microorganisms are isolated and identified, thereby permitting definitive therapy to be initiated in the patient under study and gaining valuable treatment time for the next patient the physician sees with a similar disease.

Predisposition to Thrombophlebitis

Disease with all bacteria commonly causes an associated local thrombophlebitis. This is particularly true in anaerobic bacterial pelvic disease in females, but it is also a feature accompanying anaerobic disease elsewhere. The reason for what appears to be a greater incidence of thrombophlebitis in anaerobic bacterial disease is not clear. It has been reported that certain strains of bacteroides and fusobacteria secrete a heparinase which may predispose to clotting.

One result of thrombosis and thrombophlebitis associated with anaerobic disease is an increased incidence of embolism to the portal or pulmonary venous systems. Such emboli predispose to infarcts in the liver, lung, brain, or other organs, resulting in a decreased Eh and conditions advantageous to growth of anaerobic bacteria. This is one way anaerobic disease can "metastasize" from a primary focus elsewhere in the body.

Severe septicemia from gram negative anaerobic bacteria may cause disseminated intravascular thrombosis. The mechanism is considered to be similar to that related to other gram negative bacteria, e.g., meningococci, and is thought to be mediated through endotoxin release from the bacterial cell walls. Disseminated intravascular coagulation may also be seen in severe disease due to streptococci and is not solely restricted to infections with gram negative bacteria.

Antimicrobial Therapy

Since the nature of anaerobic disease tends to predispose to abscesses and localized collections of pus in a closed space, the primary treatment is surgical. Therapy with an appropriate antimicrobial agent is a highly significant determinant in the survival of the patient. The use of an antimicrobial agent effective only against members of the family Enterobacteriaceae in patients with disease caused by both types of bacteria is associated with a much higher mortality than that seen when the agent selected is effective primarily against anaerobic bacteria.

Penicillin is useful against many species of anaerobic bacteria, but it is almost totally ineffective against the subspecies of *Bacteroides fragilis*. This limits the use of penicillin against disease likely to be caused by *B. fragilis*. One exception to this limitation is pulmonary infection. Although subspecies of *B. fragilis* are not commonly associated with anaerobic pulmonary disease, when these microorganisms are found to be the causative agent, the disease clinically responds well to penicillin.

The tetracycline group of antimicrobial agents has been used with success against anaerobic diseases for many years. Recently, however, a number of anaerobic bacteria have become resistant to tetracycline, although several derivatives, e.g., deoxycycline and minocycline, are reported to be significantly more effective in in vitro testing. The increased incidence of side effects with minocycline (e.g., vertigo) may restrict widespread use.

The two most effective antimicrobial agents available at this time for anaerobic disease are chloramphenicol and clindamycin. Both of these agents are associated with potentially serious therapeutic complications. Chloramphenicol may cause irreversible bone marrow suppression if used in excessive amounts, and clindamycin has been associated with fatal pseudomembranous enterocolitis. The pathogenesis of the pseudomembranous enterocolitis is not known, but it does not appear to be a superinfection such as that formerly seen with *Staphylococcus aureus* (see Chap. 37).

Antimicrobial Susceptibility Testing

Determining susceptibility of anaerobic bacteria to antimicrobial agents has posed a technical problem for a number of years. The most frequently used procedure, that of measuring a zone of growth inhibition around a paper disc impregnated with a known amount of antibiotic, does not have the same validity for the slowly growing anaerobic bacteria that has been shown for rapidly growing bacteria. The composition, pH, and depth of the growth medium, and the number of microorganisms inoculated have not been standardized for the anaerobic bacteria in the same manner as for rapidly growing bacteria (see Chap. 46). Information derived from testing drug susceptibility of anaerobic bacteria by measuring zone diameters on agar plates tends to vary widely from one laboratory to another.

The use of an agar growth medium containing varying dilutions of antimicrobial drugs has given results more uniform than those produced by disc diffusion. This procedure has been used at several medical centers and has proved to be reproducible and clinically useful. Because of the uniform response of many anaerobic bacteria to certain antibiotics, the suggestion has been made that routine antimicrobial drug susceptibility testing for anaerobic bacteria is not necessary and may be contraindicated. The information gained by a poorly standardized disc diffusion procedure may be misleading. Often, the rapid and specific identification of the bacterial species involved in the disease is of more help than a poorly derived susceptibility pattern.

Certain anaerobic bacteria having a slow rate of growth and fastidious culture requirement have defied all methods of susceptibility testing. Such microorganisms include species of Peptostreptococcus isolated from patients with endocarditis. Treatment of disease due to these microorganisms is usually empirical.

References

Books

Balows, A., DeHaan, R. M., Dowell, V. R., and Guze, L. B. (eds.): Anaerobic Bacteria: Role in Disease. Springfield, Illinois, Charles C Thomas, 1974.

Meynell, G. C., and Meynell, E.: Theory and Practice in Experimental Bacteriology. 2nd ed. London, Cambridge University Press, 1970.

Willis, A. T.: Anaerobic Bacteriology in Clinical Medicine. London, Butterworth and Co., 1964.

Laboratory Manuals

Dowell, V. R., and Hawkins, T. M.: Laboratory Methods in Anaerobic Bacteriology. CDC Laboratory Manual. Atlanta, Georgia, Center for Disease Control, 1974.

Holdeman, L. V., and Moore, W. E. C. (eds.): Anaerobe Laboratory Manual. Blacksburg, Virginia, Virginia Polytechnic Institute, 1972.

Original Articles

Loesche, W. J.: Oxygen sensitivity of various anaerobic bacteria. Appl. Microbiol. *18:*723, 1969.

Martin, W. J., Gardner, M., and Washington, J. A.: In vitro antimicrobial susceptibility of anaerobic bacteria isolated from clinical specimens. Antimicrob. Agents Chemother. *1:*148, 1972.

McCord, J. M., Kaele, B. B., and Fridovich, I.: An enzyme-based theory of obligate anaerobiasis; the physiological function of superoxide dismutase. Proc. Natl. Acad. Sci. USA *68:*1024, 1971.

Rosenblatt, J. E., and Schoenknicht, F.: Effect of several components of anaerobic incubation on antibiotic susceptibility test results. Antimicrob. Agents Chemother. *1:*433, 1972.

Chapter 39

DISEASES DUE TO ANAEROBIC BACTERIA

Polymicrobic Nature of Anaerobic Disease

Disease due to nonsporulating anaerobic bacteria is commonly associated with localized, necrotizing abscesses, each of which may yield from 2 to 13 different strains of bacteria. Because of the multiple species that can be isolated, the term *polymicrobic disease* is sometimes used to refer to anaerobic bacterial abscesses. Therefore, diseases caused by anaerobic bacteria are in sharp contrast to the "one microorganism–one disease" concept that characterizes many infections, such as typhoid fever, cholera, and diphtheria. Anaerobic disease commonly results from the contamination or extension of the indigenous microflora to adjacent, submucosal tissues. Improved isolation and identification techniques for anaerobic bacteria have reemphasized the need for a better understanding of the interaction of one microorganism with another. The question of which one of several bacterial strains isolated from a disease is the most significant often cannot be answered because of the complex interaction involving synergism or antagonism between strains. Such interactions are known and several have been described in the discussion of the indigenous microbial flora (see Chap. 7). Nonetheless, clinicians have been and probably will continue to be confused when trying to assess the significance of the many strains of anaerobic bacteria recovered in the laboratory.

Progress toward understanding the host-parasite interaction first requires the identification of all participating parasites. The recognition that there are five or more distinct subspecies (subsp) of *Bacteroides fragilis* has led to the finding that the most common species in terms of total numbers in the intestinal flora, *B. fragilis* subsp *vulgatus,* is associated with serious disease far less frequently than *B. fragilis* subsp *fragilis. B. fragilis* subsp *vulgatus* is the most common microorganism in the colon, while *B. fragilis* subsp *fragilis* ranks twenty-ninth in frequency (see Table 7–7). Obviously the latter microorganism, although present in fewer numbers than *B. fragilis* subsp *vulgatus,* has an enhanced ability to cause disease when compared with the other subspecies of *B. fragilis.* The nature of the factors contributing to this virulence must still be identified, but the concept that disease results from microorganisms in direct proportion to the numbers available at any one site must be firmly rejected.

Necessity for Anaerobic Bacterial Identification

The isolation and identification of different strains of anaerobic bacteria is desirable in order that appropriate therapy may be given. As mentioned in Chapter 38, many species of Bacteroides are susceptible to penicillin, but the subspecies of *Bacteroides fragilis* are not. It is important when planning therapy for patients with anaerobic disease to know that aminoglycosidic antimicrobial agents such as gentamicin are not effective against anaerobes. Treatment of a "mixed" anaerobic-facultatively anaerobic disease with an inappropriate agent such as gentamicin is associated with significantly higher mortality than therapy which includes an agent such as chloramphenicol or clindamycin. (See Case Presentation 1 at the end of this chapter.)

Diseases Caused by Non–Spore-Forming Anaerobes

Upper Respiratory Tract Infections

It is now well established that chronic disease of the paranasal sinuses may be caused by anaerobic bacteria alone or in combination with facultative anaerobic bacteria. In one study, over half of 83 patients with chronic sinusitis were found to be harboring anaerobic bacteria either in pure culture or in combination with facultative anaerobic bacteria. Peptostreptococci, *Bacteroides fragilis, Bacteroides funduliformis,* and *Bacteroides melaninogenicus* are among the most commonly isolated bacteria.

Anaerobic bacteria can be isolated from the mouth, particularly in the presence of dental caries and infection of the adjacent gingival tissues. It is probably significant that strains found in the oral cavity, including *Bacteroides melaninogenicus, Bacteroides oralis, Fusobacterium nucleatum,* and numerous species of Peptostreptococcus and Veillonella are also among the most commonly isolated anaerobic bacteria associated with pulmonary disease.

Lower Respiratory Tract Infections

Anaerobic disease of the lung may occur in one of several forms. It may be an *abscess,* defined as a solitary or dominant pulmonary cavity measuring at least 2 cm in diameter. A diffuse pulmonary infiltrate without evidence of cavitation is called *anaerobic pneumonitis,* while the term *necrotizing pneumonia* is applied to disease characterized by multiple areas of necrosis and cavitation within one or more pulmonary segments or lobes. Extension of intrapulmonary disease to the surface of the lung with involvement of the pleural space is called *empyema* and may or may not occur as a sequela to pulmonary abscess, anaerobic pneumonitis, or necrotizing pneumonia (Fig. 39–1).

The pathogenesis of these different disease processes varies, but the similarity of the bacteria isolated from most patients with anaerobic pulmonary disease to the indigenous flora of the oropharynx would support the theory that aspiration of oropharyngeal secretions is an important contributing factor. Thromboemboli from abdominal or pelvic disease have already been mentioned (see Chap. 38) and may contribute significantly to the development of an anaerobic bacterial abscess. Staphylococci are commonly associated with anaerobic pulmonary abscess and may contribute to this process by production of necrotizing toxins (see Chap. 37). The resulting ischemia provides a proper environment for growth of anaerobic bacteria, and they in turn will bring about further tissue destruction.

The microorganisms found in anaerobic pulmonary disease include *Bacteroides melaninogenicus, Fusobacterium nucleatum,* peptostreptococci, veillonella, and other anaerobic cocci. In contrast to anaerobic abscesses elsewhere in the body, surgical drainage is usually not necessary, and treatment with penicillin is adequate unless empyema is present.

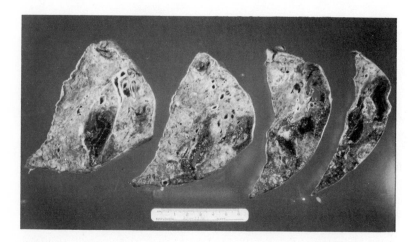

Figure 39–1. Serpiginous anaerobic bacterial abscess in the lower lobe of a lung. Extension to the pleural surface is seen in the section on the right and was associated with empyema. Culture revealed *Staphylococcus aureus* and four separate anaerobic bacterial species.

Gastrointestinal Tract Infections

In view of the large numbers of anaerobes indigenous to the gastro-intestinal tract (see Table 7–8), it is not surprising that anaerobic infections within, adjacent to, or related to disease of the gastrointestinal tract account for a significant amount of cases of clinical disease due to anaerobes. Ulceration of the gastrointestinal tract, by either inflammatory disease or malignant tumor, can provide a portal of entry, first to the regional lymphatics and later to the intravascular compartment. Septicemia from anaerobic bacteria should prompt a search for an overt or inapparent lesion of the gastrointestinal tract, such as an ulcerated tumor of the right colon, diverticulitis, or mucosal ulceration of the small intestine or colon from leukemia or lymphoma.

Anaerobic bacterial disease following intestinal surgery, ruptured appendicitis, or penetrating trauma to the intestinal tract is usually associated with multiple species of anaerobic bacteria. Contamination of poorly vascularized spaces, such as the peritoneum, with large numbers of anaerobic bacteria results in the rapid lowering of the local oxidation-reduction potential (Eh) and conditions advantageous for disease. Anaerobic disease, once established in the peritoneum, can be self-sustaining, with the Eh reaching a very low level and thereby permitting growth of even the most fastidious microorganisms. Abscesses within the peritoneal cavity or beneath the diaphragm can often be very difficult to treat unless drained surgically.

Abscesses in the liver frequently yield anaerobic bacteria when properly cultured (see Chap. 38). Inflammatory disease of the intestine or partial or complete obstruction of the biliary tract is a predisposing factor. The blood supply to the liver, predominately venous from the intestine, results in a low oxidation-reduction potential when compared to other tissues of the body with an intact blood supply. Thrombophlebitis in mesenteric or portal veins with embolism to the liver can initiate anaerobic disease and abscess formation. In addition, certain anaerobic bacteria, e.g., *Bacteroides fragilis* and *Clostridium perfringens,* have a potential advantage over other bacteria in causing infection in the liver or biliary tract in that they can grow in high concentrations of bile. This characteristic is probably of importance in the association of *C. perfringens* disease with both primary and postsurgical biliary tract infection.

Female Genital Tract Infections

Anaerobic bacteremia and septicemia are common complications of pregnancy. Septicemia may also result from induced or spontaneous abortion. Presumably, the anaerobic and facultative aerobic flora of the vagina gain entrance to the endocervical canal when the embryo or fetus and fetal membranes are being expelled. The highly vascularized endometrial surface is particularly susceptible to bacterial invasion during pregnancy, and septicemia may result. Bacteremia associated with abortion is usually transitory and clears promptly following curettage of the uterus.

In the female pelvis, anaerobic infectious disease not associated with pregnancy may cause salpingitis or result from a complication of gynecologic surgery. Careful bacteriologic study of pelvic infectious disease yields numerous microorganisms similar to those of the vagina and lower genitourinary tract of the female. The most commonly isolated bacteria are species of peptostreptococci, peptococci, and occasional species of Bacteroides and Clostridium. Contrary to previous teachings, *Neisseria gonorrhoeae* is only rarely isolated from disease involving the uterus, uterine tubes, and ovaries when careful studies for anaerobic bacteria are done.

Endocarditis

Endocarditis from anaerobic bacteria is probably more common than has been recognized in the past. Endocarditis due to anaerobic bacteria differs from that due to facultative anaerobic streptococci and other types of bacteria. Preexisting heart disease is less frequent in patients with anaerobic endocarditis, and embolic complications are more common. The oropharynx and inflammatory lesions of the gastrointestinal tract are the usual sources of infection. *Bacteroides fragilis, Fusobacterium nucleatum,* and *Fusobacterium necrophorum,* as well as *Clostridium perfringens* and other clostridial species, may cause endocarditis. *Propionibacterium acnes,* a normal inhabitant of the skin, has caused endocarditis in a number of patients following prosthetic replacement of aortic valves. Endocarditis complicating a prosthetic valve replacement may be resistant to treatment despite the use of large amounts of an appropriate antimicrobial agent (see Chap. 41). In many instances, the presenting symptoms in patients with anaerobic bacterial endocarditis are related to embolic complications (Fig. 39–2).

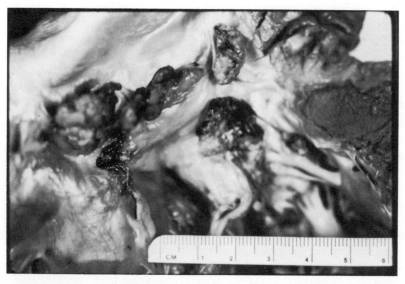

Figure 39–2. Anaerobic bacterial endocarditis with destruction of the aortic valve and colonization of the ventricular surface of the anterior mitral leaflet. Note the large friable verrucae. The patient had two anaerobic bacterial abscesses of the brain.

Central Nervous System Infections

In the brain, disease due to anaerobes may be the result of direct extension from infections in the paranasal or mastoid sinuses, causing epidural abscess or meningitis. It may also appear as a metastatic abscess from an embolus secondary to infection in the lungs or a vegetation on a heart valve. Patients with congenital heart disease who show a right to left shunt, and thereby a lowered oxygen saturation in the arterial blood, are at greater risk of developing cerebral abscesses than are normal persons. The association of recent cerebral infarction with anaerobic abscess has also been noted and is thought to reflect the decreased oxidation-reduction potential in the ischemic tissue.

Diseases Caused by Spore-Forming Anaerobes

General Characteristics

The clostridia are gram positive, spore-forming, anaerobic bacilli. Most species form spores, but some sporulate only under special conditions. Although there are more than 50 species of clostridia described and classified, disease in humans is caused by fewer than 10 to 12. Wide variation exists in the ability of different species of clostridia to tolerate oxygen. Some are considered to be aerotolerant, while others germinate and grow only under strictly anaerobic conditions.

Different species of clostridia vary widely in their ability to utilize carbohydrates and split proteins. Such characteristics are helpful in the laboratory for purposes of identification and classification, but they also aid in explaining clinical manifestations of diseases caused by individual species. *Clostridium perfringens,* the microorganism most often associated with gas gangrene, produces strong proteolytic and saccharolytic enzymes which contribute to the spread of infection. Glycogen, present in large amounts in skeletal muscle, is fermented with almost explosive formation of gas, and when coupled with collagenase and other proteolytic enzymes secreted by the microorganism, contributes to the rapid spread of disease. By contrast, *Clostridium tetani,* the microorganism that causes tetanus, has few enzymes for carbohydrate fermentation or protein degradation. Therefore, growth of *C. tetani* with production of toxin can occur without evidence of an inflammatory reaction.

Exotoxins

A characteristic of the clostridia that are pathogenic for man is the production .of one or more potent exotoxins which usually contribute significantly to the ability of these microorganisms to cause disease. Tetanus and botulism are due to a single toxin having a well-defined mode of action. Table 39–1 lists some of the exotoxins produced by different clostridia.

Clostridium perfringens produces at least 10 separate toxins which facilitate production of disease. Secretion of toxins is a highly specialized function of microorganisms in general and, in clostridia, requires a suitably low oxidation-reduction potential (Eh). As the Eh increases, toxin production will cease before death of the bacterium. This concept is important, since any mechanism that increases the oxidation-reduction potential at the site of bacterial growth will first interrupt toxin formation and then threaten the survival of the microorganism. *C. perfringens* is normally present in the gastrointestinal tract of 25 to 35 per cent of humans (see Chap. 7) and the urogenital tract of a significant number of adult females. Toxins of the clostridia are some of the most potent poisons known. Figure 39–3 lists representative toxins from animal and bacterial sources and compares their estimated potency.

TABLE 39–1. Exotoxins Produced by Principal Toxigenic Bacteria
Pathogenic for Man*

Bacterial Species	Disease	Toxin	Action
Clostridium botulinum	Botulism	Six type-specific neurotoxins	Paralytic
Clostridium tetani	Tetanus	Tetanospasmin Tetanolysin	Spastic Hemolytic cardiotoxin
Clostridium perfringens	Gas gangrene	Alpha-toxin**	Lecithinase: necrotizing, hemolytic
		Beta-toxin	
		Gamma-toxin	
		Delta-toxin	
		Epsilon-toxin	Necrotizing
		Eta-toxin	
		Theta-toxin	Hemolytic cardiotoxin
		Iota-toxin	Necrotizing
		Kappa-toxin	Collagenase
		Lambda-toxin	Proteolytic
Clostridium septicum	Gas gangrene	Alpha-toxin	Hemolytic
Clostridium novyi	Gas gangrene	Alpha-toxin	Necrotizing
		Beta-toxin	Lecithinase: necrotizing, hemolytic
		Gamma-toxin	Lecithinase: necrotizing, hemolytic
		Delta-toxin	Hemolytic
		Epsilon-toxin	Lipase: hemolytic
		Xeta-toxin	Hemolytic

*Modified from van Heyningen, W. E.: *In* Florey, H. W. (ed.): General Pathology. Philadelphia, W. B. Saunders Co., 1962, p. 754.

**The designation of toxins by Greek letters is purely arbitrary and is based on the order in which they were identified.

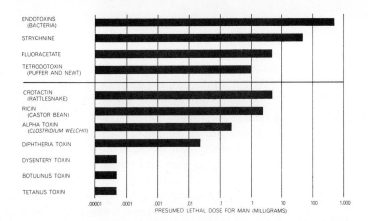

Figure 39–3. Toxicity of the bacterial toxins, including tetanus, is compared with that of other poisons. Crotactin and ricin, like the bacterial exotoxins, are simple proteins. The scale is logarithmic. The dosage figures are theoretical; they assume that the toxin is injected. (From van Heyningen, W. E.: Tetanus. Sci. Am. *218:*69, 1968. Copyright © 1968 by Scientific American, Inc. All rights reserved.)

Gas Gangrene

The classic disease caused by *Clostridium perfringens* is gas gangrene. In World War I, gas gangrene resulting from injuries associated with traumatic wounds from shell fragments was responsible for a large number of fatalities. In most cases, the wounds were contaminated with soil which had been fertilized with animal and human waste. Clinically, the presence of multiple species of clostridial spores in the soil frequently resulted in infections with more than one clostridial species, including *Clostridium novyi* and *Clostridium septicum,* as well as *C. perfringens.*

Clinical manifestations of gas gangrene are due to the vigorous utilization of glycogen and other fermentable carbohydrates, resulting in the rapid production of lactic acid and gas. Increased tissue tension from gas formation causes decreased blood flow, a lowered tissue oxidation-reduction potential, and more favorable conditions for growth of anaerobic bacteria and toxin formation. Absorption of the toxins has a profound effect on the patient and results in a marked but not well-understood "toxicity." Adequate control of disease can usually be achieved by surgical excision of tissue from accessible sites and the prompt administration of antibiotics. In more severe or generalized infections, hyperbaric therapy should be used.

Hyperbaric therapy is the exposure of the patient to increased atmospheric pressure of air or oxygen for short periods of time. This exposure does not significantly change the oxygen-carrying capacity or saturation of the red blood cells but does result in a small but significant increase in the oxygen tension of the serum and thereby lymph in the interstitial tissues. The increase in interstitial oxygen tension resulting from one or two hours in a hyperbaric chamber may be sufficient to interrupt toxin formation and microbial replication. Normal phagocytic and host defense mechanisms may then be able to control the infection. Hyperbaric chambers are not always necessary for the treatment of gas gangrene, but on occasion they can be lifesaving. Exposure to increased pressure must be carefully controlled in order to prevent untoward side effects from oxygen. When such an emergency arises, the effective use of hyperbaric chambers requires a carefully organized team approach for the proper care of the patient.

Although gas gangrene has classically been an infection associated with trauma and devitalized tissue, it is occasionally seen in hospitalized patients in situations in which necrosis, vascular insufficiency, and possible fecal contamination occur. Invasion of the bloodstream by *Clostridium perfringens* may result from ulcerating lesions of the gastrointestinal tract. As long as the microorganisms remain in the blood and do not localize at a site where there ia a low tissue oxidation-reduction potential, they will not replicate. Isolation of *C. perfringens* from skin wounds or cultures from the female genital tract in asymptomatic patients should be neither viewed with alarm nor dismissed as contaminants. Such patients should be observed carefully and given an appropriate antimicrobial agent if indicated.

Disease due to *Clostridium perfringens* also occurs at several other sites in the body; for example, *C. perfringens* may cause acute cholecystitis. The diagnosis should be considered when an x-ray of the abdomen taken when the patient is in an upright position shows a gas-fluid level in the region of the gallbladder. Care should be taken to distinguish air-fluid levels that may be present in the same area from ileus of the small intestine (which is frequently present in acute cholecystitis) or a gas bubble in the hepatic flexure of the colon. Figure 39–4 shows the typical appearance of a gas-filled gallbladder

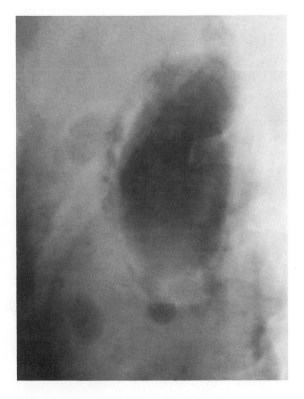

Figure 39–4. Gas-filled gallbladder. Note the extension of gas through the wall to small mucosal diverticula. Radiolucencies below the gallbladder represent accumulations of gas in the intestine.

with air outlining the thin wall and extending through small mucosal diverticula. Other gas-forming bacteria, such as species of Klebsiella and peptostreptococci, may also cause gas production. Gas gangrene may occur as a postoperative complication in patients, diabetics in particular, with amputations of extremities for peripheral arteriosclerosis. Disease under these circumstances results from decreased blood flow, decreased tissue oxidation-reduction potential, and necrosis from the surgical procedure. The micro-organism presumably was present on the skin, possibly as a contaminant from the flora of the large bowel.

Infectious complications of spontaneous or induced abortion are well known to involve *Clostridium perfringens*. Clostridial endometritis is due to a low tissue oxidation-reduction potential, endometrial necrosis, and bacterial contamination from the vagina. One of the toxins (alpha-toxin) produced by *C. perfringens* is lecithinase, which acts on the surface membrane of red blood cells. Under optimal conditions, large amounts of alpha-toxin can be secreted which may result in massive intravascular hemolysis.

Tetanus

Tetanus is a disease caused by *Clostridium tetani*, a spore-forming, gram positive, anaerobic bacillus with an ubiquitous distribution in soil fecally contaminated by man and animals. Although most cases of tetanus result from contamination of wounds by soil or objects that have been in contact with soil, tetanus may also be transmitted in drug addicts by dirty hypodermic needles or contaminated skin surfaces ("skin poppers"). *C. tetani* is considered to be part of the indigenous intestinal microbial flora of man and domestic animals. The spores are resistant to wide temperature changes and may remain viable for years in both soil and cicatrized wounds. In contrast to *Clostridium perfringens, C. tetani* requires a very low oxidation-reduction potential (Eh) for toxin production. Wounds are usually the site of infection, owing to the interruption of blood flow in traumatized tissue which results in a decreased tissue Eh. A further decrease in the Eh can occur if there are contamination and growth of facultative anaerobic bacteria. Clinical tetanus from spores, presumably introduced into wounds months or years previously, has been reported and may reflect either additional injury or continued cicatrization with a further decrease in blood supply and lowering of tissue Eh. The lack of significant numbers of proteolytic and saccharolytic enzymes in *C. tetani* tends to minimize any inflammatory reaction that may develop from germination of spores and toxin formation. This means that in occasional cases the site of infection and toxin production in patients with tetanus may not be apparent (cryptogenic tetanus).

Tetanus toxin blocks transmission of inhibiting impulses of the inter-nuncial neurons, producing prolonged muscular spasms of both the flexor and extensor muscle groups (Fig. 39–5). Inasmuch as the flexor muscles of the body are usually dominant, the patient with advanced tetanus will show generalized flexion contractures. Severe, prolonged spasm of the masseter muscle may restrict opening of the mouth and has led to the term *lock-jaw*. Progression of the disease to include the muscles of respiration may result in

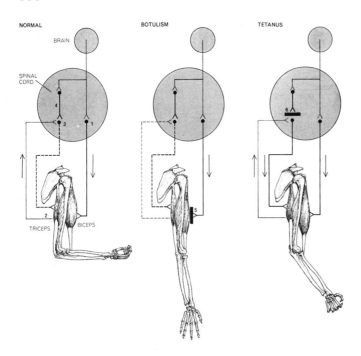

Figure 39–5. Nervous control of muscles that raise and lower the forearm is diagrammed very schematically. In a normal individual (*left*) impulses from the brain can excite a motoneuron (*1*) to cause the biceps to contract, stretching the triceps. A stretch-sensitive receptor (*2*) in the triceps would thereupon cause a triceps motoneuron (*3*) to fire and oppose the stretching — except that this firing is inhibited by impulses from an inhibitory nerve (*4*). In botulism (*center*) the neuromuscular junction is blocked (*5*), causing flaccid paralysis. In tetanus (*right*) the inhibitory impulses to the triceps motoneuron are blocked (*6*); both muscles contract, causing a spasm. (From van Heyningen, W. E. Tetanus. Sci. Am. *218*:69, 1968. Copyright © 1968 by Scientific American, Inc. All rights reserved.)

respiratory failure. In less severe cases, loss of control of pharyngeal musculature can lead to tracheal-bronchial aspiration and death from pneumonia.

Not well known in this country is the considerable worldwide mortality rate seen in neonatal tetanus. Although tetanus is not a reportable disease in many of the developing countries of the world, it has been estimated that it is one of the major causes of death from infectious disease, primarily due to neonatal and maternal infections (Fig. 39–6). Although the incidence of neonatal tetanus is low in the United States, five cases in 1971, it follows the epidemiologic pattern seen elsewhere in the world and appears in areas where there are poverty, crowded living conditions, and a lack of even minimal medical care. Neonatal tetanus usually results from the contamination of the umbilical cord of newborns with tetanus spores. In India, it has been reported that in cases of severe obstetric dystocia, packing of the birth canal with cattle dung, a practice in those regions where religious significance is assigned to cows, can result in contamination with tetanus spores of both the umbilical cord and the endometrial surface.

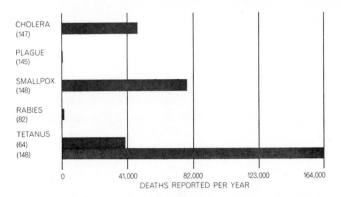

Figure 39–6. Mortality figures for five infectious diseases show smallpox as the leading killer (top five bars). The number of countries notifying or reporting deaths from each disease is shown in parentheses. If tetanus were as widely reported as smallpox, the World Health Organization estimates it would account for twice as many deaths as smallpox (bottom bar). (From van Heyningen, W. E.: Tetanus. Sci. Am. *218:*69, 1968. Copyright © 1968 by Scientific American, Inc. All rights reserved.)

Tetanus is a disease produced by an exotoxin which can be inactivated by an antitoxin. Therefore, *tetanus is a preventable disease.* Tetanus toxin can be made nontoxic by the addition of small amounts of formalin, thereby forming a toxoid. This modification does not change the antigenic capabilities of the toxin. Preparations of the toxoid are made with alum to facilitate slow absorption and prolong antigenic exposure. Current recommendations for primary immunization call for giving alum-precipitated toxoid twice, at four- to six-week intervals, followed by a "booster" 12 months later. Such a schedule will produce active immunity to the toxin; this immunity is reported to be protective for 12 to 20 years. Recent studies have shown that the routine practice of giving boosters or "recall" injections of fluid toxoid as a part of Emergency Room care following minor trauma to patients known to be adequately immunized is unnecessary. Administration of unneeded toxoid adds considerably to the incidence of allergic reactions.

Patients who develop and recover from clinical tetanus should undergo a primary immunization series with toxoid because, by getting tetanus once, these patients have demonstrated that they live and work in a manner which predisposes them to further exposure in the future. Such patients should also be immunized with toxoid, as the antigenic dose of tetanus toxin is lethal for man.

Passive protection in patients not previously immunized with toxoid can be temporarily provided by the use of antitoxin prepared from animals, usually equine or bovine. The use of antitoxin should be reserved for those patients who have not previously been given toxoid for active immunization. Hyperimmune human gamma globulin has recently been used for this purpose. Experience with the human hyperimmune gamma globulin has not shown it to be any more effective than equine antiserum in treating clinical tetanus, but it has the important advantage of eliminating serum sickness and allergic reactions to the animal serums. Benzathine penicillin, released over a 28-day period, is recommended for inactivating vegetative bacteria.

Botulism

Botulism should more properly be called an intoxication rather than an infectious disease. In most cases of botulism, the toxin is formed outside the body in food and is then ingested with the food. A number of cases of botulism resulting from skin lesions caused by *Clostridium botulinum* have recently been recognized. The pathogenesis of the disease in these cases is similar to that of tetanus.

The toxin of botulism acts at the neuromuscular junction of skeletal muscle, blocking neural transmission (Fig. 39–5). Symptoms of botulism are due to a progressive decrease of skeletal muscle function which eventually results in paralysis. The first muscles to become affected are the small muscles of the eye, larynx, and pharynx; consequently, diplopia and dysphonia are seen. Later, weakness of the extremities may appear, and impairment of the muscles of respiration may occur. Death usually is caused by cardiac arrest due to inadequate respiratory exchange.

Six serotypes of *Clostridium botulinum,* types A through F, are known. Types A and B are associated with the growth of the microorganism in home-prepared meats (the term *botulus* is from the Latin word meaning sausage) and vegetables. *C. botulinum* type C causes limberneck in fowl, and type D causes botulism in cattle but not in man. Type E botulism is most frequently found in fish or marine animals, while type F has caused disease in only two outbreaks, one from home-canned mushrooms and a second from home-prepared venison jerky. Type F *C. botulinum* has also been isolated from salmon and soil. Spores from all types of *C. botulinum* are available in the soil and may be present on plants and vegetables. The spores can be washed by rains into rivers, lakes, or the sea. Spores of *C. botulinum* are resistant to heat, and if contaminated food is not thoroughly heated during preparation, anaerobic conditions resulting from the canning procedure may allow germination, growth, and production of toxin. This is particularly dangerous in home-canned or home-prepared foods, when canning temperatures are not always carefully controlled.

Although spores of *Clostridium botulinum* are resistant to heating, the toxin is susceptible to increased temperatures and may be inactivated by heating as little as 60°C for 30 minutes. Type A *C. botulinum* is apparently more lethal than type B, as the mortality rate in patients ingesting type A toxin is 60 per cent, while in those with type B toxin it is slightly less (48 per cent).

As mentioned above, botulism caused by *Clostridium botulinum* is associated with fish and seafood products. Several outbreaks involving smoked whitefish obtained from the Great Lakes prompted investigation of the incidence of spores in fish taken from Lake Michigan. These studies showed that type E *C. botulinum* spores could be recovered from up to 13 per cent of whitefish being transferred from brine vats to smoking rooms; the presence of the spores was the result of cross-contamination with infected fish. This would indicate that the potential for clinical botulism would be considerably greater than documented cases indicate.

One interesting characteristic differentiating types A and E *Clostridium botulinum* is the minimal proteolytic activity of type E compared to that of type A. Patients will usually remember that the food tasted spoiled when food contaminated with type A *C. botulinum* has been ingested, but few patients complain of a bad taste or evidence of spoilage with type E *C. botulinum.* Bacteria belonging to type E *C. botulinum* have fewer proteolytic enzymes than those of type A and presumably produce fewer offensive end products.

Clinically, botulism caused by type E *Clostridium botulinum* presents with signs of acute gastrointestinal disease simulating intestinal obstruction. Neurologic signs may occur later and initially be overlooked owing to the intensity of the patient's vomiting and acute distress.

The diagnosis of botulism is best established by demonstration of toxin in the serum of the sick patient and in the suspected food. Even minute quantities of toxin may be detected by injecting mice with serum from patients ill with the disease or with extracts of the suspected food. The presence of toxin will be shown by the development of paralysis in the animal. The toxin type is then determined by pretreating a second set of mice with specific antiserums.

The treatment of botulism should be directed toward removing unbound toxin from the circulation with either specific or polyvalent type A, B, and E antitoxin. Because progressive disease usually causes death by paralysis of the muscles of respiration, patients with botulism must be watched carefully for need of respiratory assistance. With the exception of wound-associated botulism, the toxin is not produced within the body and antibiotics are not helpful. Heat lability of the toxin suggests that the best therapy is prevention. Heating all food at 60°C for 30 minutes or boiling for 10 minutes inactivates the toxin.

CASE PRESENTATION 1

A 62-year-old white female was admitted to the hospital complaining of polydipsia, nocturia, fever, and increasing shortness of breath of 10 days' duration. She had noted a poor appetite for the preceding eight months and had shown a 60-pound weight loss. The patient lived by herself but had moved to her daugher's apartment eight days before she was hospitalized. While living with her daugher, the patient was found to have a temperature of 101 to 102°F, for which her physician prescribed cephalexin. During this period, the patient asked her daughter about the symptoms of hemorrhoids and complained of vague discomfort in the perineal region.

Physical examination at the time of hospitalization revealed an elderly white female who appeared dehydrated and lethargic. The blood pressure was 146/90 mm Hg, and the pulse rate 126 per minute and regular. Examination of the optic fundi revealed venous congestion and hyperemia of the discs but no evidence of exudates, hemorrhages, or microaneurysms. The heart had a rapid but regular rate. No murmurs were heard. The right lung was resonant, and the left revealed coarse rales. The abdomen was soft and scaphoid, and no masses were palpable. The skin was rough and dry, although warm to the touch. Deep tendon reflexes were present and within normal limits.

At the time of hospitalization, the white blood count was 44,000 per cubic millimeter, with 76 per cent segmented neutrophils. The blood glucose was 900 mg per 100 ml, and the urine was strongly positive for reducing substances. A chest x-ray showed patchy infiltrates in the left lower lung field. The patient was started on six-hour management for what was presumed to be diabetes mellitus. On the morning of the third hospital day, she was found in a coma and had a fever of 102°F. Four blood cultures taken at that time were subsequently reported to be negative for bacteria. Because of the fever, gentamicin was added to the cephalexin the patient had been receiving. Control of the diabetes proved difficult, and on the eleventh hospital day two decubitus ulcers were noted over the sacrococcygeal region. By the thirteenth hospital day, the decubiti were associated with a fluctuant mass. This mass was surgically incised, releasing a large amount of foul-smelling, clay-colored material. Culture of the material was reported to yield beta-hemolytic streptococci. Following the incision and drainage, the patient appeared to improve, although blood glucose levels continued to show wide fluctuation, reaching 465 mg per 100 ml on one occasion. Because of a continued decline in her clinical course, the patient was transferred to a second hospital on the sixteenth hospital day.

At the time of admission to the second hospital, the patient was lethargic and responded poorly to questioning. Her temperature was 101°F; blood pressure, 85/50 mm Hg; pulse, 140 per minute; and respirations, 48 per minute. The chest was said to be clear to auscultation and percussion. The abdomen was distended, with voluntary guarding and diffuse tenderness to palpation. Examination of the gluteal region revealed a large fluctuant mass extending from the sacrococcygeal region laterally through the left gluteus maximus to the left femoral trochanter. The skin had a brownish discoloration over the mass. The white blood count was 45,000 per cubic millimeter; the blood glucose, 183 mg per 100 ml; and the blood urea nitrogen, 141 mg per 100 ml. The patient was started on six-hour management for diabetes and given 600 mg of clindamycin by intramuscular injection. Cultures were obtained from the abscess. Attempts to probe the extent of the abscess cavity were only partially successful, and the patient was scheduled for a more complete incision and drainage of the gluteal region the following morning. Approximately four hours after admission, the patient developed cardiac arrest. Resuscitation procedures were not successful.

Blood cultures taken shortly before death failed to grow bacteria, although a blood culture taken from the right ventricle at the time of autopsy grew *Clostridium perfringens*. At autopsy, a large, necrotic abscess cavity was found extending from the sacrococcyx laterally through the left gluteus maximus to the region of the left greater trochanter. The culture taken from this abscess shortly before death revealed the following:

Anaerobic bacteria (large numbers of all strains)
1. *Clostridium perfringens*
2. *Bacteriodes fragilis* subsp *vulgatus*
3. *Bacteroides fragilis* subsp *thetaiotaomicron*
4. *Bacteroides species* #1
5. *Bacteroides species* #2
6. *Bacteroides melaninogenicus*
7. *Bifidobacterium adolescentis* var *B*

8. *Peptostreptococcus anaerobius*
9. *Peptococcus prevotii*

Facultative anaerobic bacteria
1. *Streptococcus faecalis* – moderate numbers
2. *Escherichia coli* – few numbers
3. *Pseudomonas aeruginosa* – rare numbers

Fungi
1. *Candida albicans* – few numbers

The remainder of the autopsy showed multiple organizing thromboemboli with infarcts and cavity formation in the lower lobe of the right lung and the lingular portion of the upper lobe of the left lung. Focal thrombi in small vessels consistent with disseminated intravascular coagulation were found in the adrenals and kidneys.

The patient was initially hospitalized with symptoms of uncontrolled diabetes mellitus. This was evident by the history of polydipsia, nocturia, weight loss, and increasing shortness of breath. Whether she had an infection in the sacrococcygeal region at the time of admission to the first hospital is not clear, but the history of vague pain or discomfort mentioned to her daughter would suggest the possibility. It is likely that the infection in the sacrococcygeal region was the predisposing factor that precipitated diabetic coma on the third day. Severe infection in the diabetic may lead to uncontrolled hyperglycemia and coma. The presence of infarcts in both lungs, with organizing thrombi, would suggest embolization from a peripheral site. One such source could have been the gluteal abscess, although the autopsy did not provide for careful examination of veins draining from this region.

In reviewing the bacteria isolated from the sacral abscess, it is difficult to decide which one or ones of the 12 strains were responsible for the septic shock which probably caused the patient's death. *Clostridium perfringens* is known to be associated with severe infection and septicemia, but there was no evidence either before or after death to support gas or lecithinase production in the patient. Each of the other microorganisms isolated can also be associated with severe infection, but what role each played or how they may have interacted together cannot be determined in retrospect.

When the bacteria recovered from the abscess culture were tested for susceptibility to gentamicin, *Clostridium perfringens* and the Bacteroides species were found to be resistant to achievable serum levels. (See the table on the following page.)

In retrospect, if cultures for anaerobic bacteria had been obtained in the first hospital, the difficulty in bringing the patient's diabetes under control should have alerted her physicians to the significance of the underlying infection. The recognition of a polymicrobic abscess from anaerobic bacteria should have prompted more careful attention to an appropriate antimicrobial agent. Gentamicin, while a very good agent against many gram negative bacteria, is ineffective against many anaerobic bacteria. In this instance, either clindamycin or chloramphenicol would have been a better selection.

Treatment of anaerobic bacterial infections with antimicrobial agents not effective against anaerobic bacteria results in a significantly decreased survival rate of seriously ill patients. When facultative anaerobic and anaerobic bacteria are present in the same infection, survival of the patient is significantly aided when agents are employed that are selected for use against the anaerobic bacteria.

Antimicrobial Susceptibility Studies*

Microorganism	Chloramphenicol**	Clindamycin**	Penicillin**	Tetracycline**	Gentamicin**
Clostridium perfringens	8	1	1	⩽ 2	> 8
Bacteroides fragilis subsp *vulgatus*	8	1	> 4	> 16	> 8
Bacteroides fragilis subsp *thetaiotaomicron*	8	1	> 4	> 16	> 8
Bacteroides species #1 and #2	⩽ 2	⩽ 0.12	⩽ 0.03	⩽ 2	8
Bifidobacterium adolescentis var *B*	⩽ 8	⩽ 0.12	⩽ 0.03	⩽ 2	⩽ 0.25
Peptostreptococcus anaerobius	8	⩽ 0.12	⩽ 0.03	⩽ 2	4
Peptococcus prevotii	⩽ 2	⩽ 0.12	⩽ 0.03	8	1

*Minimal inhibitory concentrations.
**µg per ml.

This patient had an anaerobic bacterial infection of the skin and subcutaneous tissue called "necrotizing fascilitis." Diseases of this type are almost always due to mixed anaerobic bacterial species and are frequently associated with some underlying host defect, such as diabetes mellitus. Adequate control of infections of this type usually requires aggressive surgical incision and drainage as well as an effective antimicrobial agent.

CASE PRESENTATION 2*

On June 10, a housewife (case 1) fixed lunch for herself and two others. The lunch consisted of home-canned gefilte fish (served cold with horseradish on toast) soft drinks, and milk. Lunch was served between 2:30 and 3:00 PM. She ate two portions (approximately 100 gm each) of the gefilte fish, her employee (case 2) ate one portion, and her daughter-in-law (case 3) ate a half portion.

Case 1. Four hours after lunch, the housewife complained of headache, epigastric distress, hoarseness, and slight dyspnea. The epigastric distress continued. She vomited repeatedly and experienced dryness of the mouth, weakness, constipation, and urinary retention. Examination by a physician on the evening of June 11th revealed an anxious, moderately obese woman with labored respirations (26 per minute); a blood pressure of 80/58 mm Hg, and a pulse rate of 110 beats per minute. The pupils were equal in size but somewhat dilated; they were reactive to light. Extraocular eye movements were normal, and no facial weakness was noted. Her throat and mouth were dry, and her voice was hoarse. The chest was normal to auscultation and to

*Adapted from Armstrong, R. W., Stenn, F., Dowell, V. R., Jr., and Sommers, H. M.: Type E botulism from home-canned gefilte fish. J.A.M.A. *210:*303, 1969.

percussion. The abdomen was soft and nontender, with decreased bowel sounds. Deep tendon reflexes were normal. Because of a history of mild hypertension, the findings of tachycardia and hypotension and the history of substernal distress suggested the possibility of a myocardial infarction. The patient was therefore hospitalized.

Laboratory findings at admission included normal results from a complete blood cell count and urinalysis. Values of serum electrolytes, bilirubin, amylase, and protein determined on serum from blood drawn the morning after admission were all within normal limits. Chest and abdominal x-ray films were interpreted as normal. An electrocardiogram was unchanged from previous tracings.

The patient was treated symptomatically with antacids, nasogastric suction, and intravenous administration of fluids. On June 13th, the patient had a cardiopulmonary arrest and was resuscitated. Spontaneous respiration did not recur, and breathing was maintained on a mechanical respirator. On June 14th, no apparent benefit resulted from 80,000 units of bivalent (types A and B) and 10,000 units of type E botulism antitoxin which were administered intravenously. On June 15th, the patient died.

Autopsy showed generalized ischemic changes in the central nervous system and moderate arteriosclerosis of the coronary arteries with slight hypertrophy of the left ventricle. The liver and spleen were enlarged and hyperemic. The lungs showed pulmonary edema with focal acute bronchopneumonia.

Case 2. A 39-year-old black male was anorectic and unusually fatigued on the evening of June 10th, the date he ate the gefilte fish. The following day, recurrent vomiting, periumbilical cramping, progressive abdominal distention, constipation, and dry mouth developed. He was hospitalized shortly after midnight on June 13th. Findings of physical examination were not remarkable except for tympanites with increased bowel sounds.

Results of laboratory studies, including complete blood cell count, and levels of nonprotein nitrogen, blood glucose, serum electrolytes, and serum amylase, were normal. A roentgenogram of the abdomen showed that the small intestine was distended and had air-fluid levels. A barium enema roentgenographic study was consistent with small bowel obstruction. Attempts to pass a nasogastric tube were unsuccessful.

The patient was treated with fluids and antiemetics given intravenously; oral intake was restricted. By 12 hours after admission, abdominal distention had decreased. For the next two days, the patient complained of weakness, sore throat, dry mouth, and slightly blurred vision. No objective facial weakness, extraocular motor weakness, disturbance of accommodation, reaction to light, or changes in the pharynx could be found on reexamination. By June 17th, all symptoms had disappeared and the patient was discharged from the hospital. He did not receive botulism antitoxin.

Case 3. A 28-year-old white woman, seven months pregnant, had a brief dizzy spell several hours after eating half a portion of the gefilte fish. Late the following morning, she had another dizzy spell, followed by nausea, vomiting, profound weakness, and a slight distortion of hearing. Recovery was spontaneous, and she had no further symptoms. Two months later she gave birth to healthy twins.

Epidemiologic Investigation. The gefilte fish was the only food common to all three patients. The fish patties had been prepared from raw, unprocessed, Great Lakes whitefish purchased in a supermarket between April 18th and April 21st. Whole fish were ground at home to a fine paste on April 24th, blended with raw eggs and onions, reground, and made into patties approximately four inches in diameter. The patties were "simmered" for about four hours in a large open pot partially filled with water. Most of the patties were eaten that day; others were kept in an open dish in the refrigerator and were eaten without ill effect within a week of preparation by a dozen persons. When the patties were cooked, some were placed in a jar that had been boiled; the jar was capped immediately and put in the refrigerator. The jar was left in the refrigerator (temperature, 44°F, determined later) and was not opened until seven weeks later, when the food was eaten by the three patients as described.

Laboratory Investigation. Tests for botulinus toxin and for *Clostridium botulinum* were performed. Type E toxin was detected in the serum or plasma of the housewife (case 1) on the first, second, and third days after she ate the gefilte fish. No toxin was detected in serum samples from the other two patients. The fish patties contained 10 mouse intraperitoneal 50 per cent lethal doses (IP LD_{50}) of type E botulinus toxin per gram of food. Trypsinization of the food extract increased the toxin activity to 780 mouse IP LD_{50} per gram. Cultures of the gefilte fish patties yielded *C. botulinum* type E. Extracts taken at autopsy from portions of the patient's (case 1) myocardium, psoas muscle, kidney, brain, liver, and the proximal portion of the jejunum showed no toxin activity in mice. Type E antitoxin had been administered to the patient 10 hours prior to death, and serum obtained at autopsy neutralized type E toxin.

Type E botulism can present a confusing clinical picture in that neurologic signs may be less prominent than the acute, severe, gastrointestinal symptoms. The above case reports illustrate how the prominence of gastrointestinal symptoms in type E botulism can be confused with symptoms of bowel obstruction or myocardial infarction, thus delaying specific treatment of the intoxication.

In Case 1, hypotension, epigastric distress, and tachycardia suggested myocardial ischemia and possible myocardial infarction. In both Cases 1 and 2, severe gastrointestinal symptoms initially suggested intestinal obstruction, a characteristic of type E botulism. Another characteristic feature, urinary retention, was observed in Case 1.

These cases are noteworthy because of the lack of classic ocular and facial muscle manifestations, although transitory blurring of vision was reported in one patient, and dilated but not fixed pupils were seen in another.

Clostridium botulinum type E is widely distributed. Its spores have been demonstrated in sediment and in fish from all Northern oceans and from waterways and soils of all Northern continents, including the Great Lakes and the Atlantic, Gulf, and Pacific coasts of North America. The greatest concentration of the spores is in the sediments of shallow offshore waters, especially near the mouths of rivers. All of the major commercial fishing areas are thus well seeded with the microorganism.

The type E spores and microorganisms are mainly confined to the intestines of fish and are present in low numbers. Type E spores are relatively more heat labile than those of other *Clostridium botulinum* types, but in processing, the whole fish may become contaminated. Smoking or light cooking may not be sufficient to inactivate all spores. Of freshly smoked fish examined at one processing plant, 1 per cent contained detectable *C. botulinum.* In contrast to other varieties of *C. botulinum* type E spores germinate and produce toxin at refrigerator temperatures. Therefore, in fresh or processed fish, lethal accumulations of botulinus toxin may develop when a lightly contaminated fish is held at low temperatures under anaerobic or nearly anaerobic conditions.

Thus far the majority of reported type E botulism cases have resulted from the consumption of home-preserved fish or fish products. Because of the wide distribution of the microorganism, the potential problem of future outbreaks from commercially processed fish products exists.

References

Books

Balows, A., DeHaan, R. M., Dowell, V. R., and Guge, L. B. (eds.): Anaerobic Bacteria: Role in Disease. Springfield, Illinois, Charles C Thomas, 1974.

Willis, A. T.: Anaerobic Bacteriology in Clinical Medicine. London, Butterworth and Co., 1964.

Review Articles

Bartlett, J. G., and Finegold, S. M.: Anaerobic infections of the lung and pleural space. Am. Rev. Resp. Dis. *110:*56, 1974.

Gorbach, S. L., and Bartlett, J. G.: Anaerobic infections. N. Engl. J. Med. *290:*1177, 1237, 1289, 1974.

MacLennan, J. D.: The histotoxic clostridial infections of man. Bacteriol. Rev. *26:*177, 1962.

Original Articles

Armstrong, R. W., Stenn, F., Dowell, V. R., Ammerman, G., and Sommers, H. M.: Type E botulism from home canned gefilte fish. J.A.M.A. *210:*303, 1969.

Bartlett, J. G., Sutler, V. L., and Finegold, S. M.: Treatment of anaerobic infections with lincomycin and clindamycin. N. Engl. J. Med. *287:*1006, 1972.

Bartlett, J. G., Gorbach, S. L., Tally, F. P., and Finegold, S. M.: Bacteriology and treatment of primary lung abscess. Am. Rev. Resp. Dis. *109:*510, 1974.

Berthrong, M., and Sabiston, D. C., Jr.: Cerebral lesions in congenital heart disease. Bull. Johns Hopkins Hosp. *89:*384, 1951.

Bott, T. L., Johnson, J., Jr., Foster, E. M., et al.: Possible origin of the high incidence of *C. botulinum* type E in an inland bay. J. Bacteriol. *95:*1542, 1968.

Botulism in the United States. Review of cases 1899–1967. Center for Disease Control, Public Health Services, Department of Health, Education and Welfare, 1967.

Cherubin, C. E.: Epidemiology of tetanus in narcotic addicts. N. Y. State J. Med. *70:*267, 1970.

Edsall, G., Elliott, M. W., Peebles, T. C., et al.: Excessive use of tetanus toxoid boosters. J.A.M.A. *202:*17, 1967.

Felner, J. M., and Dowell, V. R.: Anaerobic bacterial endocarditis. N. Engl. J. Med. *283:*1188, 1970.

Frederick, J., and Braude, A. I.: Anaerobic infection of the paranasal sinuses. N. Engl. J. Med. *290:*135, 1974.

Gorbach, S. L., and Bartlett, J. G.: Anaerobic infections: Old myths and new realities. J. Infect. Dis. *130:*307, 1974.

Heineman, H. S., and Braude, A. L.: Anaerobic infection of the brain: Observations on 18 consecutive cases of brain abscess. Am. J. Med. *35:*682, 1963.

Kabat, E. A.: Uses of hyperimmune human gamma globulin. N. Engl. J. Med. *269:*247, 1963.

Levine, L., McComb, J. A., Dwyer, R. C., et al.: Active-passive tetanus immunization. N. Engl. J. Med. *274:*186, 1966.

Martin, W. J., Gardner, M., and Washington, J. A.: In vitro antimicrobial susceptibility of anaerobic bacteria isolated from clinical specimens. Antimicrob. Agents Chemother. *1:*148, 1972.

Merson, M. H., and Dowell, V. R., Jr.: Epidemiologic, clinical and laboratory aspects of wound botulism. N. Engl. J. Med. *289:*1005, 1973.

Tetanus surveillance. Center for Disease Control, Report No. 4, March, 1974.

Thadepalli, H., Gorbach, S. L., Broido, P. W., Norsen, J., and Nyhus, L.: Abdominal trauma, anaerobes, and antibiotics. Surg. Gynecol. Obstet. *137:*270, 1973.

van Heyningen, W. E.: Tetanus. Sci. Am. *218:*69, 1968.

RICKETTSIAL DISEASES

Introduction

Rickettsias* are very small coccobacilli that are obligate intracellular parasites of man and a wide variety of lower animals. Only one of many rickettsias, *Rochalimaea quintana,* has ever been cultivated on a cell-free medium.

Man is only an incidental host for most rickettsias, since the rickettsial diseases are transmitted to man by bites of a variety of arthropods, including ticks, mites, fleas, and lice. Except for epidemic typhus fever, the reservoir of rickettsial infection is lower animals or the arthropod vector. In certain arthropod vectors, e.g., ticks, the rickettsias can be transmitted transovarially from one generation to another; thus, an animal reservoir is not necessary for maintenance of the parasite in nature.

As can be noted in Table 40–1 the rickettsias are grouped together because they have in common a number of characteristics. For example, all of these microorganisms are similar in size and shape and appear as pleomorphic coccobacillary forms when viewed under the light microscope (Fig. 40–1). Electron microscopy shows greater detail (Fig. 40–2). Under natural conditions, all of the rickettsias, except that causing Q fever, occur in arthropods, either fleas, lice, ticks, or mites. The arthropod constitutes the primary means by which the rickettsial diseases are transmitted to man (see Table 40–2). In all rickettsial infections, except rickettsialpox and Q fever, agglutinating antibodies are produced to either the OX-19, OX-2, or OX-K strains of *Proteus vulgaris.* Agglutination of these Proteus strains by rickettsial antibodies is known as the Weil-Felix reaction (see Table 40–3).

---

*Order, Rickettsiales; Family, Rickettsiaceae; Tribe, Rickettsieae. There are three genera, Rickettsia, Rochalimaea, and Coxiella in the tribe Rickettsieae. In order to bring the terminology more in line with current medical usage, we are using in this chapter the general term *Rickettsia* to refer to members of all three genera.

TABLE 40-1. Rickettsial Diseases of Man*

Disease — Group and type	Agent	Geographical distribution	Natural cycle — Arthropod	Natural cycle — Mammal	Transmission to man	Serologic diagnosis — Weil-Felix reaction	Serologic diagnosis — Complement fixation
Typhus							
Epidemic	Rickettsia prowazekii	Worldwide	Body louse	Man	Infected louse feces into broken skin	Positive OX-19	Positive group- and type-specific
Brill's disease	R. prowazekii	North America, Europe	Recurrence years after original attack of epidemic typhus			Usually negative	
Endemic	R. typhi	Worldwide	Flea	Rodents	Infected flea feces into broken skin	Positive OX-19	
Spotted fever							
Rocky Mountain spotted fever	R. rickettsii	Western Hemisphere	Ticks	Wild rodents, dogs	Tick bite	Positive OX-19 OX-2	Positive group- and type-specific
North Asian tick-borne rickettsiosis	R. sibirica	Siberia, Mongolia	Ticks	Wild rodents	Tick bite	Positive OX-19 OX-2	
Boutonneuse fever	R. conorii	Africa, Europe, Middle East, India	Ticks	Wild rodents, dogs	Tick bite	Positive OX-19 OX-2	
Queensland tick typhus	R. australis	Australia	Ticks	Marsupials, wild rodents	Tick bite	Positive OX-19 OX-2	
Rickettsialpox	R. akari	North America, Europe	Blood-sucking mite	House mouse and other rodents	Mite bite	Negative	
Scrub typhus	R. tsutsugamushi	Asia, Australia, Pacific Islands	Tromiculid mites	Wild rodents	Mite bite	Positive OX-K	Positive in about 50% of patients
Q fever	Coxiella burnetii	Worldwide	Ticks	Small mammals, cattle, sheep and goats	Inhalation of dried, infected material	Negative	Positive
Trench fever	Rochalimaea quintana	Europe, Africa, North America	Body louse	Man	Infected louse feces into broken skin	Negative	Low titer

*From Davis, B. D., et al.: Microbiology. 2nd ed. Hagerstown, Maryland, Harper and Row, 1973.

TABLE 40-2. Modes of Transmission of the Principal Rickettsial Diseases*

Disease in man	Etiologic agent	Chain of transmission
Epidemic typhus	R. prowazekii	... Man → Louse → Man → Louse ...
Endemic typhus	R. typhi	... Rat → Rat flea → Rat → Rat flea → Rat ... ↓ Man
Rocky Mountain spotted fever (boutonneuse fever, other spotted fevers)	R. rickettsii	... Tick → Tick → Tick → Tick ... ↓ ↓ Dog Man ↓ Tick → Man
Scrub typhus (tsutsugamushi fever)	R. tsutsugamushi	... Mite → Field mouse → Mite → Field mouse ... ↓ Man
Rickettsialpox	R. akari	... Mite → House mouse → Mite → House mouse ... ↓ Man
Q fever	C. burnetii	... Tick → Small mammal → Tick → Cattle ... (airborne) (airborne) Man

*From Davis, B. D., et al.: Microbiology. 2nd ed. Hagerstown, Maryland, Harper and Row, 1973.

TABLE 40-3. Usual Weil-Felix Agglutination Reactions Observed in Rickettsial Diseases*

	OX-19	OX-2	OX-K
Epidemic typhus	++++	+	0
Murine typhus	++++	+	0
Spotted fever group	++++	+	0
	+	++++	0
Scrub typhus	0	0	++++
Rickettsialpox	0	0	0
Q fever	0	0	0

*From Smadel, J. E., and Jackson, E. R.: Rickettsial infections. In Lennette, E. H., and Schmidt, N. J. (eds.): Diagnostic Procedures for Viral and Rickettsial Diseases. 3rd ed. New York, American Public Health Association, 1964.

The basic lesion that occurs in all rickettsial diseases of man is a widespread peripheral vasculitis caused by the rickettsia invading endothelial cells and multiplying therein. The diseases caused by rickettsia in man are acute infectious diseases characterized by fever, headache, and a skin rash, with the exception of Q fever, in which no rash occurs. If treatment is started early enough, all of the rickettsial diseases can be controlled by optimal doses

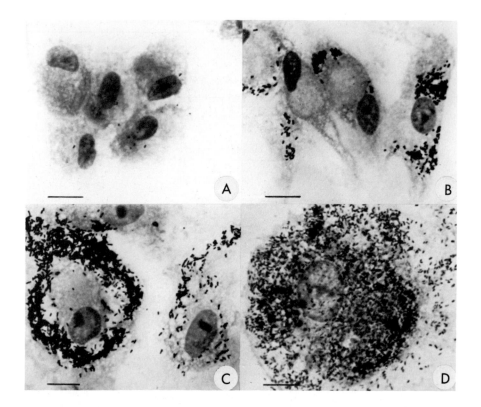

Figure 40-1. Photomicrographs of growth of *Rickettsia mooseri* in macrophages in cell culture containing normal human serum (Giménez stain). (Solid bars, 10 *μm*.) *A*, after two hours of exposure to *R. mooseri* suspension. (X 1480.) *B*, Day 3 after infection. (X 1400.) *C*, Day 6 after infection. (X 1400.) *D*, Day 6 after infection. Destruction of *R. mooseri* infected macrophage (day 6) with release of microorganisms. (X 1560.) (From Gambrill, et al.: Mechanisms of immunity in typhus infections. II. Multiplication of typhus rickettsiae in human macrophage cell cultures in the nonimmune system: influence of virulence of rickettsial strains and of chloramphenical. Infect. Immun. *8*:519, 1973.)

of antimicrobial drugs such as chloramphenicol and the tetracyclines. Table 40-1 shows that some of the rickettsias give rise to both group-specific and species-specific complement-fixing antibodies.

Morphology

The rickettsias are small nonmotile coccobacilli that vary in size from approximately 0.3 microns in width to 1 to 2 microns in length (Figs. 40-1 and 40-2). They are found, for the most part, in the cytoplasm of endothelial cells, although certain species also multiply in the nucleus. Within mammalian cells, the rickettsias structurally resemble bacteria, since what appear to be a cell wall, a cell membrane, and nuclear material can be visualized (Fig. 40-2). Polychromatic stains (Giemsa stain) are better than simple stains or the Gram stain for demonstrating rickettsias in cells.

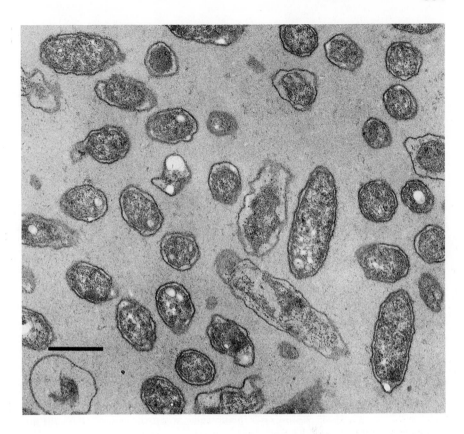

Figure 40-2. Ultrathin section through cells of *Rickettsia prowazeki* typical of those seen in the lumen of the louse midgut. (Bar, 0.5 *μm*.) (From Silverman, D. J., et al.: Infect. Immun. *10*:257, 1974.)

Physiology

For years there has been considerable controversy over whether the rickettsias were bacteria or whether they were more closely related to the larger viruses. The issue has been resolved, since it is now known that rickettsias more closely resemble bacteria not only morphologically but physiologically. Extracts of rickettsias can be shown to contain glycolytic enzymes and most of the enzymes of the Krebs cycle, as well as cytochromes. Studies have also shown that glutamate oxidation and oxidative phosphorylation are probably the principal energy-producing processes in rickettsial cells. Although they have some of the metabolic activities of bacteria, rickettsias do appear to require an outside supply of cofactors. These cofactors are provided by the infected cell. When isolated from infected cells and maintained in suspension, rickettsias are very fragile and lose cofactors very readily, apparently by diffusion. Once the rickettsias are removed from the cell they infect, viability and infectivity are lost rapidly. For this reason, man ordinarily can be infected only by direct inoculation from an infected arthropod. There is, however, one exception: *Coxiella burnetii*, the causative agent of Q fever, is very hardy and resists drying for long periods. It also resists the temperatures used for the pasteurization of milk. It is most commonly transmitted to man by the inhalation of dust containing rickettsial cells that came from soil previously contaminated by material from diseased animals.

Pathogenesis

Following the bite of an infected arthropod, the rickettsias invade the endothelial cells of blood vessels and multiply within the cells by binary fission. Rickettsias are able to penetrate in some unknown manner the membrane of the host cell and pass directly into the cytoplasm. The generation time of rickettsias within infected cells is slow, but as the numbers accumulate, endothelial cells are destroyed, probably owing to the effect of rickettsial toxin, a poorly defined toxic cell wall material. With the resulting angiitis there is accumulation of inflammatory cells, hemorrhage, and frequently widespread thrombosis. This accumulation is particularly prominent in the small blood vessels of the brain, myocardium, and skin; the latter involvement accounts for the skin rash that appears in most rickettsial diseases.

Host response to rickettsial invasion is an interesting and important study. Host defense mechanisms can have little influence on the multiplication of rickettsias within endothelial cells. When the endothelial cells are killed and the rickettsial cells are released, they can be readily phagocytized by macrophages, provided specific opsonin is present. Rickettsias, however, can penetrate the cell membrane and pass directly into the cytoplasm, where they replicate. The rickettsias grow well within macrophages under ordinary circumstances, since macrophages seem to have little capacity to cope with the rickettsias until antibody to rickettsia appears (Fig. 40–1). Once specific antibody has combined with the rickettsias, they are readily killed by macrophages. The killing takes place under these circumstances apparently because in the presence of antibody the rickettsias do not escape from the phagolysosomes and consequently are killed and degraded. In the absence of antibody, the rickettsias are apparently able to penetrate the phagolysosome membrane and pass into the cytoplasm, where they continue to replicate. The antibody within the rickettsial cell may either stabilize lysosomal membranes of the host cell or neutralize to a certain extent toxic cell wall materials that may contribute to the ability of the rickettsial cells to escape from phagolysosomes. Antibody acts to control multiplication of rickettsial cells only within phagocytic cells of the host. Antibody combined with rickettsias does not in any way interfere with the multiplication of rickettsias in nonphagocytic cells.

Thus, although antibody appears to play an important part in immunity to rickettsial disease, it is quite possible that cellular immune factors have a major if not more important role. The operation of cellular immune forces that would suppress multiplication without necessarily killing the invading parasites could better account for the fact that certain rickettsias persist in infected hosts for many years after recovery from the acute phase of a rickettsial disease.

Clinical Diseases

As already noted, the rickettsias and rickettsial diseases have in common many characteristics (see Table 40–1). However, there are distinct differences among the clinical manifestations of disease caused by different species, and the severity of the diseases in man may vary widely.

Classic Epidemic Typhus

In classic epidemic typhus, the mortality rate in uncontrolled acute disease may vary from 10 to 60 per cent, the highest mortality rate being found in people over the age of 50. After an incubation period of from 10 days to 2 weeks, the onset is usually abrupt. The initial clinical manifestations consist of severe headache and fever between 102 and 104°F; as the disease progresses, the temperature remains at a high level, frequently as high as 104 to 105°F. The headache is very severe and characteristically is not relieved by analgesics. The skin rash does not develop until about the sixth or seventh day of the illness, and appears first on the trunk, usually in the axillary area, and then spreads over the rest of the trunk and onto the extremities. The palms of the hands and soles of the feet are rarely involved. The pulse is usually rapid and weak and may be irregular. Adequate treatment with chloramphenicol or tetracyclines should be given as early in the disease as possible, and in suspected cases treatment should be initiated immediately, even though a definitive diagnosis cannot be made until later.

Brill-Zinsser Disease

Brill-Zinsser disease is essentially a recrudescence of typhus fever in a person who had the disease years before. It was first noted by Nathan Brill in 1898 in immigrants from Russia and Poland who were living in New York. Extensive epidemiologic studies on Brill's disease were made in New York in 1934 by Hans Zinsser, hence the name Brill-Zinsser disease. Clinically this disease differs from primary classic epidemic typhus. The disease is milder and has a shorter course, and frequently there is no rash. Since this disease is a recrudescence of an old infection, no arthropod vector is involved in the transmission. Usually a history of a primary attack of typhus that occurred years before can be obtained. Support of the recrudescent nature of Brill-Zinsser disease comes from the fact that the antibodies that develop are of the IgG type characteristic of the antibodies produced as a secondary immune response to antigen. In patients with classic typhus, the antibodies that first appear are IgM, as would be expected in a primary immune response.

Murine (Endemic) Typhus

The clinical manifestations of murine flea-borne typhus are similar to those of classic epidemic louse-borne typhus except that they are milder in degree and the mortality rate is much lower. This disease is found scattered throughout the world; in the United States reservoirs are found along the Atlantic seaboard and in states that border the Gulf of Mexico. The microorganisms are harbored by rats and are transmitted from rats to man by rat fleas. The microorganisms multiply in the flea without causing damage to the host and can transmit the disease to human beings when circumstances are such that persons are exposed to rat fleas in rat-infested areas; thus, the disease occurs sporadically and not epidemically. The rickettsias causing epidemic typhus fever are not transmitted transovarially from one generation of fleas to the next.

Spotted Fevers

There are a number of spotted fevers that occur in various parts of the world and are caused by closely related rickettsias. The most important one of this group, as far as the United States is concerned, is Rocky Mountain spotted fever. Although originally detected in the Rocky Mountain area, most cases of this disease now occur along the eastern seaboard (Figs. 40–3 and 40–4). The disease is transmitted by ticks and usually occurs in persons who are or have been in tick-infested areas. Clinically, the disease is characterized by sudden onset of high fever, skin rash, and headache. The symptoms may be confused with endemic typhus in those areas of the United States where both diseases occur. The rash in Rocky Mountain spotted fever, in contrast to that in typhus fever, is initially seen on the ankles and wrists and then spreads not only to the trunk but also to the palms of the hands and the soles of the feet (Fig. 40–5). Treatment consists of the administration of tetracyclines or chloramphenicol, and early therapy is essential. (See the Case Presentation at the end of this chapter.)

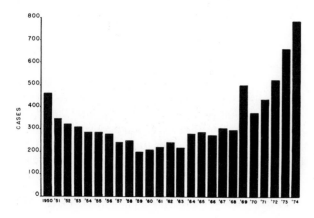

Figure 40–3. Rocky Mountain spotted fever (reported cases by year, United States, 1950 to 1974). (From Massachusetts Department of Public Health: On the Alert for Rocky Mountain spotted fever. N. Engl. J. Med. *292*:1127, 1975.)

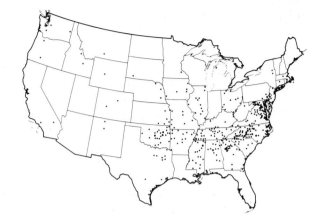

Figure 40–4. Rocky Mountain spotted fever (scatter of reported cases by county, United States, 1973.) (From Massachusetts Department of Public Health: On the Alert for Rocky Mountain spotted fever. N. Engl. J. Med. *292*: 1127, 1975.)

Scrub Typhus

Scrub typhus is a mite-borne rickettsial disease found in Southeast Asia and adjacent areas. Clinically, there is high fever and headache accompanied by lymphadenopathy and a generalized maculopapular rash. In many patients, a distinctive skin lesion, called an *eschar,* develops. This eschar appears at the site of the mite bite and increases in size; it may reach a diameter of 1 cm. The regional lymph nodes draining the eschar are usually enlarged and tender. As with some other rickettsial diseases, early treatment with tetracyclines or chloramphenicol is essential, otherwise the mortality rate may be high. The disease does not occur in the United States; however, it became a major medical problem in Allied forces in the South Pacific area during World War II.

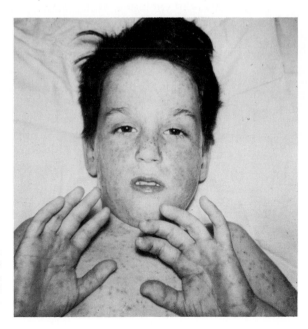

Figure 40–5. Rocky Mountain spotted fever. Typical rash occurring on the face and the palms. (From Hazard, G. W., et al.: Rocky Mountain spotted fever in the eastern United States. N. Engl. J. Med. *280:*57, 1969.)

Rickettsialpox, Q Fever, Trench Fever

Rickettsialpox, Q fever, and trench fever are rickettsial diseases in which the disease is usually fairly mild and the mortality rate very low. Rickettsialpox is transmitted to humans from the house mouse by mites. It occurs only under those conditions in which man comes into rather close contact with mice and their mites. Clinically the disease is very mild (see Table 40–1) and is frequently misdiagnosed as varicella.

Q fever is unique in that it is transmitted to man primarily by inhalation of contaminated animal products. It is apt to occur in epidemic form among slaughterhouse workers and sporadically among farmers and veterinarians. It can also be transmitted transovarially by ticks, and from ticks to man (see Table 40–1).

Trench fever is a mild louse-borne disease that was a problem among military personnel during the First World War. Since that time it has been shown to be endemic in Mexico (see Table 40–1).

Diagnosis

From the clinical standpoint, there is little to differentiate the rickettsial diseases in human beings from one another or from a number of other acute febrile conditions, although demonstration of rickettsial cells in biopsy specimens of skin lesions can sometimes be made. Therefore, in order to distinguish between the infecting rickettsial agents in human beings, attention has focused upon immunologic responses.

Rickettsias can be readily cultivated in the yolk sac of the developing chick embryo. Enormous numbers of rickettsias can be obtained in this manner, and as a result, material is now available that provides antigen for a variety of serologic tests. The most useful and most widely used serologic test has been the complement-fixation reaction.

By using the complement-fixation reaction, both group-specific and type-specific antigens have been recognized (see Table 40–1). Group-specific antigens are found in the soluble portion of the rickettsial cell, whereas the type-specific antigens appear to be associated with cell walls. The latter antigens actually are species specific and are very useful in determining the origin of some rickettsial diseases. As in the diagnosis of other diseases by serologic means, the finding of a rising antibody titer in acute phase and convalescent phase serum is desirable. In addition to complement fixation, agglutination of rickettsial suspensions and immunofluorescence tests have been employed.

Another informative serologic test is the *Weil-Felix reaction.* It was fortuitously discovered many years ago by the two for whom the test is named that antibody formed in the course of most rickettsial diseases would agglutinate certain strains of Proteus. This finding originally was interpreted as an indication of a role for the Proteus bacillus in the origin of typhus fever. Actually, these cross-reactions occur because rickettsial strains possess cell wall antigens that are similar to the polysaccharide O antigens of certain strains of Proteus. These Proteus strains are referred to as OX strains.

The reactions obtained with serum from patients with rickettsial disease, using the three Proteus strains OX-2, OX-19 and OX-K, can be of great help in differentiating certain of the rickettsial diseases from one another. Table 40–3 shows the reactions that usually occur when using these three Proteus strains. It should be kept in mind that Proteus species are indigenous to human beings and may cause infections of the urinary tract. Therefore, the presence of antibodies to Proteus OX strains is not of itself an absolute criterion for the presence of rickettsial disease.

A number of laboratory animals are susceptible to rickettsial infection, and guinea pigs, mice, and rats may be artificially infected by injection of blood from an infected patient. Protection tests using known antibody can be used, but the handling of such infected laboratory animals is risky; as a result, animal inoculation and protection tests are no longer employed for diagnostic purposes.

CASE PRESENTATION

An 11-year-old boy was admitted to the hospital because of severe headache, fever, and a rash. Three days before admission, the patient had complained of not feeling well. The following day a rash appeared on his wrists and ankles and his temperature climbed to 103.5°F. The next day rash had spread to the upper extremities and was noted on the soles of the feet and the palms of the hands. His temperature remained high, and a severe frontal headache developed. At the same time, marked tenderness of the calves and swelling of the ankles appeared, and the headache became much more severe. The headache was not relieved by aspirin. At this time a physician was consulted, and the patient was brought to the hospital.

Upon admission to the hospital the boy appeared acutely ill, with a temperature of 103.6°F. His pulse rate was 115 per minute, respirations were 34 per minute, and blood pressure was 128/66 mm Hg. Confluent erythematous macular lesions were seen upon the palms of the hands and soles of the feet, and over the lower parts of all four extremities. The lesions extended to the upper part of the extremities, and a few lesions also were seen on the abdomen and chest. In some areas, the lesions were papular, but none blanched upon pressure. Lymphadenopathy was not noted, nor was there any nuchal rigidity. The remainder of the physical examination was within normal limits except for the presence of marked tenderness when pressure was exerted on both gastrocnemius muscles.

Examination of the urine revealed no abnormalities. The white blood cell count was 11,500 cells per cubic millimeter, with 65 per cent segmented neutrophils, 5 per cent band forms, 20 per cent lymphocytes, and 10 per cent monocytes. A chest x-ray and an electrocardiogram revealed normal findings. Spinal fluid obtained by lumbar pressure was clear; the pressure was 300 mm Hg. There was slight xanthochromia. The spinal fluid contained 20 cells per cubic millimeter, mostly mononuclear cells. No microorganisms could be demonstrated upon microscopic examination.

Because of the typical distribution and appearance of the rash, the severe frontal headache, and the muscle tenderness, Rocky Mountain spotted fever was suspected. A history obtained from the parents revealed that on the previous weekend the patient had taken an overnight camping trip with several of his friends. The patient's father had supervised the trip, and according to the father the area in which they camped was known to be infested with ticks. Three of the boys, including his son, had tick bites.

Because of the high probability that the patient was suffering from Rocky Mountain spotted fever, tetracycline therapy was started immediately. Symptoms promptly abated, and the patient made a rapid and uneventful recovery. He was discharged on the fifth hospital day.

Blood for serologic tests was drawn on the first hospital day, and at the time of discharge arrangements were made to collect a second blood sample two weeks after the onset of the illness. The serum sample collected on the first hospital day (three days after the onset of the illness) was negative in both the Weil-Felix and complement-fixation tests for Rocky Mountain spotted fever. However, the second serum sample had an OX-19 agglutination titer of 1:640. The specific complement-fixation test was strongly positive. Thus, the diagnosis of Rocky Mountain spotted fever was confirmed.

Rocky Mountain spotted fever is a rickettsial disease that was first discovered in the Rocky Mountain area around the turn of the century. It remained an important disease until the late 1940s, when its incidence began to decline steadily. The disease was first recognized in the eastern part of the United States in the early 1930s. The number of cases increased until effective antibiotic therapy was discovered. However, since the late 1960s the incidence of reported cases has risen (see Fig. 40–3). Furthermore, the death rate remains apparently constant at about 5 to 7 per cent of infected patients. This constant mortality rate probably reflects the fact that the disease frequently is not detected early enough and appropriate therapy not given soon enough. This is particularly distressing, since antibiotics such as the tetracyclines or chloramphenicol can control the disease when treatment is started before the sixth day of illness. A fairly high mortality rate is a reflection of failure on the part of physicians to suspect Rocky Mountain spotted fever. Death can be avoided only by early recognition based on clinical signs and symptoms and epidemiologic considerations. High fever and a prominent skin rash that begins on the extremities and involves the palms and soles are characteristic features. Furthermore, children constitute the majority of cases. Measles, syphilis, and meningococcemia are the most frequent misdiagnoses (see Chap. 34).

Today over half of the reported cases occur in the eastern part of the United States (see Fig. 40–4). A prominent characteristic of the disease is its focal geographic nature. In the states where it is most common, small circumscribed geographic areas account for a high proportion of cases each year. In states where the incidence is low, most or all of the cases from a particular state may come from a single circumscribed area. Examples of the focal nature of the disease can be found in New York, Ohio, and Massachusetts. The disease is maintained in the ticks of these areas by transovarial transmission.

Although serologic tests can be used to diagnose the disease, they are of little help until one to two weeks after the onset of the symptoms. This is beyond the time when one can expect to obtain the maximal therapeutic effect from antimicrobial agents. The disease must be suspected initially from the clinical signs and symptoms and from epidemiologic considerations. In any patient in whom there is a likelihood of Rocky Mountain spotted fever, appropriate antimicrobial therapy should be started and a definitive diagnosis confirmed by serologic tests using appropriate paired serum.

References

Books

Beeson, P. B., and McDermott, W. (eds.): Textbook of Medicine. 14th ed. Philadelphia, W. B. Saunders Co. 1975.

Davis, B. D., Dulbecco, R., Eisen, H. N., Ginsberg, H. S., Wood, W. B., and McCarty, M.: Microbiology. 2nd ed. Hagerstown, Maryland, Harper and Row, 1973.

Hoeprich, P. D. (ed.): Infectious Diseases. Hagerstown, Maryland, Harper and Row, 1972.

Zinsser, H. (ed.): Rats, Lice and History. Boston, Little, Brown and Co., 1935.

Review Articles

Castleman, B., Scully, R. E., and McNeely, B. U.: Case records of the Massachusetts General Hospital. N. Engl. J. Med. 287:656, 1972.

Hattwick, M. A. W., Peters, A. H., Gregg, M. B., and Hanson, B.: Surveillance of Rocky Mountain spotted fever. J.A.M.A. 225:1338, 1973.

Hazard, G. W., Ganz, R. N., Nevin, R. W., Nauss, A. H., Curtis, E., Bell, W. J., and Murray, E. S.: Rocky Mountain spotted fever in the eastern United States. Thirteen cases from the Cape Cod area of Massachusetts. N. Engl. J. Med. 280:57, 1969.

Lackman, D. B.: A review of information on rickettsialpox in the United States. Clin. Pediatr. 2:296, 1963.

Massachusetts Department of Public Health: On the alert for Rocky Mountain spotted fever. N. Engl. J. Med. 292:1127, 1975

Ormsbee, R. W.: Q fever rickettsia. In Horsfall, F. L., Jr., and Tamm, I. (eds.): Viral and Rickettsial Infections of Man. 4th ed. Philadelphia, J. B. Lippincott Co., 1965, p. 1144.

Smadel, J. E., and Elisberg, B. L.: Scrub typhus rickettsia. In Horsfall, F. L., Jr., and Tamm, I. (eds.): Viral and Rickettsial Infections of Man. 4th ed. Philadelphia, J. B. Lippincott Co., 1965, p. 1130.

Snyder, J. C.: The typhus fevers. In Horsfall, F. L., Jr., and Tamm, I. (eds.): Viral and Rickettsial Infections of Man. 4th ed. Philadelphia, J. B. Lippincott Co., 1965.

Warren, J.: Trench fever rickettsia. In Horsfall, F. L., Jr., and Tamm, I. (eds.): Viral and Rickettsial Infections of Man. 4th ed. Philadelphia, J. B. Lippincott Co., 1965, p. 1161.

Original Articles

Brill, N. E.: An acute infectious disease. A clinical study based on 221 cases of unknown origin. Am. J. Med. Sci. 139:484, 1910.

Gambrill, M. R., and Wisseman, C. L., Jr.: Mechanisms of immunity in typhus infections. II. Multiplication of typhus rickettsiae in human macrophage cell cultures in the nonimmune system: influence of virulence of rickettsial strains and of chloramphenicol. Infect. Immu. 8:519, 1973.

Paterson, P. Y., and Taylor, W.: Rickettsialpox. Bull. N. Y. Acad. Med. 42:579, 1966.

Roueche, B.: The alerting of Mr. Pomerantz. In Roueche, B.: Eleven Blue Men. Boston, Little, Brown and Co., 1954.

Silverman, D. J., Boese, J. L., and Wisseman, C. L., Jr.: Ultrastructural studies of Rickettsia prowazeki from louse mid-gut cells to feces: Search for "dormant" forms. Infect. Immun. *10:*257, 1974.

Smadel, J. E.: Status of the rickettsioses in the United States. Ann. Intern. Med. *51:*421, 1959.

Tigertt, W. D., and Benenson, A. S.: Studies on Q fever in man. Trans. Assoc. Am. Physicians *69:*98, 1956.

Traub, R., and Wisseman, C. L., Jr.: Ecological considerations in scrub typhus. Bull. WHO *39:*209, 1968.

Vinson, J. W., Varela, G., and Molina-Pasquel, C.: Trench fever. III. Induction of clinical disease in volunteers inoculated with Rickettsia quintana propagated on blood agar. Am. J. Trop. Med. *18:*713, 1969.

Wisseman, C. L., Jr., Waddell, A. D., and Walsch, W. T.: Mechanisms of immunity in typhus infections. IV. Failure of chicken embryo cells in culture to restrict growth of antibody-sensitized Rickettsia prowazeki. Infect. Immun. *9:*571, 1974.

Zinsser, H.: Varieties of typhus virus and epidemiology of American form of European typhus fever (Brill's disease). Am. J. Hyg. *20:*513, 1934.

BACTERIAL ENDOCARDITIS

Introduction

Terminology

Bacterial endocarditis is an acute or chronic disease resulting from bacterial invasion of a focal area of endothelium of a heart valve leaflet or cardiac chamber, with continual shedding of the infecting microorganisms into the bloodstream. Clinical manifestations of the disease arise from widespread inflammatory and destructive changes affecting many different organ systems, especially the heart, kidneys, and brain.

Terminology pertaining to this disease often is confusing and restrictive. The qualifying adjective *bacterial* is not altogether satisfactory, since fungi, rickettsias, and spirochaetes also can cause the disease. For this reason, some physicians prefer the term *infectious* endocarditis as a more inclusive designation. The noun *endocarditis* also is too restrictive, since the site of endothelial infection occasionally may be outside the heart, e.g., coarctation of the aorta, patent ductus arteriosus, or an arteriovenous fistula located elsewhere in the circulation. Bacterial endocarditis represents more than an infectious disorder, since many of the major manifestations of the disease have an immunologic pathogenesis. One of the features of bacterial endocarditis is its persistent nature: active disease in untreated patients may last for many weeks or many months. As a result, the disease historically has been called *subacute* bacterial endocarditis or SBE. This designation, however, completely fails to recognize the fact that bacterial endocarditis may present as an acute infection of heart valves and may follow a fulminant course, ending in death in a matter of days or at the most, a week or two. In such acute forms of heart valve infections, urgent diagnostic and therapeutic decision-making is required, and effective antimicrobial therapy must be initiated without delay. For this reason, acute and subacute forms of endocarditis are discussed as separate entities in several sections of this chapter.

Aspects to be Emphasized

Descriptions of the microbiology, clinical and pathologic manifestations, and therapeutic considerations can be found in many textbooks, monographs, numerous reviews, and countless articles. Those aspects of the disease emphasized in this chapter include the following: (1) A practical clinical-etiologic classification, (2) unique host-parasite relationships with important implications for effective diagnosis and therapy, (3) new concepts concerning pathogenesis, including data implicating immunologic factors, (4) the rationale underlying antimicrobial therapy, particularly the synergistic drug effect obtained by using two antimicrobial agents in combination, and (5) prophylaxis.

Clinical-Etiologic Classification

A practical classification of bacterial endocarditis is presented in Table 41–1. The disease is divided into acute and subacute forms based on whether the clinical duration of disease is less than or more than six weeks. Considerable overlap occurs between these two forms of the disease. Nevertheless, consideration of acute and subacute forms of endocarditis as separate entities has important clinical, etiologic, and therapeutic implications.

Acute Bacterial Endocarditis

Acute bacterial endocarditis usually develops on normal cardiac valve endothelial surfaces or within two or three months after implantation of a prosthetic heart valve. The microorganisms most often responsible are gram positive cocci with a high degree of virulence that translates to rapidly evolving and often fulminating lethal infections.

Staphylococcus aureus and *Staphylococcus epidermidis* account for about 10 to 15 per cent of all cases of endocarditis, i.e., acute and subacute forms of the disease combined. Acute staphylococcal endocarditis is especially apt

TABLE 41-1. Clinical-Etiologic Classification of Acute and Subacute
Forms of Bacterial Endocarditis

Features	Acute Form of Disease	Subacute Form of Disease
Duration of disease	Less than six weeks	Six weeks or longer
Cardiovascular status	Normal heart valve or prosthetic valve implant	Rheumatic or congenital heart disease; prosthetic valve implant
Most important causative microorganisms	*Staphylococcus aureus* and *S. epidermidis* *Streptococcus pneumoniae* Lancefield Group A beta-hemolytic streptococci (*Streptococcus pyogenes*) *Neisseria gonorrhoeae* *Pseudomonas aeruginosa*	Viridans streptococci Lancefield Group D enterococci (*Streptococcus faecalis*) Anaerobic or microaerophilic streptococci
Antimicrobial therapeutic regimen	Penicillin class drug (or aminoglycoside for *P. aeruginosa* infections)	Penicillin class drug plus aminoglycoside in combination

to occur among drug abusers, e.g., heroin mainliners or skin poppers. For reasons that are not clear at present, *S. aureus* appears to have a special propensity to initiate infection of the tricuspid valve. This capacity of *S. aureus* to invade normal tricuspid endothelium transcends the fact that this microorganism is frequently introduced into the venous circulation of mainlining heroin addicts. *S. epidermidis,* although a relatively nonpathogenic staphylococcal species under ordinary circumstances, has a notorious capacity to infect recently implanted prosthetic heart valves. It is the most frequent cause of prosthetic heart valve infections occurring within two to three months after surgery.

The number of cases of endocarditis caused by *Streptococcus pneumoniae* and Group A beta-hemolytic streptococci has steadily decreased in recent decades but is still sufficient to deserve attention. Both *S. pneumoniae* and Group A streptococci have a propensity to infect aortic or mitral valves. Acute endocarditis caused by either group of microorganisms often occurs without clinical evidence of infection of other organ systems. Not uncommonly acute cardiac valve infection due to *S. pneumoniae* coincides with development of acute pneumococcal lobar pneumonia. Special emphasis must be given to the unusual capacity of *S. pneumoniae* to invade aortic valve leaflets in patients with acute pneumococcal meningitis. Attention may first be called to the previously unrecognized valve infection when a heart murmur indicative of aortic insufficiency appears during an otherwise uneventful recovery from the meningitis, or when rupture of an infected leaflet precipitates sudden congestive heart failure. Group A beta-hemolytic streptococci, and rarely Group C or G streptococci, presumably initiate valve infections in conjunction with bacteremia associated with respiratory or cutaneous infections. In contrast to the relative ease with which Group A streptococci are eradicated from the upper respiratory tract, these micro-organisms are exceedingly difficult to eradicate once they infect cardiac valves. Although invariably susceptible to penicillin, they can persist for weeks within the platelet-fibrin meshwork of valvular bacterial vegetations despite maintenance of high concentrations of this antimicrobial agent in the bloodstream. This slow and all too often incomplete elimination of streptococci within infected heart valves serves to underline the very limited capacity of infected hosts to eradicate these and other microorganisms from infected heart valves; this limited capacity of the infected host is a unique feature of bacterial endocarditis.

The sharp upturn in venereal disease in the United States in recent years has brought about the reemergence of *Neisseria gonorrhoeae* as a significant cause of acute endocarditis. The alleged predilection of this microorganism to infect the pulmonic valve has not been noted in recent years as often as it was during the 1920s and 1930s. However, the occurrence of double temperature spikes each day, as described in recently reported cases of endocarditis due to *N. gonorrhoeae,* does duplicate this feature of gonococcal endocarditis as recorded in the earlier literature.

Finally, *Pseudomonas aeruginosa* is becoming increasingly more signifi-cant as a cause of acute bacterial endocarditis in drug addicts. This is the only gram negative bacillus causing endocarditis with such frequency as to warrant inclusion in Table 41–1. The fact that other gram negative bacilli are rarely implicated in endocarditis has attracted the attention of physicians for decades. Only recently has some light been cast upon this feature of the disease (see discussion later in this chapter).

From a therapeutic standpoint, all acute forms of endocarditis listed in Table 41–1, except that caused by *Pseudomonas aeruginosa,* can be treated with large doses of either penicillin G or one of the other penicillin-class drugs. Semisynthetic penicillin derivatives such as nafcillin or methicillin are essential for the treatment of most of the staphylococcal infections that are caused by penicillinase-producing strains.

Subacute Bacterial Endocarditis

As indicated in Table 41–1, the vast majority of cases of subacute bacterial endocarditis are caused by different species of the genus Strepto-coccus. The greatest number of cases is due to the heterogeneous group of streptococci referred to as alpha-hemolytic or viridans streptococci.* These microorganisms are responsible for about 80 per cent or more of instances of subacute endocarditis; this number corresponds to approximately 50 per cent of all cases of bacterial endocarditis (i.e., the total number of patients with

---

*As already discussed in Chapter 13, a variety of different species and subspecies compose what is traditionally called the viridans streptococcus group of microorganisms. There is no species that can be designated *Streptococcus viridans* per se. The viridans group of streptococci also are referred to as alpha-hemolytic streptococci, emphasizing the type of hemolytic reaction these microorganisms give on blood agar. They are referred to in this chapter simply as "viridans streptococci."

acute and subacute forms of the disease). These relatively avirulent microorganisms presumably can colonize only endothelial surfaces previously damaged by rheumatic inflammation or altered as a consequence of abnormal cardiodynamics associated with congenital cardiac malformations.

Viridans streptococci, representing a diverse number of different species, are a major part of the normal microbial flora of the oropharynx (see Chaps. 7 and 13). They selectively colonize the periodontal tissues, where they can flourish in almost pure culture under appropriate conditions. Therefore, dental surgery or instrumentation of the upper respiratory tract, especially cleaning of the teeth or extraction of a tooth, may figure prominently in the history of many patients with subacute bacterial endocarditis due to viridans streptococci.

Lancefield Group D enterococci include several species or subspecies: *Streptococcus faecalis,* which is the type-species, *Streptococcus faecium, Streptococcus durans, Streptococcus zymogenes,* and *Streptococcus lique-faciens.* These microorganisms can be found in the normal intestinal microbial flora. In contrast to viridans streptococci indigenous to the oral cavity, *S. faecalis* and probably the other enterococci as well can infect either normal or altered endothelial surfaces and are frequently implicated in infections of implanted prosthetic valves that occur more than three months after heart surgery. In addition, *S. faecalis* also occasionally causes an acute form of endocardial infection with a clinical course as stormy and fast moving as endocarditis caused by staphylococci. The usual clinical setting of acute or subacute endocarditis due to *S. faecalis* is pregnancy or instrumentation or surgery of the genitourinary tract; therefore, older men with prostatic enlargement and urinary tract infections and young women of child-bearing age represent a high proportion of cases of enterococcal endocarditis.

Very little is known about the clinical setting of anaerobic or micro-aerophilic streptococcal endocardial infections. The relative importance of these microorganisms seems to be increasing, probably because of the greater awareness of anaerobic infections in general and ever-improving methods for isolating these microorganisms from the blood and propagating them in the clinical microbiology laboratory. It is of interest that many strains of anaerobic streptococci cannot grow at the oxidation-reduction potential of arterial blood; in theory they should not cause endocardial infections. Once these microorganisms are enmeshed in the fibrin deposits characterizing cardiac valve bacterial vegetations, however, the environment is suitable for their growth, which leads to more fibrin deposition which in turn creates a better milieu for replication.

Effective therapy for endocarditis caused by enterococci and penicillin-resistant viridans streptococci requires using two antimicrobial drugs in combination: a penicillin-class drug and an aminoglycoside antimicrobial agent. As discussed later in this chapter (see Therapy section), this drug combination has a synergistic effect on these microorganisms that translates to accelerated killing both in vitro and in vivo. Evidence is mounting in support of the theory that more rapid eradication of many penicillin-suscep-tible viridans streptococci and some strains of anaerobic-microaerophilic streptococci may also be accomplished using this type of antimicrobial drug combination.

Unique Host-Parasite Relationships

Bacteremia and Blood Cultures

Bacterial endocarditis essentially represents an infection of the intravascular compartment. Variable numbers of microorganisms are shed from the site of endothelial infection into the circulation; therefore, persistent bacteremia is a feature of the disease. Blood cultures almost always are positive in acute endocarditis, a condition in which large numbers of microorganisms are present in the bloodstream. One exception is *Neisseria gonorrhoeae*; recovery of this fastidious gram negative coccus can be a problem (see Chap. 30). In subacute endocarditis of streptococcal origin, blood cultures in 85 to 90 per cent of cases may be expected to yield the causative microorganism.

The overall high yield of positive blood cultures in both acute and subacute forms of endocarditis is fortunate on two counts. Recovery of the etiologic microorganism is the sine qua non for definitive diagnosis. Furthermore, isolation of the causative bacterium allows its antimicrobial susceptibility pattern, especially to synergistic action of combinations of antimicrobial drugs, to be determined. This is often a critical step in devising effective eradicative therapy (discussed later in this chapter).

It is important to note that relatively small numbers of bacteria are circulating in a significant proportion of patients with subacute endocarditis. Quantitative blood cultures in a large series of patients with enterococcal endocarditis have revealed that many blood samples contain only 1 to 50 microorganisms per milliliter. In light of this observation, it is crucial to use a large volume of blood for culture so that a sufficient number of infectious units will be inoculated into the culture medium to initiate growth. As discussed elsewhere (see Chap. 10), a volume of 10 ml appears to be satisfactory. In some series of patients with enterococcal endocarditis in which 10 ml of blood was routinely used for each culture, 95 per cent of all blood cultures taken yielded the causative microorganism. In another series in which 5 ml of blood was used, only 50 per cent of cultures gave positive results.

There are several explanations for persistently negative blood cultures in some patients with bacterial endocarditis. First, phagocytosis and killing of microorganisms by circulating segmented neutrophils and monocytes may prevent accumulation of numbers of viable extracellular bacteria at the time of venipuncture sufficient to initiate growth. Indeed, examination of stained smears of glutaraldehyde-fixed peripheral blood cells that have been allowed to adhere to coverslip preparations may reveal intracellular gram positive cocci in some cases of bacterial endocarditis in which blood cultures failed to show growth. Second, bacteria with defective cell walls following exposure to antimicrobial drugs may be incapable of surviving and replicating in hypo-osmolar blood culture medium. Studies to substantiate this theory and retrieve putative osmotically sensitive bacteria by using hyper-osmolar culture media have so far met with only limited success. Third, histopathologic studies have revealed that dense deposits of fibrin and platelets may constitute the outermost layers of bacterial vegetations. Conceivably in such instances bacteria are unable to enter the circulation and the disease will follow a truly "abacteremic" course.

Ineffective Host Defenses

Bacterial endocarditis, when not treated with antimicrobial drugs, is a fatal disease with rare exceptions. This is true no matter what form the disease follows and what type of microorganism is responsible. Prior to the availability of penicillin in the early 1940s, virtually all patients died. It is obvious that the host has essentially no means for sterilizing microcolonies of bacteria within a vegetation. This is true even when the causative microbes are relatively nonpathogenic microorganisms such as viridans streptococci.

The reason(s) for this completely inadequate host defense is (are) not entirely clear. The explanation usually offered is as follows. The bacterial vegetation develops among connective tissue fibers devoid of any significant blood supply. The comparatively avascular nature of the vegetation presumably prevents delivery of antibody, complement, and phagocytes within the core of the vegetation sufficient to control the growth of the microorganisms. Mention already has been made of deposits of fibrin and platelets on the outermost layers of the vegetation, including that portion in contact with the circulation. Accumulation of fibrin-platelet deposits may well prevent circulating host immune factors from penetrating the vegetation. It should be emphasized that faulty blood supply to the bacterial vegetation and enveloping layers of fibrin and platelets not only restricts passage of host immune factors but also prevents delivery of effective concentrations of antimicrobial agents to the core of the vegetation. Both of these factors, i.e., inadequate host defense and suboptimal concentrations of antimicrobial drugs within the vegetation, help explain why some cases of endocarditis are refractory to treatment and why many cases have a propensity for relapse if not treated effectively.

Pathogenesis

Development of Bacterial Vegetations

One of the most intriguing questions in bacterial endocarditis is why bacteria that happen to be in the circulation exhibit such a striking propensity to invade only certain areas of vascular endothelium. These sites of predilection usually coincide with occurrence of high pressure gradients across narrow orifices, e.g., aortic and mitral valves, coarctation of the aorta, and arteriovenous fistulae. Colonization of endothelium by microorganisms most commonly occurs at points of traumatic impact, e.g., points of closure of valve cusps. Bacterial vegetations that result usually develop on the "downstream" or low pressure side of the gradient.

Pressure gradients associated with normal or abnormal cardiac valves, as well as gradients created by congenital malformations, are believed to render endothelium more susceptible to bacterial implantation and colonization.

Special emphasis is placed on the Venturi effect, i.e., lack of lateral pressure immediately distal to the orifice through which a pressure gradient develops. Pressure and flow dynamics might allow bacteria to have more prolonged contact with endothelial cells at such sites. Lack of lateral pressure also might favor formation of fibrin-platelet thrombi that conceivably provide an especially favorable milieu for bacterial implantation and colonization. Thrombi of varying sizes are commonly found at autopsy at sites of predilection for endocarditis in normal hearts, a process termed *nonbacterial thrombotic endocarditis* or *marantic endocarditis.* These thrombi most commonly are seen in patients with advanced malnutrition or long standing, debilitating diseases characterized by "wasting." According to this line of thinking, antecedent thrombus formation is an essential initial event in the pathogenesis of bacterial endocarditis.

It should be noted, however, that bacterial vegetations can be readily produced at sites of trivial endothelial injury in experimental animals that have been given anticoagulants. In this setting, formation of even minute fibrin-platelet thrombi has been excluded. Furthermore, the thrombi not infrequently found on arterial atheromatous plaques and the mural thrombi overlying areas of subendothelial injury associated with myocardial infarction are rarely colonized by microorganisms. Indeed, those bacteria that occasionally do invade such thrombi, e.g., Salmonella species, are practically never implicated in bacterial endocarditis (see Table 41–1 and Chap. 31). In addition to thrombus formation, factors still unknown but clearly intimately related to pressure gradients must play a major role in the development of bacterial vegetations.

Another enigma of bacterial endocarditis is why different species of microorganisms are assoociated with different types of disease (see Table 41–1). Why should such relatively nonpathogenic microorganisms as viridans streptococci, which are essentially unable to produce any other disease, be responsible for most cases of subacute bacterial endocarditis? Why are gram negative bacilli so rarely implicated in view of the frequency of bacteremia due to these microorganisms? Recent studies indicate that those microorganisms most often causing endocarditis exhibit a high degree of adherence to normal human heart valves or monolayers of explanted cardiac endothelial tissue. Viewed in this light, staphylococci, streptococci, *Pseudomonas aeruginosa,* etc., which happen to be transiently present in the circulation, may preferentially bind to endothelial cells and have an advantage over *Escherichia coli, Klebsiella pneumoniae,* and other microorganisms in colonizing endothelial cells.

Although bacteria–endothelial cell adherence is an attractive idea, it does not account for occurrence of infection at specific sites of endothelium unless one assumes that endothelial receptors responsible for bacterial adherence have a remarkably restricted anatomic distribution. Moreover, if antecedent thrombus formation is important, such thrombi would be expected to "mask" receptor sites on endothlial cells and preclude specific bacterial adherence. Finally, all studies of bacterial adherence to vascular endothelium have involved normal heart valves. It would be more important to know the comparative adherence of different bacteria to endothelium that has been altered by acquired or congenital heart disease. The endothelial surface of valves afflicted by rheumatic inflammation consists not of "normal" endothelial cells but altered cells covering a connective tissue scar resulting from the underlying rheumatic disease. Conceivably viridans streptococci and enterococci may adhere to such altered endothelial cells to an even greater degree than to normal endothelial cells. Such a hypothesis, if true, would provide a plausible explanation for the prominent role of these micro-organisms in subacute forms of endocarditis.

Peripheral Manifestations of Endocarditis

The bacterial vegetation grows in size partly as a result of deposits of fibrin and platelets being added to its external surfaces. This process causes the vegetation to become large and friable. Variably sized fragments of the vegetation may break off and embolize, causing infarcts in remote tissues. If the fibrin fragments contain viable bacteria, i.e., represent septic emboli, infection at the sites of embolism may occur.

For decades the peripheral manifestations of endocarditis affecting the brain, skin, and kidneys were thought to be caused exclusively by emboli derived from the bacterial vegetation. To be sure, major embolic events can occur with catastrophic results, e.g., occlusion of a cerebrovascular artery with hemiplegia or total obstruction of a major artery with a cold, pulseless extremity. However, the peripheral manifestations specifically under discussion here are more common and more subtle in nature, and occur in a high proportion of patients. These manifestations include the following: transient focal neurologic signs frequently referred to as *toxic encephalopathy*; visible petechial or other hemorrhagic lesions occurring in the skin, conjunctivae, nail beds, or fundi; and gross or microscopic hematuria, heavy albuminuria, and diminished renal function.

Immunohistopathologic studies have revaled that these manifestations usually are not on an embolic basis with disruption of the capillary bed but result from active inflammation of small vessels, i.e., acute vasculitis. From a morphologic standpoint, the vascular inflammatory changes are often indistinguishable from those termed *hypersensitivity angiitis*. In the kidney, focal or diffuse glomerulonephritis is a frequent finding and closely resembles the acute or subacute glomerulonephritis observed in association with Group A hemolytic streptococcal infections (see Chap. 16).

Briefly, the evidence for immunologically mediated vasculitis in endocarditis is as follows:

1. Nearly two thirds of patients with the subacute form of the disease develop high titers of rheumatoid factor, an antibody restricted to IgM and directed against antigenic determinants on IgG. Rheumatoid factor is usually detected and quantitated by its capacity to agglutinate latex particles coated with normal human IgG. In this situation, the IgM rheumatoid factor is acting as an antibody reactive with IgG, which serves as the "antigen." It appears that much of this IgG antigen in patients with subacute bacterial endocarditis is in fact antibody, produced by the host in response to persistent antigenic stimulation by the microorganism responsible for the disease. In the course of continually elaborating immunoglobulins directed against the microbe, some

of the IgG molecules become altered to such an extent that they are recognized as foreign by the host. The foreign IgG molecules, although still retaining antibody activity and reacting with the microbe, serve as antigens and elicit an IgM immune response expressed as rheumatoid factor. A significantly elevated latex agglutination titer is indicative of circulating IgM antibody (rheumatoid factor), a variable portion of which is attached to IgG in the form of an immune complex. It is known that circulating IgG–IgM immune complexes can cause acute vasculitis in experimental animals.

2. In patients with evidence of glomerulonephritis, total complement activity, based on hemolytic assay, is decreased and concentrations of C3 or C4, as determined by immunologic assays, may be diminished. These complement components, as well as total complement activity, usually are increased in patients with infectious-inflammatory disorders, representing "acute phase" protein responses. Diminished total complement activity or depressed values of C3 or C4 in a patient with fever, heart murmur, and hematuria may be the initial clue to the diagnosis of bacterial endocarditis.

3. Deposits of IgG, IgM, and C3 are usually demonstrable within small blood vessels involved in peripheral manifestations of endocarditis. In one patient studied in detail at autopsy and in whom there was extensive intraglomerular deposition of IgG, the immunoglobulin was eluted from renal tissues. A significant portion of the eluted IgG was shown to react specifically with the strain of *Streptococcus faecalis* isolated from antemortem blood cultures of the patient.

It is not known whether the acute vasculitis in endocarditis results from interaction of antibody with microbial antigen deposited in peripheral tissues during bacteremia sustained over long periods of time or results from deposition of circulating immune complexes, e.g., IgG–IgM complexes or bacterial antigen-IgG complexes, at selected sites within the peripheral circulation.

Therapy

Prerequisite for Bactericidal Antimicrobial Drug Action

The inability of the host to eradicate microorganisms from endothelial vegetations (see section on Pathogenesis) places a unique emphasis on the effectiveness of antimicrobial regimens if the patient is to survive. There is virtually no other infectious disease in which such a premium is placed on the capacity of antimicrobial drugs to eliminate bacteria without assistance from the infected host.

Successful antimicrobial drug therapy for bacterial endocarditis demands close attention in order to identify a therapeutic regimen that has a bactericidal action. If there is any fact to be emphasized here, it is the woeful lack of correlation between results of in vitro antimicrobial susceptibility tests that only determine what concentration of an antimicrobial drug inhibits growth of microorganisms, i.e., the minimal inhibitory concentration (see Chap. 45), and the effectiveness of that drug in the treatment of endocarditis. In vitro tests that determine the minimum concentration having a bactericidal effect (see Chap. 45) are essential.

Antimicrobial Drug Regimens

Endocarditis Due to Streptococci

Major attention is devoted here to this type of bacterial endocarditis because questions, e.g., What drugs to use? For how long?, arise most frequently in this type.

Identification of Streptococcal Isolates. It is essential to distinguish accurately members of the viridans streptococcal group from typical Lancefield Group D enterococci as represented by *Streptococcus faecalis.* Precise identification is very important because about 85 per cent of viridans streptococcal strains and essentially all isolates of *Streptococcus bovis* (a nonenterococcal member of the Group D streptococci) are highly susceptible to penicillin. Therapy for endocarditis due to these penicillin-susceptible streptococci is less complicated and has a better outlook than that required for disease caused by penicillin-resistant *S. faecalis* (as outlined later in this section).

Hemolytic reactions on blood agar by different strains of non–Group A streptococci vary considerably and may be difficult to interpret (see Chap. 13). Many other determinant characteristics, i.e., growth in selective media, hydrolysis of different carbohydrates, reactivity with Lancefield precipitating antisera, and in vitro susceptibility to different antimicrobial drugs, are therefore used for identification and speciation of streptococci.

Determination of Penicillin-Susceptibility of Streptococcal Isolates. Of equal importance to accurate identification of streptococci is their precise penicillin susceptibility, as determined by tube dilution assays (see Chap. 45). Streptococcal isolates with penicillin minimum inhibitory concentrations of 0.1 to 0.5 units per ml (0.6 to 0.3 μg per ml) are arbitrarily classified as penicillin susceptible. Streptococci with penicillin minimum inhibitory concentrations greater than 0.5 units per ml (0.3 μg per ml) are designated as penicillin resistant. All enterococcal strains are penicillin resistant, and from 1 to 25 units or more of penicillin is required for inhibition of growth. Most strains are inhibited by 6 to 12 units per ml. About 15 per cent of the strains of viridans streptococci exhibit comparable degrees of penicillin resistance, further illustrating the heterogeneity of the viridans streptococcal group of microorganisms.

Therapy for Penicillin-Resistant Streptococcal Infections. Endocarditis infections caused by penicillin-resistant streptococci (as defined previously) must be treated with a combination of a penicillin-class drug and an aminoglycoside antimicrobial agent. The combination employed most often is penicillin plus streptomycin. These two drugs are used even though the clinical microbiologic laboratory antimicrobial susceptibility data reveal that the streptococcal isolate is resistant to both of these drugs when tested individually but is susceptible to representative members of other antimicrobial drug classes. The combination of penicillin and streptomycin exerts a synergistic bactericidal effect on about two thirds of penicillin-resistant streptococcal strains. By synergistic effect is meant a bactericidal action greater than would be expected by the sum of each drug alone (see Chap. 44).

The basis for this synergism is illustrated in Figure 41–1. Penicillin in concentrations readily achieved in vivo causes the cell wall of enterococci to

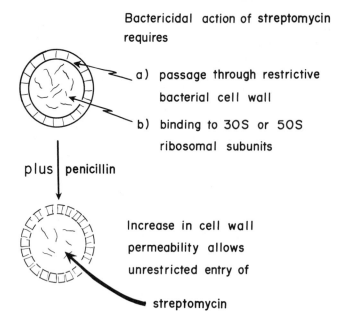

Bactericidal action of streptomycin requires

a) passage through restrictive bacterial cell wall

b) binding to 30S or 50S ribosomal subunits

plus | penicillin

Increase in cell wall permeability allows unrestricted entry of

streptomycin

Figure 41–1. Schematic representation of postulated synergistic bactericidal activity of penicillin plus streptomycin for enterococci.

become more permeable. Increased permeability of the cell wall allows streptomycin to enter the bacteria and bind to the 30S and 50S ribosomal subunits, resulting in a potent bactericidal effect. It is the bactericidal activity of the streptomycin that accounts for the capacity of this combination of antimicrobial drugs to eradicate enterococcal infections. Enterococcal isolates reportedly can be screened to determine in advance which strains will be susceptible to a synergistic action of penicillin and streptomycin; strains inhibited by 2000 μg per ml of streptomycin alone usually are susceptible to accelerated bactericidal action of penicillin plus streptomycin; those strains that are not inhibited by this high concentration of streptomycin are not susceptible.

Strains of enterococci not susceptible to synergistic killing with penicillin and streptomycin combinations usually can be readily killed if gentamicin is substituted for streptomycin in the combination. Antimicrobial drugs other than penicillin that also prevent cell wall formation, such as vancomycin, can be used with any one of the aminoglycoside antimicrobial agents to obtain a synergistic action.

Irrespective of what particular drug combination is used, treatment of penicillin-resistant streptococcal endocarditis almost invariably must be given for a period of at least six weeks if cure is to be anticipated. Recent case reports suggest that this period of therapy may be shortened to a month or even less when using a drug combination of gentamicin and penicillin;

however, additional experience with this drug combination is required before the six-week rule warrants revision.

Therapy for Penicillin-Susceptible Streptococcal Infections. Endocarditis due to penicillin-susceptible viridans streptococci and *Streptococcus bovis* can be treated with penicillin alone for six weeks. Preferably, a combination of penicillin and streptomycin can be used for two or three weeks. The success of this short-term treatment regimen for endocarditis caused by penicillin-susceptible streptococci has been demonstrated many times over in large series of cases. Recent studies in vitro and in experimental animals have shown that penicillin-streptomycin combinations indeed exert a synergistic bactericidal effect on many strains of penicillin-susceptible viridans streptococci.

Patients with a history indicative of severe penicillin allergy and in whom use of penicillin or any penicillin-class drug is contraindicated can be effectively treated with vancomycin in combination with an aminoglycoside antimicrobial drug.

Endocarditis Due to Other Microorganisms

Staphylococcal infections are treated with semisynthetic penicillinase-resistant derivatives of penicillin until in vitro testing demonstrates that the strain in question is penicillin susceptible. Treatment should be continued for six weeks. Relapse and the necessity for retreatment, with increased risk of irreversible valve damage, usually are the price paid for shorter courses of therapy.

Pseudomonas aeruginosa infections can be extremely refractory to treatment. Experience is limited and no guidelines for therapy can be spelled out at present. Aminoglycoside antimicrobial agents clearly are the pivotal drugs in those patients who have survived.

Adjuncts to Antimicrobial Therapy

Surgical excision of an infected valve or prosthetic valve implant is indicated in the following situations: (1) when medical therapy with antimicrobial drugs clearly has failed, and (2) when a valve leaflet ruptures or an infected prosthetic implant becomes displaced, resulting in congestive heart failure that is unresponsive to the usual medical therapy. Increasing experience with combined medical-surgical approaches to endocarditis indicates that valves should be replaced much earlier than judged advisable in the past and when the patient is still a good operative risk (see Case Presentation 1 at the end of this chapter).

Life-threatening peripheral manifestations of bacterial endocarditis, e.g., lateralizing neurologic signs, may respond dramatically to the use of corticosteroids for a few days because of the capacity of these drugs to reduce the inflammation associated with acute vasculitis. If the causative microorganism has been identified and is known to be susceptible to the antimicrobial drug regimen being employed, short-term use of corticosteroids will not interfere with eradicating the infection.

Prophylaxis

Details concerning the rationale for the methods of administering antimicrobial drugs to patients with congential or rheumatic valvular heart disease and who are at increased risk of acquiring bacterial endocarditis can be found in a statement published under the auspices of the American Heart Association. In this statement, mention is also made of procedures known to precipitate transitory bacteremia. Two points should be emphasized here. First, patients receiving long-term daily penicillin by mouth to prevent recurrences of rheumatic fever may harbor large numbers of penicillin-resistant viridans streptococci in their oropharynxes. To prevent the occurrence of bacterial endocarditis in such patients, erythromycin instead of parenteral injections of penicillin should be used for two or three days prior to surgery or other procedures involving the upper respiratory tract, especially dental manipulation. Second, instrumentation or surgery involving the gastrointestinal or genitourinary tract may cause bacteremia due to penicillin-resistant enterococci. Prophylaxis in patients in whom transitory bacteremia due to enterococci may be anticipated should receive both a penicillin class drug and an aminoglycoside antimicrobial drug for two or three days.

CASE PRESENTATION 1

A 39-year-old white male was hospitalized during the early evening of December 2. The patient had been found totally disoriented and thrashing around in his bed by a friend and was brought to the hospital by ambulance. The friend who accompanied the patient believed that the patient was a drug abuser.

Major physical findings included a temperature of 104.8°F (rectally), a pulse of 126 per minute, a blood pressure of 130/60 mm Hg, and respirations, 24 per minute. The patient was acutely ill and disoriented with respect to time, place, and person. His pharynx was very erythematous but no exudates were observed. His neck was resistant to dorsiflexion. Numerous petechial lesions, 1 to 3 mm in size, were noted over both lower legs. There was an area of ischemic necrosis involving the medial aspect of the right great toe.

Laboratory data included a total leukocyte count of 11,000 per cubic millimeter, with 63 per cent mature segmented neutrophils and 24 per cent band forms; urine showed 2+ albumin.

The diagnosis made at the time of admission was acute meningococcal septicemia and meningitis. A lumbar puncture was performed and revealed turbid cerebrospinal fluid containing 13,000 leukocytes per cubic millimeter, 100 per cent of which were segmented neutrophils; the glucose level was 67 mg per 100 ml and protein was 40 mg per 100 ml. A simultaneously performed blood glucose was 108 ml per 100 ml. A Gram stained smear of the cerebrospinal fluid revealed no evidence of microorganisms. Antimicrobial therapy with large doses of intravenous nafcillin was initiated promptly.

Twenty-four hours after hospitalization, the clinical microbiology laboratory reported that a gram positive coccus was growing in two blood cultures that had been taken prior to initiation of antimicrobial therapy; hemolytic streptococci were also noted on the blood agar plate streaked with a pharyngeal swab specimen. On December 4, the bacterial isolate from the blood cultures was reported to be a Group A streptococcus, as was the hemolytic streptococcus isolated from the oropharynx. The spinal fluid culture remained sterile.

On December 6, a widening pulse pressure and a soft blowing diastolic murmur heard best along the lower left border of the sternum provided compelling clinical evidence for acute endocarditis of the aortic valve due to Group A hemolytic streptococci.

Despite intensive therapy initially with nafcillin and subsequently with penicillin G (when the blood isolate was identified), the patient remained febrile, showed evidence of increasing aortic insufficiency, and developed congestive heart failure. The congestive heart failure soon proved refractory to medical management. On Dec. 28, therefore, serious consideration was given to surgical implantation of a prosthetic aortic valve. Cardiac surgery was deferred, however, because it was felt that the patient would not survive the operation. The patient was found dead, lying in his bed, during the morning of January 2.

Autopsy revealed large vegetations on two aortic cusps and several perforations of the involved valve leaflets. Appropriately stained sections of the valvular vegetations revealed innumerable gram positive cocci; unfortunately, no cultures were made of the involved valves or vegetations. Microscopic sections of the aortic valve subsequently revealed that the acute bacterial infection was largely confined to the leaflets and did not encroach significantly on the base of the valves.

The clinical presentation strongly suggested acute meningococcal disease. The cutaneous lesions were consistent with meningococcemia, and initial evaluation of the patient revealed classic signs of meningitis. The admitting physician believed this patient's disease was of meningococcal origin. The history of drug abuse and more detailed physical exmination of the extremities, which revealed sclerosed veins, provided strong evidence that the patient was a heroin mainliner. Therefore, the attending physician felt that septicemia due to microorganisms indigenous to the skin or commonly only associated with skin trauma must be included in the differential diagnosis. In accordance with this line of thinking, therapy with nafcillin was initiated. This antimicrobial agent was selected because it would be effective against a penicillinase-secreting staphylococcus as well as a penicillin-susceptible staphylococcus, meningococcus, and streptococcus. Without detailed serotyping of the blood and oropharyngeal isolates of the Group A streptococcus, it is impossible to determine whether or not the strain in question was one frequently associated with skin infections (see Chap. 36). However, the frequency of bacteremia in mainlining drug addicts would support the notion that the streptococcus causing the infection of the aortic valve originally was part of the microbial flora of the skin rather than the oropharynx.

Clinical signs of meningitis unaccompanied by evidence of bacterial infection of the leptomeninges (normal cerebrospinal fluid glucose concentration and a failure to observe microorganisms in the Gram stained smear or isolate any microorganisms from the fluid on culture) is a not infrequent set of findings in patients with bacterial endocarditis. It is not clear whether the clinical and laboratory abnormalities in this patient represented vasculitis of the central nervous system or embolization by fragments of the bacterial vegetation to the brain, with microinfarcts occurring close to the meninges and eliciting the inflammatory changes noted in the cerebrospinal fluid.

The autopsy findings emphasize the indolent nature of streptococcal infections when they involve cardiac valves. It is worth noting that in retrospect an earlier consideration of heart surgery and decision to excise the infected and damaged aortic valve and implant an aortic prosthetic device might well have proved lifesaving. This therapeutic approach would have corrected the congestive failure, thereby buying more time for intensive antimicrobial drug therapy to eradicate whatever residual infection might still have existed at the site of valve extirpation. Lack of invasion of the bases of the aortic valves by bacteria suggests that in this case there was little danger that the prosthetic valve would have become infected, as often occurs when it is necessary to sew the valve ring into an already infected field.

Mention should also be made of the failure carefully to collect appropriate autopsy tissue specimens for detailed microbiologic study. This is a not uncommon error of omission. In this case, it prevented the physicians from learning whether viable Group A streptococci still existed within the bacterial vegetation after four and one half weeks of intensive therapy with nafcillin and penicillin G. The presence of bacteria in histologic sections gives no information concerning this important point.

CASE PRESENTATION 2*

A 61-year-old white female was hospitalized because of persistent fever of four months' duration. Past history revealed that seven months previously the patient had undergone an uneventful routine cholecystectomy and ventral hernia repair. Bladder catheterization was not required following surgery. Her postoperative course was complicated by development of a wound infection from which a non–Group A beta-hemolytic streptococcus was cultured. At the time of discharge from the hospital, the wound was no longer draining and the patient was afebrile. Approximately three weeks later the patient developed a fever spiking to 101 to 103°F daily, accompanied by night sweats, chills, and bilateral flank pain. She was told by her physician that she had a urinary tract infection and was treated with a "sulfa drug" for a few weeks and then received several courses of "expensive antibiotics" because of the persistent low grade fever and night sweats. During the month preceding her second hospitalization, increasing dyspnea on exertion, together with severe weakness, was noted. There was no history of rheumatic fever or cardiac disease; no dental work had been performed within the past two years.

---

*This case was originally reported as one of the first patients to be cured of enterococcal endocarditis following treatment with a combination of vancomycin and streptomycin. (From Westenfelder, G. O., Paterson, P. Y., Reisberg, B. E., and Carlson, G. M.: Vancomycin-streptomycin synergism in enterococcal endocarditis. J.A.M.A. *223:*37, 1973. Copyright 1973, American Medical Association.)

At the time of the patient's second hospital admission, physical examination revealed the following: temperature, 102°F; pulse rate, 120 per minute; blood pressure, 160/40 mm Hg; and respirations, 20 to 24 per minute. The patient appeared pale and acutely ill; she was slightly obese. Several petechial lesions were observed over the lower legs; the retina of the left eye had a Roth spot. The lungs were clear. The heart was grossly enlarged to the left. A grade III/VI aortic blowing decrescendo diastolic murmur, together with a grade II/VI aortic systolic ejection murmur, was readily heard along the left sternal border. Splenomegaly was present, and the edge of the spleen was felt 3 cm below the left costal margin.

Initial laboratory work revealed the following: hematocrit, 33 ml per 100 ml; and total leukocyte count, 5700 cells per cubic millimeter, with 76 per cent segmented neutrophils, 3 per cent immature neutrophils, 17 per cent lymphocytes, and 4 per cent monocytes. The urine contained 15 to 20 erythrocytes per high power field but otherwise was within normal limits; no bacteria were evident in the urine. During the next few days, three of six blood cultures that had been collected during the first 48 hours of hospitalization were reported to have yielded a gram positive coccus identified as an enterococcus and confirmed to be a Group D enterococcus by the Lancefield precipitin technique. The blood culture isolate was speciated and eventually was reported as *Streptococcus faecalis*. In vitro antimicrobial susceptibility tests revealed a penicillin minimal inhibitory concentration of 3.13 units per ml and a streptomycin minimal inhibitory concentration of greater than 100 μg per ml. A latex fixation test for rheumatoid factor was positive in a titer of 1:640; total serum complement activity was 18 units per ml (normal 40 to 50 units per ml). The patient was started on a therapeutic regimen of penicillin plus streptomycin.

This is a fairly typical presentation of subacute bacterial endocarditis caused by *Streptococcus faecalis*. Note that there was no past history of cardiac disease, and no mention was made of a heart murmur at the time of surgery. Presumably, therefore, the enterococcal infection in this patient developed on a normal aortic valve, a situation that appears to occur in nearly 40 per cent of patients with enterococcal valve infection.

The microorganism responsible for the wound infection may well have been a Group D enterococcus. A small percentage of enterococcal strains give a beta-hemolytic reaction on blood agar (see Chap. 13). The wound infection may have been the source of the bacteremia that resulted in heart valve colonization and initiation of the bacterial vegetation. In retrospect, a greater effort should have been made to identify the streptococcus isolated from the surgical wound infection.

The clinical illness that developed following the patient's initial discharge from the hospital may have been an acute urinary tract infection with pyelonephritis, as suggested by the high fever, chills, and bilateral flank pain. It is noteworthy that the patient could provide no information as to whether her urine contained "pus cells" or bacteria at this time, implying that detailed study of her urine may not have been carried out. In any event, the evolving illness soon acquired many of the clinical hallmarks of bacterial endocarditis. Since the etiologic agent proved to be *Streptococcus faecalis*, a not infrequent cause of urinary tract infections (see Chaps. 27 and 28), it is reasonable to assume that urinary tract infection and bacteremia due to this microorganism were the initial events leading to infection of the aortic valve.

The several months that elapsed between the estimated time of onset of bacterial endocarditis and the definitive diagnosis of the disease as confirmed by positive blood cultures is not unusual. All too often, the subtle manifestations of the disease, many of which divert attention away from the heart, lead to delay that can stretch into many months. Repetitive courses of suppressive but not eradicative antimicrobial therapy cause further postponement of inclusive evaluation of a persistent febrile disorder. The extensive use of antimicrobial drugs also may account for the fact that negative blood cultures are obtained, creating more delay in the determination of the true nature of the underlying disease.

At the time of rehospitalization, the patient had cardinal manifestations of bacterial endocarditis of the subacute form, i.e., fever, anemia, and wide pulse pressure indicative of aortic insufficiency, which was almost certainly caused by valve destruction and malfunction secondary to the bacterial vegetations. The cutaneous manifestations of the disease probably reflect underlying immunologically mediated small vessel inflammation. The same no doubt holds for the vascular lesion in the left eye, viz., the Roth spot. The microscopic hematuria accompanied by markedly depressed serum complement activity almost certainly is indicative of subacute focal or diffuse glomerulonephritis, a type of renal lesion found in a high proportion of patients with subacute endocardial infections. The strongly positive test for rheumatoid factor provides additional support for the diagnosis of subacute bacterial endocarditis and offers evidence for the theory that immunologic mechanisms play an important role in the pathogenesis of this disease.

Definitive diagnosis was established by isolation of a Group D enterococcus identified as *Streptococcus faecalis*. Although the enterococcus was resistant to penicillin and streptomycin, both drugs were selected for initial antimicrobial therapy; the use of this combination is consistent with attempts to achieve a maximal synergistic bactericidal effect capable of eradicating the bacteria from the heart valve. One would have liked to know the exact streptomycin minimal inhibitory concentration, since that information might have allowed the attending physician to predict in advance whether or not the penicillin-streptomycin combination would exert a synergistic effect on the enterococcal strain causing infection in this patient.

References

Book

Kerr, A.: Subacute Bacterial Endocarditis. Springfield, Illinois, Charles C Thomas, 1955.

Review Articles

Kaye, D.: Changes in the spectrum, diagnosis and management of bacterial and fungal endocarditis. Med. Clin. North Am. *57:* 941, 1973.

Paterson, P. Y.: Bacterial endocarditis prophylaxis. *In* Matson, J. M., and Wannamaker, L. W. (eds.): Streptococci and Streptococcal Diseases: Recognition, Understanding and Management. New York, Academic Press, 1972.

Weinstein, L., and Schlesinger, J. J.: Pathoanatomic, pathophysiologic and clinical correlations in endocarditis. N. Engl. J. Med. *291:*892, 1122, 1974.

Original Articles

Austrian, R.: Pneumococcal endocarditis, meningitis and rupture of aortic valve. Arch. Intern. Med. *99:*539, 1957.

Beeson, P. B., Brannon, E. S., and Warren, J. V.: Observations on the sites of removal of bacteria from the blood in patients with bacterial endocarditis. J. Exp. Med. *81:*9, 1945.

Bell, E. T.: Glomerular lesions associated with endocarditis. Am. J. Pathol. *8:*639, 1932.

Belli, J., and Waisbren, B. A.: The number of blood cultures necessary to diagnose most cases of bacterial endocarditis. Am. J. Med. Sci. *232:*284, 1956.

Carruthers, M. M., and Kanokvechayant, R.: Pseudomonas aeruginosa endocarditis. Report of a case, with review of the literature. Am. J. Med. *55:*811, 1973.

Durack, D. T., and Petersdorf, R. G.: Chemotherapy of experimental streptococcal endocarditis. I. Comparison of commonly recommended prophylactic regimens. J. Clin. Invest. *52:*592, 1973.

Durack, D. T., Pelletier, L. L., and Petersdorf, R. G.: Chemotherapy of experimental streptococcal endocarditis. II. Synergism between penicillin and streptomycin against penicillin-sensitive streptococci. J. Clin. Invest. *53:*829, 1974.

Garrison, P. K., and Freedman, L. R.: Experimental endocarditis. I. Staphylococcal endocarditis in rabbits resulting from placement of a polyethylene catheter in the right side of the heart. Yale J. Biol. Med. *42:*394, 1970.

Gutman, R. A., Striker, G. E., Gilliland, B. C., and Cutler, R. E.: The immune complex glomerulonephritis of bacterial endocarditis. Medicine *51:*1, 1972.

Harder, E. J., Wilkowske, C. J., Washington, J. A., II, and Geraci, J. E.: Streptococcus mutans endocarditis. Ann. Intern. Med. *80:*364, 1974.

Hunter, T. H., and Paterson, P. Y.: Bacterial endocarditis. DM, pp. 1–48, November, 1956.

Keslin, M. H., Messner, R. P., and Williams, R. C., Jr.: Glomerulonephritis with subacute bacterial endocarditis. Immunofluorescent studies. Arch. Intern. Med. *132:*578, 1973.

Kirby, W. M. M.: Antibiotic synergism against enterococci. J. Infect. Dis. *122:*462, 1970.

Koenig, M. G., and Kaye, D.: Enterococcal endocarditis. Report of nineteen cases with long-term follow-up data. N. Engl. J. Med. *264:*257, 1961.

Levy, R. L., and Hong, R.: The immune nature of subacute bacterial endocarditis (SBE) nephritis. Am. J. Med. *54:*645, 1973.

Mandell, G. L., Kaye, D., Levison, M. E., and Hook, E. W.: Enterococcal endocarditis. An analysis of 38 patients observed at the New York Hospital – Cornell Medical Center. Arch. Intern. Med. *125:*258, 1970.

Messner, R. P., Laxdal, T., Quie, P. G., and Williams, R. C., Jr.: Rheumatoid factors in subacute bacterial endocarditis – bacterium, duration of disease or genetic predisposition? Ann. Intern. Med. *68:*746, 1968.

Moellering, R. C., Jr., Watson, B. K., and Kunz, L. J.: Endocarditis due to Group D streptococci. Comparison of disease caused by Streptococcus bovis with that produced by the enterococci. Am. J. Med. *57:*239, 1974.

Moellering, R. C., Jr., and Weinberg, A. N.: Studies on antibiotic synergism against enterococci. II. Effect of various antibiotics on the uptake of ^{14}C–labelled streptomycin by enterococci. J. Clin. Invest. *50:*2580, 1971.

Neefe, L. I., Chretien, J. H., Delaha, E. C., and Garagusi, V. F.: Streptococcus mutans endocarditis. Confusion with enterococcal endocarditis by routine laboratory testing. J.A.M.A. *230:*1298, 1974.

Paterson, P. Y., and Maden, G. M.: Occurrence and erythromycin susceptibility of penicillin-resistant viridans streptococci in rheumatic fever patients on oral penicillin prophylaxis. Antimicrob. Agents Chemother. *8:*323, 1968.

Phair, J. P., Klippel, J., and Mackenzie, M. R.: Antiglobulins in endocarditis. Infect. Immun. *5:*24, 1972.

Powers, D. L., and Mandell, G. L.: Intraleukocytic bacteria in endocarditis patients. J.A.M.A. *227:*312, 1974.

Reyes, M. P., Palutke, W. A., Wylin, R. F., and Lerner, A. M.: Pseudomonas endocarditis in the Detroit Medical Center, 1969–1972. Medicine *52:*173, 1973.

Sande, M. A., and Irvin, R. G.: Penicillin-aminoglycoside synergy in experimental Streptococcus viridans endocarditis. J. Infect. Dis. *129:*572, 1974.

Sprunt, K., Redman, W., and Leidy, G.: Penicillin resistant alpha streptococci in pharynx of patients given oral penicillin. Pediatrics *42:*957, 1968.

Tan, J. S., Terhune, C. A., Jr., Kaplan, S., and Hamburger, M.: Successful two-week treatment schedule for penicillin-susceptible Streptococcus viridans endocarditis. Lancet *2:*1340, 1971.

Watanakunakorn, C.: Penicillin combined with gentamicin or streptomycin: synergism against enterococci. J. Infect. Dis. *124:*581, 1971.

Watanakunakorn, C.: Streptococcus bovis endocarditis. Am. J. Med. *56:*256, 1974.

Werner, A. S., Cobbs, C. G., Kaye, D., and Hook, E. W.: Studies on the bacteremia of bacterial endocarditis. J.A.M.A. *202:*199, 1967.

Westenfelder, G. O., Paterson, P. Y., Reisberg, B. E., and Carlson, G. M.: Vancomycin-streptomycin synergism in enterococcal endocarditis. J.A.M.A. *223:*37, 1973.

Special Statement for Physicians

Prevention of Bacterial Endocarditis. A statement for physicians and dentists prepared by the Rheumatic Fever Committee and the Committee on Congenital Cardiac Defects of the Council on Rheumatic Fever and Congenital Heart Disease of the American Heart Association. (Committee members: Taranta, A., and Manning, J. A. – Chairmen; Ayoub, E. M., Gordis, L., Kaplan, E. L., Krause, R. M., Jackson, W. H., Milland, H. D., Paterson, P. Y., Perry, L. W., Zimmerman, R. L., Goldberg, S. J., Jesse, M. J., Malm, J. R., Ongley, P. A., Rashkind, W. J., Ritter, D. C., Robinson, S. J., and Talner, N. S.) American Heart Association, 44 East 23rd St., New York, New York, 10010. Revised statement 1972, available on request.

Chapter 42

ZOONOSES

Introduction

The zoonoses include a large number of infectious diseases of lower animals which are transmissible to man. Table 42-1 lists some of the more common zoonoses found in the Western Hemisphere. The table includes only selected diseases caused by bacteria, viruses, and rickettsiae. This table could be expanded greatly if numerous, less common diseases were included. In addition, there are a large number of fungal and animal parasite diseases of lower animals which could be added. However, it is not our intent to provide complete coverage of this large subject. Rather, we wish to bring out the nature of the public health and clinical problems that arise because of the occurrence of large reservoirs of disease and infection in both wild and domestic lower animals. More complete lists of zoonotic diseases can be found in *Infectious Diseases* by Paul Hoeprich and *A Manual of Tropical Medicine* by Hunter et al (See References).

An infectious agent may be transmitted from animal to man in a variety of ways. The following are a few examples: direct contact with diseased animal flesh (tularemia); drinking of cow's milk or goat's milk (tuberculosis and brucellosis, respectively); inhalation of dust particles contaminated by animal excreta or products (Q fever, anthrax); eating of insufficiently cooked infected flesh (anthrax, trichinosis); the bite of insect vectors such as mosquitoes, ticks, fleas, mites, or biting flies, (equine encephalomyelitis, Rocky Mountain spotted fever, plague, scrub typhus, and tularemia, respectively); and the bite of a diseased animal (rabies). Table 42-1 provides further information on transmission of infection from animals to man.

Because they live in greater proximity to man, domestic animals are the more common source of zoonoses. For example, at one time tuberculosis of

TABLE 42-1. Review of Bacterial, Viral, and Rickettsial Diseases of Animals Which Can Be Transmitted to Man

Disease	Etiologic Agent	Common Animal Host	Usual Method of Human Infection
Anthrax	Bacillus anthracis	Cattle, horses, sheep, swine, goats, dogs, cats, wild animals, birds	Inhalation or ingestion of spores; direct contact
Brucellosis	Brucella melitensis, B. abortus, B. suis	Cattle, goats, swine, sheep, horses, mules, dogs, cats, fowl, deer, rabbits	Milk; direct or indirect contact
Cat-scratch fever	Unknown	Cats, dogs	Cat or dog scratch
Colorado tick fever	Arbovirus	Squirrels, chipmunks, mice, porcupines	Tick bite
Cowpox	Cowpox virus	Cattle, horses	Skin abrasions
Herpes B viral encephalitis	Herpesvirus simiae	Monkeys	Monkey bites; contact with material from monkeys
Encephalitis (California)	Arbovirus	Rat bites, squirrels, horses, deer, hares, cows	Mosquito
Encephalitis (St. Louis)	Arbovirus	Birds	Mosquito
Encephalomyelitis (eastern equine)	Arbovirus	Birds, ducks, fowl, horses	Mosquito
Encephalomyelitis (Venezuelan equine)	Arbovirus	Rodents, horses	Mosquito
Encephalomyelitis (western equine)	Arbovirus	Birds, snakes, squirrels, horses	Mosquito
Glanders	Pseudomonas mallei	Horses	Skin contact; inhalation
Listeriosis	Listeria monocytogenes	Sheep, cattle, goats, guinea pigs, chickens, horses, rodents, birds, crustaceans	Unknown
Lymphocytic choriomeningitis	Arbovirus	Mice, rats, dogs, monkeys, guinea pigs	Inhalation of contaminated dust; ingestion of contaminated food
Mediterranean fever (boutonneuse fever, African tick typhus)	Rickettsia conorii	Dog	Bite of tick
Melioidosis	Pseudomonas pseudomallei	Rats, mice, rabbits, dogs, cats	Arthropod vectors, water, food
Orf (contagious ecthyma)	Virus	Sheep, goats	Through skin abrasions

TABLE 42-1. Review of Bacterial, Viral, and Rickettsial Diseases of Animals Which Can Be Transmitted to Man *(Continued)*

Disease	Etiologic Agent	Common Animal Host	Usual Method of Human Infection
Pasteurellosis	Pasteurella multocida	Fowl, cattle, sheep, swine, goats, mice, rats, rabbits	Animal bite
Plague (bubonic)	Yersinia pestis	Domestic rats, many wild rodents	Flea bite
Q fever	Coxiella burnetii	Cattle, sheep, goats	Inhalation of infected soil and dust
Rabies	Rabies virus (Rhabdovirus group)	Dogs, bats, opposums, skunks, foxes, cats, cattle	Bite of rabid animal
Rat bite fever	Spirillum minus	Rats, mice, cats	Rat bite
Rat bite fever	Streptobacillus moniliformis	Rats, squirrels, weasels, turkeys	Rat bite
Relapsing fever (borreliosis)	Borrelia sp.	Rodents, porcupines, opposums, armadillos, ticks, lice	Bite of tick or louse
Rickettsialpox	Rickettsia akari	Mice	Bite of mite
Rocky Mountain spotted fever	Rickettsia rickettsii	Rabbits, squirrels, rats, mice, groundhogs	Tick bite
Salmonellosis	Salmonella sp. (except S. typhosa)	Foul, swine, sheep, cattle, horses, dogs, cats, rodents, reptiles, birds, turtles	Direct contact; food
Scrub typhus	Rickettsia tsutsugamushi	Wild rodents, rats	Bite of mite
Tuberculosis	Mycobacterium bovis	Cattle, horses, cats, dogs	Milk; direct contact
Tularemia	Francisella tularensis	Wild rabbits, most other wild and domestic animals	Direct contact with infected carcass, usually rabbit; tick bite, biting flies
Typhus fever (endemic)	Rickettsia mooseri	Rats	Flea bite
Vesicular stomatitis	Virus (rhabdovirus group)	Cattle, swine, horses	Direct contact
Weil's disease (leptospirosis)	Leptospira interrogans	Rats, mice, skunks, opposums, wildcats, foxes, racoons, shrews, bandicoots, dogs, cattle, swine	Through skin, drinking water, eating food
Yellow fever (jungle)	Yellow fever virus	Monkeys, marmosets, lemurs, mosquitoes	Mosquito

cattle was a very common source of tuberculosis in human beings. At present, in the United States at least, because of the practice of pasteurizing milk and a program which has almost eliminated tuberculous cattle, bovine tuberculosis in man is very rare. Plague, a disease transmitted by fleas and endemic in domestic rats in some Asian and African seaports, has been eliminated in the rat populations of the seaport cities of the United States by vigorous anti-rat and anti-vector programs. Plague in the United States is now endemic in wild rodent populations in the western states, and the disease occurs sporadically in human beings who accidentally have contact with diseased rodents.

Other important infectious diseases of domestic animals transmissible to man are anthrax, brucellosis, salmonellosis, rabies, leptospirosis, Q fever, psittacosis, and trichinosis.

Persons in certain occupations have a greater risk of acquiring certain animal diseases. Farmers and veterinarians who work directly with animals are at greater risks. Slaughterhouse workers also have a greater chance of contracting a disease such as Q fever since they work in an environment conducive to the inhalation of material contaminated with *Coxiella burnetii.* Workers handling hides and wool have an increased chance of getting anthrax, since these materials may harbor spores of *Bacillus anthracis.*

Diseases of wild animals that are transmissible to man tend to occur more sporadically, since close contact is less frequent. In addition, certain persons are more prone to contract some of these diseases. For example, although tularemia can be transmitted to man by ticks or biting flies, it is most frequently seen in hunters who have killed infected wild rabbits, skinned them, and then handled the infected flesh. Certain infectious diseases of birds are transmitted by mosquitoes (arbovirus encephalitides) and may occur in epidemic proportion in human beings. Such epidemics are usually preceded by an epidemic in birds, following which a domestic animal, e.g., the horse, becomes infected; finally man, either simultaneously or later, also becomes infected.

The methods for the control of diseases in domestic animals that are transmissible to man can be listed as follows:

1. Slaughter of diseased and infected animals to eliminate tuberculosis.
2. Pasteurization of milk to eliminate tuberculosis and brucellosis.
3. Adequate cooking of meat before eating to eliminate trichinosis.
4. Vector control, i.e., control of fleas with insecticides, to eliminate endemic typhus.
5. Raising the level of resistance of animals by vaccination, i.e., vaccination of dogs against rabies.

None of the above can, except in isolated instances, be applied to the control of infectious diseases of wild animals that are transmissible to man. Here, avoidance of exposure to bites of wild animals and protection from arthropods that bite become most important. In addition, handling of carcasses of dead wild rodents should be avoided.

The following brief case presentations are provided to show the scope of the zoonoses problem in the United States today (all of the cases occurred in the United States in 1972 and 1973) and to indicate the types of clinical situations that may be encountered. Since many of these diseases are seen rarely, the major problem for the physician is to consider the possibility of one of the zoonoses when he examines an ill patient. In this age of very rapid transportation, a clue to proper diagnosis frequently can be gained from a careful history. A person may contract a disease today in Africa and not become ill until next week in Chicago.

CASE PRESENTATION 1 — AFRICAN TICK TYPHUS*

On June 16, 1973, a 53-year-old woman in Rhode Island became ill with an influenza-like illness characterized by fever (temperature 101°F), malaise, myalgia, headache, and rhinitis; she also had 13 painful skin lesions on her forearms, thighs, and popliteal areas which were erythematous and raised with a pustular center. She did not have a cough or conjunctivitis. Two days later she visited a local hospital clinic. The lesions were approximately 1 cm in diameter, erythematous, and indurated, with a central, grayish area; no adenopathy was present. The patient was treated symptomatically and placed on oral oxacillin for the infected skin lesions. By June 23, her condition was improving; however, the skin lesions had a black, necrotic center, and a generalized skin rash had developed which ranged from confluent, macular, erythematous areas to discrete, papular, erythematous lesions.

On June 26, the patient reported that between June 1 and 13 she had visited with friends in Koof Natal, South Africa, and that she had just received a cable stating that her hostess had African tick typhus. The patient did not recall receiving any tick bites during her visit to South Africa, although she did spend one day riding in a jeep in a game reserve and had been in her hosts' garden.

When this information was received, the patient had almost fully recovered, but her antibiotic therapy was changed to oral tetracycline. Immunofluorescent antibody titers were 1:160 for both Rocky Mountain spotted fever and African tick typhus in both serum specimens. These results are compatible with a diagnosis of African tick typhus.

African tick typhus, South African tick bite fever, and boutonneuse fever are synonyms for the disease caused by *Rickettsia conorii*, a microorganism endemic in Africa, the Mediterranean Basin, and India. The clinical picture seen here is typical; fever and an initial lesion (tache noire) followed by a maculopapular rash. Various tick species act as vectors, and treatment is similar to that for Rocky Mountain spotted fever (chlortetracycline or chloramphenicol). Alertness to the patient's recent travel history is important in making an early diagnosis. As in this case, even immunologic studies may not differentiate between the closely related members of the spotted fever group of rickettsiae (see Chap. 40).

---

*From Center for Disease Control, Morbidity and Mortality Weekly Report, Vol. 22, No. 42, 1973.

CASE PRESENTATION 2 – BRUCELLOSIS*

Between February and March, 1973, two outbreaks of brucellosis associated with exposure to Mexican cheese were reported in Colorado and Texas; each is summarized below.

Outbreak 1. On February 19, 1973, a 24-year-old woman was hospitalized in Denver, Colorado, with a three-week history of fever, chills, night sweats, and generalized abdominal and low back pain. One week prior to admission, she had had bitemporal headache, dark urine, and watery diarrhea. On February 16, she had been examined in the emergency room of the hosptial; her hematocrit was 32, and her white blood cell count was 4900 with atypical lymphocytes.

On admission, she had tachycardia and a rectal temperature of 40.9°C; other physical findings included a soft systolic murmur at the cardiac base, mild lower quadrant abdominal tenderness, hepatosplenomegaly, and bilateral costovertebral angle tenderness. Her hematocrit was 28 and hemoglobin 8.4 gm per 100 ml and she had evidence of disseminated intravascular coagulation without bleeding. Liver function tests and electrolytes were normal; her white blood count was 2700.

A serum specimen taken on February 20 showed a brucella agglutination titer of 1:3200, and a blood culture was positive for *Brucella melitensis*. Following treatment with ampicillin, kanamycin, and tetracycline, she has remained asymptomatic.

On March 13, the 24-year-old sister of this patient was admitted to the same hospital and gave a two-week history of head cold and fever. The week prior to admission, she had experienced a dry, nonproductive cough, bitemporal headache, nausea, vomiting, and mild generalized arthralgia; she had also had occasional night sweats, fever, and chills.

On admission, her temperature was 38.6°C orally, and her pulse rate was 120 per minute. She had inspiratory rales over the left lower lobe and a soft systolic murmur at the cardiac base; otherwise, the physical examination was normal. Chest x-ray revealed a left lower lobe infiltrate. Her hematocrit was 28 and hemoglobin 9.7 gm per 100 ml with normal clotting tests. A serum specimen obtained on March 15 showed a brucella agglutination titer of 1:320. She was treated with kanamycin and is presently asymptomatic.

The household contacts of these two patients were subsequently examined; the husband, daughter, and brother of the first patient were asymptomatic, and a serum specimen from the brother was negative for brucella antibodies. The husband and daughter of the second patient were also asymptomatic, but her mother-in-law reported having fever and chills in late February and had been treated with a one-week course of tetracycline by her private physician. Serum specimens from the husband and daughter were negative; the mother-in-law's serum had a brucella agglutination titer of 1:320.

Epidemiologic investigation revealed that the mother-in-law of the second patient had purchased goat cheese at a market in Juarez, Mexico, and

---

*From Center for Disease Control, Morbidity and Mortality Weekly Report, Vol. 22, No. 23, 1973.

that this cheese had subsequently been eaten by several members of the two families. Both sisters gave a history of eating the cheese, but the mother-in-law denied eating it.

Outbreak 2. In March, 1973, three members of a family living in El Paso, Texas, became ill with brucellosis; *Brucella melitensis* was isolated from the blood of one child, and all symptomatic individuals had elevated brucella agglutinin titers. Seven other family members were asymptomatic and had negative titers. Cheese purchased at a Juarez, Mexico, market had been eaten by all members of the family in the three weeks prior to onset of symptoms in the three ill persons.

Three additional cases of brucellosis were reported from El Paso between January and April, 1973; one was in a person who had eaten cheese purchased in Mexico.

Brucellosis in the United States today occurs predominantly in workers in the livestock and meat processing industries; in recent years, about 15 per cent of reported cases have been associated with the ingestion of presumably unpasteurized dairy products. Of the 190 reported cases in 1971, 19 were associated with Mexican cheese or dairy products, and two persons were infected after ingestion of Italian dairy products. The persons with brucellosis in the two outbreaks reported here have in common a history of exposure to cheese purchased in Juarez, Mexico, early in 1973. An inquiry regarding exposure to such food is definitely indicated in investigating cases of brucellosis.

CASE PRESENTATION 3 – BUBONIC PLAGUE*

Between July 6 and 7, 1973, a 9-year-old girl from near Payson, Arizona, became ill with headache, fever, and right axillary lymphadenopathy. Four days later, she developed what appeared to be a metastatic anterior chamber endophthalmitis. A blood specimen obtained on July 11 yielded a gram-negative organism identified in the Arizona State Laboratory on July 19 as *Yersinia pestis.* This identification was corroborated by the Plague Section, Vectorborne Diseases Branch, Bureau of Laboratories, CDC, in Fort Collins, Colorado.

During the two weeks before diagnosis of her illness was confirmed, the patient was treated with various antibiotics and topical eye drops. Initial specific antibiotic therapy for *Yersinia pestis* was started July 19 and included parenteral tetracycline and chloramphenicol eye drops. She had also been started on a short course of streptomycin sulfate to help resolve the possible anterior chamber septic endophthalmitis and marked lymphadenitis.

She improved generally, and her axillary bubo diminished since specific therapy was instituted. Her ocular problems also showed considerable improvement, although her pupil remained markedly dilated.

Initial epidemiologic investigation suggests she was exposed near her mountain cabin home. *Yersinia pestis* was detected in the animals of this area

---

*From Center for Disease Control, Morbidity and Mortality Weekly Report, Vol. 21, No. 10, 1972.

in February, 1972 when a single plague case resulted from direct contact with a wild lynx. A serologic survey of wild carnivore populations in 1971 showed widespread intensive plague activity on the Coconino Plateau and in contiguous ecologically similar areas immediately north of the site where this case apparently originated.

CASE PRESENTATION 4 — HUMAN PLAGUE*

On June 2, 1973, a 64-year-old resident of Lincoln, New Mexico, traveling through Brownfield, Texas became ill with fever and general malaise. The following day he was admitted to a Brownfield hospital with a temperature of 103°F, nausea, weakness, and lower extremity myalgia. No lymphadenopathy or abnormal lung findings were apparent. On the second day of hospitalization, blood specimens were positive for gram-negative organisms, and the patient was begun on chloramphenicol and gentamicin. Identification of *Yersinia pestis* was performed by the Center for Disease Control Bureau of Laboratories.

The patient's general condition improved rapidly following antibiotic therapy, although fever persisted for 10 days; his clinical course was punctuated by an episode of pulmonary edema. Persistent pulmonary infiltrates were thought to be related to congestive heart failure rather than to true plague pneumonia. He was discharged after a two-week hospitalization and is presently asymptomatic.

Epidemiologic investigation by the Texas State Department of Health revealed that the patient had spent most of the previous month at his brother's ranch in Lincoln, New Mexico, where he had handled dead mice; he did not recall being bitten by fleas. During the two days immediately preceding his illness, the patient had been traveling in Texas. He spent one night on a ranch in Plano, Texas, but had no contact with rodents there.

On the basis of the usual two- to seven-day incubation period in humans, and this patient's history of animal contact, it is assumed that he was exposed to plague in New Mexico.

Sylvatic plague has been reported in most New Mexico counties in recent years, but not from the Plano, Texas, vicinity. The last human case in the Lincoln, New Mexico area was reported in 1949.

CASE PRESENTATION 5 — TULAREMIA*

Seven cases of tularemia have recently been reported to the Center for Disease Control among fishing companions in Oklahoma and three among

---

*From Center for Disease Control, Morbidity and Mortality Weekly Report, Vol. 22, No. 32, 1973.

family members in Missouri. The clinical histories and the epidemiologic investigations of these cases are described below:

Oklahoma

Case 1. On April 9, 1973, a 24-year-old man in Oklahoma became ill with a high temperature, backache, and sore throat which lasted for three days. He did not seek medical attention or report for serologic testing.

Case 2. On April 10, a 43-year-old man had the abrupt onset of fever (temperature 103°F) and frontal headache and noted a weeping lesion on his right palm. Two days later he complained of a tender lump in the right axillary region. Because of continued fever and progressive weakness, he was hospitalized on April 18. A chest x-ray revealed bilateral patchy infiltrates. His fever defervesced following treatment with streptomycin and tetracycline, and a chest x-ray on May 31 showed complete resolution of the pulmonary infiltrate.

Case 3. On April 11, a 23-year-old man had the sudden onset of fever, headache, and mild, right-sided pleuritic pain. Physical examination revealed bilateral cervical lymphadenopathy but no ulcerative skin lesions. On May 21, he was hospitalized for an unrelated problem, and a chest x-ray showed an infiltrate surrounding a 1 cm X 1 ½ cm cavitary lesion in the right upper lobe and right sided hilar adenopathy. Sputum examinations were negative for acid-fast bacilli, and an intermediate strength tuberculin skin test was negative. The patient had not taken tetracycline as prescribed by his physician; a chest x-ray on July 5 showed minimal resolution of the cavitary lesion.

Case 4. This 27-year-old man developed sore throat, fever, headache, and muscle and joint pain on April 11. Bilateral cervical and right axillary lymphadenopathy were noted by his physician. No skin ulcerations were present. A chest x-ray showed no pulmonary abnormalities. He improved following treatment with streptomycin.

Although *Francisella tularensis* was not cultured from blood specimens from any of the men, two of the three tested had a 4-fold or greater rise in tularemia agglutinin titers, and one had a single high convalescent titer.

Epidemiologic investigation revealed that on April 7 Case 1 had killed a wild rabbit with a stick in Tulsa County, Oklahoma, while on a fishing trip with Cases 2, 3, and 4. Cases 1 and 3 subsequently dressed the rabbit, which was then cooked over an open fire. Cases 1, 3, and 4 ingested some of the cooked rabbit. Case 2 tasted the meat but did not swallow it because he did not like the taste. All four men handled the rabbit entrails, which were used as fishing bait. None of the men reported exposure to ticks during their outing.

Missouri

On December 27, 1972, two brothers, age 9 and 12, killed a sitting rabbit with a BB gun. Three days later the 12-year-old boy became ill with severe headache, and on the following day he was admitted to a local hospital with a temperature of 103°F. Both the brother and the boys' mother, who had assisted in cleaning the rabbit, experienced similar symptoms. The mother had an indurated cutaneous lesion on the middle finger of her left hand and generalized lymphadenopathy. All three persons responded clinically to tetracycline and chloramphenicol.

On January 9, the Missouri Division of Health Laboratory reported that the 9-year-old boy had a bacterial agglutination titer of 1:2560 and his brother and mother had agglutination titers of 1:1280 against *Francisella tularensis.*

Both of these outbreaks of tularemia involved contact with tissues of recently killed rabbits infected with *Francisella tularensis.* High attack rates of tularemia have been reported previously in the southern Mississippi Valley, where cases are often associated with tick bites or direct contact with tissues from infected rabbits.

If the cavitary lesion in the third Oklahoma case is due to tularemia, this represents a rare pulmonary finding.

CASE PRESENTATION 6 — HERPES B ENCEPHALITIS*

On April 13, 1973, a 28-year-old research assistant in California became ill with right-sided paresthesia, sore throat, and low-grade fever. On April 19, he had anorexia, stiff neck, and difficulty concentrating and moving his right fingers and was hospitalized. His temperature rose to 103°F, and on April 22 he had bladder paralysis. His electroencephalogram became diffusely abnormal but a brain scan and a carotid arteriogram were normal. Serial spinal taps showed normal pressure, but moderate lymphocytosis and increased protein.

The patient was diagnosed as having encephalitis due to herpesvirus B *(Herpesvirus simiae,* monkey B virus). By May 1, he had bilateral paralysis and a respiratory arrest, and a tracheostomy was performed. Human plasma containing herpesvirus B antibody was supplied by the Center for Disease Control but was not administered since his condition had stabilized; he steadily improved until late June when recovery was nearly complete.

No viruses could be isolated from stool, urine, throat washing, or cerebrospinal fluid specimens, but serologic tests at the California Regional Primate Research Center, Davis, California, and at the State Viral and Rickettsial Disease Laboratory confirmed the diagnosis.

The patient worked regularly with rhesus monkeys (*Macaca mulatta*) in the laboratory; 9 of the 26 monkeys to which he was exposed were found to have herpesvirus B antibody, indicative of latent infection.

A total of 24 cases of monkey B virus infection have been reported throughout the world, half from the United States. Of the 24 patients 23 had encephalitis, and 18 died. Of the 5 survivors, 3 had serious neurologic sequelae, 1 was expected to recover completely, and this case had a documented full recovery. Of the 17 cases for which information is available, 14 had received a bite or scratch wound, 1 had a history of a

---

*From Center for Disease Control, Morbidity and Mortality Weekly Report, Vol. 22, No. 40, 1973.

puncture with a contaminated needle, 1 had been cut on 2 occasions by glass from monkey tissue cell culture, and 1 had no reported prior injury. The mechanism for infection in this case is unknown.

Monkey B virus is most commonly found in rhesus, cynomolgus, and bonnet macaque monkeys. These monkeys are often used in laboratories, and the rarity of this disease despite frequent human contact with infected monkeys suggests a high degree of resistance to the pathogenic effects of this virus.

CASE PRESENTATION 7 – RABIES*

On September 7, 1973, a 26-year-old man in Kentucky developed bilateral paresthesia and pain in his ears, headache, sore throat, and anorexia. These symptoms persisted and later were accompanied by fever, difficulty in swallowing, confusion, and tremor. On September 10, he was admitted to the Clark County Hospital in Winchester, Kentucky, with a temperature of 105°F, nuchal rigidity, confusion, agitation, and spasmodic tremors.

Because of continuing deterioration of his condition, the patient was transferred to St. Joseph's Hospital in Lexington. Physical examination on admission revealed a temperature of 105°F, dysarthria, dysphagia, pharyngeal paralysis, and drooling. Stimulation of the patient precipitated spasms with spontaneous flexion of all extremities. A lumbar puncture revealed no marked abnormalities.

On September 14, the patient had pharyngeal and laryngeal spasms, subsequent cyanosis, and suffered a respiratory arrest; he was resuscitated immediately.

The next day the patient's family offered the additional history that he had been bitten on the right ear by a bat in mid-August. The bat had escaped, and the patient had not sought medical care. On the basis of the epidemiologic and clinical data, the diagnosis of rabies was entertained.

Over the next few days, the patient lapsed into a coma. Neurologic examination revealed intermittent right lower motor neuron facial paralysis, generalized hyporeflexia, and response to only deep pain. No other focal abnormalities were present. Initially the patient was treated with diphenylhydantoin, diazepam, and chlorpromazine. Once the coma ensued, the sedatives were discontinued.

Proteinuria, hypothermia, and hypoxia subsequently developed. Despite intensive respiratory care which included ventilatory support by a volume-cycled respirator, antibiotics, postural drainage, use of bronchodilators, and vigorous suctioning, hypoxemia persisted. Serial chest x-rays revealed a progressive diffuse interstitial pattern. In spite of the use of continuous positive pressure breathing, pulmonary compliance and oxygenation deteriorated. On September 22, pneumothorax developed, and the patient had a cardiorespiratory arrest and died.

---

*From Center for Disease Control, Morbidity and Mortality Weekly Report, Vol. 22, No. 39, 1973.

The diagnosis of rabies was confirmed ante mortem from corneal smears that were positive by the direct fluorescent antibody technique. Rabies virus was subsequently isolated from a sputum specimen obtained on September 20 and from brain tissue obtained post mortem.

Two bats captured near the patient's home and tested for rabies were negative. However, wildlife rabies, including bat rabies, is known to be endemic in this area of Kentucky.

CASE PRESENTATION 8 — RELAPSING FEVER*

In July, 1973, two epidemiologically related cases of relapsing fever were reported to the Center for Disease Control from Georgia and Arizona; these cases and a subsequent investigation for additional cases are summarized below.

Georgia

On June 22, 1973, a 12-year-old girl from Atlanta, Georgia, became ill with chills, headache, and fever (temperature 104°F) which lasted three days. After the fever subsided, the girl felt completely well, but on July 4, she had a febrile episode of two days' duration. On July 11, she consulted a local physician; physical examination was normal, and no therapy was instituted. On July 12, her temperature rose briefly to 104°F. On July 19, she had another episode of fever and returned to her physician. Loosely coiled spirochetes were noted on a peripheral blood smear taken while she was febrile, and she was placed on tetracycline therapy.

The patient and her parents had vistited several western National Parks between June 17 and 21. On June 18, they had stayed in an old wooden cabin on the North Rim of the Grand Canyon. The girl and her father carried firewood into the cabin, but they noticed no ticks and gave no history of tick bites.

Arizona

On July 4, 1973, a 20-year-old desk clerk at North Rim Lodge, Grand Canyon National Park, Arizona, developed an acute illness characterized by headache, fever, chills, and myalgia. Diagnositc studies performed during this four-day hospitalization at a local hosptial were unrevealing, and he was discharged, having improved on no antibiotic therapy. A clinical relapse with fever (temperature 103.8°F) and severe prostration occurred on July 13, and the patient was admitted to another hospital. Routine studies on admission, including urinalysis, electrolytes, BUN, bilirubin, and SGOT, were considered normal. A complete blood cell count revealed a hemoglobin of 14.5 gm per 100 ml, white blood cell count of 7200, and a normal differential count. A peripheral blood smear was noted to contain numerous spirochetal organisms consistent with a diagnosis of relapsing fever. Oral tetracycline therapy was initiated with rapid clinical improvement, and the patient has subsequently remained asymptomatic.

---

*From Center for Disease Control, Morbidity and Mortality Weekly Report, Vol. 22, No. 29, 1973.

Epidemiologic investigation on July 21, revealed that 46 of 290 employees and their family members living at the park had experienced similar illnesses in the preceding month. No apparent temporal clustering was noted, with sporadic cases occurring throughout the period June 15–July 18, 1973. Mouse inoculation studies on blood specimens from 10 individuals with most recent symptoms revealed all 10 to be infected with Borrelia organisms. The rustic cabins where the patients resided were scattered throughout the North Rim Park area and included standard and deluxe cabins, mens' and womens' employee dormitories, and the ranger housing area. A preliminary survey of South Rim employees revealed no cases of a clinically similar illness.

CASE PRESENTATION 9 – PET MONKEY–ASSOCIATED TUBERCULOSIS*

On October 23, 1973, a pet stump-tail macaque monkey (*Macaca arctoides*) was taken to a veterinarian in Seattle, Washington, because of a persistent cough. The animal was found to be tuberculin-positive and had evidence of nodular lesions in the right lung on chest x-ray. The monkey was sacrificed and a necropsy performed; granulomatous lesions were found in its lung, liver, spleen, and one lymph node. *Mycobacterium tuberculosis* was isolated from the lung.

On October 31, all five members of the family who owned the monkey were tuberculin tested with 5 TU PPD and found to be negative. However, in December, a skin test on the 9-year-old son showed a 40 mm reaction, and the 18-year-old daughter had a 12 mm reaction in January, 1973. The other family members were still negative at this time. Both siblings were placed on isoniazid chemoprophylaxis.

Investigation revealed that this monkey (A) had been bought by the Washington family on October 9, 1972. Prior to purchase, it has been kept by several different California residents. It was one of two stump-tail macaque monkeys (A and B) purchased by two different individuals from an Inglewood, California, pet shop in 1969. In March 1971, both monkeys were sold to a third person. The new owner had been hospitalized with active tuberculosis in May, 1970, and *Mycobacterium tuberculosis* had been isolated from his sputum.

At the time monkeys A and B were purchased by the new owner, he had a third stump-tail macaque monkey (C) that had been purchased as an infant in early 1970. At the time the new owner was hospitalized, monkey C was tuberculin tested and found to be negative. On retesting in August and October, 1970, monkey C was tuberculin-positive and had a positive chest x-ray. The owner refused to dispose of it. During the period March–November, 1971, the three monkeys were housed in the same outdoor cage; in November, monkeys A and B were boarded at the home of another family. Monkey C died of tuberculosis on March 18, 1972, and *Mycobacterium tuberculosis* was isolated from its tissues. Monkey B died in June, 1972, of

---

*From Center for Disease Control, Morbidity and Mortality Weekly Report, Vol. 22, No. 17, 1973.

undetermined causes. A necropsy was not performed, but the animal had a history of cough. Monkey A was later sold to the Washington Family.

Based on available evidence, it is likely that monkey C acquired tuberculosis from its owner in 1970 and subsequently infected monkeys A and B. In turn, monkey A infected the Washington patients.

This episode illustrates the transmissibility of *Mycobacterium tuberculosis* between primates, both human and nonhuman. Tuberculosis in nonhuman primates may be acquired from either a human or an animal source, often spreads rapidly between animals, and may be transmitted to human contacts. Tuberculosis in nonhuman primates may cause significant economic losses to laboratories, zoos, and the pet trade and presents a definite hazard to human health.

CASE PRESENTATION 10 – BAT CAVE–ASSOCIATED HISTOPLASMOSIS*

On February 10, 1973, a healthy 18-year-old girl from north central Florida was admitted to the University of Florida Medical Center in severe respiratory distress. Therapy with supplemental oxygen, systemic cortico-steroids, and ventilatory assistance was initiated for presumed influenza pneumonia. On the third hospital day, the patient's mother related the occurrence of a respiratory illness in several of her daughter's friends, three of whom had been recently hospitalized elsewhere. Subsequently, *Histoplasma capsulatum* was cultured from a bone marrow aspirate.

On further questioning, it was learned that between January 1 and 21, 1973, the patient and 28 members of a church-sponsored youth group, 21 males and 8 females, had explored a bat-infested limestone cave in Suwannee County, Florida. They had entered the cave on one or two occasions for approximately 30 minutes. Attempting to encourage the bats to fly, the youths had thrown soil from the cave floor at them. Upon experiencing mild shortness of breath in the dusty atmosphere, several of the explorers left the cave.

Twenty-three of the 29 spelunkers were subsequently identified as infected, for an attack rate of 79 per cent. Predominant symptoms were cough, fever, night sweats, dyspnea on exertion, malaise, and chest congestion. Illness became evident between 6 and 44 days after exposure. Intradermal histoplasmin tests on 24 of the spelunkers revealed that 15 of 18 reporting illness and 3 of 6 reporting no illness had 10 mm induration or greater at 48 hours. Sera from 26 of the 29 explorers were examined for histoplasmin precipitin bands; 11 of the 20 persons reporting illness that were sampled and 2 of the 6 persons reporting no illness had positive m band precipitins. Yeast form complement fixation tests performed on 10 of the 20 persons reporting illness revealed titers of 1:32 in all 10; titers in the 6 persons reporting no illness were not detectable. One convalescent serum from a patient reporting illness demonstrated a histoplasmin titer of 1:32. Chest

*From Center for Disease Control, Morbidity and Mortality Weekly Report, Vol. 22, No. 15, 1973.

roentgenograms demonstrated a diffuse miliary infiltrate compatible with acute pulmonary histoplasmosis in 14 of 17 people reporting illness and in 1 of 3 who were clinically well. Histoplasmin skin test surveys of 103 local residents revealed indurations of 10 mm or greater in 7 (7 per cent). Histoplasmin and yeast form complement fixation titers on each of 110 sera obtained from local residents were negative.

Histoplasmosis is most prevalent in the Mississippi and Missouri River valleys. Contact with soil containing an accumulation of either bat or bird excreta is usually required for acquisition of histoplasmosis, and recent evidence suggests that bat habitats are infested with *Histoplasma capsulatum* (see Chap. 26).

Histoplasmosis in humans has been reported from Florida on only two previous occasions, and both cases were associated with exploration of bat caves; however, the outbreak presented here is the largest known instance of cave-associated histoplasmosis in the state. The data suggest that bat caves infected with *Histoplasma capsulatum* are a significant source of infection primarily for subjects who explore them.

CASE PRESENTATION 11 – HUMAN ORF MIMICKING CUTANEOUS ANTHRAX*

In January, 1973, two sisters ages 12 and 18 from Napa County, California, developed vesiculo-papular lesions of the fingers one to two weeks after acquiring young lambs. The lambs which had vesicular and scabby lesions about the mouth failed to thrive and were killed and buried. Lesions on the girls' fingers became more severe; each patient had two raised, mildly tender, nonpustular, granulomatous papules, with a dry scab over the center and a red indurated border. One also developed lesions typical of erythema multiforme on the affected hand and arm. Neither girl had systemic symptoms of regional adenopathy. Anthrax was suspected, and erythromycin and later penicillin were administered without apparent effect. Cultures yielded no pathogens.

Review of these cases by the Infectious Disease staff, California State Department of Public Health, indicated the most likely diagnosis was contagious pustular dermatitis of sheep (orf, sore mouth, contagious ecthyma). Scrapings of the lesions were obtained for electron microscopy at the State Viral and Rickettsial Disease Laboratory. The diagnosis was confirmed by finding typical particles of orf virus within a few hours after obtaining specimens. On February 21, sera were collected from both patients. A 1:8 complement fixation titer against orf was present in the 18-year-old and a 1:4 titer in the 12-year-old.

Contrary to the reported benign nature of human orf, this is the second report in the literature of erythema multiforme as a sequel to orf. In 1972, four human orf cases were reported to the Center for Disease Control from

---

*From Center for Disease Control, Morbidity and Mortality Weekly Report, Vol. 22, No. 12, 1973.

four states — Illinois, Michigan, New Mexico, and New York. Three cases were associated with sheep and one with goats. Three of the cases reported had a complement fixation titer of 1:8. Orf virus was isolated from primary ovine kidney cell cultures in one case; no isolation attempts were made in the other three cases. The National Animal Disease Laboratory of the United States Department of Agriculture considers a complement fixation titer of 1:8 diagnostic for the disease in sheep. One of the four patients had a generalized vesiculo-papular rash, involving the axilla, groin, face, abdomen, arms, legs, shoulder, and feet. The other three patients had a single circumscribed lesion described as vesicular or granulomatous; two had axillary lymphadenopathy.

As demonstrated by this report, orf should be considered in the differential diagnosis when subcutaneous anthrax is suspected.

CASE PRESENTATION 12 – EPIDEMIC RINGWORM*

Between August 26 and October 10, 1972, 25 cases of dermatophytosis occurred among 109 students at an elementary school in Greenwood, Nebraska. Cases were evenly distributed in all grades, kindergarten through 6. Two culture surveys were conducted, and *Microsporum canis* was isolated on Sabourard's agar from four children of two families.

Lesions were confined primarily to the trunk, neck, face, and upper limb areas, but 3 (12 per cent) of the 25 cases also developed scalp lesions later in the course of their illness. A school-based treatment program utilizing topical application of Tinactin was effective in controlling spread of infection and transmission to others.

Epidemiologic investigation revealed that the first three cases occurred in children of the same family who formerly had 16 cats. Fifteen of the 16 had clinical ringworm with typical areas of alopecia about the head and neck region. The cats were destroyed on the recommendation of the family physician and veterinarian before the investigation.

Another family, whose three children (two of whom were positive for *Microsporum canis* in the school survey) had skin lesions, had acquired a kitten in late August, 1972. This kitten was also disposed of prior to the investigation. Other children who were culture-positive had two cats and one dog at home; cat had typical ringworm lesions (not cultured) that developed after this child and another sibling became infected, suggesting the possibility of person to cat transmission.

CASE PRESENTATION 13 – SHELLFISH–ASSOCIATED HEPATITIS **

On July 30–31, 1971, 12 persons attended a family reunion in Cape Cod, Massachusetts. Five persons subsequently became ill with hepatitis between

---

*From Center for Disease Control, Morbidity and Mortality Weekly Report, Vol. 22, No. 4, 1973.

**From Center for Disease Control, Morbidity and Mortality Weekly Report, Vol. 21, No. 2, 1972.

August 9 and September 5. Their symptoms included malaise, anorexia, and mild icterus. All patients had abnormal liver function tests. Serologic testing for hepatitis associated antigen performed on one patient was negative. All patients recovered uneventfully. The patients' family members received gamma globulin; no secondary cases occurred.

All patients denied a history of exposure to hepatitis, blood transfusions, parenteral drug use, and recent foreign travel. At the reunion, however, the patients had shared one meal together at which only steamed clams were served. Six persons ate the clams, and five subsequently became ill. The person who ate clams but did not become ill received gamma globulin soon after the first cases were recognized. The six persons who did not eat clams remained well.

The clams had been purchased from a merchant in nearby Chatham, Massachusetts, and prepared at home. They were added to a pot of boiling water, heated until they opened, and then served. The original source of the clams could not be determined, since the merchant purchases his clams from many sources. No other outbreaks of possible shellfish-associated hepatitis have been reported in Massachusetts.

The occurrence of five cases of hepatitis within a four-week period, the high attack rate (five of six) for those eating the steamed clams, and the zero attack rate for those who did not, suggest a common-source outbreak of shellfish-associated hepatitis. Since the large shellfish-associated hepatitis outbreaks of the early and mid 1960's, only small sporadic outbreaks, such as this one, have been reported to the Center for Disease Control. This is the first report of an outbreak of viral hepatitis attributed to the ingestion of only steamed clams.

When clams are steamed only until the shells open, the internal temperature is not high enough to inactivate the infectious agent of hepatitis. The minimum period of steaming needed to ensure safety has not been determined, but the temperature of boiling water for 20 minutes was effective in early studies of the temperature stability of the hepatitis agents.

CASE PRESENTATION 14 – SALMONELLOSIS*

On August 14, 1971, a 37-year-old man from Mobile, Alabama, had onset of high fever, explosive diarrhea, and persistent vomiting; he was hospitalized that day. Stool specimens sent to the State Health Laboratories were cultured and yielded *Salmonella typhimurium*. The patient was treated with ampicillin (500 mg four times a day). He made an uneventful recovery and was discharged on August 27. Two subsequent cultures of stool specimens in November and December, 1971 were negative.

An epidemiologic investigation revealed that a recently purchased Amazon parrot belonging to the patient's family had died with severe gastroenteritis on August 14. The carcass of the parrot was submitted to the

---

*From Center for Disease Control, Morbidity and Mortality Weekly Report, Vol. 20, No. 52, 1972.

State Health Laboratories and found to be positive for *Salmonella typhimurium.* The rest of its food was fed to the family's pet chipmunk which subsequently became drowsy and had slight diarrheaa; it died on August 19. No specimens from the chipmunk or the parrot food were available for culture.

Stool specimens were obtained from the patient's wife and four children. Three of the children were found to have asymptomatic *Salmonella typhimurium* infections. These children and the patient had fed and handled the parrot, suggesting that it was the original source of infection. Samples of parrot food and cage droppings from two other parrots at the pet store where the family's bird had been purchased were also obtained. Cultures of these were negative for enteric pathogens.

CASE PRESENTATION 15 – TRICHINOSIS*

Between January 14 and 29, 1973, 15 of 25 members of four families in West Point, Nebraska, became ill with fever (93 per cent), diarrhea (73 per cent), muscle aches (67 per cent), periorbital edema (53 per cent), and headache (47 per cent) (Table 42-2). Three of the ill persons were hospitalized: one with pneumonia and severe muscle aches, one with nephritis, and one with evidence of myocarditis and central nervous system symptoms. Using the trichinosis bentonite flocculation test, titers were observed in 12 of the 15 ill individuals. Of 11 persons on whom data were available, 10 had white blood cell counts $\geq$ 10,000, and 11 had eosinophilia. All ill persons were diagnosed as having trichinosis and were treated with thiabendazole; some also received steroids. There were no deaths. A survey of other household members of the four families identified three children with trichinosis bentonite flocculation titers but no signs or symptoms of illness.

Epidemiologic investigation revaled that on December 26, 1972, family 1 had butchered two brood sows and one beef animal and two days later had made sausage. The ingredients were equal portions of ground beef and pork, salt, pepper, monosodium glutamate, and saltpeter. The mixture was packed in natural casing, was not smoked, and hung dry until January 6, 1973, when it was divided between families 1 and 2.

On January 7, family 2 sponsored a card party, invited two other couples from families 3 and 4, and served the sausage uncooked. Five members of these three families subsequently became ill with trichinosis (Fig. 42–1). In addition, all members of family 1 and children of family 2 ate sausage in their school lunches and at other meals during the week of January 7. In all, 15 (75 per cent) of 20 persons who ate the sausage became ill, and none of 5 persons who did not eat the sausage became ill. Samples of the remaining sausage and of pork chops from the same carcass were tested; all were positive for *Trichinella spiralis* larvae.

Further investigation revealed that family 1 had a drove of 30 brood sows and approximately 300 barrows and gilts. On February 21, 1973, all 30 sows

*From Center for Disease Control, Morbidity and Mortality Weekly Report, Vol. 22, No. 23, 1973.

TABLE 42-2. Signs and Symptoms in 15 Persons with Trichinosis, West Point, Nebraska (January–February, 1973)*

Sign or Symptom	Patients with Sign or Symptom		Sign or Symptom	Patients with Sign or Symptom	
	Number	Per Cent		Number	Per Cent
Fever	14	93	Chills and Sweating	3	20
Diarrhea	11	73	Fainting and Vertigo	2	13
Muscle Aches	10	67	Hair Loss (late)	2	13
Weakness	10	67	Cramps	1	7
Periorbital Edema	8	53	Nausea	1	7
Headache	7	47	Myocarditis	1	7
Weight Loss	5	34	Pneumonia	1	7
Facial Edema	4	27	Nephritis	1	7

*From Center for Disease Control, Morbidity and Mortality Weekly Report, Vol. 22, No. 23, 1973.

were bled; subsequent bentonite flocculation titer results were negative. Between February 21 and 28, eight adult rats (*Rattus norvegicus*) were trapped, and tongue-diaphragm tissues were submitted for larval studies; these results were also negative. A history of the operation revealed no previous garbage feeding practices and generally a "closed" herd management for the past several years, ruling out possible trichinae exposure at another location.

In this outbreak, the infection in the swine was most likely acquired on the farm, and the source of infection is presumed to have been an infected wild animal. With garbage-fed pigs diminishing as a source of trichinosis in man in the United States, the occurrence of *Trichinella spiralis* in wild animals has gained significance in the evaluation of the disease. Unfortunately, with the exception of extensive studies in Iowa and Alaska, little attention has been given to the relationship of wildlife and the perpetuation of trichinosis among farm-raised swine in this country.

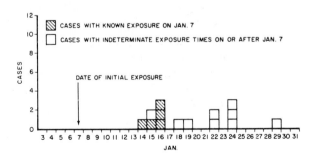

Figure 42-1. Trichinosis cases by date of onset (date of onset for one case unknown) in West Point, Nebraska, January, 1973. (From Center for Disease Control, Morbidity and Mortality Weekly Report, Vol. 22, No. 23, 1973.)

References

Books

Hoeprich, P. D.: Infectious Diseases. Hagerstown, Maryland, Harper and Row, 1972.

Hull, T. G.: Diseases Transmitted from Animals to Man. 3rd ed. Springfield, Illinois, Charles C Thomas, 1947.

Hunter, G. W., Frye, W. W., and Swartz-Welder, J. C.: A Manual of Tropical Medicine. 4th ed. Philadelphia, W. B. Saunders Co., 1966.

Seamer, J. (ed.): Safety in the Animal House. London, Laboratory Animals Ltd., 1972.

Symposium Volume

Perkins, F. T., and O'Donoghue, P. N. (eds.): Hazards of Handling Simians. Proceedings of the 29th Symposium Organized by the Permanent Section for Microbiological Standardization of the International Association of Microbiological Societies. London, Laboratory Animals Ltd., 1969.

Chapter 43

INFECTION IN THE COMPROMISED HOST

Introduction

Host Defense: The Critical Issue

In the initial chapters of this book (Chaps. 2 and 3) the overriding importance of host defense mechanisms as determinants of microbial infection and disease has been emphasized. The point has been made that the issue of clinical well-being as opposed to disease is decided in most instances by the collective defenses of the host rather than the virulence of potential invading microorganisms. Considerable attention has been devoted to deficiency in or malfunctions of host phagocytic action. The importance of antibody synthesis and mobilization of cell-mediated immune responses in allowing either exogenous microorganisms or the host's own indigenous microbial flora to breach normal anatomic surfaces and organ system barriers and cause disease has been stressed.

Since before the turn of this century much has been learned concerning the many virulence factors that endow pathogenic microorganisms with disease-producing capacity. Only in the past 20 or 30 years, however, has it

701

been appreciated to what degree altered host defense mechanisms predispose every host to develop infectious diseases. There are many types of altered host defense: genetic, acquired, secondary (to other diseases) and, especially important, iatrogenic. It is as though *any* diminution in *any* host defense system "opens the door" to microbial invasion and disease. This seems to be true irrespective of whether the microorganism is a "classic" pathogen or a member of the host's own normal microbial flora with relatively low virulence under ordinary circumstances.

Compromised Host Defenses: A Price of Medical Advances

The point has been underscored in the very first portion of this book (Chap. 1) that virtually every medical advance causes some unwanted blunting of host defense mechanisms. Specific examples are (1) the many indwelling tubes that constitute the support system to which all seriously ill patients invariably are attached as soon as they enter a modern hospital, (2) implanted bypass tubes and prosthetics which, being foreign bodies, will predispose to infection, and (3) the increasing use of ever more potent drugs designed expressly to suppress or diminish the normal inflammatory and immune response of the host.

On balance, the net result all too often is a markedly reduced number of segmented neutrophils, inadequacy of macrophage function, and decreased antibody formation or suppressed cellular immune reactions. Collectively, these host responses are crucial for resistance to infection.

The main purpose of this chapter is to highlight briefly compromised patients whose defenses have been blunted in various ways, largely through the utilization of current therapeutic modalities of one kind or another. Specific types of infection all too often are the consequence of application of such therapeutic regimens. The primary cause of the initial loss of resistance in the host usually is an underlying disease of a noninfectious nature. The precipitating cause of the ensuing infection is frequently the specific treatment the patient receives for the primary disorder, i.e., the "medical advance."

Rather than attempt to cover the multitude of different types of infections that reportedly can occur in compromised hosts, "opportunistic microbes" that commonly are implicated in specific clinical situations are discussed in this chapter. In this way, the altered microbe-host interrelationships will be better understood.

Patients with Compromised Defense Mechanisms

Table 43–1 lists a number of factors that may compromise host defenses. The major explanation for increased susceptibility to infection, together with specific examples of common forms of infection that may be anticipated, also is given. An inspection of Table 43–1 reveals that knowledge of the type of compromised host enables one to predict frequently what type of infectious process is most likely to occur. Although this statement is an oversimplification of what happens in practice, it has sufficient validity to help the

TABLE 43–1. Patients with Compromised Defenses at Increased Risk of Infection

Predisposing Factors	Basis for Increased Susceptibility to Infections	Most Common Types of Infection
Indwelling catheters or implanted devices	Foreign body	Abscess; bacteremia
Allograft recipients (renal, heart, bone marrow)	Diminished cell-mediated immunity	Pneumonia; urinary tract infection; bacteremia
Extensive skin burns	Diminished cell-mediated immunity; ? impaired antibody production	Pseudomonas (*Pseudomonas aeruginosa*) bacteremia
Absence or malfunction of the spleen (splenectomy; sickle cell anemia)	Impaired IgM antibody synthesis	Pneumococcal (*Streptococcus pneumoniae*) bacteremia and meningitis
Bone marrow failure	Agranulocytosis; neutropenia	Bacteremia; pneumonia; urinary tract infection
Malignant disorders (hematoproliferative states; solid tumors)	Diminished or absent cell-mediated immunity; neutropenia; impaired antibody synthesis	Bacteremia; pneumonia; urinary tract infection

physician to be on the alert for specific forms of infectious diseases. In addition, if the physician knows the most likely microorganism(s) responsible for fever and other signs of infection in a certain patient, he can move through differential diagnostic and therapeutic decision-making in an expeditious fashion.

Foreign Bodies

Indwelling intravenous or other types of catheters or surgically implanted prosthetic devices represent foreign bodies that, in ways which still remain unclear, allow microorganisms to gain a foothold in the host with comparative ease. Since the compromise in defense is localized at the site of the foreign body, focal suppuration with abscess formation is the most common type of infection. Spread of the infecting microbes into the bloodstream not infrequently is a life-threatening complication.

Allograft Recipients

Recipients of allografts, irrespective of the type of donor cells or tissue, must be given immunosuppressive and anti-inflammatory drugs or they will reject the allograft. Treatment regimens are designed to retard or abolish most cell-mediated immune responses that otherwise would jeopardize survival of the allograft. By suppressing these cell-mediated immunologic defenses, the stage is set for a multitude of infectious complications. These complications often appear as an undifferentiated pulmonary infiltrative process, as urinary tract infections (especially in renal allograft recipients), or as bacteremia.

Extensive Skin Burns

Patients with extensive burns of the skin uniformly exhibit a predisposition to infection with *Pseudomonas aeruginosa*. Bacteremia with septic shock due to this microorganism all too often follows local infection at burn sites. The first clinical indication is greenish discoloration of the burn dressings due to pigments produced by a majority of strains of Pseudomonas. The reason for a markedly increased susceptibility of burned patients to Pseudomonas microorganisms is not clear. Following extensive second or third degree burns, experimental animals demonstrate a marked decrease in their capacity to exhibit delayed-type hypersensitivity responses. Little evidence has accrued so far suggesting that depression in such cell-mediated immune responsiveness is accompanied by comparable reduction in antibody production. This question deserves more attention than it has received, in light of the major role of antibody in host defense against pseudomonas infections. Antibody reactive with *P. aeruginosa* appears to act as an opsonin, augmenting and accelerating uptake and intracellular destruction of the bacteria by neutrophils and the reticuloendothelial system. Antibody also may act as antitoxin, neutralizing the toxic active site(s) on the lipid moiety of gram negative bacterial lipopolysaccharide.

Altered Splenic Function

Complete loss of splenic function (e.g., removal of the spleen because of trauma or for purposes of "staging" in Hodgkin's disease) or the gradual loss of splenic function in association with disease (e.g., multiple splenic infarcts in sickle cell anemia) appears to result in decreased production of IgM-type antibodies. This class of immunoglobulin is synthesized in splenic lymphoid tissues. IgM antibody with complement is of particular importance in opsonizing pneumococci and plays a central role in the rapid phagocytosis of these bacteria by neutrophils or mononuclear phagocytes. Patients with splenic malfunctions or the absence of the spleen may have an unduly high incidence of bacteremia and meningitis due to *Streptococcus pneumoniae.*

Bone Marrow Failure

Bone marrow failure from any cause inevitably leads to decline in all formed elements of the blood. Because of their exceptionally short half life, a decline in segmented neutrophils occurs early; leukopenia may progress to an almost total lack of demonstrable neutrophils, i.e., agranulocytosis. Patients with agranulocytosis are prone to a variety of infections caused by both gram positive and gram negative microorganisms. Bacteremia, pneumonia, and urinary tract infections are the most frequent clinical consequences of the increased susceptibility to infection in these patients.

Malignancies

Any malignant process leads to some degree of lowered host defense. Depending on the nature of the malignant disease, any of the major host defenses may be breached, singly or collectively. For example, patients with either solid epithelial tumors or lymphocytic hematoproliferative disorders tend to have diminished cell-mediated immune responses. Conversely, patients with acute leukemia usually exhibit markedly reduced numbers of circulating segmented neutrophils. Increased susceptibility to infection in patients with malignant disease, irrespective of type, usually is manifested by bacteremia, pneumonia, or urinary tract infections.

Opportunistic Microorganisms Associated with Certain Compromised Host Defenses

Table 43–2 lists a limited number of specific microorganisms that commonly cause infection in certain compromised hosts. Some of these microbes may cause disease in apparently healthy individuals, as well as in patients with patently evident altered defense capabilities. Other microorganisms listed, e.g., *Propionibacterium acnes* and *Pneumocystis carinii,* cause infections *only* in clinical situations involving compromised hosts and in this sense are true "opportunists."

TABLE 43–2. Specific Opportunistic Microorganisms Commonly Causing Infectious Diseases in Association with Selected Clinical Settings Involving Compromised Host Defenses

Specific Opportunistic Microorganisms	Clinical Settings Associated with Compromised Host Defense Mechanisms
Staphylococcus aureus and S. epidermidis	Indwelling intravenous polyethylene catheters; implanted prosthetic heart valve(s); ventriculoatrial catheter shunt for hydrocephalus
Streptococcus pneumoniae	Absence of spleen or abnormal splenic function; multiple myeloma
Pseudomonas aeruginosa	Leukopenia (agranulocytosis) associated with malignant tumors and hematoproliferative disorders or bone marrow failure
Serratia marcescens	Extended or permanent urinary catheterization
Listeria monocytogenes	Hematoproliferative disorders; newborn or elderly patient
Nocardia asteroides	Immunosuppressed allograft recipient
Mycobacteria	Prolonged use of corticosteroid; immunosuppressed patient
Propionibacterium acnes	Implanted prosthetic heart valve
Cryptococcus neoformans	Hodgkin's disease and other forms of lymphoma
Aspergillus sp.	Implanted prosthetic heart valve; immunosuppressed allograft recipient
Candida albicans	Implanted prosthetic heart valve; immunosuppressed allograft recipient
Toxoplasma gondii	Pregnancy; immunosuppressed allograft recipient
Pneumocystis carinii	Immunosuppressed allograft recipient
Herpes simplex virus	Immunosuppressed allograft recipient
Varicella-zoster virus	Hodgkin's disease and other hematoproliferative malignant disorders; immunosuppressed allograft recipient.
Cytomegalovirus	Blood transfusions; immunosuppressed allograft recipient

Staphylococci

Both *Staphylococcus aureus* and *Staphylococcus epidermidis* have a characteristic propensity for invading skin and adjacent tissue at the sites of indwelling polyethylene intravenous catheters. Within 48 to 72 hours, relatively large numbers of staphylococci are demonstrable at the site of insertion of these foreign bodies. Gross evidence of infection becomes more frequent the longer the catheters remain in place. The skill with which the catheters are initially inserted appears to be an important determinant of infection. Catheters placed and cared for by experienced members of an IV team are less likely to develop infections than those placed by house officers. S. aureus and especially S. epidermidis are respected for their capacity to colonize and infect prosthetic cardiac heart valves. Antimicrobial prophylactic regimens are recommended for patients undergoing open heart surgery and artificial valve implantation, in order to prevent or suppress staphylococcal bacteremia during surgery and to eradicate any staphylococci that may have colonized the prosthesis during, or for a period of a week or so following, surgery.

Streptococcus pneumoniae

Mention already has been made of the frequency of infection due to Streptococcus pneumoniae in patients with decreased splenic function. Increased risk of pneumococcal bacteremia in experimental animals and man is known to be present for approximately 12 to 18 months following splenectomy. This appears to be the time necessary for IgM antibody synthesis to be taken over by other lymphoid tissue so that the host once again is able to opsonize encapsulated pneumococci.

Patients with multiple myeloma frequently can be shown to have deficient antibody production. Presumably for this reason they are at increased risk of developing pneumococcal infection. In contrast to the pattern of infection with Streptococcus pneumoniae in patients with splenic defects (see Table 43–1), patients with multiple myeloma usually present with pneumococcal pneumonia, as opposed to bacteremia or meningitis.

Pseudomonas aeruginosa

Pseudomonas aeruginosa has a unique capacity to invade the bloodstream in the patient with leukopenia, i.e., agranulocytosis. The concentration of circulating neutrophils below which the risk of pseudomonas bacteremia rises precipitously is in the range of 500 to 1000 neutrophils per cubic millimeter. P. aeruginosa has the ability to invade the endothelial cell lining of major blood vessels. Such foci develop further, causing vasculitis and thrombosis, and serve as a source for continued reentry of the microorganisms into the circulation. The mortality rate of leukopenic patients with P. aeruginosa bacteriemia is extremely high, approximately 80 to 85 per cent.

Most Pseudomonas species, including Pseudomonas aeruginosa, have relatively simple nutritional requirements and can replicate in medicinal solutions such as procaine and benzalkonium chloride. Instruments or endoscopes stored in such solutions may become heavily contaminated.

Serratia marcescens

Serratia marcescens was once considered a harmless microorganism devoid of disease-producing capacity. Some strains produce a bright red pigment; in years past such strains were used as "marker bacteria" in studies utilizing human volunteers. For example, large numbers of Serratia microorganisms were applied to the gingiva of volunteers to establish that tooth extraction may be followed by a transitory bacteremia. In other studies, the pigmented strains provided data concerning specific pathways whereby bacteria residing on the perineum or periurethral area gained access to the bladder in patients with indwelling urinary catheters. Today, *S. marcescens* is a respected "opportunist"; it is not infrequently the source of bacteremia in patients with indwelling polyethylene intravenous catheters and may be the cause of persistent urinary tract infection. The latter type of opportunistic infection is common in patients with spinal cord injury who have need of a urinary drainage system.

An ominous feature of those strains of *Serratia marcescens* currently responsible for many intrahospital infections is their resistance to antimicrobial drugs. Such strains may be susceptible only to gentamicin or a more toxic member of the aminoglycoside class of drugs. Recently, infection due to *S. marcescens* has been reported in which the strain was resistant to *all* available antimicrobial agents. In patients with this type of infection, bacteremia cannot be treated with any effective antimicrobial regimen and the patients often die. The occurrence of Serratia strains resistant to many drugs suggests plasmid or episomal transfer (see Chap. 31).

Listeria monocytogenes

Infections due to *Listeria monocytogenes* may occur in patients with hematoproliferative disorders or in patients at extremes of the life span. Both newborns and elderly patients not infrequently have either immature or partially impaired immune responses, especially involving thymic-dependent lymphoid cells. Infection may be first detected as septicemia, especially in newborns, perhaps reflecting the presence of this microorganism in the microbial flora of the uterine cervix. Meningitis due to *L. monocytogenes* may be seen in both infants and patients with leukemia. A Gram stained cerebrospinal fluid sediment may reveal small gram positive bacilli that resemble, and may be confused with, diphtheroids. They must be identified following isolation by culture.

Nocardia asteroides

Despite the fact that *Nocardia asteroides* is a true bacterium, the acid-fast staining characteristic of many strains, together with other characteristics, has led for years to the erroneous classification of this microorganism as a fungus. Since it may be acid-fast at times, it may be confused with mycobacteria in stained smears or tissue sections. However, *N. asteroides* causes a totally different type of disease consisting of extensive abscess formation, especially in the lung, the organ usually initially infected. Spread of the microorganisms from the lung to the bloodstream often results in metastatic cerebral abscesses. In many patients with nocardiosis, skin lesions can also be found. Often, these skin lesions drain material that can be cultured and found to contain the microorganisms. This finding is sometimes the first clue that the patient has systemic infection due to *N. asteroides.* Nocardia infections appear to be especially prone to occur in patients who are on long-term immunosuppressive drug therapy to maintain allograft function.

Mycobacteria

Introduction of corticosteroids during the early 1950s was followed by numerous reports suggesting that some of these anti-inflammatory agents can activate latent *Mycobacterium tuberculosis* and lead to active tuberculosis. Currently, physicians prescribe antituberculous therapy for patients with positive tuberculin skin tests when such patients are to be started on long-term steroid therapy. Infection due to *M. tuberculosis* as well as other mycobacteria appears to be occurring with increased frequency in patients on immunosuppressive therapy and in patients who have congenital immunologic defects of thymic-derived lymphoid tissues, e.g., severe combined deficiency disease.

Propionibacterium acnes

Infection due to *Propionibacterium acnes* or other Propionibacterium species appears to be uniquely associated with implanted prosthetic heart valves. Microorganisms similar to Propionibacterium species, often termed *diphtheroids,* are part of the normal microbial flora of the skin and are not uncommonly isolated from blood cultures. Therefore, the presence of *P. acnes* in multiple blood cultures is required for documentation of sustained bacteremia due to this microbial species in a patient with an artificial heart valve and, by inference, infection of the valve (see Chaps. 10 and 41).

Cryptococcus neoformans

Infection with *Cryptococcus neoformans* has long been known to be associated with Hodgkin's disease and other forms of malignant lymphoma. In fact, infection with *C. neoformans* in conjunction with malignancy occurs to such an extent that some investigators have raised a question of an etiologic relationship between the two. The cloacae of pigeons appears to be an important if not the major reservoir for this fungus. Dissemination of *C. neoformans* via the fecal droppings of pigeons and subsequent infection of the lower respiratory tract by inhalation of aerosols containing viable *C. neoformans* cells is believed to be the most frequent mode of infection in man (see Fig. 43–1).

Hematogenous spread of *Cryptococcus neoformans* from the lungs leads to metastatic infection of various organ systems, especially the central nervous system. Signs of a slowly evolving meningitis are the usual clinical presentation of cryptococcal infection, particularly in the patient with some

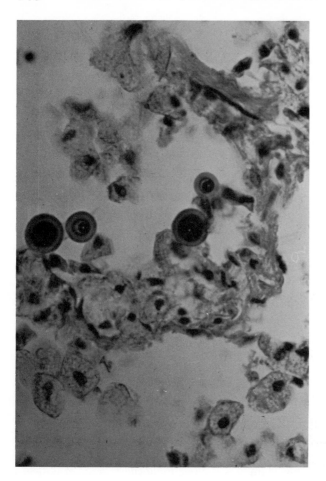

Figure 43-1. A section of a lobe of the lung removed at the time of surgical exploration for a presumed malignancy involving the lower right lung of a middle-aged male with a history of heavy cigarette smoking. Morphologic details of the cryptococcal yeast cells are seen especially well with the methenamine-silver stain used in this instance. The patient made a complete and uneventful recovery. Lack of demonstrable involvement of any other organ system led to a decision to withhold treatment with amphotericin B after the diagnosis of cryptococcal infection of the lung was established postoperatively. Fungi identified as *Cryptococcus neoformans* were isolated from the surgically removed lung specimen. The only evidence of altered host defense in this patient was a persistently low serum concentration of gamma globulin.

form of malignant lymphomatous disease. Cerebrospinal fluid abnormalities may be indistinguishable from those associated with meningitis caused by *Mycobacterium tuberculosis* (see Chap. 33). Budding yeast cells seen in India ink preparations, i.e., negative stains of cerebrospinal fluid sediments, constitute compelling evidence of cryptococcal meningitis (see Fig. 43–2 and Chap. 10). A relatively sensitive latex agglutination test has proved useful for detecting and quantitating cryptococcal capsular polysaccharide antigen in cerebrospinal fluid, serum, urine, and other body fluids. The presence of demonstrable antigen may be invaluable if the microorganism is not revealed in India ink preparations or if cultures of cerebrospinal fluid are negative. Hematogenous spread of *C. neoformans* to the kidney may occur, with subsequent development of chronic pyelonephritis. Therefore, the demonstration of yeast cells in the urine should establish a diagnosis of disseminated cryptococcal disease.

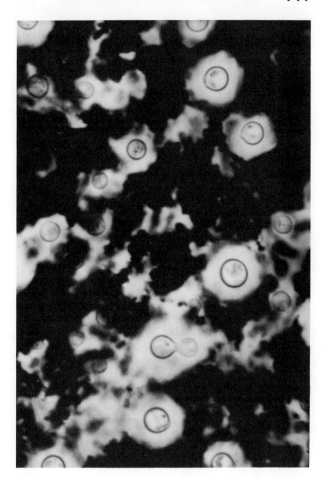

Figure 43-2. Cerebrospinal fluid sediment (from a 36-year-old male) mixed with India ink illustrates heavily encapsulated yeast cells, one of which is in the process of budding. Clinical signs of meningitis prompted hospitalization of this patient. Initial cerebrospinal fluid findings included a total cell count of 340 cells per cubic millimeter; glucose was 32 mg per 100 ml and protein was 128 mg per 100 ml. Culture of the cerebrospinal fluid yielded a yeast identified as *Cryptococcus neoformans.* The history revealed that eight months previously the patient had received a renal allograft for endstage chronic glomerulonephritis. Allograft function had been maintained by an immunosuppressive regimen consisting of azathioprine and prednisone.

Aspergillus species

Infection of prosthetic heart valves with *Aspergillus fumigatus* or other Aspergillus species, as well as pulmonary infection due to these microorganisms in immunosuppressed patients, is becoming sufficiently common to warrant mention. Definitive diagnosis is difficult. Blood cultures are often negative despite extensive growth of the fungus on the implanted prosthetic heart valve. Sputum cultures yielding Aspergillus species may not be indicative of infection of the lower respiratory tract, since the fungus may be found as part of the normal oropharyngeal flora in certain patients.

Candida albicans

Invasion of host tissues by *Candida albicans,* with subsequent candidemia and dissemination of the fungus to multiple organ systems, may occur in patients who (1) have an underlying malignant disease, usually hemato-proliferative disease, (2) are receiving intensive treatment with cortico-steroids, and (3) are undergoing extensive therapy with multiple antimicrobial agents. The difficulty of establishing a definitive diagnosis of disseminated candidiasis by blood cultures or the problem of interpreting a single, positive blood culture out of many taken would appear to be partially resolved by a recently reported new diagnostic technique. Using gas chromatographic analysis of blood samples, characteristic "fingerprints" of *C. albicans* cell wall constituents have been described in a high proportion of patients with disseminated candidiasis in whom the diagnosis was subsequently established by positive blood cultures obtained antemortem or by isolation of the yeast from autopsy specimens (see Chap. 10).

Toxoplasma gondii

There are two clinical settings in which infection due to *Toxoplasma gondii* may be anticipated: (1) the pregnant woman, in whom a variable degree of immunosuppression appears to develop as indicated by reduced immune responsiveness, and (2) the patient receiving immunosuppressive drugs in order to maintain the function of an allograft. Toxoplasmosis also occurs in patients who have a preference for eating raw or partially cooked meat. The appearance of *T. gondii* in meat reflects the widespread presence of this protozoan microorganism in sheep and other animal species used as food sources. Active infection often mimics infectious mononucleosis, with fever, generalized adenopathy, splenomegaly, and perhaps a fleeting maculopapular cutaneous eruption. The blood smear shows an increased percentage of lymphoblastoid mononuclear cells. A significant clinical concern is activation of latent *T. gondii* during pregnancy and consequent intrauterine infection of the fetus. This may result in congenital infection involving the choroid and central nervous system.

Pneumocystis carinii

Considerable debate surrounds the question as to how best to classify *Pneumocystis carinii*. Many investigators believe it is a protozoan, while other workers prefer to place it in an unclassified category. The microbe presumably colonizes a high proportion of healthy individuals early in life but does not disclose its presence until there is some compromise in host defense. Pulmonary infection is the most common clinical expression of active infection due to *P. carinii* and presents as a bilateral interstitial pulmonary infiltration, which progresses rapidly and severely reduces gas exchange. The hypoxia is responsible for many of the symptoms. *P. carinii* cannot be cultured on an artificial medium, and a diagnosis depends on demonstrating the microorganisms morphologically in appropriately stained tissue or body fluid specimens (Fig. 43-3). Pulmonary pneumocystosis is one of the most frequent causes of unilateral or bilateral pulmonary densities in patients with an allograft who develop fever and other manifestations of infectious disease.

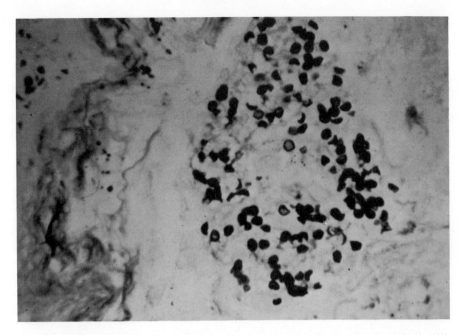

Figure 43–3. Lung tissue obtained at thoracotomy; biopsy sections stained with methenamine-silver. Structures indistinguishable from *Pneumocystis carinii* can be seen lying in the periphery of the alveolus. Although the life cycle of *P. carinii* is not completely known, cysts first appear within alveolar septal cells, usually without appreciable host inflammatory response. Maturing trophozoites break out of the cysts and spill into the alveolus, leaving behind partially collapsed, crescent-shaped cysts. The cysts and free trophozoites almost invariably are found amid a protein and lipid-rich coagulum that originates, at least in part, from disintegration of the cysts. It is at this point that the host begins to respond with an influx of the mononuclear inflammatory cells. The microorganisms are rarely seen in sputa specimens and only rarely visualized in transtracheal aspirates.

The patient in this instance was a 43-year-old female with a renal allograft maintained for one and one half years by intensive immunosuppressive drug therapy. Rapidly progressive bilateral lower lung densities accompanied by pleural effusions, rising fever, and increasing nonproductive cough and dyspnea led to hospitalization and intensive diagnostic work-up. Open lung biopsy was carried out 72 hours after careful microscopic examination and culture of sputa and lower respiratory tract secretions obtained by translaryngeal aspiration and endo-bronchial brushing provided no explanation of the pulmonary process. The patient was given a 10-day course of pentamidine. She responded well and there was complete clearing of the lung infiltrates and disappearance of all other signs of lower respiratory tract infection.

Rapid diagnosis is imperative, since the disease often has a fatal outcome if untreated. Reasonably effective treatment is available in the form of pentamidine isethionate.

Opportunistic DNA Viruses

Three DNA viruses commonly cause infection in patients receiving intensive or long-term immunosuppressive therapy or who have malignant lymphomas or other hematoproliferative diseases. These viruses are herpes simplex virus, varicella-zoster virus, and cytomegalovirus. All three viruses are capable of producing disseminated disease with pulmonary involvement as a common feature. Cutaneous disease may be an extensive and conspicuous manifestation of disseminated infection due to herpes simplex and varicella-zoster viruses (Fig. 43–4). Cytomegalovirus can produce a systemic illness simulating infectious mononucleosis; it has all the features of the latter disease except the production of heterophil antibodies, an important differential diagnostic point. Cytomegalovirus disease may also occur in otherwise healthy young adults. Multiple blood transfusions, particularly in association with the use of an extracorporeal pump in open heart surgery, are especially apt to induce systemic cytomegalovirus infection, viz., the so-called post-perfusion syndrome.

Diagnostic Approaches and Considerations

The diagnosis of infection in the compromised host is often hindered because of the suppression of certain host responses. Diminished cellular exudation and decreased diapedesis of leukocytes often cause late-appearing or atypical clinical manifestations of disease. Not infrequently, classic physical findings may be totally lacking. Appreciable delay in reaching a provisional or definitive diagnosis may result in the patient becoming

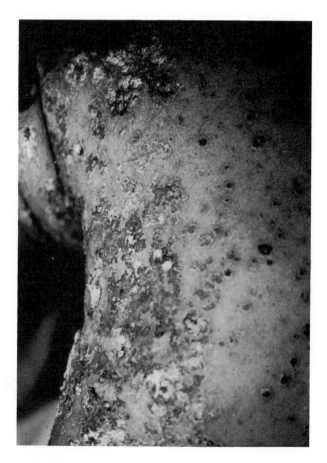

Figure 43–4. Extensive cutaneous eruption associated with dissemination of varicella-zoster viral infection in a 28-year-old male with a diagnosis of lymphosarcoma, established four months previously by lymph node and bone marrow biopsies. Treatment with cyclophosphamide and prednisone had been initiated three months prior to development of shingles, i.e., a cutaneous vesicular and pustular eruption confined to a few dermatomes of the back and stopping abruptly at the midline. A few days following the appearance of shingles, however, the cutaneous eruption became generalized; a chest roentgenogram revealed a pulmonary density in the left lower lung field. Aspiration of fluid from one of the cutaneous vesicles revealed cells containing prominent intranuclear inclusion bodies. Varicella-zoster virus was isolated by inoculating appropriate tissue culture lines with some of the vesicular fluid.

moribund by the time the correct diagnosis is revealed. At this point, specific therapy is of little use. This is a tragic outcome for patients with infections that, when treated early, are potentially reversible or capable of being eradicated with appropriate antimicrobial drugs. The lesson to be learned is the need for a persistent, aggressive diagnostic approach from the moment there is serious question of infection. In addition to utilization of all available serologic, microbiologic, cultural, and roentgenographic-radioisotopic procedures already discussed in this and other chapters, a number of noninvasive or invasive procedures may be employed. Diagnosis of certain infections, e.g., *Pneumocystis carinii* infections, that requires morphologic demonstration of the responsible microorganisms, is often impossible without securing tissue specimens for histopathologic studies.

One of the most common sites for infection in the compromised host is the lungs. The clinical setting usually involves a patient receiving intensive immunosuppressive drug therapy who develops fever, an increasing respiratory rate, and evidence of hypoxia in conjunction with progressive bilateral pulmonary infiltrates. Sputum cultures usually reveal normal microbial flora; blood cultures show no growth. In such a situation, the diagnostic possibilities and therapeutic approaches are numerous, and therapy should not be based merely on a clinical impression. The most direct approach is utilization of various procedures in the following order: (1) translaryngeal aspiration of lower respiratory secretions (see Chaps. 10 and 19); (2) endobronchial brushing, especially if done with a directable catheter under radiologic control; (3) percutaneous lung biopsy if the patient is not too hyperpneic to hold his breath momentarily; or (4) limited thoracotomy with open biopsy of the lung. It cannot be stressed enough that if temporization and procrastination are allowed to substitute for an aggressive diagnostic approach, by the time it is obvious that a diagnostic lung biopsy is mandatory, the patient's condition is often so precarious that he is no longer a suitable candidate for the procedure. An opportunity to uncover a potentially reversible infectious process is lost forever.

Therapeutic Approaches

Therapeutic approaches are designed not only to suppress growth of or eradicate the causative microorganism but also, if possible, to provide the patient with the defense mechanism that is needed. Antimicrobial drugs used in combinations are frequently synergistic in their action on some opportunistic microorganisms. Examples of such combinations include (1) erythromycin plus penicillin for accelerated clearance of *Listeria monocytogenes,* (2) carbenicillin plus cephalothin or gentamicin for bacteremia due to *Pseudomonas aeruginosa,* and (3) cycloserine or some other inhibitor of bacterial cell wall synthesis, e.g., ampicillin, plus a sulfonamide derivative for treatment of nocardiosis or local infection due to *Nocardia asteroides.* Even brain abscess due to *N. asteroides* has now been cured without the need of neurosurgical intervention by using long-term antimicrobial drug therapy involving at least two drugs shown to exert a synergistic action on *N. asteroides* in vitro.

Increasing evidence suggests that transfusion of large numbers of neutrophils provided by clinically well donors may be a useful therapeutic adjunct to treatment of leukopenic patients with infection, especially in those with bacteremia due to *Pseudomonas aeruginosa.*

Transfer factor is a dialyzable low molecular weight immunologic product of circulating peripheral blood lymphocytes that is induced by and specifically reactive with certain antigens to which the patient has been sensitized in the past. Transfer factor is thought to be responsible in large part for the development of the delayed-type cutaneous hypersensitivity to a wide variety of microbial antigens. This type of immune response is generally believed to be implicated in host defense against infections caused by facultative or obligate intracellular microorganisms. For these reasons, efforts have been made to provide patients who are demonstrably anergic with transfer factor in an attempt at immunologic reconstitution. In such instances, transfer factor, together with antimicrobial therapy directed at the underlying causative microorganism, is injected at frequent intervals. Double-blind studies concerning the efficacy of transfer factor therapy are in progress on a worldwide scale in patients with coccidioidomycosis, candidiasis, and leprosy.

The use of antiserum, prepared in human volunteers immunized with gram negative bacillary lipopolysaccharide, has already been mentioned in connection with hope for improvement in the therapeutic approach to gram negative bacillary sepsis, especially that caused by *Pseudomonas aeruginosa.* Recent studies involving experimental animals indicate that the polysaccharide lipid A core of endotoxin produced by widely diverse gram negative bacterial genera contains at least one common antigenic determinant. It would now appear feasible to consider the use of antiserum against endotoxin core as an adjunct to immunotherapy for gram negative bacterial infections.

Prophylaxis of infection in patients undergoing therapy that might predictably and variably compromise their host defenses has received increasing attention. Specific approaches include: (1) placement of patients in a protected environment, such as that provided by laminar flow systems that interpose an air barrier between the patient and exogenous microorganisms in his immediate vicinity, (2) extensive use of nonabsorbable antimicrobial drugs to reduce or abolish enteric microbial flora and thereby decrease the likelihood of infection developing from microorganisms within the gastrointestinal tract, (3) immunization with vaccines such as the heptavalent *Pseudomonas aeruginosa* lipopolysaccharide preparation (this pseudomonas vaccine has proved effective in reducing the incidence of pseudomonas infections in patients with cancer who are receiving various forms of cytolytic and immunosuppressive drug regimens), (4) injections of gamma globulin at appropriate intervals to decrease or prevent acquisition of infection due to hepatitis virus A, which can be a very serious infection in hosts lacking normal defense mechanisms, and (5) prophylactic antimicrobial drug regimens *if* directed against a specific microorganism, such as *Staphylococcus aureus* or *Staphylococcus epidermidis,* and used for a relatively short period of time following surgical implantation of a prosthetic device (e.g., heart valve, Holter ventriculoatrial bypass).

References

Review Articles

Lawrence, H. S.: Selective immunotherapy with transfer factor. Clin. Immunobiol. *2:*116, 1974.

Lawrence, H. S.: Transfer factor in cellular immunity. Harvey Lec. *68:*239, 1974.

McGee, Z. A., Schaffner, W., and Koenig, M. G.: Superinfection in lymphoreticular diseases. Ann. Rev. Med. *22:*25, 1971.

White, A., and Crowder, J. G.: Pseudomonas diseases. Adv. Intern. Med. *20:*23, 1975.

Original Articles

Biggar, W. D., Bogart, D., Holmes, B., and Good, R. A.: Impaired phagocytosis of pneumococcus type 3 in splenectomized rats. Proc. Soc. Exp. Biol. Med. *139:*903, 1972.

Goffinet, D. R., Glatstein, E. J., and Merigan, T. C.: Herpes zoster-varicella infections and lymphoma. Ann. Intern. Med. *76:*235, 1972.

Goldstein, E., and Hoeprich, P. D.: Problems in the diagnosis and treatment of systemic candidiasis. J. Infect. Dis. *125:*190, 1972.

Goodman, J. S., Kaufman, L., and Koenig, M. G.: Diagnosis of cryptococcal meningitis. Value of immunologic detection of cryptococcal antigen. N. Engl. J. Med. *285:*434, 1971.

Graw, R. G., Jr., Herzig, G., Perry, S., and Henderson, E. S.: Normal granulocyte transfusion therapy. Treatment of septicemia due to Gram-negative bacteria. N. Engl. J. Med. *287:*367, 1972.

Hoeprich, P. D., Brandt, D., and Parker, R. H.: Nocardial brain abscess cured with cycloserine and sulfonamides. Am. J. Med. Sci. *255:*208, 1968.

Hoeprich, P. D.: Chemoprophylaxis of infection in patients receiving steroids, irradiation and cytotoxic agents. Med. Times *97:*133, 1969.

Krick, J. A., Stinson, E. B., and Remington, J. S.: Nocardia infection in heart transplant patients. Ann. Intern. Med. *82:*18, 1975.

Meyer, R. D., Young, L. S., Armstrong, D., and Yu, B.: Aspergillosis complicating neoplastic disease. Am. J. Med. *54:*6, 1973.

Miller, G. G., Witwer, M. W., Braude, A. I., and Davis, C. E.: Rapid identification of Candida albicans septicemia in man by gas-liquid chromatography. J. Clin. Invest. *54:*1235, 1974.

Remington, J. S.: The compromised host. Hosp. Practice *7:*59, 1972.

Reynolds, D. W., Stagno, S., Hosty, T. S., Tiller, M., and Alford, C. A., Jr.: Maternal cytomegalovirus excretion and perinatal infection. N. Engl. J. Med. *289:*1, 1973.

Reynolds, H. Y., Levine, A. S., Wood, R. E., Zierdt, C. H., Dale, D. C., and Pennington, J. E.: Pseudomonas aeruginosa infections: Persisting problems and current research to find new therapies. Ann. Intern. Med. *82:*819, 1975.

Robboy, S. J., and Vickery, A. L., Jr.: Tinctorial and morphologic properties distinguishing actinomycosis and nocardiosis. N. Engl. J. Med. *282:*593, 1970.

Rodriguez, V., and Bodey, G. P.: Bacterial infections in immunosuppressed patients: diagnosis and management. Transplant Proc. *5:*1249, 1973.

Schimpff, S., Serpick, A., Stoler, B., Rumack, R., Mellin, H., Joseph, J. M., and Block, J.: Varicella-zoster infection in patients with cancer. Ann. Intern. Med. *76:*241, 1972.

Schimpff, S. C., Greene, W. H., Young, V. M., Fortner, C. L., Jepsen, L., Cusack, N., Block, J. B., and Wiernick, P. H.: Infection prevention in acute nonlymphocytic leukemia. Laminar air flow room reverse isolation with oral, nonabsorbable antibiotic prophylaxis. Ann. Intern. Med. *82:*351, 1975.

Walzer, P. D., Perl, D. P., Krogstad, D. J., Rawson, P. G., and Schultz, M. G.: Pneumocystis carinii pneumonia in the United States. Epidemiologic, diagnostic and clinical features. Ann. Intern. Med. *80:*83, 1974.

Western, K. A., Perera, D. R., and Schultz, M. G.: Pentamidine isethionate in the treatment of Pneumocystis carinii pneumonia. Ann. Intern. Med. *73:*695, 1970.

Ziegler, E. J., Douglas, H., Sherman, J. E., Davis, C. E., and Braude, A. I.: Treatment of E. coli and Klebsiella bacteremia in agranulocytic animals with antiserum to UDP-GAL epimerase-deficient mutant. J. Immunol. *111:*433, 1973.

X

ANTIMICROBIAL THERAPY

Chapter 44

MOLECULAR BIOLOGY OF SENSITIVITY AND RESISTANCE TO ANTIMICROBIAL AGENTS

Introduction

Just prior to the outbreak of the First World War, a noteworthy statement of the principles of chemotherapy was made. Ehrlich defined the essential qualities needed for a useful chemotherapeutic drug as two in number: (1) an *affinity* between some part of the drug and a receptor possessed by the parasite, and (2) a *toxic potential* of the drug which is capable of destroying the (viability of the) parasite once the binding has occurred. Although the language used by Ehrlich is somewhat old fashioned by today's standards, his analysis is as fresh and compatible with current biology as anything now being written. However, the disciplines of biochemistry, microbiology, and pharmacology, with their subdivisions into molecular biology, biophysics, etc., had to be developed before the basic tools necessary to understand drug action could become available. The rate limiting process has not been any major deficiency in our concepts but in our knowledge of biochemical detail.

The treatment of infectious diseases with antibiotics has been one of the major practical miracles of modern medicine. The course of history has seen incredible ravages caused by relatively few infectious agents. For instance, even a cursory look at the history of western Europe and England shows that from time to time whole populations were nearly eliminated or suddenly greatly reduced. These people were victims of cholera, typhus, plague, and other infectious agents which are now treatable with antimicrobial agents or preventable by immunization. The effect of these virulent infectious agents on our social, religious, economic, political, and cultural development is beyond comprehension. We cannot know what the world would be like today had even an empirical knowledge of antibiotics been available a few centuries ago. Similarly, we now face a different problem which paradoxically is caused in part by the availability of antibiotics. What will our civilization be like now that we are able to produce and potentially keep alive more people than we can feed? The antibiotic age illustrates an old principle concerning the balance of nature. Whenever the system is perturbed — in this case by the development of new knowledge that helps maintain or extend human life — a new equilibrium is achieved to return the system to a balance. We do not yet see the final effect of antibiotics on society, and it may never be possible to separate the effect of their availability from that of other modalities of medicine.

Basic Principles

Before an antibiotic can act it must first interact with some part of a parasite or a pathogenic microorganism in a human or animal host. This interaction may be less specific than the binding implied in Ehrlich's definition. The interaction may be initiated by a specific active transport process of the cell that serves to increase the intracellular "free" concentration of the antibiotic above that which would be achieved by passive diffusion. The intracellular concentration of the antibiotic is determined by the balance of influx and efflux, and no specific binding of the drug to any intracellular components need be assumed. The consequences of the high intracellular concentration of the antibiotic eventually will be expressed by a specific interaction of the drug molecule with some enzyme, a subcellular component of the cell, etc.

The explanation of how any given antibiotic acts ultimately involves one or more very specific biochemical or biophysical events in the invading bacterial or fungal cell. Successful chemotherapy requires that the metabolic process to be attacked in the microorganism be as different as possible from that of the animal host. Obviously it is a clinical failure to kill or inhibit the growth of the microorganism at the cost of the patient's life or continued well-being. Some antibiotics (e.g., streptomycin and other aminoglycosidic antibiotics, chloramphenicol) are toxic to the host as well as to the microorganism, and the real damage that is or may be done to the patient by the antimicrobial agent must be balanced against the degree of danger to his life posed by the microorganism. Many of today's physicians are not well informed about these risks, and casually use antibiotics when their need is not established. The choice of relatively toxic drugs is frequently inappropriate and their use without adequate supervision potentially dangerous (see Chaps. 1 and 46).

A discussion of the biochemical basis of the *mode of action* of the clinically used antibiotics depends on understanding some fundamental processes in the human host. *Resistance* to the effect of an antibiotic, either as a constitutive property of the microorganism before it infects a host or as a complication which suddenly appears during a course of therapy with an antibiotic, is also explainable in highly specific biochemical terms. Resistance to specific antimicrobial agents is reviewed below.

The purpose of this chapter is to discuss the biochemical basis of susceptibility (sensitivity) and resistance to some commonly used antibiotics. There are a variety of specific ways by which an antimicrobial agent may inhibit a microorganism. These are reviewed later. However, there are only three general ways by which a microorganism can *resist* an antibiotic, and these constitute the basic reasons why a particular antimicrobial agent may not inhibit the growth of a microorganism that is isolated from a patient.

1. *The antibiotic may be unable to reach the potential target site of its action.* In a mutant some change in the physiology of the cell following a biochemical change to that cell may increase the difficulty of the drug reaching the site of action.

2. *The pathogenic agent may possess some biochemical mechanism (enzyme) that acts to reduce or eliminate the toxic potential of the antibiotic.* In a mutant an increased level of enzymatic activity or even a new mechanism for inactivating the drug may develop. Examples are (1) beta lactamases that cleave penicillins and cephalosporins to inactive components, (2) acylases that acetylate chloramphenicol to yield inactive derivatives, and (3) enzymes that inactivate aminoglycosides by phosphorylation, adenylation, acetylation, etc.

3. *The pathogenic agent may have evolved biochemically in such a way that the target site for the antibiotic as determined with other cells no longer accommodates the drug, and no productive (toxic) interaction occurs.* In the mutant cell this change in the biochemistry of the target site occurs during the time period of observation or of treatment of the patient. Examples are cells which become resistant to erythromycin, lincomycin, streptomycin, etc.

All three mechanisms for blocking the action of an otherwise active antibiotic or for acquiring resistance to it are known. To understand them it is necessary to know the biochemical basis for the mode of action of the drug. In particular, this is essential if resistance is related to a change at the cellular target of the antibiotic. It is necessary to consider here a number of the salient facts known about the antibiotics currently useful in medicine. These are discussed in the remaining portion of this chapter. The general organization follows the known (or presumed) major biochemical target for each antibiotic or class of antibiotic if a large number of chemically related drugs have the same or similar targets. The ways in which an antibiotic may disturb the physiology of a parasitic or pathogenic agent are almost infinite. Any single enzyme or structure in the living cell can potentially be affected and rendered incapable of fulfilling its normal function. In spite of this tremendous range of potential target sites for antibiotics, those most used in human and veterinary medicine fall into well-defined categories of action, and only a few critical areas of microbial physiology are affected. These areas are mostly concerned with the genetic replication of the cell (transcription), the expression of that genetic information into functional proteins (translation), and the assembly or function of critical cell components such as the bacterial cell wall or membranes.

It should be noted here that there is a major difference between human eukaryotic cells and the usual bacterial or fungal antagonist. In contrast to the latter, the human cell possesses mitochondria, and although the argument as to their origin is not settled, these semiautonomous organelles have many of the characteristics of bacteria. Their nonchromosomal genetic material is similar to that of bacteria and their apparatus for transcription and translation of mitochondrial DNA and RNA is also similar. Thus, although many of the useful antibiotics to be mentioned attack some part of the bacterial or fungal cell which is fundamentally different from anything in the human host, there is a real potential for some damage to human cells via the mitochondria they possess. The toxic action of chloramphenicol on mammalian cells is perhaps related to its ability to permeate the mitochondrial membrane and interfere with mitochondrial protein synthesis. A chemically different drug, erythromycin, which has a very similar target site and mode of action, is seemingly unable to cross the mitochondrial membrane and, thus, erythromycin shows little, if any, toxicity to human cells. Subtle factors of this sort account for many of the anomalies connected with the practical use of antibiotics.

Mode of Action of Major Antimicrobial Agents Used in Clinical Medicine

Thousands of antimicrobial agents are known and have been derived either from natural selection procedures or from chemical routes. Of these, a large number have been tested for potential clinical application. Unfortunately, the vast majority have not proved useful, often because the agent is too toxic to be employed as a selective chemotherapeutic agent. In pharmacologic terms, this means that the therapeutic index (ratio of the curative to the toxic dose) is unfavorable. Many of the toxic antibiotics have been thoroughly studied by those interested in the mechanisms of microbial physiology and chemotherapy. Detailed chapters on some of these clinically useless drugs are to be found in reference works (see References, especially Gottlieb and Shaw, 1967; and Corcoran and Hahn, 1975).

The intent of this chapter is to focus on a limited number of examples of drugs that are used today in clinical practice. In cases in which a large variety of agents with the same basic structure and mode of action are available to the physician, e.g., semisynthetic penicillins, cephalosporins, and aminoglycosides, only a few representative examples are discussed. Some of the clinical differences within closely related groups of antimicrobial agents have been discussed elsewhere (see Chaps. 45 and 46).

The organization of this section follows the current opinion regarding the major target of action of the antimicrobial agent. It must be kept in mind that the presence of a drug causes both primary and secondary biochemical changes in a microbial cell, and it is often difficult to separate one group of changes from the other. Perhaps the best example of confusion regarding a primary mode of action for a clinically important antibiotic group is that seen with streptomycin and the other aminoglycosides. The results of a tremendous amount of work have finally suggested strongly that the primary effect of streptomycin is to inhibit ribosomal-dependent protein synthesis. However, evidence also exists that would place the primary action at the level of an interference with messenger RNA function.

Inhibitors of Bacterial Cell Function

An antimicrobial agent may affect either the function or the structure of a bacterial cell. Although the function of a structurally normal cell may be inhibited in almost an infinite number of ways, it is convenient to categorize the inhibitors as (1) inhibitors of nucleic acid synthesis or function, (2) inhibitors of protein synthesis, (3) inhibitors of the normal functioning of the plasma membrane, and (4) inhibitors of the function of a specific microbial enzyme or enzyme system. Useful antimicrobial agents are known which fit into each of these four categories.

Antimicrobial Agents That Affect DNA and RNA

Many drugs are known which are potent inhibitors of some phase of transcription and translation, the complex series of reactions by which the DNA of a parent cell is copied prior to cell division and directs the formation of RNA species which are needed for the synthesis of cellular proteins, cofactors, substrates, etc. A large number of potent antibiotics are known which inhibit transcription. However, relatively few antibiotics of this type are in clinical use, probably because the biochemistry of transcription in bacteria is not sufficiently different from that in the human host cells to permit a very favorable therapeutic index with this class of drug. Agents such as the actinomycins are too toxic to be of much use as antimicrobial drugs in humans. They are used occasionally as antitumor agents but are cited here as an example of drugs showing the high toxicity associated with so many inhibitors of transcription. In clinical medicine, the most useful antibiotics which do affect DNA transcription are the rifamycins (rifampin) and nalidixic acid. Rifampin is an inhibitor of DNA-dependent RNA polymerase, and this enzyme system in bacteria is sufficiently different from that in mammalian cells to permit selective chemotherapy. Nalidixic acid also inhibits DNA replication without seriously affecting mammalian cells.

Rifamycins (Rifampin, Ansamacrolides). There are a large number of rifamycin antibiotics, mostly of semisynthetic origin. The class comprises other chemically similar structures (streptovaricins, tolypomycins, etc.) and has been given the generic name *ansamacrolide.* This term should *not* be confused with the macrolides, e.g., erythromycin. The two classes of antibiotics are chemically very different, and their modes of action differ as well. The original rifamycins as isolated from *Streptomyces mediterranei* were not well absorbed and were not very active. Chemical modification of the structures has led to several series of semisynthetic derivatives with high antimicrobial potency and excellent therapeutic indices. The actions of these drugs are somewhat varied, but the most useful one and that for which the best known derivative, rifampin, is marketed is a rather specific inhibitor of *Mycobacterium tuberculosis.* The current therapy for tuberculosis has been greatly improved by the availability of rifampin (see Chap. 24).

The rifamycins (rifampin) are very specific inhibitors of RNA polymerase (Fig. 44–1). Moreover, it is specifically the bacterial DNA-dependent RNA polymerase which is affected. Neither DNA-dependent DNA synthesis in bacteria nor nuclear DNA-dependent RNA synthesis by eukaryotic cells is inhibited. This explains the selective toxicity of rifampin toward bacterial cells. Rifampin can inhibit RNA synthesis in the mitochondria of human cells, but the drug appears to be relatively impermeable to the mitochondrion. Rifampin occasionally causes hepatotoxicity, which could be related to an effect on mitochondrial RNA replication. Rifampin specifically inhibits bacterial RNA polymerase by binding to the *beta* subunit of the core enzyme of the polymerase. The initiation phase of RNA synthesis is blocked by this drug, and if RNA synthesis has begun prior to the addition of the rifampin there is no inhibition of the remaining steps in the synthesis of RNA.

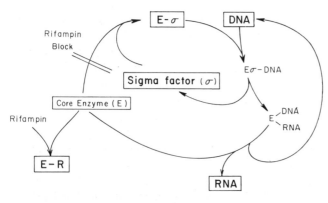

Figure 44-1. Diagrammatic illustration of the way in which rifampin inhibits DNA-dependent RNA synthesis in bacteria. The core enzyme (E) normally forms a complex with the sigma factor (σ) before binding to the DNA template to form an active enzyme capable of synthesizing RNA. Once RNA synthesis is complete, the core enzyme and sigma factor are released and each returns to the pool of "free" subunits. With rifampin present, a complex between the antibiotic and the core enzyme is formed, and the abnormal complex (E-R) is incapable of forming the core enzyme–sigma factor aggregate that is required for binding with DNA and leads to active synthesis of RNA.

Nalidixic Acid. Nalidixic acid (Fig. 44–2), a rather simple compound made by chemical means, is an inhibitor of DNA replication in bacterial cells. It fails to inhibit DNA transcription in mammalian cells. It apparently can inhibit mitochondrial DNA replication, but the drug is usually relatively nontoxic, perhaps because it fails to reach significantly high concentrations in plasma and other body compartments. It is, however, concentrated in the urine, where it reaches effective therapeutic levels. The exact target of nalidixic acid action is still in dispute. It is safe to say that its primary effect in the intact living bacterium is a prompt, selective, and reversible block in DNA synthesis. This block occurs with many types of DNA replication, including normal duplication of DNA as necessary for cell duplication, the repair of DNA which normally occurs after damage by ultraviolet light, and the replication seen with some viruses.

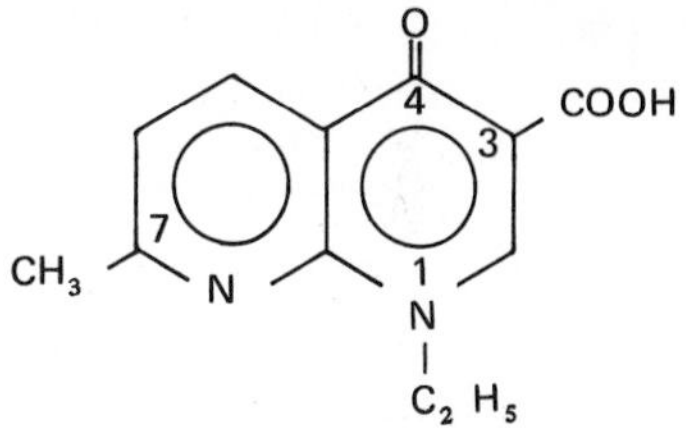

Figure 44–2. Structure of nalidixic acid.

Inhibitors of Protein Synthesis

A rather large group of useful antimicrobial agents interfere with protein synthesis in bacteria. Since this process differs in a few essential details from that in eukaryotic (mammalian) cells, it is a good target for chemotherapy. In particular, the ribosomal subunits involved in messenger RNA translation in bacterial systems are smaller (30S and 50S) than those involved in mammalian translation (40S and 60S, respectively). Figure 44–3 illustrates the essential steps in the formation of the 70S ribosome in bacterial systems and will be referred to as each antimicrobial drug is discussed.

Aminoglycosidic Antibiotics (Streptomycin, Neomycin, Kanamycin, Gentamicin, etc.). A large number of antibiotics are included under the term *aminoglycosides.* Their common denominator structurally is the presence of a cyclohexane ring with basic (amino or guanidino) groups in the 1 and 3 positions (Fig. 44–4). In naturally occurring structures, the other positions have hydroxyl groups, with the exception of C-2, which sometimes has only hydrogen atoms. Different residues (sugars, including basic sugars) are attached by other links to the free hydroxyl groups; thus, a great variation in overall structure is possible; e.g., the streptomycin group differs greatly from the more recently introduced gentamicins, tobramycins, etc. The mode of action of each of the aminoglycosides is believed to be roughly similar and is discussed here in terms of streptomycin, the longest used aminoglycosidic antibiotic and the substance whose action has been the most intensely studied. Streptomycin is one of the oldest antibiotics known, and it is still

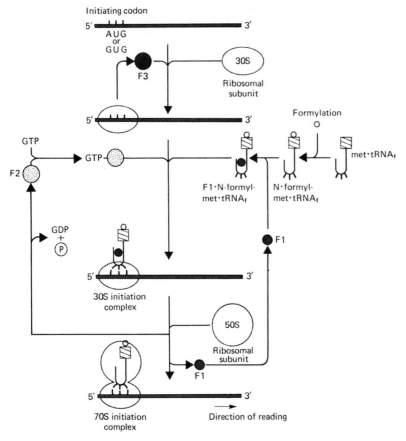

F1 [MW 8000] probably involved in binding 50S to 30S initiation complex.
F2 [MW 75,000] probably involved in binding N-blocked amino acyl tRNA.
F3 [MW 30,000] probably binds 30S ribosomal subunit to mRNA.

Figure 44–3. Diagrammatic view of the initiation process in bacterial protein synthesis. (From Watson, J. D.: Molecular Biology of the Gene. 2nd Ed. Copyright © 1970 by J. D. Watson; W. A. Benjamin, Inc., Menlo Park, California.)

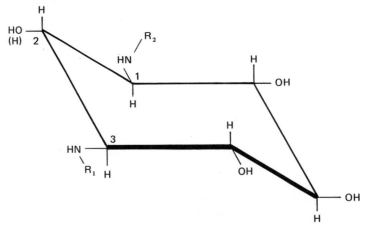

Figure 44–4. Structure of the substituted streptamine (or 2-deoxystreptamine) moiety present in all aminoglycoside antibiotics (R_1 and R_2 = basic amino or guanidino groups).

used extensively today. It has a broad spectrum of action, but resistance in bacteria readily develops (see below). In addition, this and other aminoglycosidic antibiotics are selectively toxic to the cranial nerve (eighth) responsible for hearing and equilibrium.

The various actions of streptomycin on both in vivo and in vitro protein synthesis in bacteria are well described. A large number (10 or more) of rather different effects have been noted, and the problem is to distinguish between primary and secondary actions. The primary effect of streptomycin is thought to be interference with 30S ribosomal unit function and its ability to form an initiation complex with messenger RNA, an aminoacyl transfer RNA species, and the various initiation factors (see Fig. 44–3).

Another property of streptomycin and most but not all aminoglycosides is the ability to induce misreading of the codons in messenger RNA, thereby producing mistakes in the translated product. These mistakes have been blamed for the killing effect of streptomycin, gentamicin, etc. However, this is not in agreement with the conclusion that the primary action of streptomycin on bacterial protein synthesis is an inhibition of 30S ribosomal unit function.

There is a protein component in the 30S ribosomal unit that determines the degree of sensitivity to streptomycin, and mutants which lack this protein are resistant to streptomycin.

Tetracyclines. These are broad-spectrum antibiotics with a complex ring system (Fig. 44–5). The tetracyclines form an insoluble complex with many metal ions, and poor absorption of orally administered tetracyclines from the gastrointestinal tract may be caused by their interaction with calcium or other salts that are present in food.

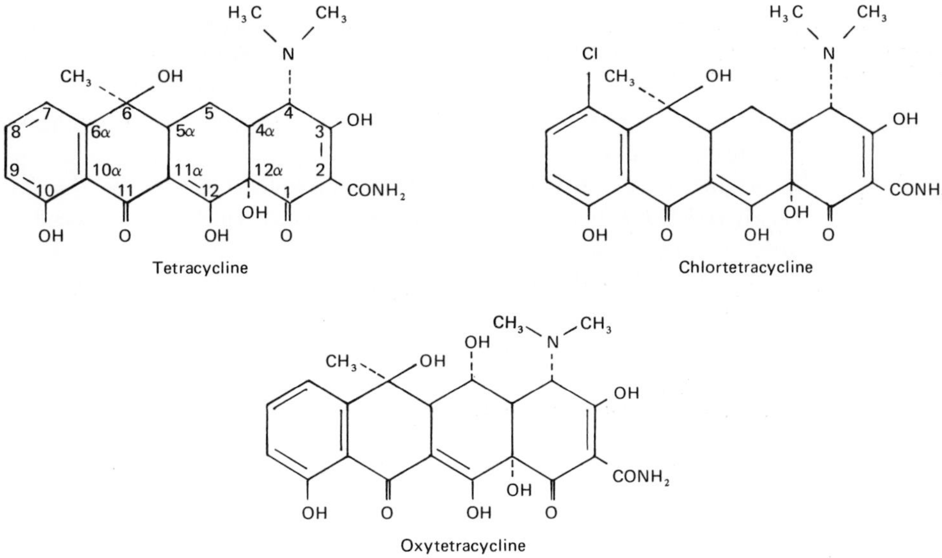

Figure 44-5. Chemical structures of the three major tetracycline antibiotics.

The tetracyclines inhibit protein synthesis at the ribosomal level. They act on both bacterial and mammalian ribosomes but have their greatest action on the 30S subunit of bacterial systems. The tetracyclines apparently do not block formation of the 30S ribosome–messenger RNA complex, but they probably do interfere with aminoacyl transfer RNA attachment to the 30S initiation complex (see Fig. 44–3).

Macrolide Antibiotics. The so-called macrolides are a very large group of antibiotics produced primarily by the genus Streptomyces. Their common structural denominator is a large lipid ring (inner ester or lactone, chemically termed a *macrolide*). The 14- and 16-membered macrolide antibiotics are the macrolides most studied and used in both human and veterinary antibacterial chemotherapy. Erythromycin and oleandomycin, which are quite similar in structure, are examples of the 14-membered group. The 16-membered macrolides (tylosin, members of the leucomycin complex including derivatives such as josamycin, niddamycin, maridomycin, etc.) have lactones different from the 14-membered macrolides, and although the sugars they possess are identical or similar to those of the erythromycin type (14-membered), the mode of structural attachments is different. Currently, the 16-membered macrolide antibiotics are not used in clinical practice in the United States. However, cross-resistance between some of them (e.g., tylosin) and erythromycin has been noted, and the very heavy use of tylosin in veterinary medicine poses a potential problem for human therapy. Consequently, the use of tylosin has been severely restricted in the United Kingdom, although no such action has been taken in the United States. The 16-membered macrolides are also used for the treatment of humans in Japan and the Orient. Therefore one should be aware of their existence and the possibility that exposure of the microbial population to these agents, even if in animals used for food, may increase clinical resistance to erythromycin.

It is essential to note here that, in addition to the so-called ansamacrolides already discussed, a second and quite different type of antimicrobial agent is also classified with the macrolides. These other macrolide drugs are antifungal agents and have no antibacterial effects. They are structurally quite different from erythromycin and have a very different mode of action. Two of them, amphotericin B (candicidin) and nystatin, are used in human chemotherapy and are discussed briefly below.

Erythromycin. Erythromycin A (erythromycin) is one of the four closely related antibiotics of the macrolide class which are produced by *Streptomyces erythraeus*. Erythromycin, whose structure is shown in Figure 44–6, has been in clinical use since the 1950s. It is a nontoxic antibiotic effective mainly against gram positive bacteria and certain strains of mycoplasma and is structurally very similar to oleandomycin.

All of the studies done on the mode of action of erythromycin lead to the conclusion that its primary action is to inhibit RNA-dependent protein synthesis in bacteria. Protein synthesis in so-called resistant bacteria (e.g., gram negative microorganisms such as *Escherichia coli*) is also sensitive to erythromycin, but these insensitive strains of bacteria are limited in their ability to accumulate erythromycin at the target site of its action. Erythromycin inhibits protein synthesis in a very specific way. It first binds to a 50S ribosomal subunit (see Fig. 44–3) and then remains attached to this

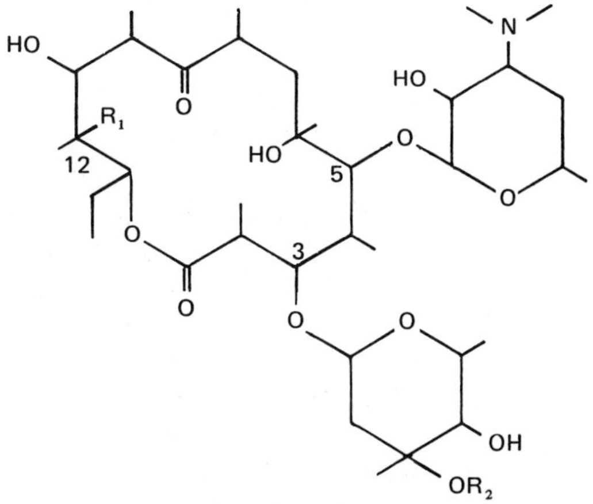

		R₁	R₂
Erythromycin	A	OH	Me
	B	H	Me
	C	OH	H
	D	H	H

Figure 44–6. The erythromycins.

unit when the functional 70S monosome is formed (including the polysomes in which many monosomes are simultaneously translating a molecule of messenger RNA). A single molecule of erythromycin binds to each 50S unit; this same stoichiometry has been noted in all macrolide antibiotics studied. The exact stage of protein synthesis which is inhibited by the bound erythromycin is not completely understood. However, the observed effect is a slowdown or stoppage in the translation of messenger RNA into functional protein molecules. The effect of erythromycin is reversible; thus, if the concentration of the drug is low and the duration of contact with the bacterium short, a bacteriostatic action is seen. The bacterial cell may be killed if contact is prolonged and the concentration of erythromycin is high.

Studies of bacterial resistance to erythromycin have failed to give any evidence supporting the fact that bacteria can enzymatically change the structure of the antibiotic. However, there is some evidence to show that resistant strains of bacteria are impaired in their ability to accumulate erythromycin. This effect may be secondary to the proven changes in the bacterial ribosome (50S subunit) which occur when a mutational event leads to a reduction in the sensitivity of the bacterial cell to erythromycin. In the cases studied, the binding constant for the erythromycin and the 50S ribosomal subunit is sharply reduced after the occurrence of such a mutation.

A second and somewhat unusual pattern for the development of resistance to erythromycin and other macrolide antibiotics has also been described. It is one in which exposure of a sensitive strain of a bacterium to *subinhibitory* concentrations of erythromycin induces resistance to much higher concentrations of the antibiotic. If the erythromycin is removed completely from the growth medium for the newly resistant bacteria, bacteria rapidly revert to the sensitive state. It is not certain that this phenomenon of "inducible resistance" is very common or if, indeed, it presents a clinical problem. However, the use of erythromycin at subinhibitory concentrations may prove to be dangerous.

Lincomycin. Lincomycin is a relatively new antimicrobial agent which has been shown to inhibit bacterial protein synthesis in a manner very similar to that of erythromycin. Lincomycin is produced by *Streptomyces lincolnensis* and has a structure seemingly quite different from erythromycin (Fig. 44–7). The activity of lincomycin is greatest against gram positive microorganisms, although a semisynthetic 7-chloro derivative (clindamycin) demonstrates increased potency against some gram negative strains. The mode of action of the lincomycins is so similar to that of erythromycin that sensitive biochemical measurements have been necessary to show that there are differences. Lincomycin binds to the 50S ribosomal subunit, and both biochemical and genetic evidence strongly suggests that the binding site overlaps but is not identical with that of erythromycin. Lincomycin does not bind to the ribosome as tightly as does erythromycin, but once bound it may be a more potent inhibitor of bacterial protein synthesis. There is an antagonism between erythromycin and lincomycin (see below) that is explainable on the basis that erythromycin can displace the more potent lincomycin from its binding site on the ribosome. Although originally believed to be as nontoxic as erythromycin, lincomycin, especially clindamycin (the 7-chloro derivative), may cause pseudomembranous colitis. For this reason, clindamycin should not be used for general prophylaxis or the treatment of minor infections.

Chloramphenicol. Chloramphenicol is a broad-spectrum antibiotic produced by *Streptomyces venezuelae* and, more practically, by total chemical synthesis. It has a simple structure (Fig. 44–8) but possesses two relatively unusual features, an aromatic nitro group and a dichloroacetyl side chain. Of four possible stereoisomers, only one possesses antibacterial

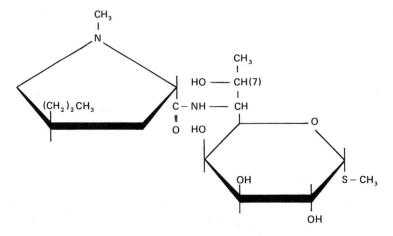

Figure 44–7. Structure of lincomycin.

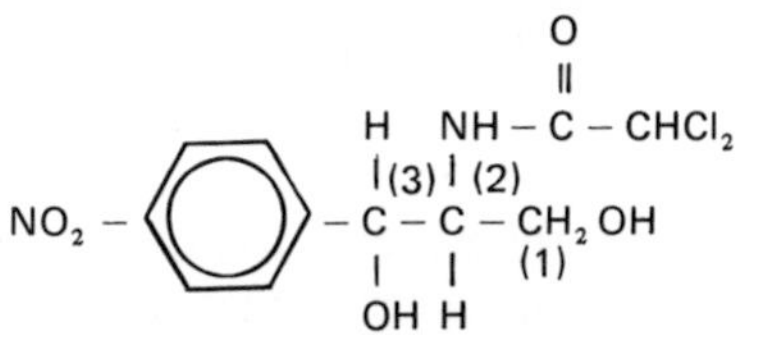

Figure 44–8. The structure of chloramphenicol.

activity. Both the nitro group and the dichloroacetyl residue may be replaced by some other groupings with substantial retention of biologic activity.

Chloramphenicol has always been an attractive antibiotic, and it still enjoys a large degree of support from certain clinicians, especially for hospital use. It is probably the most controversial antimicrobial drug in common use, because of its known tendency to produce highly toxic symptoms, including blood dyscrasias, aplastic anemia, and depression of bone marrow function. These dangers must be balanced against the broad spectrum of activity of chloramphenicol and the ability it possesses to inhibit the growth of most bacteria, rickettsiae, and chlamydiae (microorganisms of the psittacosis-lymphogranuloma group). It should be used with great caution, and most physicians believe that it should be administered only under adequate hospital supervision, including frequent tests for changes in the hematopoietic system.

Of all the known inhibitors of protein synthesis in bacteria, chloramphenicol has most likely been studied in the greatest detail. Nonetheless, its precise mode of action remains in doubt. It clearly inhibits the function of the 50S ribosomal subunit by first binding to this particle. The binding is quite weak when compared with that of either erythromycin or lincomycin. There may be some overlap of the binding sites for these three antimicrobial agents, although studies performed with clinically significant concentrations of the drugs suggest that the binding of erythromycin and chloramphenicol is additive and that the two drugs have a synergistic effect. At higher concentrations, mutual interference between erythromycin and chloramphenicol occurs.

The toxicity of chloramphenicol, when compared with that of erythromycin and lincomycin, is probably due to the ability of chloramphenicol to penetrate the eukaryotic cell and, in particular, the mitochondria. Here it probably inhibits mitochondrial protein synthesis and thus is toxic to the host as well as to the infectious microorganism.

Resistance to chloramphenicol is well documented and is related to enzymes (either constitutive or induced) that inactivate the drug primarily by acetylation of the two free hydroxyl groups present in the molecule (discussed later in this chapter).

Antimicrobial Agents That Affect Function of Bacterial Cytoplasmic Membrane

A large number of antimicrobial agents affect the function of the cytoplasmic membrane of bacteria. The problem with most of these drugs is that toxicity occurs not only in the bacterial cytoplasmic membrane but also in erythrocyte membranes and the membranes of other cells in the human host. Thus, for the most part, these agents are of no clinical utility. A few of these antimicrobial agents are used when the mode of application may be topical, and occasionally they are administered by infusion into closed compartments (joints, etc.).

Gramicidins and Tyrocidins.   These are cyclic oligopeptides whose exact structures reflect the amino acids available to the producing microorganism at the time of their synthesis. They are highly charged molecules, and the mode of their action is believed to be that of a cationic detergent. In the presence of gramicidins or tyrocidins the permeability of the bacterial cell membrane is seriously affected. Many secondary changes follow this primary action.

Amphotericin B and Nystatin.   These antimicrobial agents are also members of the macrolide groups (discussed earlier), but as stated previously, they are chemically quite different from erythromycin. Structurally, they have a lipid ring much larger than the 14-membered ring of erythromycin (Fig. 44–9), and their mode of action is completely different from that of

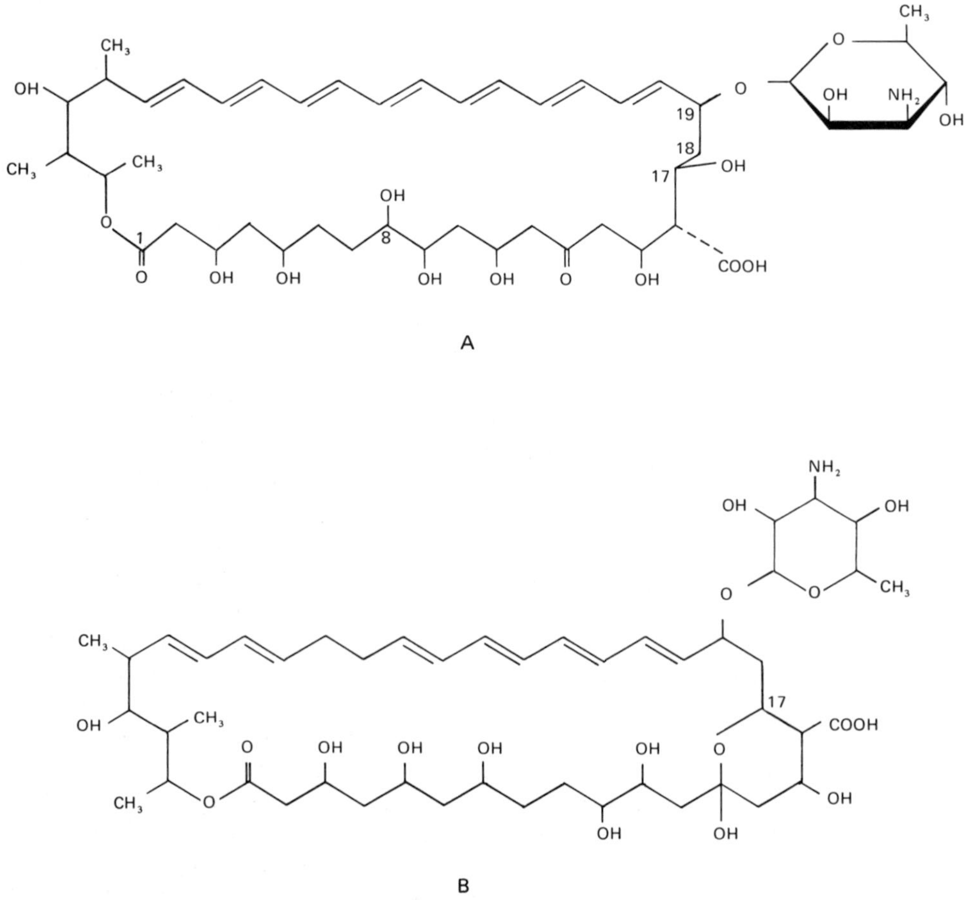

Figure 44–9. Structure of amphotericin B (*A*) and nystatin (*B*).

erythromycin. Neither amphotericin B (candicidin) nor nystatin is an antibacterial agent. Each demonstrates instead an antifungal activity and is included among the very few systemic antifungal agents available for clinical use; however, these two agents are toxic to the human host and must be used with care (see Chap. 26).

The biologically active antifungal macrolides such as amphotericin B and nystatin possess a number of conjugated carbon-carbon double bonds in their structure. These macrolides are, for this reason, quite unstable to both ultraviolet light and mild chemical reagents. It is also believed that the polyene system (this group of antibiotics is often termed the *polyene macrolides*) is responsible for the known mode of action of these drugs. Those that are active are capable of forming tight complexes with certain sterols, e.g., cholesterol and ergosterol. Cholesterol is an essential component of mammalian cell membranes, and ergosterol plays a similar role in the fungal plasma membrane. Bacteria lack sterols in their plasma membranes, thereby explaining the selective action of these agents against human and fungal cells.

Once the amphotericin B or nystatin molecule has complexed with ergosterol from the fungal membrane, the properties of the membrane are seriously altered. The membranes become "leaky," and the normal gradients of ions and other metabolites cannot be maintained, leading to the killing of the fungal cell. Since these antimicrobial agents remove cholesterol from the human host cell membranes, there is the possibility of toxicity.

Inhibitors of Microbial Enzyme Systems

There are many individual enzymes and complexes of enzymes in bacterial cells. It is only recently that systematic screening for inhibitors of many of these enzymes has begun. It is not difficult to find such inhibitors, but many are too toxic to be useful as antimicrobial agents. A few inhibitors of this type have been very useful in medicine and deserve mention. Perhaps the most important example is the sulfonamides (sulfanilamide, etc.).

Sulfonamides. Introduced into therapy in the mid-1930s, the sulfa drugs were the first useful antimicrobial agents. They were found to be active against a wide range of bacteria, but their main success was in the treatment of streptococcal infections and pneumococcal pneumonia. The antibiotics discovered since then have a greater use in chemotherapy because of their higher potency and the fact that bacteria readily develop resistance to sulfonamides. However, sulfonamides are still widely used in the treatment of urinary tract infections and certain forms of meningitis, and in veterinary medicine. Many derivatives of the sulfonamides have been prepared and a few are employed in the treatment of highly selective infections; e.g., diaminodiphenylsulphone (dapsone) is used in the treatment of leprosy. The structures of representative sulfonamides are shown in Figure 44–10.

The mode of action of sulfonamides is rather clearly defined. Paraaminobenzoic acid (PAB) is a component of tetrahydrofolic acid, the carrier of one-carbon units in metabolism. The structure and shape of the sulfonamides closely resemble those of para-aminobenzoate, and these drugs inhibit the formation of folic acid (the non-reduced form of tetrahydrofolic

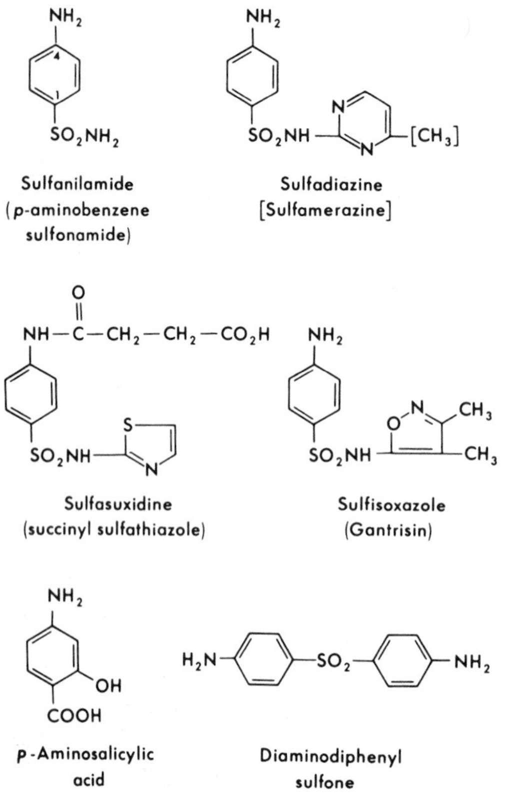

Sulfanilamide
(p-aminobenzene sulfonamide)

Sulfadiazine
[Sulfamerazine]

Sulfasuxidine
(succinyl sulfathiazole)

Sulfisoxazole
(Gantrisin)

p-Aminosalicylic acid

Diaminodiphenyl sulfone

Figure 44-10. Sulfonamides and other PAB analogues. (From Davis, B. D., et al.: Microbiology. 2nd Ed. Hagerstown, Maryland, Harper and Row, 1973.)

acid) because they are a competitive inhibitor of the para-aminobenzoate moiety which must be incorporated into the tetrahydrofolate structure if an active cofactor is to be made (Fig. 44–11).

Para-Aminosalicylic Acid (PAS). This drug is not a general antimicrobial agent but has a specific inhibitory effect on the tubercle bacillus. It has often been used as one of a combination of drugs in the treatment of tuberculosis. The action of para-aminosalicylate is believed to be the same as that of the sulfonamides, but the reasons for selectivity with respect to different microorganisms are not known.

Trimethoprim. This substance is not used alone as an antibiotic, but it seems to have a synergistic effect when used in combination with sulfonamides and some inhibitors of cell wall formation, e.g., vancomycin (discussed later in this chapter). Trimethoprim, like the sulfonamides, is a drug which inhibits a step in folic acid metabolism (Fig. 44–11). It inhibits the activity of the reductase enzyme, which converts the inactive folic acid into the biologically active tetrahydro form.

Isonicotinic Acid Hydrazide (INH). This is one of the most important drugs used in the chemotherapy of tuberculosis. It is usually given in combination with streptomycin and para-aminosalicylate; however, with the availability of rifampin, this particular combination is being changed or modified (see Chap. 24). Despite the importance of isonicotinic acid hydrazide, its mode of action is virtually unknown.

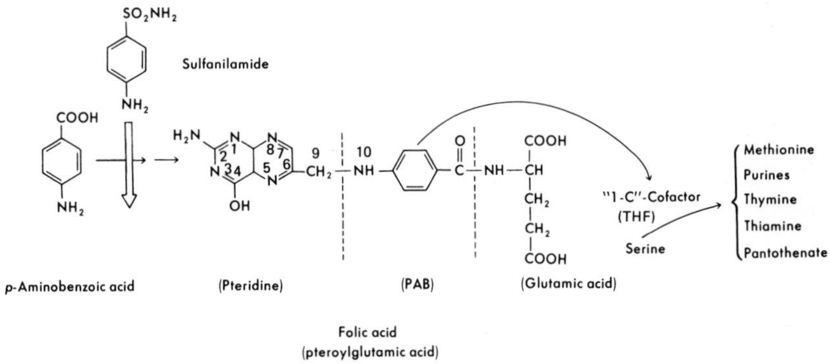

Figure 44-11. Metabolism affected by sulfonamides. (From Davis, B. D., et al.: Microbiology. 2nd Ed. Hagerstown Maryland, Harper and Row, 1973.)

Antibiotics That Affect Bacterial Cell Wall Synthesis

Perhaps the best known example of how an antibiotic may selectively inhibit an infectious cell without harming the human host is certain agents that affect the formation of the bacterial cell wall. Mammalian cells completely lack a cell wall, a semirigid (basketlike) structure possessed by most bacteria. Thus, an agent which prevents the normal synthesis of a bacterial cell wall cannot be expected to affect any related biochemical process in the human host. The natural and semisynthetic penicillins – the cephalosporins, vancomycin, bacitracin, cycloserine, etc. – have been remarkably effective antibiotics and they act in exactly this way. They selectively inhibit bacterial cell wall formation without an appreciable concomitant toxic effect on the human host (vancomycin may be toxic to humans but for other reasons). To understand this action, it is necessary first to learn the structures (which differ widely) of the cell walls found in disease-producing bacteria and then to define in detail the specific step in which penicillin intervenes.

Penicillin is a competitive inhibitor of a normal substrate, peptide-linked D-alanyl-D-alanine, which participates in a cross-linking reaction that confers rigidity on the cell wall. When penicillin is administered, this cross-linking reaction does not take place and the bacteria are unstable and subject to osmotic shock; they do not survive except under very specific conditions. A corollary to this established effect of penicillin is that mature cells already having a fully fashioned cell wall should be immune to this antibiotic, and such is the case. Fortunately, in most clinical infections the causative bacteria must multiply in order to be a danger; thus, the possibility that only mature cells would be present is not a real concern. The penicillin and cephalosporin antibiotics, therefore, are effective in preventing rapid or uncontrolled proliferation of the bacteria.

Penicillins

The first antibiotic produced by a microorganism and used successfully to treat man (in March, 1941) was penicillin (Fig. 44–12). The activity of the

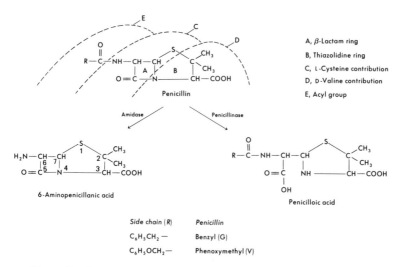

A, β-Lactam ring

B, Thiazolidine ring

C, L-Cysteine contribution

D, D-Valine contribution

E, Acyl group

Side chain (R)	Penicillin
$C_6H_5CH_2$ —	Benzyl (G)
$C_6H_5OCH_2$ —	Phenoxymethyl (V)

Figure 44–12. Structure of some penicillins and diagrammatic indication of the different parts of the antibiotic and the way in which enzymes may inactivate the molecule. (From Davis, B. D., et al.: Microbiology. 2nd Ed. Hagerstown, Maryland, Harper and Row, 1973.)

natural penicillins against gram positive microorganisms is high and their toxicity is low; however, allergic reactions are fairly common. The naturally produced penicillins are a mixture of compounds that have the same beta-lactam ring system but varying side chains (the R group in Fig. 44–12). Penicillin G (benzyl penicillin) is produced in nearly pure form if the Penicillium species manufacturing the penicillins is provided with phenyl-acetic acid. The side chain (R group) may vary widely with retention of useful biologic activity. Variation in the chemical nature of the side chain is achieved by "feeding" different organic acids to the Penicillium species making the penicillin or by utilizing a chemical reaction between acids and 6-aminopenicillanic acid (Fig. 44–13); the latter is the more effective method. The aim of variation in the side chain is threefold: (1) to increase the stability of the beta-lactam ring system to acid, thus improving oral dose effectiveness; (2) to change the spectrum of antimicrobial action, and (3) to increase resistance to beta-lactamase (penicillinase) action, which renders penicillins ineffective. The beta-lactamases are widespread and occur naturally in many bacteria. Their activity may increase suddenly following mutation or as a result of the infectious transfer of extrachromosomal DNA.

At least 10,000 biosynthetic and semisynthetic penicillins have been made, but only a few are in clinical use. Penicillin V (phenoxymethyl-penicillin), ampicillin (alpha-aminobenzylpenicillin), and methicillin (2,6-dimethoxycyclohexylpenicillin) are probably the best known. Ampicillin, in particular, is interesting, as it has substantial activity against gram negative microorganisms but reduced activity toward many gram positive cells. Methicillin and cloxacillin show stability toward some forms of penicillinase (beta-lactamases).

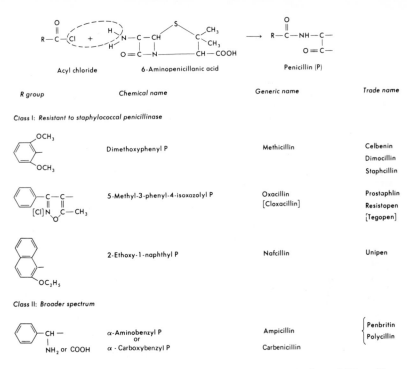

Figure 44-13. Formation and structure of some semisynthetic penicillins. (From Davis, B. D., et al.: Microbiology. 2nd Ed. Hagerstown, Maryland, Harper and Row, 1973.)

The mode of action of the penicillins is well understood. Penicillin inhibits the formation of the bacterial cell wall by growing cultures of sensitive bacteria. An important part of the cell wall is the so-called peptidoglycan, which is a polymeric structure of a glycan (alternating neutral and basic sugars in linear array) that is cross-linked in all possible dimensions through polypeptide chains (Fig. 44–14). The exact composition of the polypeptide bridges varies from one strain of bacteria to another, but a common feature of their biosynthesis is a transpeptidation reaction in which a D-alanine moiety is removed from a pentapeptide, terminating in the sequence D-alanyl-D-alanine. The reaction consists of an exchange between the potential alpha-amino group of the released D-alanine molecule and that of a glycine residue at the terminus of a polypeptide originating from a different strand of the peptidoglycan (Fig. 44–15). The result is the linking together of two different strands of peptidoglycan. This linkage can occur between peptidoglycan strands lying in the same plane, and the result would be the creation of a two dimensional polymer much like a layer of thin fabric. The same sort of cross-linkage between peptidoglycan polymers in different planes gives a three-dimensional structure with great strength. Penicillin acts as a structural analogue of the D-alanyl-D-alanine moiety in the pentapeptide parts of the peptidoglycan (nascent peptidoglycan), and it reacts with the transpeptidase to inactivate the enzyme (Fig. 44–16).

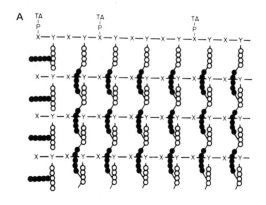

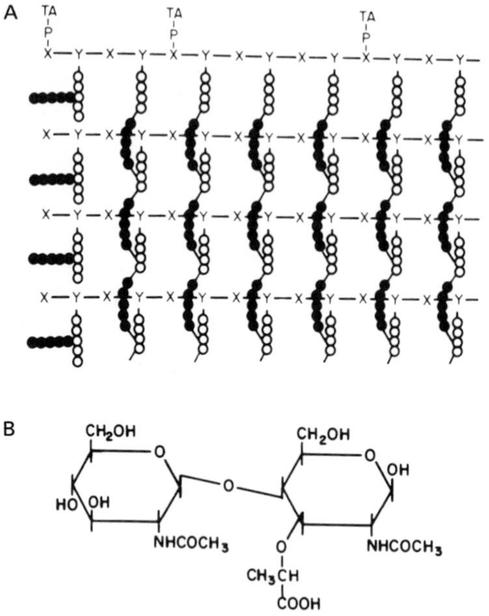

A

B

Figure 44–14. Structure of the peptidoglycan of the cell wall of *Staphylococcus aureus*. *A*, In this representation, X (acetylglucosamine) and Y (acetylmuramic acid) are the two sugars in the peptidoglycan. Open circles represent the four amino acids of the tetrapeptide. L-alanyl-D-γ-glutamyl-L-lysyl-D-alanine. Closed circles are pentaglycine bridges which interconnect peptidoglycan strands. The nascent peptidoglycan units bearing open pentaglycine chains are shown at the left of each strand. TA-P is the teichoic acid antigen of the organism which is attached to the polysaccharide through a phosphodiester linkage. *B*, The structures of X, *N*-acetylglucosamine and Y, *N*-acetylmuramic acid, which are linked by β, 1 → 4 linkages and alternate in the glycan strand. (From "The actions of penicillin and other antibiotics on cell wall synthesis." by Jack L. Strominger. Johns Hopkins Med. J. *133*:63–81, 1973. Copyright © The Johns Hopkins University Press.)

UTP + N-acetylglucosamine-1-P

→ P P

UDP-GlcNAc

phosphoenolpyruvate ⟶

UDP-GlcNAc-pyruvate enol ether

⟶ TPNH

UDP-MurNAc

— L-alanine

ATP — D-glutamic acid

— L-lysine

UDP-MurNAc-L-Ala-D-γ-Glu-L-Lys

L-alanine

D-alanine

— ATP

ATP

D-alanyl-D-alanine ⟶

UDP-MurNAc-L-Ala-D-Glu-L-Lys-D-Ala-D-Ala
(UDP-acetylmuramyl-pentapeptide)

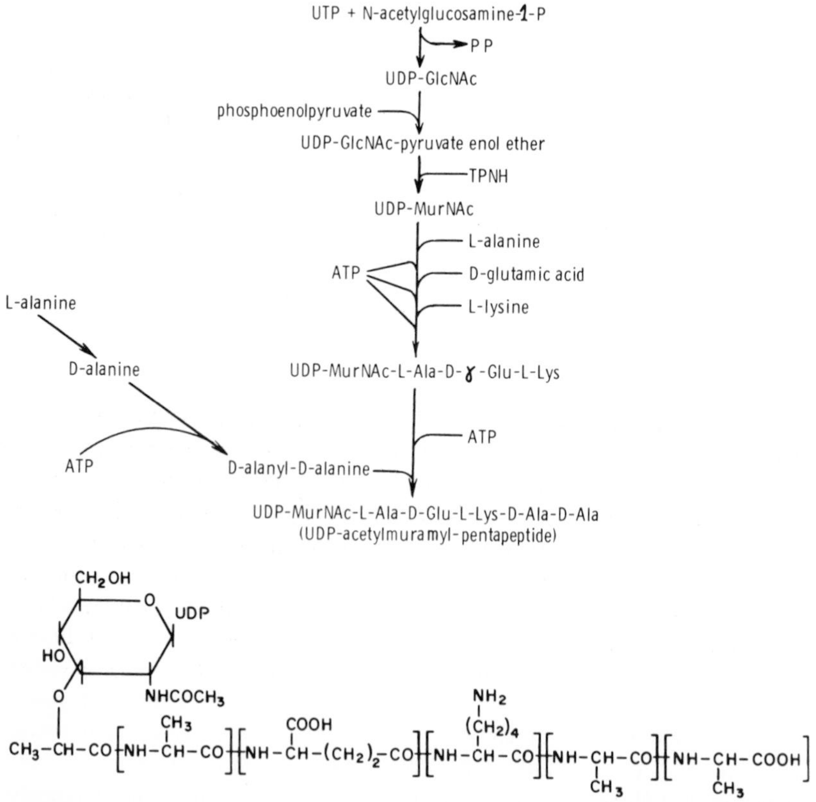

Figure 44–15. The first stage of cell wall synthesis: formation of UDP-*N*-acetylmuramyl-pentapeptide (structure shown). (From "The actions of penicillin and other antibiotics on bacterial cell wall synthesis." by Jack L. Strominger. Johns Hopkins Med. J. *133*:63–81, 1973. Copyright © The Johns Hopkins University Press.)

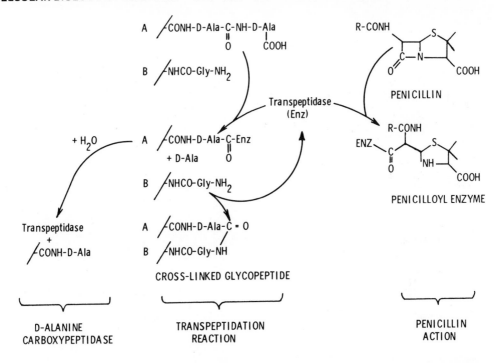

Figure 44–16. Proposed mechanism of inhibition of transpeptidation by penicillins. *A* represents the end of the main peptide chain of the glycan strand. *B* represents the end of the pentaglycine substituent from an adjacent strand. If the acyl enzyme intermediate can react with water instead of the acceptor (left), the enzyme would be regenerated and the substrate released. The overall reaction would be the hydrolysis of the terminal D-alanine residue of the substrate (D-alanine carboxypeptidase activity). Such a reaction could be an "uncoupled transpeptidation" reaction, but it also seems likely that carboxypeptidation (left) and transpeptidation (center) reactions can be catalyzed by separate proteins, perhaps using similar mechanisms. (From "The actions of penicillin and other antibiotics on bacterial cell wall synthesis." by Jack L. Strominger. John Hopkins Med. J. *133*:63–81, 1973. Copyright © The Johns Hopkins University Press.)

Cephalosporins

These agents are chemically similar to the penicillins, but the beta-lactam ring system is fused to a six-membered heterocyclic ring rather than to a five-membered ring as in the case of the penicillins (Fig. 44–17). The side chain is the major variable in the structure of the cephalosporins. Cephalosporin C occurs naturally, while cephaloglycin, cephalothin, and cephaloridine are prepared by partial chemical synthesis. Enzymatic inactivation by beta-lactamases occurs frequently, as it does in the penicillins, and one aim of structural modification is to produce lactamase-resistant cephalosporins.

The mode of action of the cephalosporins is essentially the same as that of the penicillins.

D-Cycloserine

This substance is a broad-spectrum antibiotic with a very simple structure (Fig. 44–18). It is more active against gram positive than gram negative microorganisms and has a significant inhibitory effect on *Mycobacterium*

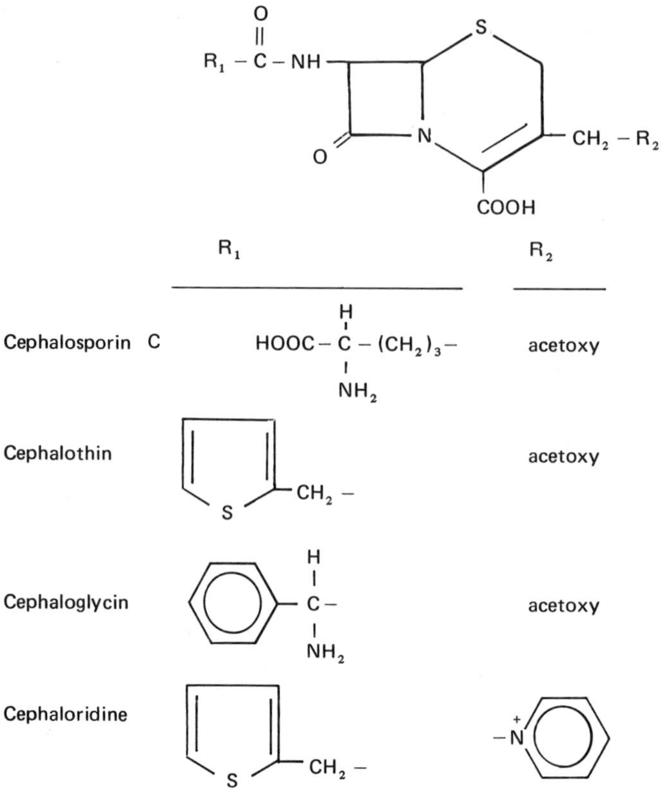

	R$_1$	R$_2$
Cephalosporin C	HOOC–C–(CH$_2$)$_3$– with H above and NH$_2$ below	acetoxy
Cephalothin	thiophene-CH$_2$–	acetoxy
Cephaloglycin	phenyl–C– with H above and NH$_2$ below	acetoxy
Cephaloridine	thiophene-CH$_2$–	–N$^+$ pyridinium

Figure 44–17. Structures of some cephalosporins.

tuberculosis. The usefulness of cycloserine is limited in that many bacteria rapidly acquire resistance to the drug. However, it is employed in combination with other agents, e.g., penicillin, streptomycin, tetracycline, and chloramphenicol.

The action of D-cycloserine is specifically aimed at interference with the synthesis of the D-alanyl-D-alanine dipeptide, a process necessary for the biosynthesis of the UDP-muramyl-pentapeptide involved in the formation of the cell wall of bacteria (Fig. 44–16). Both of the enzymes involved, the

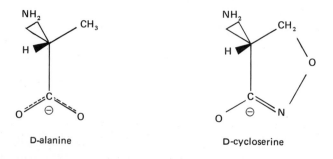

D-alanine   D-cycloserine

Figure 44–18. Structure of D-cycloserine and a comparison with D-alanine.

L-alanine racemase and the D-alanyl-D-alanine synthetase, are inhibited by cycloserine. The inhibition, which is competitive in nature, is caused by a very close structural similarity between D-cycloserine and D-alanine.

Bacitracin

The bacitracins are antimicrobial agents produced by *Bacillus licheniformis.* They are a mixture of peptides, and the A form is the most important. Bacitracin A inhibits the growth of many gram positive bacteria and also strains of Neisseria. The Group A streptococci are more sensitive to bacitracin than are the strains of all other streptococcal groups. Bacitracin prevents the formation of the bacterial cell wall by inhibiting one of the steps occurring within the plasma membrane of the bacteria. It is in the plasma membrane that the muramyl pentapeptide intermediates are metabolized while attached to a polyisoprenoid alcohol carrier (undecaprenyl alcohol). The muramyl pentapeptide is first formed in the cytoplasm of the cell, where the carrier is the nucleotide uridine diphosphate (UDP). As the UDP-muramyl-pentapeptide enters the plasma membrane, there is an exchange reaction in which uridine monophosphate (UMP) is exchanged for a unit of undecaprenyl phosphate (Fig. 44–19). The latter carrier is produced from the

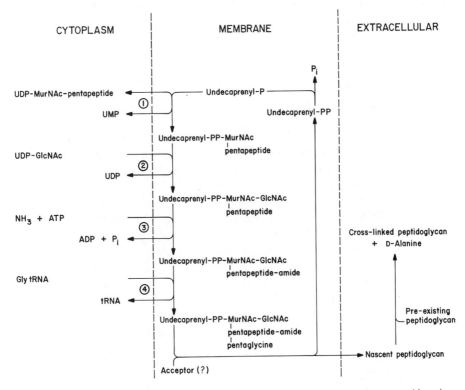

Figure 44–19. Biosynthesis of the bacterial cell wall, with emphasis on the steps taking place in the bacterial plasma membrane (reactions 1 to 4) where a lipid carrier (undecaprenyl alcohol) is involved. Reaction 1 is prevented by bacitracin, while vancomycin and ristocetin affect some step later in the scheme (step 3 or 4 ?). (Diagram prepared by Francis C. Neuhaus, Department of Biochemistry and Molecular Biology, Northwestern University, Evanston, Illinois.)

diphosphate form of undecaprenyl alcohol. Bacitracin specifically prevents the formation of undecaprenyl phosphate from the pyrophosphate precursor. It is interesting to note that bacitracin inhibits this reaction in a manner quite different from the mechanism by which penicillin inhibits a later stage in the formation of the cell wall. Penicillin is a competitive inhibitor of the enzyme (transpeptidase) involved at its target, while bacitracin acts by complexing the substrate undecaprenyl pyrophosphate at the site of its action.

Vancomycin and Ristocetin

These agents are complex glycopeptides with unknown structures. Both are occasionally toxic, and at present only vancomycin is used with any frequency in human chemotherapy. The toxicity, when noted, is quite variable and includes "renal irritation." When impaired renal function exists in a patient receiving vancomycin, higher than normal levels of the drug occur in the serum; these higher levels may be responsible for toxic effects, including damage to the eighth cranial nerve.

Vancomycin and ristocetin are inhibitors of the formation of a normal bacterial cell wall. The specific target is quite different from that of the penicillins and cephalosporins and is somewhat like that ascribed to bacitracin. The most accepted theory is that vancomycin and ristocetin bind substrates involved in the metabolism of the undecaprenyl-muramyl-penta-peptide after its formation from UDP-muramyl-pentapeptide and undecap-renyl phosphate (Fig. 44–19). The action occurs within the plasma membrane of the susceptible bacteria.

Effects of Two or More Antimicrobial Agents in Combination

From a theoretical point of view, two or more antimicrobial agents having different modes of action could augment each other's effect (*synergism*) or, contrarily, they might interfere with each other (*antagonism*). Synergism is somewhat the easier condition to understand. If the two (or more) drugs have different targets for their action, and if neither is able to inhibit completely the growth of the cell, the combined action of both may well be enough to produce complete bacteriostasis or a bactericidal result. A second possible advantage of using two or more agents is that if resistance to one develops during chemotherapy, it is not statistically likely to develop for the other agent(s) (see Chaps. 34 and 41).

Synergistic Effect Between Two Antimicrobial Agents

A synergistic effect between two antibiotics has been documented in a number of cases, some of which have been mentioned previously. For example, in the combination of a sulfonamide with trimethoprim the first agent blocks the biosynthesis of folic acid and the second drug interferes with its reduction to the biologically active tetrahydro form (Fig. 44–20). In this instance, both drugs have a closely related target. Perhaps more effective

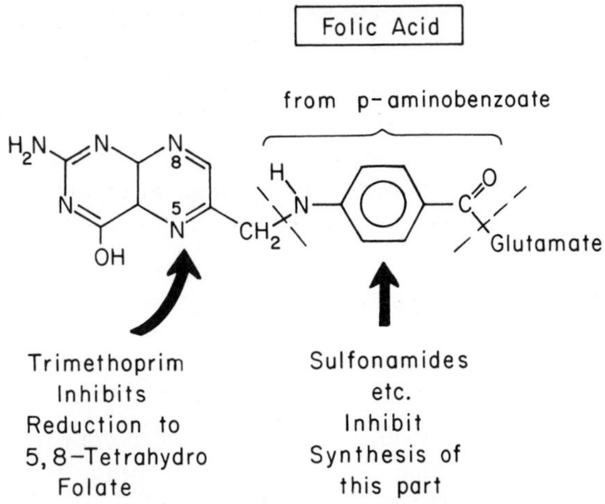

Folic Acid

from p-aminobenzoate

Figure 44-20. Biosynthesis of tetrahydrofolate in bacteria with an indication of the sites of inhibition produced by sulfonamides and trimethoprim. (From Burroughs Wellcome Co. Bulletin SE-19R 5M, November, 1973.)

Trimethoprim
Inhibits
Reduction to
5, 8–Tetrahydro
Folate

Sulfonamides
etc.
Inhibit
Synthesis of
this part

combinations from both a theoretical and practical viewpoint involve drugs with two quite dissimilar sites of action. Trimethoprim, which inhibits an intracellular enzyme, and penicillin, cephalosporin, or vancomycin, which inhibits cell wall formation, are good examples of pairs of antibiotics with rather different actions, and these combinations are used occasionally. One would predict that other combinations, e.g., an inhibitor of protein synthesis (streptomycin, gentamicin, tetracycline, erythromycin, etc.) and a cell wall inhibitor such as penicillin or cephalosporin, might also prove useful; in fact, this type of combination has been shown to be beneficial in the treatment of endocarditis caused by *Streptococcus faecalis*. In this condition, the use of penicillin or vancomycin with an aminoglycosidic antibiotic such as streptomycin or gentamicin is necessary for a successful cure. The penicillin seems to change the cell wall of the *S. faecalis* so that higher concentrations of streptomycin accumulate within the microorganism. Similar synergistic actions of an aminoglycosidic antibiotic with penicillin are seen in strains of Listeria. In certain enterococci that are resistant to streptomycin or kanamycin, gentamicin forms a synergistic combination with penicillin, showing that subtle differences can exist between members of the same class of antibiotic (see Chap. 41).

The Food and Drug Administration has, at times, encouraged and then discouraged the use of combinations of antimicrobial drugs. Combined therapy has been recognized as necessary for some diseases, notably tuberculosis (see Chap. 24), but as a general method of treatment it has not been popular.

Antagonistic Effect Between Two or More Antimicrobial Agents

In contrast to the advantages of using certain drugs in combination, the possibility exists that some drugs can interfere with each other's action. It is usually difficult to predict and often impossible to explain such antagonism. A detailed knowledge of the mode of action of each drug and, in particular, an insight into its pharmacokinetic behavior are necessary for a complete understanding. For example, erythromycin and lincomycin may show some mutual antagonism (see section on Inhibitors of Bacterial Cell Function), and a possible explanation depends on their very similar modes of action and relative differences in potency and binding affinities with respect to the 50S ribosomal subunit of an infectious microorganism.

Biochemical Mechanisms of Resistance to Antimicrobial Agents

It is impossible to separate the important aspects of the sensitivity of microorganisms to antibiotics from their resistance to them. The approach of this chapter has been to consider both sides of the problem at the same time. The basic statement of the ways in which resistance of a microorganism to an antimicrobial agent may be expressed has been given in the section on Modes of Action. The purpose of this section is to review some aspects of the mechanisms by which those changes may occur in a microorganism.

Mutation or Natural Selection

The fact that resistance to chemotherapeutic drugs occurs has been known at least since the time of Ehrlich. The current view of how resistance may appear in a large population of microbial cells exposed to an antimicrobial agent is rather simple: If, in that large population of cells, there are a few genotypically resistant cells (possessing constitutive resistance to the drug in question), the ability of those cells to grow in the presence of the antibiotic leads to a new population of progeny which are mostly of the resistant genotype (Fig. 44–21). The question of how the few genotypically resistant cells arise is related to the process of general microbial mutagenesis. Many agents, e.g., radiation and ultraviolet light, lead to more or less spontaneous genetic change of the chromosomal DNA, or spontaneous chemical change of the DNA may occur as a result of any of the chemical or physical

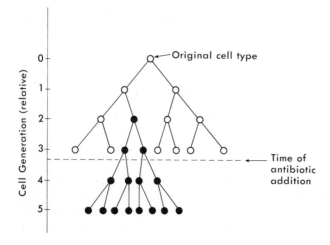

Figure 44–21. Diagrammatic picture of the emergence of an antibiotic-resistant microbial population originating from a spontaneous mutation whose multiplication is favored by the presence of an antibiotic (○ = sensitive cells; ● = resistant cells).

forces to which a cell is subject. These mutational changes may take place in either the presence or absence of an antimicrobial agent, and single-point mutations occur (e.g., in *Escherichia coli*) at about the rate of one per 10^5 to 10^7 cells per cell division. If a change leads to resistance to an antimicrobial agent, the resistance may appear in either of two ways: (1) If the change is specifically related to the drug (e.g., if it increases the amount of an enzyme such as beta-lactamase, which can hydrolyze penicillin), a high level of resistance may suddenly be seen. (2) If the genetic change is only indirectly related to the biochemical action of the antibiotic, small increases in resistance may occur, but if these small increases appear several times with the same microbial population, a gradual development of a much greater resistance to the drug may be seen. Both types of changes occur with most of the common antibiotics.

Transformation, Transduction, or Conjugation

In contrast to the relatively simple single-point mutation of a bacterial chromosome just referred to (in which a single nucleotide base is altered), there are several ways in which larger pieces of new or foreign DNA may be introduced into a microbial cell. If these code for enzymes that affect antibiotic sensitivity, profound changes in resistance may result.

Transformation. Exposure of a microbial cell to DNA isolated from a different species affords the possibility that some of this DNA will enter the viable cell and be incorporated into its chromosomes. The process operates with relatively low efficiency, and the foreign DNA must come from a strain of microorganism with which it has something in common. This mechanism for changing the antibiotic sensitivity of microbial populations is probably not of great clinical importance, although it has been used often by research workers to introduce antibiotic resistance markers into laboratory strains of microorganisms.

Transduction. Phage particles of both gram positive and gram negative cells may enter receptive phage-sensitive cells of related microbial strains. The DNA of the infectious phage can be inserted into the bacterial genome, and, once there, it replicates with the bacterial DNA. If the phage DNA codes for proteins that confer drug resistance, then this action can be a mechanism by which the infected cell suddenly acquires resistance to an antimicrobial agent. It is an observed fact that such phage DNA may simultaneously carry resistance determinants for more than one antibiotic, and this explains the sudden appearance of resistance to two or more antibiotics, often those which are unrelated to each other in terms of structure or mode of action.

Conjugation or the Transfer of Episomes, Plasmids, or Resistance Transfer Factors Bearing Antibiotic Resistance Determinants from One Cell to Another. Most of our information regarding the transfer of resistance determinants by conjugation has come from careful study of some outbreaks of dysentery that occurred in Japan a few years ago. The infectious agents were Shigella species, and initially these were sensitive to the commonly used antibiotics. However, the sudden appearance of resistance to several antibiotics was noted. While researching the mechanisms involved, it was discovered that the pattern of antibiotic resistance acquired by the Shigella species was similar to that possessed by some *Escherichia coli* strains in the patients. It was found subsequently that certain of the *E. coli* strains were able to infect the Shigella species by a process involving direct transfer of DNA from the *E. coli* to the Shigella via a connecting *pilus,* or tubular connection. The ability of a microbial cell to take part as either the donor or recipient in this process is related to its sexuality, and the whole matter is complicated. The terminology used is often that employed in describing bacterial sex factors, but in the context of antibiotic resistance the term *resistance transfer factor* (RTF or RTR) is more often used. The DNA transmitted from one cell to the other is called an *episome* or a *plasmid,* and once it enters a recipient cell it may persist and be replicated separately from the chromosomal DNA. It occasionally may fuse with the chromosome, and the resultant altered chromosome will replicate as a unit. In any event, this infectious process is another method by which DNA may enter a microbial cell that is sensitive to a number of antibiotics, leading to the simultaneous acquisition of resistance to several antibiotics. How often this process operates in the clinical situation is not clear, but it is a mechanism which can cause severe complications in chemotherapy (see Chap. 31).

Specific Examples

There are many ways in which the action of a specific antimicrobial agent may be nullified so that a cell which was at one time sensitive to a certain drug becomes either totally or relatively resistant to that same drug. A few of the more interesting cases are discussed here.

Permeability Changes. An example of a change in microbial cell permeability which leads to antibiotic resistance is that involving the tetracyclines. Normally, the tetracyclines are transported into cells by an ATP-dependent process. A resistance transfer factor that confers resistance to tetracyclines leads to a reduced accumulation of tetracycline in the cells. A similar situation is seen with the accumulation of erythromycin, which is sharply reduced in mutants of *Bacillus subtilis* showing a relative resistance to this macrolide antibiotic. This phenomenon is doubtlessly widespread and pertains to other antibiotics as well.

Chemical Modification. A large number of specific examples are known in which an enzyme system will modify the structure of an antibiotic from a biologically active inhibitor to an innocuous agent. In addition to beta-lactamases that hydrolyze penicillins and cephalosporins, the aminoglycosidic antibiotics are particularly susceptible to such change. The changes which occur include phosphorylation, adenylation, and acetylation of appropriate hydroxyl groups in the aminoglycoside structure. Much of the research in this area is directed toward the synthesis of new aminoglycosides that are incapable of being enzymatically modified. The widely used antibiotic chloramphenicol possesses two hydroxyl groups, and stepwise inactivation of chloramphenicol occurs by the acetylation of these two groups, leading first to a 3-acetyl derivative and finally to a 1,3-diacetyl form of chloramphenicol (see Fig. 44-8).

Modification of Target Site. This is probably a common mechanism for the acquisition of resistance to an antibiotic. The best studied example is that seen with streptomycin. A specific protein moiety of the 30S ribosomal subunit is a major determinant of the overall sensitivity of the whole cell to streptomycin, and mutation can lead to an alteration in this protein or its complete deletion from the 30S unit. These changes are associated with a reduced sensitivity to streptomycin.

A similar situation exists with the use of erythromycin. Two sorts of changes in the structure of 50S ribosomal subunit are correlated with reduced sensitivity to the drug. In one, an alteration in an RNA component of the 50S unit is associated with reduced sensitivity to erythromycin. This change apparently may be introduced into the cell by any of the mechanisms previously mentioned or in a quite novel fashion by induction of an enzyme system caused by subinhibitory concentrations of erythromycin itself. The induced enzyme system (a methylase that modifies an adenine base in the RNA moiety) persists only as long as the erythromycin is present. In its absence, the cells lose the methylase and revert to their original sensitive state. Still another mechanism for modification of the target site for erythromycin is seemingly like that seen with streptomycin. A protein component of the 50S unit is altered or lost following mutation, and the 50S unit that is formed has a reduced affinity for erythromycin.

References

Books

Corcoran, J. W., and Hahn, F. E. (eds.): Antibiotics. Volume II. Mechanism of Action of Antimicrobial and Anti-Tumor Agents. New York, Springer-Verlag, 1975.

Davis, B. D., Dulbecco, R., Eisen, H. N., Ginsberg, S., Wood, W. B., Jr., and McCarty, M.: Microbiology. 2nd ed. Hagerstown, Maryland, Harper and Row, 1973.

Franklin, T. J., and Snow, G. A.: Biochemistry of Antimicrobial Action. New York, Academic Press, 1971.

Gale, E. F., Reynolds, P. E., Cundliffe, E., Richmond, M. H., and Waring, M. J.: The Molecular Basis of Antibiotic Action. New York, John Wiley & Sons, 1972.

Gottlieb, D., and Shaw, P. D. (eds.): Antibiotics. Volume I. Mechanism of Action. New York, Springer-Verlag, 1967.

Original Articles

Benveniste, R., and Davies, J.: Mechanisms of antibiotic resistance in bacteria. Annu. Rev. Biochem. *42:*471, 1973.

Watanabe, T.: Infectious drug resistance. Sci. Am. *217:*19, 1967.

Chapter 45

DRUG SUSCEPTIBILITY TESTING IN VITRO: MONITORING OF ANTIMICROBIAL THERAPY

Introduction

The development of antimicrobial chemical agents in the 1930s opened a new and successful approach to the control of bacterial and fungal infections. The ability to predict a favorable clinical response to the use of an antimicrobial agent by in vitro testing can be of great help in treating serious infections. Guidance in the selection and monitoring of antimicrobial therapy can be gained through in vitro testing.

The susceptibility of many microorganisms, e.g., Group A beta-hemolytic streptococci, to specific antimicrobial agents is well known and need not be tested. However, microorganisms not having known, stable susceptibility patterns should always be tested in order to save time that might otherwise be used in awaiting the patient's clinical response. Variation in susceptibility of microorganisms to different antimicrobial agents may be caused by mutation, transmissible episomes coding for drug resistance or by induction of beta-lactamase enzymes. The use of in vitro testing can rapidly separate resistant from susceptible variants, facilitating the selection of effective agents.

The selection of an antimicrobial agent for therapy depends on several factors, including the mode of action of the agent, the optimal method of administration, the rate of excretion, and the degree of binding to serum proteins. The microorganism involved and the site of infection, whether a carbuncle, an abdominal abscess, or a superficial urinary tract infection, are significant factors. It should be remembered that the most important factor in recovery from infection is the status of the patient's immune system.

Methods for Antimicrobial Susceptibility Testing

In most instances, antimicrobial susceptibility testing is directed toward correlating in vitro susceptibility of a microorganism to clinically achievable levels of antimicrobial agents. This is usually done by incorporating antimicrobial agents in a culture medium and then determining if the microorganism is inhibited from growing or is killed at different concentrations of the test agent. Although there are a number of variations on this principle, most susceptibility testing is carried out either by one of two "dilution" methods or by measuring a zone of growth inhibition of the test microorganism surrounding a paper disc containing the antimicrobial agent. Certain of the advantages and disadvantages of these procedures are listed in Table 45–1.

TABLE 45–1. Antimicrobial Susceptibility Tests

Property	Type of Susceptibility Test		
	Dilution		Agar Disc Diffusion
	Broth	Agar	
Will give minimal inhibitory concentration	+	+	−
Can be used to determine lethal action of antimicrobial agent	+	−	−
Accurate to within ± 1 dilution	+	+	−
Requires relatively little effort (cost)	−	+*	+
Information about a large number of microorganisms easily obtainable	−	+	+
Contamination easily recognized	−	+	+

*Will depend on number of isolates.

Broth and Agar Dilution

Quantitative susceptibility testing is performed by making twofold dilutions of the test antimicrobial agent in a culture medium, either broth or agar, inoculating a standard number of microorganisms, and incubating for 18 hours. The amount of the test agent that will inhibit visible growth of the microorganism is called the *minimal inhibitory concentration*. If the culture medium is a broth, subcultures from tubes showing inhibition of growth after 18 hours are made to a medium free of antimicrobial agents and reincubated for an additional 18 hours to determine the minimal lethal concentration. The *minimum lethal concentration* is defined as the smallest concentration of antimicrobial agent which on subculture either fails to show growth or results in a 99.9 per cent decrease of the initial inoculum. Colloquial use has termed antimicrobial agents that have a minimum lethal concentration the same as, or within one dilution of, the minimum inhibitory concentration as "lethal" or "bactericidal" agents, while antimicrobial agents showing more than a one or two dilution difference between the minimal inhibitory concentration and the minimum lethal concentration are called "bacteriostatic."

Although both broth and agar dilution methods for susceptibility testing of antimicrobial agents will provide the minimal inhibitory concentration of agents, only the broth dilution test can be used to determine the minimal lethal concentration. Broth dilution studies have traditionally been carried out by the serial twofold dilutions of a single antimicrobial agent to produce 8 to 10 separate concentrations. The technical effort necessary to obtain minimal inhibitory and lethal concentrations by this technique has limited its use to special problems, e.g., susceptibility testing for isolates from patients with endocarditis. The development of automatic dilution devices has now made plastic microtiter trays containing serial twofold dilutions of six to eight different antimicrobial agents readily available, suggesting that broth dilution susceptibility data will be widely available in many hospitals within a few years.

Agar dilution susceptibility testing is easily adapted to multiple bacterial or fungal isolates by use of a replicator device. This device, called the "Steers replicator," will inoculate 32 to 36 cultures to a single culture plate (Figs. 45–1 and 45–2). Although serial twofold dilutions of the antimicrobial agent can be made, it is also possible to select concentrations of drug to bracket the

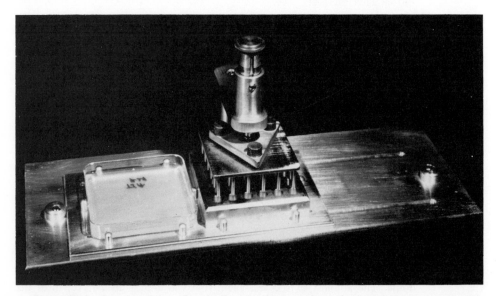

Figure 45–1. Steers replicator. Standardized broth suspensions of microorganisms are placed in wells beneath the inoculating pins. The inoculation head is dipped into the wells and the agar plate moved to the right beneath the inoculating head. The inoculation head is lowered so that the pins touch the culture medium and deliver a defined number of microorganisms to the medium.

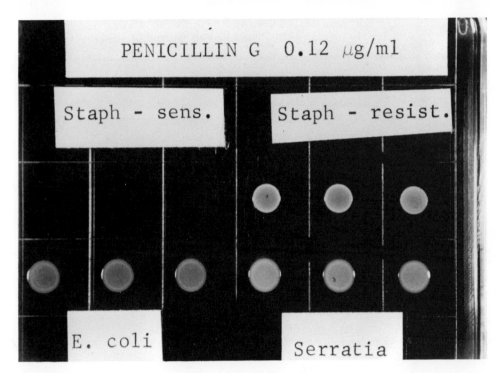

Figure 45–2. Four different bacterial strains inoculated in triplicate to a culture medium containing 0.12 μg per ml of penicillin G. Growth, indicating resistance to this concentration of penicillin, is seen by all strains except a penicillin-sensitive *Staphylococcus aureus.*

clinically useful range. Meaningful information on the minimal inhibitory concentrations of a large number of microorganisms can be determined using only two to five concentrations of the test agent (see Table 45–2). Inadvertent contamination of the test inoculum, an error that may produce a misleading result, is more easily recognized with agar than broth dilution tests.

Disc-Agar Diffusion

Perhaps the most widely used method for antimicrobial susceptibility testing is disc-agar diffusion. Susceptibility testing by this method consists of exposing a pure culture of the test microorganism on an agar culture medium to a filter paper disc containing a known amount of an antimicrobial agent. Once the antimicrobial disc has been placed on the agar, diffusion of the agent from the disc produces a variable concentration of the agent that in turn inhibits susceptible microorganisms until a critical population is reached. At this point, further bacterial multiplication is no longer inhibited. Variations in the lag phase of growth, generation time of the test microorganism, molecular weight, electrical charge and diffusion rate of the agent, and size of the test inoculum all contribute to the size of the zone of growth inhibition surrounding the disc (Fig. 45–3).

TABLE 45–2.   Antimicrobial Agents and Concentrations Tested
(Agar Dilution Method)

Antimicrobial Agent	Concentrations (in μg/ml)									
Ampicillin					2		8	16			
Carbenicillin									50	100	200
Cephalothin				.5	2		8	16			
Chloramphenicol					2		8	16			
Clindamycin			.12		1	4					
Erythromycin				.5	2		8				
Gentamicin			.25		1	4	8				
Kanamycin						4	8	16			
Nafcillin			.12	.25	1	4					
Nalidixic Acid									64	128	256
Nitrofurantoin									64	128	256
Oxacillin			.12	.25	1	4					
Penicillin G	.03	.06	.12		1	4					
Polymyxin B						4	8				
Streptomycin					2		8	16			
Tetracycline HCL					2		8	16			

Criteria have been established to relate the diameter of the zone of growth inhibition found on disc-agar diffusion susceptibility tests to the minimal inhibitory concentration as determined by either broth or agar dilution. An inverse linear relationship exists between the minimal inhibitory concentration and the zone of inhibition resulting from many antimicrobial agents and rapidly growing bacteria. The larger the inhibitory zone, the lower the corresponding minimal inhibitory concentration. This inverse relationship has made possible the construction of regression lines and the correlation of zones of inhibition with the minimal inhibitory concentration (Fig. 45–4). When clinically achievable levels of the test antimicrobial agent are correlated with the minimal inhibitory concentrations, broad guides of clinical susceptibility or resistance can be deduced. Information of this type is available for a large number of antimicrobial agents (see Table 45–3).

Interpretation of Results

The interpretation and significance of in vitro susceptibility tests are usually based on the assumption that the administration of an antimicrobial agent will achieve a serum level from one- to fivefold greater than the minimal

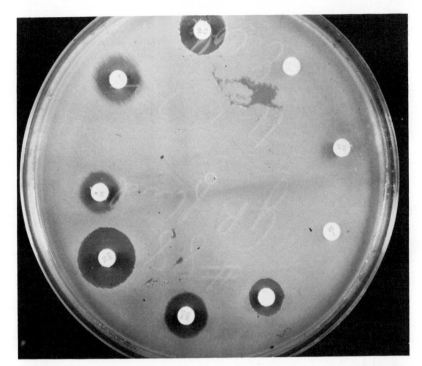

Figure 45–3. An agar plate inoculated with *Escherichia coli* shows a series of paper discs containing different antimicrobial agents. The size of the zone of growth inhibition is measured and the susceptibility of the microorganism is determined by reference to an interpretive chart (see Table 45–3).

inhibitory concentration. The wide range of protein binding by some agents suggests that even this range is not sufficient (see the section on Protein Binding later in this chapter). In reporting the results of susceptibility tests by disc-agar diffusion, three terms are used, *susceptible, intermediate* or *indeterminate susceptibility,* and *resistant. Susceptible* indicates that an infection with the test microorganism will likely respond to the usual dose of an antimicrobial agent recommended for that microorganism. The term

Figure 45–4. Results of tube-dilution and single-disc tests of 108 strains of staphylococci. The correlation was good in 105 instances. (From Bauer, A. W., et al.: Single-disc antibiotic sensitivity testing of staphylococci. Arch. Intern. Med. *104:*208, 1959. Copyright 1959, American Medical Association.)

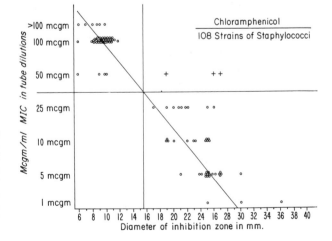

TABLE 45–3. Zone-Size Interpretive Standards and Approximate MIC Breakpoints for the Disc Diffusion Technique*

Antimicrobial Agent	Disc Potency	Inhibitory Zone Diameter (to nearest mm)			Approx. MIC Breakpoint	
		Resistant	Intermediate	Susceptible	Resistant	Susceptible
Penicillin G and ampicillin	10 units 10 µg.					
Staphylococci		20 or less	21–28	29 or more	Penase†	≤ 0.1 µg./ml.
Enterobacteriaceae and enterococci		11 or less	12–13	14 or more	≥ 32 µg./ml.	≤ 5–15 µg./ml.**
Other organisms		11 or less	12–21	22 or more	≥ 32 µg./ml.	≤ 1.5 µg./ml.
Methicillin	5 µg.	9 or less	10–13	14 or more		≤ 2.5 µg./ml.
Nafcillin or oxacillin	1 µg.	10 or less	11–12	13 or more		≤ 0.6 µg./ml.
Vancomycin	30 µg.	9 or less	10–11	12 or more		≤ 5 µg./ml.
Cephalothin	30 µg.	14 or less	15–17	18 or more	≥ 32 µg./ml.	≤ 10 µg./ml.
Cephalondine	30 µg.	11 or less	12–15	16 or more	≥ 40 µg./ml.	≤ 10 µg./ml.
Carbenicillin	50 µg.					
Pseudomonas sp		12 or less	13–14	15 or more	≥ 250 µg./ml.	≤ 125 µg./ml.
Proteus and E. coli		17 or less	18–22	23 or more	≥ 32 µg./ml.	≤ 16 µg./ml.
Polymyxin B††	300 units	8 or less	9–11	12 or more	≥ 50 units/ml.	
Chloramphenicol	30 µg.	12 or less	13–17	18 or more	≥ 25 µg./ml.	≤ 12.5 µg./ml.
Tetracycline	30 µg.	14 or less	15–18	19 or more	≥ 12.5 µg./ml.	≤ 4 µg./ml.
Erythromycin	15 µg.	13 or less	14–17	18 or more	≥ 8 µg./ml.	≤ 2 µg./ml.
Lincomycin	2 µg.	9 or less	10–14	15 or more	≥ 8 µg./ml.	≤ 2 µg./ml.
Clindamycin	2 µg.	11 or less	12–15	16 or more	≥ 8 µg./ml.	≤ 2 µg./ml.
Kanamycin	30 µg.	13 or less	14–17	18 or more	≥ 25 µg./ml.	≤ 6 µg./ml.
Neomycin	30 µg.	12 or less	13–16	17 or more		≤ 10 µg./ml.
Streptomycin	10 µg.	11 or less	12–14	15 or more	≥ 15 µg./ml.	≤ 6 µg./ml.
Gentamicin	10 µg.	12 or less	13–14	15 or more	> 12.5 µg./ml.	≤ 6 µg./ml.
Sulfonamides ‖	300 µg.	12 or less	13–16	17 or more	> 35 mg.%††	≤ 10 mg.%††
Nitrofurantoin ‖	300 µg.	14 or less	15–18	19 or more	> 100 µg./ml.	≤ 25 µg./ml.
Nalidixic acid ‖	30 µg.	13 or less	14–18	19 or more	> 12.5 µg./ml.	≤ 12.5 µg./ml.

*From Gavan, T. L.: In vitro antimicrobial susceptibility testing. Med. Clin. North Am. 58:493, 1974. Prepared by NCCLS Subcommittee on Antimicrobic Susceptibility Testing.

†Penicillinase-producing staphylococci.

**MIC dependent upon dilution method used.

††Polymyxin B diffuses poorly in agar and the accuracy of the diffusion method is thus less than with other antibiotics. Resistance is always significant, but when treatment of systemic infections due to susceptible strains is considered, it is wise to confirm the results of a diffusion test with a dilution method.

§300 µg. or 250 µg. sulfonamide discs can be used with the same standards of zone interpretation (MIC values are for sulfamethizole).

‖Urinary tract infections only.

resistant is used for those agents that do not inhibit the test microorganism within the range of achievable blood levels. The term *intermediate* or *indeterminate susceptibility* is reserved for microorganisms that may respond to an agent if large doses are used or when other measures are taken to optimize the mode of treatment. The term *indeterminate susceptibility* is best used in the interpretation of small differences in zone sizes that may result from technical variability.

A somewhat similar set of interpretative categories was recommended in 1971 by an international collaborative study on antimicrobial susceptibility testing. This report recommended a fourth category to include the situation in which a favorable in vivo response was probable in the treatment of localized infections at sites where the agent could be concentrated by physiologic processes or local application. This would include the concentration of antimicrobial agents in the urine, achieving manyfold the levels found in serum. Such a category would also apply to antimicrobial agents in ointments that can be employed in local skin infections (see Table 45–4).

TABLE 45–4. Categorization of Antimicrobial Susceptibility*

Group 1

Should include high degrees of bacterial susceptibility that make in vivo response probable when patients with mild to moderately severe systemic infections are treated with the usual dosage of antimicrobial agent. This would be the oral route when applicable (e.g., ampicillin). Group 1 can be defined as "sensitive" without further qualification.

Group 2

Should include degrees of susceptibility that make in vivo response probable in systemic infections when the antimicrobial agent is given in high dosage or up to the limits of toxicity.

Group 3

Should include degrees of susceptibility that make in vivo response probable in the treatment of localized infections at sites where the agent can be concentrated by physiologic processes or local application, e.g., the urinary tract or application of an ointment to a local skin infection.

Group 4

Should include microorganisms of a degree of resistance that makes in vivo response improbable. This group can be designated as "resistant."

*Adapted from Ericsson, H. M., and Sherris, J. C.: Antibiotic sensitivity testing. Report of an international collaborative study. Acta Patholog. Microbiol. Scand. [B] *217*(Suppl. 217): 1, 1971.

The standardized disc-agar diffusion susceptibility test (also known as the Bauer-Kirby test) is a simple procedure and is widely used by many clinical laboratories. In 1972, the simplicity and reproducibility of the disc-agar diffusion susceptibility testing led to the recommendation by the Food and Drug Administration that the test be used as the only means for reporting antimicrobial agent susceptibilities when employing the disc-agar diffusion method.

Although disc-agar diffusion susceptibility testing provides good reproducibility in separating susceptible from resistant microorganisms, the zones of inhibition for many microorganisms fall into the narrow indeterminate zone where results often produce interpretations different from those of dilution tests. A recent study has indicated that comparison of zones of inhibition against a number of aminoglycoside antimicrobial agents did not show good regression curves between disc-agar diffusion and dilution studies for determination of *susceptibility,* although the ability to detect *resistance* was good (see Fig. 45–5). With increasing recognition of the limitations of disc-agar diffusion susceptibility testing, it is likely that improved technical innovations and competence will provide ready access to susceptibility results in minimal inhibitory and minimal lethal concentrations. The increased amount of detailed information that can now be made available on minimal inhibitory and lethal concentrations of antimicrobial agents may pose a

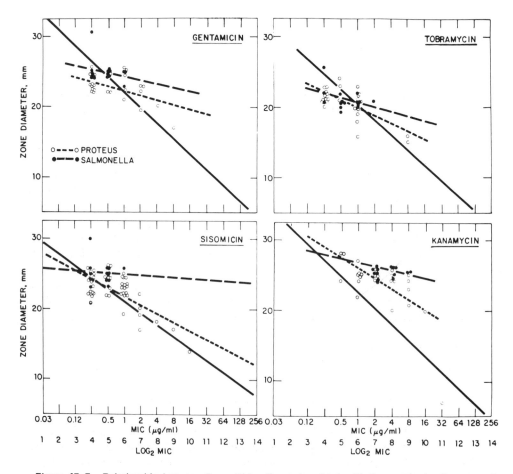

Figure 45–5. Relationship between Bauer-Kirby disc test and tube-dilution results for Proteus and Salmonella strains. Solid lines are calculated regression lines for all bacterial species; broken lines are calculated lines for Proteus and Salmonella species. (From Waitz, J. A.: Interrelationships between disc and tube dilution sensitivity tests for the aminoglycoside antibiotics gentamicin, kanamycin, sisomicin, and tobramycin. Antimicrob. Agents Chemother. *4:*445, 1973.)

problem of interpretation for many physicians. The data concerning the mechanism of action, the amount to be given for different types of infection, the mode of administration, the achievable blood levels, and the degree of protein binding contribute to the increasing need for a separate infectious disease specialist.

Indications for Susceptibility Testing

Testing of all bacterial isolates for antimicrobial susceptibility is neither necessary nor desirable. Alpha-hemolytic streptococci, normally present in the throat, should not be tested for drug susceptibility. Similarly, as mentioned previously, there is no reason to test the susceptibility of Group A beta-hemolytic streptococci to penicillin.

The staphylococci are a group of microorganisms on which antimicrobial susceptibility testing should always be done. The recognition of resistance to penicillin and other antimicrobial agents is of significant therapeutic importance. Members of the family Enterobacteriaceae exhibit extensive variation of susceptibility, related in part to the presence or action of transferable episomes. Occasionally, susceptibility studies should be repeated on microorganisms isolated at intervals during therapy to monitor for the induction of resistance. The appearance of an episome-carrying variant of the same microorganism or replacement by a similar but drug-resistant strain can alter the course of an infection.

It should be remembered that the Bauer-Kirby disc-agar diffusion susceptibility test has been standardized only for rapidly growing micro-organisms such as those of the family Enterobacteriaceae and staphylococci. The determination of antimicrobial susceptibility to more fastidious and slowly growing bacteria, including *Haemophilus influenzae, Neisseria gonorrhoeae* and anaerobic bacteria, requires more exacting test conditions than are provided by the Bauer-Kirby method. In most instances, it is not necessary to test such strains for drug susceptibility, but the appearance of ampicillin-resistant strains of *Haemophilus influenzae* and the increasing penicillin resistance of certain strains of *Neisseria gonorrhoeae* require that facilities be available to carry out such studies if clinical evidence of resistance is suggested. Susceptibility testing for fastidious microorganisms is done by a dilution procedure, varying the culture media, drug concentrations, and incubation conditions as indicated.

Selection of Antimicrobial Agents for Susceptibility Testing

During the past 20 years there have been numerous antimicrobial agents introduced that differ from the original by only slight chemical modifications. The modified forms may provide superior resistance to degradation by gastric acid, improved gastrointestinal absorption, or slower renal excretion. In vitro testing of microorganisms for susceptibility to closely related antimicrobial agents is usually not affected by the chemical modifications. For this reason it is not necessary to test microorganisms against more than one tetracycline, one cephalosporin, or one penicillinase-resistant penicillin. The number of different types of antimicrobial agents necessary for susceptibility testing of either gram negative or gram positive bacteria can then be reduced to no more than six or eight. Additional agents can be added for microorganisms isolated from the urinary tract where concentration of the agent in the urine makes it active at this site but not elsewhere in the body. In vitro susceptibility studies should not be reported when inappropriate or when they may represent an artifact of the testing process. Since nalidixic acid is not present in therapeutic levels until it is concentrated and excreted by the kidney, it is meaningless to report the susceptibility of a microorganism to this agent unless it is isolated from the urinary tract. The routine reporting of antimicrobial susceptibility to dangerous or seldom used toxic agents, e.g., vancomycin or chloramphenicol, should be discouraged in order to prevent inappropriate use. This does not mean that the laboratory should discontinue susceptibility testing of these agents, only that care should be exercised in the "drug-bug" combinations reported. Table 45–5 lists currently available antimicrobial agents appropriate for susceptibility testing of either gram positive or gram negative bacteria when isolated from different sites of the body.

TABLE 45–5. Suggested Antimicrobial Agents to be Tested Against
Bacterial Isolates from Clinical Specimens

Microorganisms from Any Source

*Staphylococcus aureus, Staphylococcus epidermidis and
nonenterococcal streptococci*
Cephalothin
Clindamycin
Erythromycin
Gentamicin
Nafcillin
Oxacillin
Penicillin G

Enterococcus (Lancefield Group D streptococci)
Ampicillin
Erythromycin
Gentamicin
Penicillin

Pseudomonas aeruginosa
Carbenicillin
Gentamicin
Polymyxin B
Tobramycin

*Pseudomonas species and other nonfermentative gram
negative bacteria*
Carbenicillin
Chloramphenicol
Gentamicin
Kanamycin
Polymyxin B
Tetracycline
Tobramycin

Isolates from Urine

Proteus species
Ampicillin
Carbenicillin
Cephalothin
Gentamicin

TABLE 45–5. Suggested Antimicrobial Agents to be Tested Against
Bacterial Isolates from Clinical Specimens *(Continued)*

Kanamycin
Nalidixic Acid
Nitrofurantoin
Sulfamethoxizole/trimethoprim combination
Other gram negative bacilli
  Ampicillin
  Carbenicillin
  Cephalothin
  Gentamicin
  Nalidixic Acid
  Nitrofurantoin
  Sulfamethoxizole/trimethoprim combination
  Tetracycline HCL
  Tobramycin

Throat, Sputum, General Culture Isolates
Gram positive cocci
  Cephalothin
  Clindamycin
  Erythromycin
  Gentamicin
  Nafcillin
  Oxacillin
  Penicillin G
Gram negative bacilli other than proteus and pseudomonas
  Ampicillin
  Carbenicillin
  Cephalothin
  Gentamicin
  Kanamycin
  Tetracycline HCL
  Tobramycin
Pseudomonas aeruginosa
  Carbenicillin
  Gentamicin
  Polymyxin B
  Tobramycin
  Any other effective drug
Pseudomonas species and other nonfermentative gram negative bacteria
  Carbenicillin
  Chloramphenicol
  Gentamicin
  Kanamycin
  Polymyxin B
  Tetracycline
  Tobramycin
Proteus
  Ampicillin
  Carbenicillin
  Cephalothin
  Gentamicin
  Kanamycin
  Tobramycin

Blood and Cerebrospinal Fluid Isolates

As in Throat, Sputum, General Culture Isolates, plus chloramphenicol

Salmonella and Shigella Isolates
  Ampicillin
  Chloramphenicol
  Streptomycin
  Tetracycline HCL

In Vitro Studies for Antimicrobial Synergism

Occasionally it is necessary to determine the susceptibility of bacteria or fungi to the synergistic action of two antimicrobial agents. The determination of synergism is particularly useful when treating patients with endocarditis caused by *Streptococcus faecalis*. Optimal treatment of endocarditis caused by this microorganism requires the use of cell wall inhibiting antimicrobial agents, such as penicillin or vancomycin, with an aminoglycoside, usually either streptomycin or gentamicin, to inhibit protein synthesis. The method for studying synergism by in vitro tests involves a cross-titration of tube-dilution susceptibility tests. This will give the minimum combination of both agents resulting in the inhibitory and lethal concentrations to the microorganisms. The end point may then be reported either as minimal inhibitory or lethal concentrations of the different combinations, or as the log decrease in viable microorganisms plotted against time. Assuming no host defect in cellular phagocytic or immune mechanisms, combinations of agents sufficient to result in a 99.9 per cent decrease in the number of inoculated microorganisms will be sufficient to bring about a prompt clinical response. Figure 45–6 illustrates an in vitro test for synergistic action of ampicillin and gentamicin against *S. faecalis* (see also Chaps. 41 and 44).

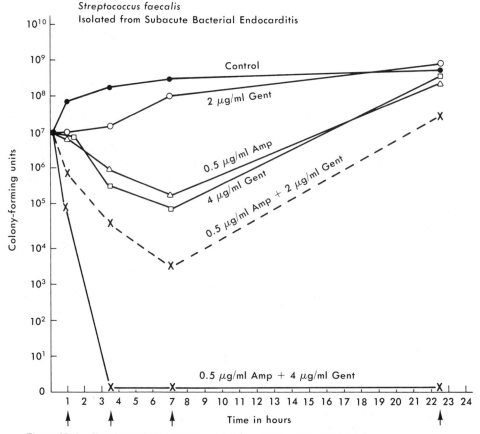

Figure 45–6. Test for antimicrobial synergism (ampicillin with gentamicin).

Protein Binding of Antibiotics

It has been known since 1946 that many antimicrobial agents bind reversibly to serum proteins in varying amounts. The binding of serum proteins results in both free and bound components that make up the total serum level. Binding of most antimicrobial agents occurs to the albumin fraction, but erythromycin binds to alpha-1-globulin. Protein binding is of clinical significance because only the unbound portion of the drug is available for antimicrobial effect and diffusion into the interstitial tissues. The free and bound portions of the antimicrobial agents are in equilibrium, and in this manner binding fulfills a storage function, preventing rapid excretion by glomerular filtration (Fig. 45-7). The effect of protein binding on the minimal inhibitory concentration of penicillin and the duration of efficacious clinical levels of the drug is illustrated in Figure 45-8, in which the minimal inhibitory concentration is compared, using both 95 per cent human serum and a broth culture medium. Two findings are significant: (1) the minimal inhibitory concentration is much higher when determined in serum, and (2) the period when there is a serum concentration equal to or greater than the minimal inhibitory concentration for the microorganism is much shorter when measured in serum than in broth. Table 45-6 lists the protein binding of various penicillin derivatives. The variations noted reflect differences in the measuring technique. The degree of protein binding with individual antimicrobial agents will vary between sera of different animals. Therefore, studies of protein binding for drugs used in humans can be done only with human serum shown to be free of antimicrobial activity.

The degree of protein binding of antimicrobial agents influences the partition of the antimicrobial agent between the blood, interstitial tissue, and the site of infection, since the gradient of drug concentration is related to the amount of free agent in the serum (see Fig. 45-7). The peak level of the drug at the site of infection rarely exceeds the peak level of free drug in the blood and usually reaches a maximum sometime later than the peak in the serum. The effective delivery of an antimicrobial agent to the site of an infection depends on the presence of an intact vascular system. The presence of necrosis with interruption of the capillary network (abscess) may inhibit this

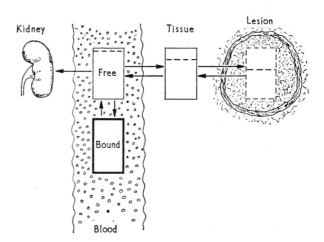

Figure 45-7. Protein binding of drugs. (From Crofton, J.: Some principles in the chemotherapy of bacterial infections. Br. Med. J. 2:209, 1969.)

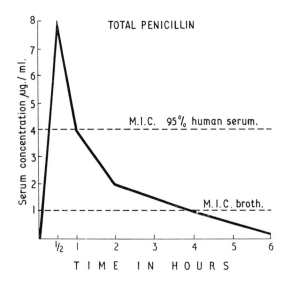

Figure 45–8. Total penicillin concentration and minimal inhibitory concentration (MIC) value in broth and 95 per cent human serum. (From Knudsen, E. T.: Interpretation of assay values. *In* Therapy with the New Penicillins. Proceedings of a conference held at the Apothecaries' Hall, London, June, 1964.)

TABLE 45–6. Human Serum Protein Binding of Various Penicillins*

Agent	Per Cent Bound (Range)
Benzylpenicillin	49 – 68
Phenoxymethylpenicillin	74 – 83
Phenethicillin	71 – 83
Methicillin	28 – 49
Oxacillin	86 – 93
Cloxacillin	89 – 95
Dicloxacillin	89 – 96
Nafcillin	69 – 89
Ampicillin	10 – 21

*Adapted from Warren, G. H.: The prognostic significance of penicillin serum levels and protein binding in clinical medicine. A review of current studies. Chemotherapia *10:*339, 1965/66.

delivery and the diffusion of the agent, offering the invading microorganism protection from effective levels of the drug. Conversely, the active inflammatory process resulting from acute inflammation with vascular dilatation and increased permeability can aid in the accumulation of agents at sites of infection, e.g., meningitis. Figures 45–9 and 45–10 illustrate the relationship between serum and interstitial fluid levels of a moderately and highly protein-bound penicillin. Data from these experiments are summarized in Table 45–7, confirming in vivo the in vitro tests of protein binding for ampicillin and nafcillin.

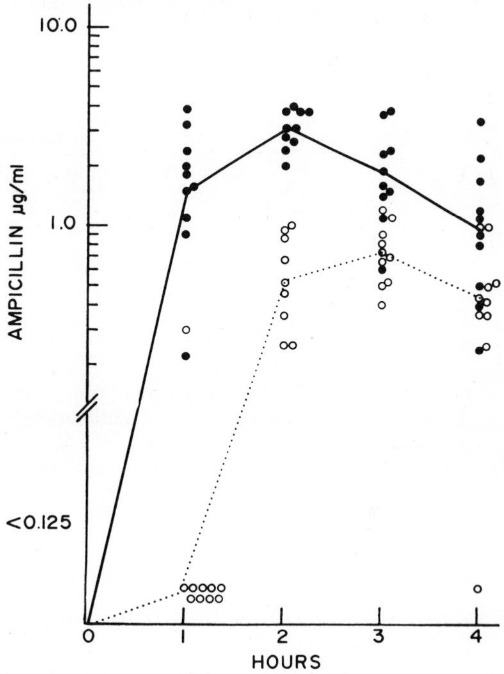

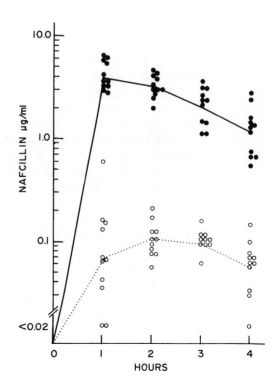

Figure 45–9. Ampicillin concentrations in serum and skin-window interstitial fluid after oral administration of 1 gm of ampicillin. ● = serum; ○ = skin-window interstitial fluid; ——— = mean values of serum; • • • = mean values of skin-window interstitial fluid. (From Tan, J. S., Trott, A., Phair, J. P., et al.: A method for measurement of antibiotics in human interstitial fluid. J. Infect. Dis. *126:*492, 1972.)

Figure 45–10. Nafcillin concentrations in serum and skin-window interstitial fluid after intramuscular administration of 500 mg nafcillin. ● = serum; ○ = skin-window interstitial fluid; ——— = mean values of serum; • • • = mean values of skin-window interstitial fluid. (From Tan, J. S., Trott, A., Phair, J. P., et al.: A method for measurement of antibiotics in human interstitial fluid. J. Infect. Dis. *126:*492, 1972.)

TABLE 45-7. Relationship between Binding to Protein and the Ratio of Antibiotics in Skin-Window Interstitial Fluid to those in Serum*

Antibiotic	Skin-window to serum ratio				Bound to protein (%)
	1 hr	2 hr	3 hr	4 hr	
Ampicillin	−†	0.17	0.39	0.46	18–29
Penicillin G	0.093	0.174	0.209	0.212	59–65
Penicillin V	0.071	0.24	0.21	–	80
Nafcillin	0.016	0.035	0.045	0.042	89–90

*Modified from Tan, J. S., Trott, A., Phair, J. P., et al.: A method for measurement of antibiotics in human interstitial fluid. J. Infect. Dis. *126*:492, 1972.

†No detectable antibiotic activities in the majority of skin-window fluid specimens.

Assay of Antimicrobial Agents in Serum and Other Body Fluids

Occasionally it is helpful to determine the total amount of antimicrobial agent in serum, cerebrospinal fluid, urine, or other types of clinical specimens. Requests to assay the total amount of an antimicrobial agent in serum are usually restricted to those drugs exerting a significant nephrotoxic or similar toxic action, such as gentamicin. Assay for antimicrobial agents can be done by chemical, biologic, enzymatic, or immunologic (often radio-immunoassay) procedures. Sulfonamide compounds are the only anti-microbial agents readily measured by chemical means.

The simplest and most commonly used method for measuring most antibiotics is a biologic assay based on the principle of inhibition of bacterial growth by different concentrations of test agent. A microorganism suscepti-ble to the agent to be assayed is incorporated in an agar culture plate. A series of small metal cups are placed on the surface of the agar and filled with measured amounts of the test specimen to be assayed. Because of the variation of protein binding and other factors that can influence the activity of antimicrobial agents, standard concentrations of the test agent are prepared in a medium similar to the test substrate but known to be free of antimicrobial activity, e.g., serum or cerebrospinal fluid. The substrate containing the known amounts of test agent, along with the unknown specimen to be tested, is then placed in similar metal cups in quadruplicate. During incubation, the antimicrobial agent diffuses from the cup, resulting in a zone of growth inhibition proportional to the concentration of the test agent in the cup. Zones of inhibition for the reference standards are measured, and the mean is determined for the four zones and plotted on semi-log graph paper. The zones of inhibition surrounding the four cups containing the test specimen are then measured, the mean determined, and the concentration of antimicrobial agent in the specimen read from the curve. This procedure has been a standard method of measuring drug levels for many years and is known as the *cup-plate method*. Recent modifications of this procedure have led to the use of paper discs instead of metal cups, preincubated seed plates, and rapidly growing strains of microorganisms yielding results within four to six hours (Figs. 45–11 and 45–12). The accuracy of "cup-plate" biologic assays is approximately ± 10 per cent, well within the limits necessary for clinical usefulness.

Occasionally the patient may be under treatment with several antimicrobial agents but a serum level is needed for only one. If gentamicin is the agent to be measured and is present in the serum specimen along with cephalothin, the biologic assay as described above will be of little value, as cephalothin has a smaller molecular weight and will diffuse more rapidly than gentamicin, producing a larger zone of inhibition than that produced by gentamicin alone. When more than one antimicrobial agent is present in a sample, it may be possible to inactivate some agents by adding enzymes such as penicillinase or cephalosporinase. When enzymatic inactivation of antimicrobial agents cannot be done, it may be possible to use a test microorganism that is sensitive to the agent to be measured but resistant to other commonly used agents. For example, there is a strain of *Staphylococcus epidermidis* that is resistant to all antimicrobial agents but gentamicin.

Recently the development of a radioimmunoassay procedure for gentamicin has offered another approach for assay of antimicrobial agents.

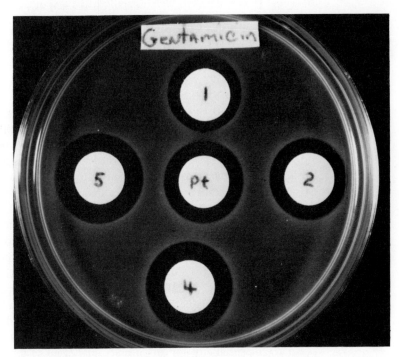

Figure 45–11. Serum assay for gentamicin. Serum from the patient is placed on the center disc while control serum containing 1, 2, 4, and 5 μg per ml of gentamicin are placed peripherally. The zone of inhibition around each disc is measured after incubation. Owing to small differences in the size of zones, the test is run in quadruplicate and the mean zone plotted (see Fig. 45–12).

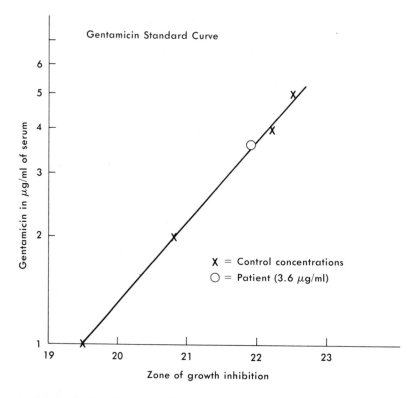

Figure 45–12. The mean inhibitory zones determined from quadruplicate control concentrations in serum are plotted to establish a standard curve. The test serum concentration is then read from this curve.

Although rapid and specific, the simplicity and ease of biologic procedures will probably limit the wide use of radioimmunoassay for this purpose.

Perhaps of greater interest has been the development of highly specific assays for certain of the aminoglycoside antimicrobial agents (gentamicin-kanamycin-tobramycin) based on inactivating enzymes isolated from transmissible episomal resistance factors. A number of enzymes have been isolated that have been found to inactivate different antimicrobial agents at specific sites. Isolation and purification of these enzymes has led to a rapid four-hour assay using radioactive isotopes. Aminoglycosides are strongly basic compounds that will bind quantitatively to cation exchange paper (phosphocellulose) at any pH between 5 and 9. By using ^{14}C-ATP or ^{14}C acetyl coenzyme A, the transfer of a ^{14}C AMP or ^{14}C acetate moiety to any aminoglycoside in the presence of a suitable inactivating enzyme can readily be detected. It is possible to measure as little as 10 ng of an aminoglycoside by assaying the antibiotic in the presence of the appropriate enzyme. This procedure has the advantage of specificity for an antimicrobial agent in the presence of more than one agent but has the disadvantages of limited availability of the inactivating enzymes and the requirement of expensive isotope counting devices. Table 45–8 lists different types of enzymes that inactivate antimicrobial agents (see also Chap. 44).

TABLE 45–8. Enzymes Inactivating Antimicrobial Agents Determined by
R Factors*

Enzyme	Substrate
Beta-lactamase	Various penicillins
Chloramphenicol acetylase	Chloramphenicol
Streptomycin phosphotransferase	Streptomycin
Streptomycin adenylate synthetase	Streptomycin, spectinomycin
Kanamycin phosphotransferase	Kanamycin, neomycin B, paromomycin
Kanamycin acetyltransferase	Kanamycin, neomycin B
Gentamicin adenylate synthetase	Gentamicin, kanamycin
Gentamicin acetyltransferase	Gentamicin, sisomicin, tobramycin

*Adapted from Davis, B. D., et al.: Microbiology. 2nd ed. Hagerstown, Maryland, Harper and Row, 1973.

Determination of Antimicrobial Activity

The use of assay procedures for monitoring the treatment of a patient with bacterial endocarditis by measuring the total amount of penicillin or other highly protein-bound antimicrobial agent in serum is usually inappropriate. Measuring the actual free and protein-bound portions of antimicrobial agents is a research procedure. While the determination of the serum concentration of the unbound portion of an antimicrobial agent may tell the physician whether he has achieved a level consistent with the minimal inhibiting concentration for the infecting microorganism, the correlation of total serum levels of highly protein-bound agents with minimal inhibitory concentrations of infecting microorganisms may be grossly misleading. In addition to an antimicrobial drug, there may be numerous other antibacterial substances in the blood, including serum bactericidal activity, circulating opsonins and specific antibody, lysozyme, beta lysin, and other poorly defined components. All of these substances contribute to the total antimicrobial effect of the serum. Within a few days after the onset of an infection, normal humoral and cellular immunologic mechanisms respond to the microbial challenge with varying degrees of effectiveness. Subinhibitory levels of antimicrobial agents that ordinarily would not be lethal for a microorganism may now contribute a deciding effect in the control of infection. In vitro experiments have shown that sublethal concentrations of different penicillins render certain strains of *Staphylococcus aureus* more vulnerable to lysozyme than if penicillin had not been present. Conversely, small amounts of certain antimicrobial agents may protect microorganisms from normal host defense mechanisms. Chloramphenicol, if present in small amounts in a mixture of human serum and gram negative bacteria, can reduce the normal bactericidal effect of the serum, presumably by partial inhibition of bacterial metabolism.

Perhaps the most useful test for following patients with severe infection who are on antimicrobial therapy is to measure the inhibitory or lethal action of serial twofold dilutions of the patient's serum, cerebrospinal fluid, urine, or other specimen against a standard inoculum of the microorganism causing the infection. This test is sometimes called the *bactericidal activity test* but is more properly referred to as the *antimicrobial activity test* inasmuch as it can be used against both bacteria and fungi. The purpose of the antimicrobial activity test is to measure the net effect of all factors in the test specimen, e.g., serum, cerebrospinal fluid, urine, and so forth, including all antimicrobial agents present, against the infecting microorganism.

Antimicrobial activity levels have been used most often to follow the treatment of patients with bacterial endocarditis. Empirically, it has been found that serum lethal levels of 1:8 or greater have been associated with favorable outcomes, while serum lethal levels lower than 1:8 are associated with less favorable results. The test has also been found to be useful in determining the effectiveness of different modes of therapy for many other types of infection. With the exception of patients with respiratory tract infections, if the peak inhibitory titer (serum taken shortly after the administration of the antimicrobial agent) was 1:8 or greater, the infection was cured in 80 per cent of a large series of patients with cancer. Response to therapy in patients with urinary tract infections correlated best with the inhibitory level found in the urine; clinical cure was observed in 90 per cent of patients whose urine inhibited growth of the infecting microorganism with dilutions of 1:4 or better. Determination of serum or urine antimicrobial inhibitory levels early in the course of infection can allow for adjustment of therapy.

When performing the antimicrobial activity test it should be remembered that normal serum contains antimicrobial substances and may have a lethal activity in dilutions of 1:4 to 1:8. Because of normal or recently augmented host antimicrobial activity, it is best to compare dilutions of the patient's serum both before and after starting therapy. Serum specimens should be drawn before starting therapy on all patients with serious infections and kept frozen so that they may be used as a control. To perform the test, two serum samples are drawn — one within 30 to 60 minutes following the administration of the antimicrobial agent and the second just prior to giving the next dose. This will provide a "peak" and "trough" level, thereby giving the therapeutic range occurring in the patient. The test sera are diluted in human serum free of antimicrobial activity. A known number of the patient's microorganisms are added to the diluted serums and the inhibitory levels determined after 18 to 20 hours of incubation. The serum lethal levels are determined 18 to 20 hours later by subculture (Fig. 45–13).

The advantage of following therapy by antimicrobial activity levels rather than concentrations of antimicrobial agents is illustrated in Figures 45–14 and 45–15. Cefazolin and cephaloridine are two members of the cephalosporin group of antimicrobial agents. Advertisements tell the physician of the increased serum concentrations that can be achieved with cefazolin when compared to other members of the cephalosporin group of antibiotics. Total serum concentrations of cefazolin and cephaloridine that were injected into volunteers are shown in Figure 45–14. Cefazolin has clearly higher levels. When serum inhibitory and lethal levels were determined with the same serum, cephaloridine showed significantly greater lethal activity against a sensitive strain of *Staphylococcus aureus* than did cefazolin, despite the

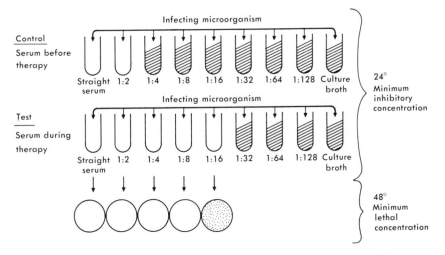

Figure 45–13. Serum antimicrobial activity. *Principle:* The test determines the maximum dilution of serum that will show bacteriostatic or lethal activity against an infecting microorganism. Serum taken before and during antimicrobial therapy will define the in vivo effect of an agent against the infecting microorganism. (The test can also be used with cerebrospinal fluid, urine, or other types of clinical specimens.) *Interpretation:* Serum minimum inhibitory concentration = 1:16; serum minimum lethal concentration = 1:8.

higher serum concentration of the latter (Fig. 45–15). Although not all the reasons for this difference are known, serum protein binding of cefazolin is significantly higher (81 per cent) than that of cephaloridine (24 per cent). It must be emphasized that serum assay and activity levels are not the only considerations when choosing an antimicrobial agent. In this example, the nephrotoxic action of cephaloridine would place it far down the list of alternative agents. The selection of any antimicrobial agent should be based on careful evaluation of the patient's needs and the characteristics of individual antimicrobial agents.

Figure 45–14. Mean concentration of antibiotic in the serum of 10 subjects after intramuscular injection of 500 mg of cefazolin or cephaloridine. The vertical bars represent standard error of the mean. (From Bergeron, M. G., Brusch, J. L., Barza, M., et al.: Bactericidal activity and pharmacology of cefazolin. Antimicrob. Agents Chemother. *4:*396, 1973.)

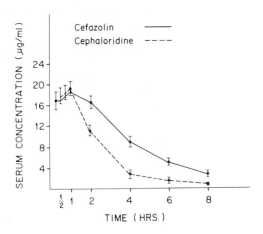

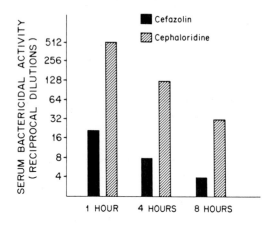

Figure 45–15. Mean serum bactericidal activity against a penicillin-sensitive *Staphylococcus aureus* in 10 subjects after intramuscular injection of 500 mg of cefazolin or cephaloridine. (From Bergeron, M. G., Brusch, J. L., Barza, M., et al.: Bactericidal activity and pharmacology of cefazolin. Antimicrob. Agents Chemother. *4:*396, 1973.)

References

Books

Balows, A. (ed.): Current Techniques for Antibiotic Susceptibility Testing. Springfield, Illinois, Charles C Thomas, 1974.

Gavan, T. L., Cheatle, E. L., and McFadden, H. W.: Antimicrobial Susceptibility Testing. Chicago, American Society of Clinical Pathologists, 1971.

Grove, D. C., and Randall, W. A.: Assay Methods of Antibiotics. A Laboratory Manual. New York, Medical Encyclopedia, 1955.

Sherris, J. C.: Laboratory tests in chemotherapy. *In* Lennette, E. H., Spaulding, E. H., and Truant, J. P. (eds.): Manual of Clinical Microbiology. 2nd ed. Washington, D. C., American Society for Microbiology, 1974.

Original Articles

Bauer, A. W., Kirby, W. M., and Sherris, J. C.: Antibiotic susceptibility testing by a standardized single disc method. Am. J. Clin. Pathol. *45:*493, 1966.

Benveniste, R., and Davies, J.: Mechanism of antibiotic resistance in bacteria. Annu. Rev. Biochem. *42:*471, 1973.

Ericsson, H. M., and Sherris, J. C.: Antibiotic sensitivity testing. Report of international collaborative study. Acta Pathol. Microbiol. Scand. [B] *217*(Suppl. 217):1, 1971.

Food and Drug Administration: Federal Register. *37:*20525, 1972.

Gavan, T. L.: In vitro antimicrobial susceptibility testing. Clinical implications and limitations. Med. Clin. North Am. *58:*493, 1974.

Jawetz, E.: Combined antibiotic action: Some definitions and correlations between laboratory and clinical results. Antimicrob. Agents Chemother. *7:*203, 1967.

Klastersky, J., Danean, D., Swings, G., and Weerts, D.: Antibacterial activity in serum and urine as a therapeutic guide in bacterial infections. J. Infect. Dis. *129:*187, 1974.

Marymont, J. H., Jr., and Wentz, R. M.: Serial dilution antibiotic sensitivity testing with the microtiter system. Am. J. Clin. Pathol. *45:*548, 1966.

Sabath, L. D., Casey, J. I., Ruch, P. A., Stampf, L. L., and Finland, M.: Rapid microassay of gentamicin, kanamycin, neomycin, streptomycin and vancomycin in serum or plasma. J. Lab. Clin. Med. *78:*457, 1971.

Schlichter, J. G., and MacLenn, H.: A method of determining the effective therapeutic level in the treatment of subacute bacterial endocarditis with penicillin. Am. Heart J. *34:*209, 1947.

Smith, D. H., Van Otto, B., and Smith, A. L.: A rapid chemical assay for gentamicin. N. Engl. J. Med. *286:*583, 1972.

ANTIMICROBIAL THERAPY

Introduction

With the introduction of sulfonamides in the early 1930s and penicillin in 1942, the end of life-threatening bacterial infections was thought to be at hand. This early optimism quickly faded. Antimicrobial agents have not played a major role in the prevention of infection. Presently, an increasing population of elderly patients, the development of extensive life-saving surgical procedures and supportive care, and the prolongation of life in patients with various illnesses leading to temporary or permanent suppression of natural host defense contribute to the fact that infection continues to play a major role in morbidity and mortality (see Chap. 43).

Antimicrobial agents themselves may predispose to the development of bacterial infections when given to patients with viral infections, especially measles and influenza. When used improperly, they often mask the true nature of the infectious process and in this manner prolong the patient's illness.

To use antimicrobial agents intelligently, the practitioner of medicine should be thoroughly familiar with the various classes of antimicrobial agents, their spectrum of activity, and the mechanisms of action, metabolism, elimination, and adverse side effects. It is the purpose of this chapter to discuss some of the factors that should be taken into consideration when selecting and using antimicrobial agents.

Antimicrobial Agents Effective Against Gram Positive Bacteria

As a guide to the treatment of patients with bacterial infections, it is useful to subdivide antimicrobial agents into two major groups: (1) those agents that are most effective in the treatment of infections produced by gram positive bacteria, and (2) those agents whose activity is directed primarily against gram negative bacteria.

This somewhat artificial subdivision is clinically useful, for frequently the initial choice of an antimicrobial agent must be made on the basis of an appropriately obtained Gram stain, or the result of preliminary culture from which microorganisms can be classified only on the basis of their staining reaction and microscopic appearance. If necessary, therapy may be modified or changed 24 to 48 hours later, when final identification and antimicrobial susceptibilities are known. The usefulness of this approach is illustrated in the following case history.

A 21-year-old male heroin addict was admitted to the hospital because of fever (104°F), shaking chills, and a swollen, painful left knee. Physical examination was normal with the exception of the left knee, which was markedly swollen, erythematous, and painful to palpation and passive movement. Needle aspiration of the knee joint revealed creamy, thick, yellow fluid which contained 145,000 segmented neutrophils per cubic millimeter and numerous gram positive cocci in clusters. On the basis of the Gram stain, antimicrobial therapy was begun with a penicillinase-resistant semisynthetic penicillin administered intravenously. Culture of the aspirated synovial fluid, reported 48 hours later, revealed a heavy growth of *Staphylococcus aureus* sensitive to 0.06 μg per ml of penicillin G. On the basis of this culture report, aqueous penicillin G was substituted for the initial penicillinase-resistant semisynthetic penicillin started on admission. Recovery was prompt and uneventful.

Within each class of antimicrobial agents, e.g., the cephalosporin group, there may be one or more derivatives effective against both gram positive and gram negative bacteria. The cephalosporins are mentioned in both this section of the chapter and the section dealing with antimicrobial agents effective against gram negative bacteria.

Table 46-1 lists antimicrobial agents used primarily in the treatment of infections produced by gram positive bacteria. Anaerobic bacteria (both gram positive and gram negative), with the exception of *Bacteroides fragilis,* are sensitive to penicillin G and are therefore included in this table. *Neisseria meningitidis* and *Neisseria gonorrhoeae,* although gram negative cocci, fall into a special category in that they are sensitive to agents (i.e., penicillin, ampicillin) used primarily in the treatment of gram positive bacterial infections, as well as those used in the treatment of gram negative bacterial infections (i.e., chloramphenicol, tetracycline). All other microorganisms listed are gram positive.

Antimicrobial Agents Effective Against Gram Negative Bacteria

A wide variety of antimicrobial agents are now available for the treatment of infections produced by gram negative bacteria. The susceptibility of gram negative bacteria to various antimicrobial agents is much less predictable than

TABLE 46-1. Antimicrobial Agents Used in Treatment of Infections
Produced by Gram Positive Bacteria

Antimicrobial Agent (Class)	Primary Agent in the Treatment of Infection Produced by:	Secondary Agent in the Treatment of Infection Produced by:

Penicillins
 Penicillin G
	Staphylococcus aureus, Staphylococcus epidermidis (non-penicillinase producing)
	 Streptococcus pneumoniae
	 Streptococcus
	   Lancefield Groups A–F†
	   Viridans group
	   (alpha-hemolytic, non–Lancefield
	   groupable streptococci)
	 Clostridia–all species
	 *Neisseria gonorrhoeae**
	 *Neisseria meningitidis**
	 Corynebacterium diphtheriae
	 Actinomyces israelii
	 Anaerobic bacteria–all types except
	   *Bacteroides fragilis** subspecies	

Penicillinase-resistant penicillins	*Staphylococcus aureus, Staphylococcus epidermidis* (penicillinase producing)	*Streptococcus pneumoniae*
		 Streptococcus
		   Lancefield Groups A–F†
		   Viridans group (alpha-hemolytic, non–Lancefield groupable streptococci)

Cephalosporins		*Staphylococcus aureus, Staphylococcus epidermidis*
		 Streptococcus pneumoniae
		 Streptococcus
		   Lancefield Groups A–F†
		   Viridans group (alpha-hemolytic, non–Lancefield groupable streptococci)
		 Peptostreptococcal species

Erythromycin	*Corynebacterium diphtheriae*	*Staphylococcus aureus, Staphylococcus epidermidis*
		 Streptococcus pneumoniae
		 Streptococcus
		   Lancefield Groups A–F
		   Viridans group (alpha-hemolytic, non–Lancefield groupable streptococci)
		 Peptostreptococcal species
		 Clostridia–all species

Clindamycin Lincomycin	*Bacteroides fragilis**	Same as erythromycin Anaerobic bacteria*
Vancomycin		*Staphylococcus aureus, Staphylococcus epidermidis* Enterococcal species (Lancefield Group D streptococci) *Streptococcus faecalis*

*See text for gram negative microorganisms included in this table.

†Enterococcal species (Lancefield Group D streptococci) usually treated in combination with streptomycin or gentamicin.

that of the gram positive bacteria. Definite changes in antimicrobial susceptibility have occurred with time. In addition, considerable variation in antimicrobial susceptibility may be found in different institutions. Because of this variability that occurs with time and geographic location, it is important for the practicing physician to have knowledge of the susceptibility patterns to gram negative bacteria that prevail in the institution or community in which he practices.

Table 46-2 lists antimicrobial agents frequently used in the treatment of infections produced by gram negative bacteria. It must be pointed out that this is only a guide to initial therapy. Final selection of an antimicrobial agent will depend on the microorganism isolated, the antimicrobial susceptibility, and the patient's response to therapy.

When several agents are effective against the same bacteria, those agents that are the least toxic or are most effective are listed as the primary agent.

Route of Administration

Once it has been decided that an antimicrobial agent is indicated, the most effective route of administration must be determined. Patients not requiring hospitalization are usually treated with oral antimicrobial agents. One of the primary considerations in choosing an oral antimicrobial agent is whether or not it is well absorbed from the gastrointestinal tract. For example, nafcillin, oxacillin, cloxacillin, and dicloxacillin are all semi-synthetic, penicillinase-resistant penicillins that can be given orally. Of these four penicillins, cloxacillin and dicloxacillin are the agents most effectively absorbed and produce the highest blood levels. When given by mouth, nafcillin is partially degraded by acid in the stomach, and its absorption is erratic. Blood levels of orally administered nafcillin are therefore the lowest of the four agents. Oxacillin occupies a position between these two extremes.

Antimicrobial agents should be administered parenterally to seriously ill patients. All too often, associated nausea, vomiting, delayed gastric emptying, or diarrhea impedes or delays absorption of orally administered agents in the seriously ill patient. In addition, parenteral administration frequently permits quantities of an antimicrobial agent to be given that are much larger than could be tolerated by mouth. It is often failure to achieve adequate circulating blood levels (and secondarily, tissue levels) rather than an incorrect choice of antimicrobial agent that results in failure to control the infection.

Penetration of Antimicrobial Agents into Body Compartments

There are multiple potential spaces and membrane-limited compartments within the body that may be involved in an infectious process. Since these cavities or potential spaces are avascular, antimicrobial agents must first traverse the lining membranes and then by diffusion pass into the space itself. The following factors influence the concentration of an antimicrobial agent within a closed space: (1) concentration of the agent in the blood — the higher the concentration, the greater the gradient; (2) molecular size; (3)

TABLE 46-2. Antimicrobial Agents Used in Treatment of Infections
Produced by Gram Negative Bacteria

Antimicrobial Agent (Class)	Primary Agent in the Treatment of Infection Produced by:	Secondary Agent in the Treatment of Infection Produced by:
Penicillins Ampicillin	*Salmonella typhimurium* and *Salmonella enteritidis* Shigella sp., *Escherichia coli, Proteus mirabilis, Haemophilus influenzae*	
Carbenicillin	*Pseudomonas aeruginosa** *Proteus rettgeri, Proteus morganii,* and *Proteus vulgaris* (indol-positive species)	
Cephalosporins	*Klebsiella pneumoniae*	*Escherichia coli* *Proteus mirabilis*
Tetracyclines	*Vibrio cholerae* Moraxella sp.; Mima sp. Brucella sp.	Enterobacter species, *Escherichia coli,* *Klebsiella pneumoniae,* Proteus sp.†
Aminoglycosides Streptomycin	*Yersinia pestis, Francisella tularensis*	
Kanamycin	*Proteus morganii, Proteus rettgeri,* (indol-positive species)	*Serratia marcescens*
	Klebsiella pneumoniae	*Providencia stuartii* and *Providencia alcalifaciens*
Gentamicin	*Pseudomonas aeruginosa* *Serratia marcescens* *Providencia stuartii* and *Providencia alcalifaciens*	Enterobacter sp. *Proteus rettgeri, Proteus morganii,* and *Proteus vulgaris* (indol-positive species)
Chloramphenicol	*Salmonella typhosa*	Shigella species *Haemophilus influenzae,* *Neisseria meningitidis,* *Bacteroides fragilis,* all subspecies
Polymyxin B and E**		*Escherichia coli* *Pseudomonas aeruginosa*
Sulfonamides	*Escherichia coli, Proteus mirabilis†*	

*Often in combination with gentamicin
†Usually limited to urinary tract infections
**Polymyxin E (Colistin)

degree of protein binding — only that portion of the drug which is unbound is free to diffuse across the limiting membrane (see Chap. 45); (4) degree of lipid solubility — diffusion is enhanced by high lipid solubility; (5) presence and strength of ionic charge — those agents which carry a strong electrical charge diffuse poorly; and (6) presence of inflammation — the inflammatory reaction usually favors increased passage of antimicrobial agents into membrane-limited compartments.

The pleural, peritoneal, and pericardial cavities are examples of potential body spaces that may be involved in an active inflammatory process. When inflammation exists, antimicrobial agents given parenterally are almost always found to be present in therapeutic concentration in the pleural, peritoneal, or pericardial fluid.

In patients with septic arthritis, the inflammatory reaction present in the synovial membrane allows antimicrobial agents to readily enter synovial fluid. The amount of antimicrobial agent in synovial fluid closely approximates the amount present in the serum. Often there may be a lag of 30 to 60 minutes between the peak synovial fluid concentration of the drug used and the peak serum concentration. The failure to take into consideration the lag in peak joint fluid activity, along with the small doses used in the past, led to the erroneous concept of the need for direct instillation of antimicrobial agents into the joint to achieve therapeutic concentrations. In light of recent experience and measured synovial fluid levels of antimicrobial agents following parenteral administration, this practice is no longer considered necessary.

Direct instillation of an antimicrobial agent into a joint or a pleural or peritoneal cavity may be harmful. High concentrations of certain antimicrobial agents injected directly may induce an inflammatory reaction producing a chemical synovitis or serositis. Direct instillation of an aminoglycoside or polymyxin antibiotic into the peritoneal cavity may lead to respiratory paralysis by producing a curare-like blockade at the myoneural endplate. Less frequently, similar complications may follow rapid intravenous administration of these agents.

It should be emphasized that along with antimicrobial therapy, adequate and sufficient drainage of loculated, extensive, or a rapidly accumulating inflammatory exudate is mandatory. Improving local circulatory conditions through drainage permits better penetration of antimicrobial agents into a closed space. Microorganisms that are relatively dormant in abscesses because of adverse local environmental conditions of low pH, metabolic inhibitors, and proteolytic enzymes become metabolically active and begin to multiply following drainage of accumulated exudate. During this period of renewed metabolic activity and growth, microorganisms are more susceptible to the action of antimicrobial agents. Phagocytosis by polymorphonuclear leukocytes is also enhanced by the improved local conditions following drainage.

In the treatment of bacterial or fungal meningitis, it is imperative to attain adequate antimicrobial activity in the cerebrospinal fluid. Fortunately, in the presence of active inflammation of the meninges, antimicrobial agents that ordinarily do not enter the cerebrospinal fluid in significant amounts attain therapeutic concentrations (see Table 46-3). The presence of fever also may increase the passage of drug into the cerebrospinal fluid because of vasodilation and increased cerebral blood flow. The lower concentration of protein in the cerebrospinal fluid as compared to plasma results in less drug bound to protein and therefore proportionately greater activity of the total amount of the agent present. For those antimicrobial agents capable of diffusing across the meninges with or without the presence of inflammation, the amount present in the cerebrospinal fluid is directly related to the serum

TABLE 46-3. Relative Diffusion of Antimicrobial
Agents Into Cerebrospinal Fluid

Good Without Inflammation	Good in Presence Of Inflammation	Minimal to Poor With Inflammation	None, Even With Inflammation
Sulfadiazine	Penicillin G	Tetracycline	Polymyxin B
Chloramphenicol	Ampicillin	Streptomycin	Colistin
	Carbenicillin	Kanamycin	Vancomycin
	Methicillin	Gentamicin	
	Oxacillin	Amphotericin B	
	Nafcillin		
	Cephaloridine		

concentration. In order to increase the diffusion gradient and thereby increase the amount of drug in the cerebrospinal fluid, all antimicrobial agents should be administered intravenously in maximum amounts. With time, and as the patient improves, there is a tendency to reduce the amount of antimicrobial agent given, or to administer it by a route other than intravenously. It must be recognized that as the patient improves, meningeal inflammation is also subsiding and less drug will enter the cerebrospinal fluid. For this reason the antimicrobial agent used should be continued intravenously in maximal dosage for the duration of therapy.

Occasionally, when meningitis is produced by gram negative bacilli resistant to chloramphenicol, ampicillin, or carbenicillin, intrathecal administration of gentamicin or polymyxin B must be given to achieve therapeutic activity in cerebrospinal fluid. This is necessary because gentamicin enters the cerebrospinal fluid in minimal amounts even in the face of inflammation, while polymyxin B does not enter at all.

Antimicrobial Therapy and its Relation to Renal Function

With few exceptions, renal excretion is the major pathway for the elimination of antimicrobial agents from the body (see Table 46-4). By virtue of renal concentrating mechanisms, antimicrobial agents predominantly eliminated by the kidneys are present in the urine in concentrations that greatly exceed serum concentrations, even in patients with moderate renal impairment. For example, 500 mg of ampicillin given orally produces a peak serum concentration of 5 to 8 μg per ml. Simultaneous urine concentrations may reach 850 to 2000 μg per ml. The very high concentrations present in the urine make it possible to treat urinary tract infections produced by microorganisms resistant to peak serum concentrations but sensitive to the increased amount of antimicrobial agent present in the urine. Similarly, dosages of antimicrobial agents lower than would ordinarily be used in the treatment of systemic infections may be utilized in treating infections of the urinary tract. For example, if carbenicillin is used in treating infection produced by *Pseudomonas aeruginosa* outside the urinary tract, 25 to 30 gm is the usual daily dosage. Since carbenicillin is excreted by the kidneys and is present in the urine in extremely high concentrations, the same micro-organism, if confined to the urinary tract, may be successfully treated with 4 to 6 gm of carbenicillin per day.

Certain antimicrobial agents, such as nitrofurantoin, methenamine mandelate (mandelamine), nalidixic acid, and cephaloglycin, are found in adequate antibacterial concentration only in the urine. Since the serum antimicrobial activity produced when these agents are given is negligible, they

TABLE 46–4. Dosage Schedule and Renal Excretion of Antimicrobial Agents

Drug	% Bound To Serum Protein	Half Life (T 1/2, hrs)	Renal Excretion (% of dose given)	Drug Administration Time Interval Related To Renal Impairment (Hours)*			
				Normal	*Mild*	*Moderate*	*Severe*
Penicillin G	65	0.5	75–90	4–6	Same	Same	6–12
Ampicillin	20–25	0.5–1	60–75	4–6	Same	Same	8–12
Methicillin	38	0.5–1	67–75	4–6	Same	Same	8–12
Oxacillin	92	0.5	56	4–6	Same	Same	8–12
Nafcillin	89	0.5–1		4–6	Same	Same	8–12
Cloxacillin	94–95	0.5–1	62	6–8	Same	Same	8–12
Dicloxacillin	96–98	0.7	73	6–8	Same	Same	12–18
Carbenicillin	50	0.5–1	75–85	4	Same	6	8–12
Sulfadiazine	32–56	17	50–85	6	6–8	Avoid	Avoid
Tetracycline	25–30	6–8	60	6	12	12-24	Avoid
Chlortetra-cycline	50–70	5.6	18	6	12	12-24	Avoid
Oxytetracycline	20–25	10	70	6	12–24	Avoid	Avoid
Cephalothin	60–65	0.5–0.85	60–90	4–6	6–8	8–12	12–24
Cephaloridine	20	1.5	75–100	6–8	8–12	Avoid	Avoid
Cephalexin	15	1	90	6	6–12	8	12–24
Cefazolin	84–86	1.8–2.2	70–100	4–6	6–8	8–12	12–24
Chloram-phenicol	60	1.6–3.3	5–10	6–8	6–8	6–8	6–8
Erythromycin		1.5	5–10	6–8	6–8	6–8	6–8
Streptomycin	25–40	2–4	50–90	12	12–24	24–36	42–72
Kanamycin	Low	3–4	80	12	12–24	Serum Cr × 9	
Gentamicin	30	2.5	80–100	8	12–24	Serum Cr × 9	
Vancomycin	10	6	80	6–8	24–72	Avoid	Avoid
Polymyxin B		6	60	6–12	12–24	Avoid	Avoid
Colistin		2–3	65	6–12	12–24	Avoid	Avoid
Lincomycin	80–90	4.5	10–15	6	6	6	8–12
Clindamycin	80	3	10–15	6–8	6–8	6–8	6–8

*Mild renal impairment = Creatinine Clearance (Ccr) 60 to 80 ml per minute. Moderate impairment = Ccr 20 to 60 ml per minute. Severe impairment = Ccr 20 ml or less per minute.

should not be used in the initial therapy of pyelonephritis because of the possibility of an inadequate effect should there be an associated bacteremia.

For certain antimicrobial agents, the pH of the urine is extremely important in determining the resultant antimicrobial activity. An acid pH is required for the conversion of methenamine mandelate (mandelamine) to formaldehyde. An acid pH also increases the antimicrobial activity of nalidixic acid and tetracycline. Conversely, the antimicrobial activity of the aminoglycoside antibiotics is increased in the presence of an alkaline urine.

Administration of antimicrobial agents to patients with impaired renal function is a difficult problem. The problem becomes more critical when the agent used is also nephrotoxic. With the rise in incidence of hospital-acquired gram negative bacterial infections over the past decade there has been a concomitant increase in the use of aminoglycoside antibiotics. The aminoglycosides are eliminated almost exclusively by renal excretion. As a class, the aminoglycosides possess a narrow therapeutic to toxic ratio. Excessive serum concentrations of these agents may occur as a result of diminished renal excretion, leading to further renal impairment and possible eighth nerve damage. In contrast, if the serum level is too low, the concentration of the drug is insufficient for adequate antibacterial activity. Other antimicrobial agents are also potentially nephrotoxic if present in excessive concentrations. They include the sulfonamides, polymyxins, vancomycin, cephaloridine, and amphotericin B.

Fortunately, several classes of antimicrobial agents can be used in full or slightly modified dosage even in the presence of mild to moderate renal dysfunction. These include the penicillins, cephalosporins (except cephaloridine), chloramphenicol, erythromycin, lincomycin, and clindamycin. Care must be taken when large doses of penicillin G and carbenicillin are used in patients with diminished renal function. Generalized seizures secondary to direct stimulation of the central nervous system may occur.

For those antimicrobial agents that possess potentially serious nephrotoxic effects, alterations must be made in either the dose or the time interval between doses if normal serum concentrations are to be maintained. To meet this need several different regimens have been devised. These are outlined and discussed below.

1. *Administration of antimicrobial agents according to assessment of renal function as mild, moderate, or severe impairment.*

For purposes of this discussion, mild impairment of renal function is defined as a creatinine clearance between 60 and 80 ml per minute. Moderate impairment is present if the creatinine clearance is 20 to 60 ml per minute, and severe impairment is present if the creatinine clearance is less than 20 ml per minute. Depending on the assessment of the patient's renal dysfunction into one of these three categories, the usual maintenance dose is given but the time interval between doses is increased (see Table 46-4).

2. *Determination of the time interval between doses in patients with impaired renal function as a function of serum creatinine.*

Impaired renal function is reflected by a rise in serum creatinine. For the most part, the rise in serum creatinine parallels the fall in creatinine clearance. Certain classes of antimicrobial agents, such as the aminoglycosides, are excreted predominantly by glomerular filtration. Thus, as the glomerular filtration falls (as determined by creatinine clearance, and reflected by the serum creatinine), the amount of aminoglycoside excreted is proportionally less. From the relationship between serum creatinine and the elimination of gentamicin and kanamycin in patients with impaired renal function a constant has been calculated. This constant, which is equal to 9, if multiplied by the serum creatinine, determines the time interval in hours between maintenance doses of gentamicin and kanamycin. For example, a patient whose serum creatinine is 4 mg per 100 ml would receive a dose of gentamicin (9 X 4) every 36 hours.

3. *Retaining the normal time interval between doses, but reducing the amount given based on the calculation of the elimination constant.*

This last method requires knowledge of the elimination constant of a drug (the rate at which a drug is eliminated) at various creatinine clearances. In most cases of drugs excreted by the kidneys this proves to be a straight line relationship. For practical purposes the rate of elimination in the normal and anephric state is plotted on left and right ordinates, and a straight line drawn connecting these two points. The elimination constant for any creatinine clearance can then be determined (see Fig. 46-1). The dose to be given is then calculated or, when nomograms exist, read directly. In this approach the antimicrobial agent is given at the normal time interval, but the dose administered is appropriately reduced.

In order to ensure prompt attainment of adequate antibacterial activity in patients with renal failure, the first dose given to the patient (the loading dose) is usually one half to two thirds the total daily dosage in all of the outlined schemes.

The three regimens just outlined have limitations. All work best if the patient's renal function is stable. Unfortunately, this is usually not the case with hospitalized patients whose renal function may change dramatically over a short period of time. Alternative pathways for drug elimination (i.e., hepatic) may be more efficient in some patients than others, depending on the underlying or associated disease. The previously mentioned regimens are only guidelines, for there is considerable variability in excretion of drugs in patients with renal impairment, even though the degree of impairment as measured by serum creatinine or creatinine clearance may be the same.

Assaying the serum for the amount of antimicrobial agents present is a great aid in making individual dosage adjustments and correcting for patient variability. Serum assay is especially helpful when patients with impaired renal function are receiving aminoglycoside antibiotics. It is now possible to determine within two to six hours the actual amount of antimicrobial agent present in the serum. (see Chap. 45). Many of these assays are inexpensive and can easily be performed in the hospital microbiology laboratory. By combining one of the above dosage regimens with periodic serum assay, potentially toxic antimicrobial agents can be given with a greater margin of safety.

Adverse Reactions to Antimicrobial Agents

Antimicrobial agents, like all drugs, are capable of producing adverse effects. Before prescribing any antimicrobial agent, the physician should

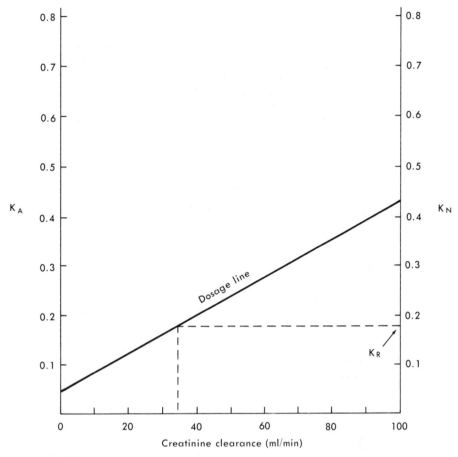

Figure 46-1. K_A = elimination constant of the antimicrobial agent in the anephric patient. K_N = elimination constant of the antimicrobial agent in the normal patient. To determine the elimination constant at any intermediate creatinine clearance, a perpendicular line is drawn to the dosage line and then to the right ordinate. The dose to be given is calculated by $D_R = D_N \cdot \dfrac{K_R}{K_N}$, where D_R = dose to be given, D_N = dose given to a normal patient, and K_R = elimination constant determined from the graph. See text. (Modified from Dettli et al.: Drug dosage in patients with impaired renal function. Postgrad. Med. J. *46* (Suppl.):32, 1970.)

know not only its beneficial properties but also any untoward effects. With this knowledge, potentially harmful effects can be anticipated and corrected before they pose a danger to the patient. The major adverse reactions to antimicrobial agents are discussed below. The list is by no means inclusive. Any agent may be capable of producing multiple adverse reactions.

Allergic or Hypersensitivity Reactions

The most serious reactions to antimicrobial agents are those that are mediated by allergy or hypersensitivity. Anaphylaxis and angioneurotic edema are immediate-type reactions that may be life threatening if not rapidly reversed. Reactions occurring after the first 24 hours may present in a variety of ways. Urticaria, erythema multiforme, erythema nodosum, rashes of almost any type, exfoliative dermatitis, aplastic anemia, Coombs' positive hemolytic anemia, allergic purpura, pulmonary infiltrates, serum sickness, and drug fever have all been reported in patients receiving antimicrobial therapy. Drug fever is a poorly defined reaction, and is especially confusing since the temperature graph may be either continuously elevated or occasionally "spiking" in character. This frequently suggests to the physician the development of a new infection or the presence of cryptic abscess and therefore the need for continued antimicrobial therapy. (See the Case Presentation at the end of this chapter.)

Reactions Related to Dosage and Time

A wide variety of adverse drug reactions appear to be related to high circulating levels of the antimicrobial agent or prolonged duration of administration. In these instances the antimicrobial agent is injurious not only to the infecting microorganism but to the host as well. For this reason these reactions are frequently referred to as "toxic" reactions. An example of toxicity to both the infecting microorganism and the host is the effect produced by amphotericin B, a commonly used antifungal agent. Amphotericin B binds to the sterols in the fungal cell membrane, producing damage and lysis of the fungus. Unfortunately amphotericin B may produce similar damage by binding to the sterols present in the renal tubules or lysosomes of the host, resulting in tubular necrosis and atrophy.

Cells of different organs vary in their susceptibility to toxic effects of antimicrobial agents. This variability may be due to either higher concentrations of the agent present in certain organs or of structural or metabolic differences. Frequently the reasons for toxic reactions to antimicrobial agents are unknown.

Mention has already been made of the renal toxicity possible from aminoglycoside and polymyxin antibiotics. Vestibular dysfunction, partial hearing loss, or complete deafness may occur following prolonged administration of aminoglycoside antibiotics and vancomycin, especially when circulating levels are high. These eighth nerve changes may be permanent, for unlike liver or renal tubular cells, when specialized nerve cells are irreversibly damaged, they are incapable of regenerating.

Hepatic injury may be produced by many antimicrobial agents. Those agents metabolized by the liver or concentrated in the bile are most frequently implicated. This includes erythromycin, especially erythromycin estolate and tetracycline. Tetracycline, when administered in large doses, (2 gm or more per day), may be hepatotoxic to pregnant women and, indeed, several fatalities have been reported. For this reason, tetracycline should not be used in the treatment of infectious complications of pregnancy. Several antituberculous drugs are also potentially hepatotoxic. In order of frequency of potential hepatotoxicity they are isoniazid, para-aminosalicylic acid, and rifampin. Patients receiving isoniazid should be monitored by monthly liver enzyme and bilirubin determinations. In many of the previously mentioned adverse hepatic reactions, hypersensitivity to the agent is believed to play an important role.

Antimicrobial agents may also produce bone marrow suppression or selectively depress any one of the formed blood cells. It is often difficult to differentiate the changes produced by the agent from those of the disease process itself. Chloramphenicol may produce bone marrow suppression by two separate mechanisms. Aplastic anemia, the most serious consequence of chloramphenicol administration, appears to be mediated by hypersensitivity. Total suppression of the bone marrow has been reported following the ingestion of a single capsule. Fortunately, aplastic anemia rarely occurs — once in every 60,000 to 100,000 courses of therapy. More commonly, toxic reactions to chloramphenicol are manifested by a gradual fall in the circulating neutrophils, red blood cells, and platelets, or by any one of these elements selectively. If chloramphenicol is promptly discontinued, these changes in the formed elements of the bone marrow are reversible. It is thought that this reaction is best explained by a time-dose relationship.

Reactions Secondary to Change in the Indigenous Microflora

Administration of antimicrobial agents results in changes in the ecology of the normal microflora and favors proliferation of microorganisms resistant to the agent given. A rare example of the consequence of altered microbial flora may be seen in patients who undergo abdominal surgery and are given tetracycline or chloramphenicol, both capable of producing marked changes in the host intestinal flora. In these patients, staphylococci resistant to tetracycline or chloramphenicol may colonize and proliferate in the large bowel, producing dysentery characterized by blood and mucus. This serious complication is called *staphylococcal pseudomembranous enterocolitis* and if unrecognized, may lead to death. A similar clinical syndrome may occur in patients who are treated with clindamycin, especially following oral administration. There is no adequate explanation for the pseudomembranous enterocolitis produced by clindamycin. Changes in bowel flora have not been implicated. Suppression of normal intestinal flora may also interfere with vitamin K absorption and result in a secondary depletion of vitamin K-dependent clotting factors. This effect is further magnified in patients receiving oral anticoagulants.

Reactions Secondary to Drug Interaction

Only recently has attention been drawn to the possible adverse effect produced by the interaction of drugs with each other and the host. This includes interaction between not only various antimicrobial agents but other therapeutic agents as well. The adverse reaction may be based on the physicochemical properties of the antimicrobial agent. Tetracycline, for example, may be chelated by bivalent cations such as Ca++ and Mg++. Concomitant oral administration of antacid or milk will therefore decrease absorption of tetracycline from the intestine.

Several drugs share a common metabolic pathway in the host, and when both are administered they may compete for the same enzyme system. One such example is chloramphenicol, which will increase the half life of barbiturates, diphenylhydantoin, coumadin, and tolbutamide by competition for the same hepatic inactivating enzymes. Similar metabolic competition exists between isoniazid and diphenylhydantoin, and between sulfonamide and tolbutamide. Interactions of this type should be considered when therapy with more than a single drug is necessary.

Competition for binding sites on serum albumin may also result in untoward reactions. Sulfonamides displace bilirubin bound to serum albumin, a fact which may become quite important in the newborn infant. If the infant has developed hemolytic anemia because of maternal blood group incompatibility or has a marked degree of physiologic jaundice, there may already be an elevated bilirubin level. If sulfonamides are given, bilirubin is displaced by preferential binding of the sulfa to albumin, and more unbound bilirubin is available to diffuse into the central nervous system, increasing the potential for the development of kernicterus.

Reactions Secondary to Host-Drug Interaction

Adverse reactions to antimicrobial agents may occasionally develop because the host lacks or is temporarily deficient in a specific enzyme system. Acute hemolytic anemia may be induced by the administration of nitrofurantoin, chloramphenicol, or sulfonamides to patients who lack glucose-6-phosphate dehydrogenase. Newborn infants, especially premature infants, have a relative deficiency of glucuronyl transferase in the liver and do not effectively conjugate chloramphenicol with glucuronic acid. The excessive concentrations of chloramphenicol resulting from this deficiency lead to the *gray syndrome*. This syndrome consists of vomiting, rapid irregular respirations, ashen-gray color, flaccidity, and finally vascular collapse. If chloramphenicol must be used in the newborn, the dosage should be limited to no more than 25 mg per kilogram per day.

Alternative Therapy in the Penicillin-Allergic Patient

Penicillin, or one of the semisynthetic derivatives, is the most effective antibiotic for infections produced by gram positive bacteria and by a select number of gram negative microorganisms (see Table 46-1). For minor infections such as streptococcal pharyngitis or gonococcal urethritis, equally effective alternatives are available. In patients with subacute bacterial endocarditis produced by members of the viridans group of streptococci or enterococci, penicillin in combination with streptomycin or gentamicin constitutes the most effective antimicrobial therapy. Patients who give a history of allergy to penicillin should be carefully evaluated to determine if true penicillin hypersensitivity exists. If a minor allergic reaction occurred in the distant past, or if the allergic reaction was ill defined, patients may frequently be able to receive penicillin after proper evaluation. A more pressing problem arises in the patient who presents with a life-threatening illness such as bacterial meningitis, when time does not permit an adequate evaluation for penicillin allergy. An alternative antimicrobial agent must be selected immediately. A similar need exists for the patient with an unsuspected penicillin allergy who develops an immediate reaction to the first dose of penicillin.

A guide to alternative therapy in the penicillin-allergic patient is outlined in Table 46-5. Patients who are not progressing as expected or who are not responding to adequate alternative therapy should be evaluated by an allergist to determine if penicillin allergy exists, and if it does, to consider the possibility of desensitization. In Table 46-5 cephalothin appears at times as an alternative drug. It must be mentioned that some patients who are allergic to penicillin may also manifest an allergic reaction to cephalothin because of the structural similarities between these two drugs. The physician who

TABLE 46-5. Alternative Therapy in the Penicillin-Allergic Patient

Disease	Alternative Drug	Adult Dose (Route and Duration)
Group A streptococcal infection	Erythromycin	500 mg 4×/day PO (10 days)
Gonococcal urethritis (uncomplicated)	Tetracycline	500 mg 4×/day PO (5 days)
	Spectinomycin	2 gm. IM one dose
Pneumococcal pneumonia	Erythromycin	500 mg 4×/day IV. Switch to PO as soon as possible (7–10 days)
	Clindamycin	300 mg 4×/day IV or IM. May switch to PO (7–10 days)
	Cephalothin	75 mg/kg/day IV (7–10 days)
Meningitis caused by *Streptococcus pneumoniae, Neisseria meningitidis, Haemophilus influenzae*	Chloramphenicol	50–100 mg/kg/day IV. Switch to PO as soon as possible (7–10 days)
Subacute bacterial endocarditis caused by *Streptococcus viridans* group (penicillin sensitive)	Vancomycin or cephalothin plus streptomycin	30 mg/kg/day IV (4 weeks) 100–150 mg/kg/day IV (4 weeks) 500 mg 2×/day IM (4 weeks)
Enterococcal species (Lancefield Group D streptococci) and other species of penicillin-resistant streptococci	Vancomycin plus streptomycin or gentamicin (if necessary)	30 mg/kg/day IV (6 weeks) 30 mg/kg/day IM (6 weeks) 3–5 mg/kg/day IM (6 weeks)
Staphylococcal septicemia (with or without endocarditis)	Vancomycin or cephalothin	30 mg/kg/day IV (6 weeks) 100–200 mg/kg/day IV (6 weeks)

PO, by mouth; IM, intramuscular; IV, intravenously.

chooses to use cephalothin must be aware of this possibility. He should be present when the first dose is given and be ready to institute immediate therapy if a serious allergic reaction develops.

Prophylactic Use of Antimicrobial Agents

The role of antimicrobial agents in the prevention of infection has been steeped in controversy since they were first used for this purpose. Despite the administration of antimicrobial agents it is impossible to prevent all the infectious complications attendant to major surgery, organ transplantation, the compromised host, or viral illness.

When the purpose of prophylaxis is limited and well defined, a much greater chance for success exists. Thus, the spread of Group A streptococcal infection can be halted in closed populations by the prophylactic administration of benzathine penicillin G to all persons at risk (see Chap. 15). Contacts of patients with syphilis or gonorrhea can be prevented from developing clinical disease by penicillin prophylaxis. The risk for patients with rheumatic heart disease who are undergoing dental procedures of developing subacute streptococcal endocarditis is minimized by prophylactic administration of penicillin or erythromycin (see Chap. 41). The chances of contracting malaria are reduced for travelers in endemic areas if they receive primaquine-chloroquine prophylaxis.

There is no doubt that the physician, in his zeal to protect his patient from infection, utilizes antimicrobial prophylaxis too freely. Antimicrobial agents have been found to be ineffective in preventing the following types of infection:

1. Infection in the unconscious patient.
2. Urinary tract infection following insertion of a Foley catheter.
3. Infection following most routine surgical procedures.
4. Bacterial superinfection in patients with viral illness.

When prophylactic antimicrobial therapy has been used indiscriminately in an attempt to prevent all possible infectious complications, an even higher infection rate may result. When the infection rate has remained constant, careful inspection often reveals that the microorganisms now isolated are more resistant to antimicrobial agents and more difficult to eradicate.

CASE PRESENTATION

A 48-year-old male was admitted to the hospital because of fever (103.6°F), shaking chills, and a dense right upper lobe pulmonary infiltrate. The patient had a history of heavy alcoholic consumption for many years. Gram stain of a sputum specimen revealed numerous gram negative bacilli and many segmented neutrophils. Sputum and one of three blood cultures obtained on admission grew *Klebsiella pneumoniae* within 24 hours. On further study the Klebsiella microorganisms isolated from both the blood and sputum were found to be susceptible to cephalothin, 8 μg per ml, kanamycin, 4 μg per ml, and gentamicin, 2 μg per ml. After the initial sputum and blood cultures were obtained, the patient was treated with cephalothin, 2 gm intravenously every six hours. The patient improved considerably over the next seven days. His temperature ranged between 99.6 and 100.8°F. On the tenth hospital day, auscultation of the patient's lungs revealed improved breath sounds and a decrease in rales heard over the right upper lobe. Chest x-ray showed a resolving pneumonia. On the eleventh day of hospitalization, the patient's temperature began to spike to 102 to 103°F. A repeat physical examination and chest x-ray were unchanged from the day before. Because of the rise in fever and the suspicion by the house staff that they may be missing a distant focus of *Klebsiella pneumoniae* infection, kanamycin, 500 mg intramuscularly every 12 hours, was added to the patient's ongoing cephalothin therapy. The patient's elevated temperature persisted over the next three days. After consultation and reevaluation on the fifteenth day it was decided that the patient's pneumonia was continuing to improve and that his elevated temperature was most likely due to cephalothin-induced drug fever. All antibiotics were discontinued and the patient became afebrile over the next 36 hours.

References

Books

Cluff, L. E., Caranasos, G. J., and Stewart, R. B.: Clinical Problems with Drugs. Philadelphia, W. B. Saunders Co., 1975.

Goodman, L. S., and Gilman, A.: The Pharmacological Basis of Therapeutics. New York, The Macmillan Co., 1970, pp. 1154–1343.

Hoeprich, P. D.: Infectious Diseases. New York, Harper and Row, 1972, pp. 177–222.

Kagan, B. M. (ed.): Antimicrobial Therapy. 2nd ed. Philadelphia, W. B. Saunders Co., 1974.

Original Articles

Bartlett, J. G., Sutter, V. L., and Finegold, S. M.: Treatment of anaerobic infections with lincomycin and clindamycin. N. Engl. J. Med. *287*:1006, 1972.

Bennett, W. M., Singer, I., and Coggins, C. H.: Guide to drug usage in adult patients with impaired renal function. J.A.M.A. *223*:991, 1973.

Boston Collaborative Drug Surveillance Program: Drug-Induced Deafness. J.A.M.A. *224*:515, 1973.

Chan, R. E., Benner, E. J., and Hoeprich, P. D.: Gentamicin therapy in renal failure: A nomogram for dosage. Ann. Intern. Med. *76*:773, 1972.

Christensen, L. K., and Skovsted, L.: Inhibition of drug metabolism by chloramphenicol. Lancet *2*:1397, 1969.

Cutler, R. E., Gyselynck, A. M., Fleet, P., and Forrey, A. W.: Correlation of serum creatinine concentration and gentamicin half-life. J.A.M.A. *219*:1037, 1972.

Dettli, L., Spring P., and Habersang, R.: Drug dosage in patients with impaired renal function. Postgrad. Med. J. *46*(Suppl):32, 1970.

Finland, M., and Hewitt, W. (ed.): Second international symposium on gentamicin. An aminoglycoside antibiotic. J. Infect. Dis. *124*(Suppl. 1):1, 1971.

Jackson, G. G.: Prospective from a quarter century of antibiotic usage. J.A.M.A. *227*:634, 1974.

Kagan, B. M., Fannin, S. L., and Bardie, F.: Spotlight on antimicrobial agents – 1973. J.A.M.A. *226*:306, 1973.

Kirby, W. M. M. (ed.): Symposium on carbenicillin: A clinical profile. J. Infect. Dis. *122*(Suppl. 1):1, 1970.

Kluge, R. M., Standiford, H. C., Tatem, B., Young, V. M., Schimpff, S. C., Green, W. H., Calia, F. M., and Hornick, R. B.: The carbenicillin-gentamicin combination against

Pseudomonas aeruginosa. Correlation of effect with gentamicin sensitivity. Ann. Intern. Med. *81*:584, 1974.

Kovnat, P., Labovitz, E., and Levison, S. P.: Antibiotics and the kidney. Med. Clin. North Am. *57*:1045, 1973.

Levine, B. B.: Immunologic mechanisms of penicillin allergy. A haptenic model system for the study of allergic diseases in man. N. Engl. J. Med. *275:*1115, 1966.

Marsh, D. C., Matthew, E. B., and Persellin, R. H.: Transport of gentamicin into synovial fluid. J.A.M.A. *228*:607, 1974.

McHenry, M. C., Gavan, T. L., Gifford, R. W., Jr., Geurkink, N. A., Ommen, R. A. V., Town, M. A., and Wagner, J. G.: Gentamicin dosages for renal insufficiency adjustments based on endogenous creatinine clearance and serum creatinine concentration. Ann. Intern. Med. *74*:192, 1971.

Parker, R. H., and Schmid, F. R.: Antibacterial activity of synovial fluid during therapy of septic arthritis. Arthritis Rheum. *14*:96, 1971.

Rahal, J. J.: Treatment of gram-negative bacillary meningitis in adults. Ann. Intern. Med. *77*:295 1972.

Wallerstein, R. O., Condit, P. K., Kasper, C. K., Brown, J. W., and Morrison F. R.: Statewide study of chloramphenicol therapy and fatal aplastic anemia. J.A.M.A. *208*:2045, 1969.

Warner, W. A., and Sanders, E.: Neuromuscular blockade associated with gentamicin therapy. J.A.M.A. *215*:1153, 1971.

Weinstein, L., and Kaplan, K.: The cephalosporins. Microbiological, chemical, and pharmacological properties and use in chemotherapy. Ann. Intern. Med. *72*:729, 1970.

Westenfelder, G. O., and Paterson, P. Y.: Life-threatening infection. Choice of alternative drugs when penicillin cannot be given. J.A.M.A. *210*:845, 1969.

INDEX

NOTE: Page numbers in *italic* type indicate illustrations;
(t) indicates Table.